PRACTICAL DECISION MAKING
IN
HEALTH CARE ETHICS

PRACTICAL DECISION MAKING

IN

HEALTH CARE ETHICS

CASES AND CONCEPTS

THIRD EDITION

Raymond J. Devettere

GEORGETOWN UNIVERSITY PRESS / Washington, D.C.

Georgetown University Press, Washington, D.C. www.press.georgetown.edu
© 2010 Georgetown University Press. All rights reserved. No part of this book may be reproduced or utilized in any form or by any means, electronic or mechanical, including photocopying and recording, or by any information storage and retrieval system, without permission in writing from the publisher.

Devettere, Raymond J.
    Practical decision making in health care ethics: cases and concepts / Raymond J. Devettere.—3rd ed.
        p. ; cm.
    Includes bibliographical references and indexes.
    ISBN 978-1-58901-251-6 (pbk. : alk. paper)
    1. Medical ethics.   2. Medical ethics—Case studies.   3. Decision making.
I. Title.
[DNLM: 1. Ethics, Medical.   2. Bioethical Issues.   3. Decision Making. W 50 D491p 2009]
R724.D48   2009
174.2—dc22

2009009046

⊗ This book is printed on acid-free paper meeting the requirements of the American National Standard for Permanence in Paper for Printed Library Materials.

15 14 13 12 11 10 09   9 8 7 6 5 4 3 2
First printing

Printed in the United States of America

For Paula

It is a characteristic of reason to proceed from general principles to particular conclusions. Nonetheless, speculative reason does this one way, and practical reason another. Speculative reason is chiefly concerned with necessary things which cannot be otherwise than they are, and so truth is found without diminution in the particular conclusions just as in the general principles. But practical reason is concerned with things which can be otherwise than they are, and this includes human behavior, and thus, even if there is some force in the general principles, the more you descend to the particular conclusions, the greater is their failure.

THOMAS AQUINAS, *Summa Theologiae*, I II, q. 94, a.4, 13th century

In short, our moral discourse . . . involves the concept of an objectively or absolutely valid moral action-guide, and our moral judgments and decisions claim to be parts or applications of such an action-guide.

WILLIAM FRANKENA, *"The Principles of Morality,"* 1973

Whereas young people can become proficient in geometry and mathematics, we do not find young people proficient in prudential reasoning. The reason is that prudential reasoning is about particular cases, and knowledge about particulars comes from experience.

ARISTOTLE, *Nicomachean Ethics*, 1142a12–16, 4th century B.C.E.

The argument aims eventually to be strictly deductive. . . . Clearly arguments from such premises can be fully deductive, as theories in politics and economics attest. We should strive for a kind of moral geometry with all the rigor which this name connotes.

JOHN RAWLS, *A Theory of Justice*, 1971

Contents

Preface to the Third Edition   xiii

Introduction   xv

ONE
What Is Ethics?   1
Defining Ethics, Two Kinds of Ethics, Historical Versions of the Ethics of
Obligation, Moral Reasoning and the Theories of Obligation, Contrasting
the Ethics of Obligation with an Ethics of the Good, Retrieving the Ethics
of the Good, Bioethics Today, Suggested Readings

TWO
Prudence and Living a Good Life   20
The Good We Seek, Happiness, Moral Virtue, Prudence, Suggested
Readings

THREE
The Language of Health Care Ethics   47
Distinctions That Can Mislead, Helpful Distinctions, Suggested Readings

FOUR
Making Health Care Decisions   70
Complexity of Health Care Decisions, Decision-Making Capacity,
Informed Consent, Advance Directives, The Patient Self-Determination
Act, The Case of Hazel Welch, Final Reflections, Suggested Readings

FIVE
Deciding for Others   99
Becoming a Proxy, Standards for Making Proxy Decisions, Deciding for
Older Children, Deciding for the Mentally Ill, Deciding for Patients of
another Culture, Final Reflections on Deciding for Others, Suggested
Readings

SIX

Determining Life and Death   121

The Classical Conceptual Framework, A New Conceptual Framework,
When Does One of Us Begin? When Does One of Us Die? Recent
Controversies over Determining Death, Ethical Reflections, Suggested
Readings

SEVEN

Life-Sustaining Treatments   150

Ventilators, The Case of Karen Quinlan, The Case of Brother Fox, The
Case of William Bartling, The Case of Helga Wanglie, The Case of
Barbara Howe, Dialysis, The Case of Earle Spring, Surgery, The Case of
Rosaria Candura, Other Life-Sustaining Treatments, Suggested Readings

EIGHT

Cardiopulmonary Resuscitation   181

Terminology, A Brief History of Resuscitation Attempts, The
Effectiveness of Attempting CPR, Learning to Withhold CPR, Important
Ethical Elements for a DNR Policy, Lingering Questions about DNR
Orders, The Case of Maria M, The Case of Shirley Dinnerstein, The Case
of Catherine Gilgunn, Suggested Readings

NINE

Medical Nutrition and Hydration   202

The Techniques and Technologies, Conceptualizing Medical Nutrition
and Hydration, The Case of Clarence Herbert, The Case of Claire
Conroy, The Case of Elizabeth Bouvia, The Case of Nancy Cruzan, The
Case of Terri Schiavo, An Emerging Controversy: The Vatican and
Feeding Tubes, Ethical Reflections, Suggested Readings

TEN

Reproductive Issues   232

Contraception and Sterilization, Artificial Reproductive Techniques,
Cloning, Surrogate Motherhood, Ethical Reflections, Suggested Readings

ELEVEN

Prenatal Life   263

Abortion, Moral Issues of Abortion, RU-486, Maternal-Fetal Treatment
Conflicts, The Case of Angie, Ethical Reflections, Suggested Readings

TWELVE

Infants and Children   286

Historical Background, A Sampling of Neonatal Abnormalities, Special
Difficulties in Deciding for Neonates and Small Children, The *Baby Doe*
Regulations, The Case of Baby Doe, The Case of Baby Jane Doe, The
Case of Danielle, The Case of Baby K, The Case of Ashley, Infant
Euthanasia in the Netherlands, Suggested Readings

THIRTEEN

Euthanasia and Physician-Assisted Suicide 321

Historical Overview, Recent Developments, Physician-Assisted Suicide and State Laws, Physician-Assisted Suicide and the Constitution, Relevant Distinctions, Moral Reasoning and Euthanasia, Reasons for Euthanasia and Physician-Assisted Suicide, Reasons against Euthanasia and Physician-Assisted Suicide, The Story of a Landmark Physician-Assisted Suicide, The Case of Diane, Concluding Reflections, Suggested Readings

FOURTEEN

Medical Research 357

Notorious Examples of Questionable Ethics in Research, Reactions to the Questionable Medical Research, Research on Embryos, Research on Fetuses, Research on Minors, Research in Developing Countries, Two Cases of Controversial HIV/AIDS Research in Developing Countries, Other Special Populations in Research, Animals and Medical Research, Suggested Readings

FIFTEEN

Transplantation 394

Transplantation of Organs from Dead Human Donors, The Case of Jamie Fiske, The Case of Jesse Sepulveda, Transplantation of Organs from Living Human Donors, Transplantation of Organs from Animals, The Case of Baby Fae, Implantation of Artificial Hearts, Suggested Readings

SIXTEEN

Medical Genetics 420

Genetic Testing, A Case of Concern about Cancer, Genetic Screening, Genetic Research on Humans, The Case of Jesse Gelsinger, Genetic Enhancement, Human Genome Project, Suggested Readings

SEVENTEEN

Social and Political Issues 458

Paying for Health Care, Legislation and the "Futility" Debate, The Case of Sun Hudson, The Case of Emilio Gonzales, Experimental Drugs for Dying Patients, The Case of Abigail Burroughs and the Abigail Alliance, Seeding Trials and Ghostwriters, Suggested Readings

Glossary 485

Index of Cases 493

Index 495

Preface to the Third Edition

THE THIRD EDITION has added important new cases that have arisen since the last edition and attracted national interest, among them the stories of Terri Schiavo, Jesse Gelsinger (the first death caused by genetic research), Barbara Howe (a multiyear dispute between the family and Massachusetts General Hospital over withdrawing life-sustaining treatment), Ashley and the Ashley Treatment (surgery and treatment to sterilize and stunt the growth of a female child with encephalopathy), Sun Hudson (removal of a child's life-sustaining treatment against the wishes of his mother in accord with the Texas Advance Directives Act), Abigail Burroughs and the Abigail Alliance (efforts to force the FDA and pharmaceutical companies to release unapproved drugs for dying patients), and more examples of controversial HIV/AIDS research in Africa.

The third edition also contains most of the case studies in the earlier editions, including the classic cases that have shaped American bioethics (e.g., those of Quinlan, Conroy, Bouvia, Wanglie, Cruzan, Baby M, Baby Doe, Baby K, and Baby Fae). In addition, new topics in the third edition include the partial birth abortion law (upheld in *Gonzales v. Carhart*, 2007), embryonic stem cell research, infant euthanasia in the Netherlands, recent Vatican instructions on feeding tubes, organ donation after cardiac death, new developments in artificial hearts, clinical trials developed by pharmaceutical companies to market new drugs ("seeding trials"), and ghostwritten scientific articles published in major medical journals. One new chapter has been added to the third edition, chapter 17, which replaces the chapter on managed care in the second edition. It treats the ethical aspects of several social and political issues in American health care.

The bibliographic essays at the end of each chapter have been retained and updated, although now the reader has access through powerful search engines to a vast trove of relevant and updated bibliographic references as well as abstracts and full texts of journal articles online. In addition, the reports of the National Bioethics Advisory Commission (NBAC) that existed from October 1995 until October 2001 are available free at bioethics.georgetown.edu/nbac, and the reports of the President's Council on Bioethics (PCB) that was announced in August 2001 and ended its work in June 2009 are also available free at bioethics.gov. The NIH's National Center for Biotechnology Information (NCBI) has developed and manages a free digital archive of the biomedical and life sciences that includes many articles on bioethics published in various scientific journals. It can be accessed at pubmedcentral.ncbi.nih.gov/sites/entrez?db = pmc. Many articles are free as soon as they are published; others become available some months after publication. One can search the site by topic, by author, or by journal title. Many other online sites have helpful articles and can be found with the help of Google. Examples include the American Medical Association's *Journal of Ethics* at virtualmentor.ama.assn.org and the Hastings Center's *Bioethics Forum* at thehastings center.org/bioethicsforum.

In order to maintain consistency of vocabulary throughout the book, the translations of Aristotle and Aquinas are my own, although I was aided immensely by several standard translations of Aristotle's *Nicomachean Ethics*. Especially helpful was J. Tricot's richly annotated and textually faithful translation titled *Éthique à Nicomaque* (Paris: J. Vrin, 1983) as well as two English translations: the second edition of Terence Irwin's translation and notes (Indianapolis: Hackett Publishing Company, 1999) and Christopher Rowe's translation with commentary by Sarah Broadie (New York: Oxford University Press, 2002).

I am indebted also to fellow members of both the Ethics Committee and the Institutional Review Board at Newton–Wellesley Hospital for many thoughtful dialogues on ethics in clinical settings; to countless students over many years at Emmanuel College, Boston College, and Tufts Medical School for their interest and questions during our classes and seminars; and to anonymous readers at Georgetown University Press for their helpful comments on the text.

This book is not intended to be exhaustive. It reviews many of the current topics in health care ethics, but it does not cover all of them. However, it does provide the reader with a decision-making approach, the virtue of prudential reasoning, that can readily be extended to other issues of moral concern not treated in the text.

Aristotle noted in his *Nicomachean Ethics* (1141b14–22) that prudence, while needing some knowledge of what is good for human life in general, focuses primarily on the particulars of real life and on the particular knowledge the person needs to make good decisions in the concrete situation. In his thirteenth century *Commentary* (section 1194) on this text, Thomas Aquinas reinforced Aristotle's emphasis on the practical side of prudence by taking a rather startling position. Aquinas argued: If a person of moral integrity had to choose one of the two kinds of moral knowledge (general or particular), it would be better to have the knowledge of particulars than the knowledge of generalities.

In other words, for a person of moral character the particular insights and deliberations of prudence, the cognitive virtue of decision making, in each actual situation are more important for deciding what helps him live a good life and what enhances the common good than are the moral generalities captured in moral laws and moral principles, rules, and rights, and even in the moral virtues themselves. This preference for the priority of the virtue of prudential reasoning about particulars may be an important moral insight. In any event, it sets the tone for this book, and distinguishes it from most other texts in bioethics.

Introduction

THIS BOOK OFFERS an alternative approach to health care ethics. The field is currently dominated by ethical theories centered on obligation and duty. These theories make moral principles the centerpiece: they propose a set of general action-guiding principles, rules, and rights that we apply to particular situations to determine what we are obliged to do. Sometimes the principles and rules are derived from ethical theories, sometimes from experience, sometimes from an equilibrium of both theory and experience, sometimes from what some call a universal "common morality," but it is always the principles and rules that occupy the central position in these moral philosophies.

The ethics proposed in this book is not an ethics of obligation and duty determined by principles, rules, and rights. It is an ethics of personal well-being and fulfillment. These theories make the good life—my good life—the centerpiece: they propose a process of prudential reasoning to determine what habits, feelings, and behaviors in the various situations of life will fulfill the goal we all ultimately share—living a fulfilled and happy life. The ethics proposed in this book is a virtue ethics.

Interest in virtue-based ethics, both on the general level and in particular domains such as health care, has continued to grow steadily in the past few decades. However, many modern accounts of virtue ethics consider the virtues chiefly as character traits, dispositions, or habits—the moral virtues. This book follows Aristotle and focuses more on the pivotal *intellectual* virtue of prudence, the virtue of ethical decision making. Prudence is not, for Aristotle, a character trait, disposition, or habit but the wisdom to figure out what to do to move toward a good life when we are faced with personal choices involving what is truly good or bad in our lives, and with political choices involving what is truly good or bad for the common good. Prudence is the decision-making virtue for both personal and political practical matters. It is about making good choices for our lives and for the common good.

Aristotle (384–322 B.C.E.) grew up in Macedonia but lived most of his life in Athens, although he never enjoyed the privileges of Athenian citizenship. He accomplished an extraordinary amount of scientific and philosophical research during his lifetime and lectured on many topics, including ethics. Some of his lectures on ethics comprise the first major books in our culture devoted exclusively to ethics—the *Nicomachean Ethics* and the *Eudemian Ethics*.

Aristotle's work is impressive because it was extraordinarily profound. It has also proven relevant far beyond its original cultural milieu. Sixteen hundred years after Aristotle, for example, Thomas Aquinas (1224–74) embraced Aristotle's approach in ethics and saw no trouble integrating it with his religious faith and Christian theology. Today, seven hundred years later, we may be able to retrieve something of value from the ethics of Aristotle and Aquinas.

This book will attempt such a retrieval in reference to health care ethics. It does not, however, pretend to explain the ethics of Aristotle or of Aquinas, nor is it a defense of their ethical positions. Rather, the intention is to capture the fundamental intuition of these ethicists and to approach the moral issues of contemporary health care ethics in their philosophical spirit. This move is motivated by the conviction that ethics is more about the virtues than about our obligations, more about flourishing than about duties. Implied in this preference is the idea that fulfilling moral obligations and duties, although necessary, is simply not sufficient to bring happiness and to make any human life a truly good and noble life.

There are, of course, serious obstacles confronting any attempt to retrieve an older ethics. Some problems are textual: we do not have any original manuscripts, so the oldest texts that we do have are hand-made copies and not always consistent. Some problems are cultural: one reason we cannot fully understand older texts is that we do not share the cultural context in which they were produced.

Some problems are linguistic: most people cannot read Aristotle's Greek or Aquinas's Latin and must rely on translations. Translations can be notoriously misleading. For example, H. Rackham's translations of both the *Nicomachean Ethics* and the *Eudemian Ethics* in the Loeb Classical Library editions render Aristotle's key phrase *kata ton orthon logon* as "according to the right principle," thus giving the incorrect impression that the ethics of Aristotle is an ethics of principles in the same way as modern deontological and utilitarian ethics are ethics of action-guiding principles. Aquinas's translation of this phrase as "according to right reason" (*secundum rectam rationem*) is accurate. The point is worth noting because both Aristotle and Aquinas went to extraordinary lengths to show that right reason in ethics is prudential reasoning, a reasoning quite unlike principle-based reasonings.

Finally, some problems are philosophical: philosophers have always differed and undoubtedly will always differ over how we should understand the moral philosophies of Aristotle and Aquinas. There is no definitive interpretation of their doctrines, and sometimes their texts give rise to conflicting positions. Unfortunately, they are not here to explain their ideas to us. In many ways, then, the moral philosopher influenced by the texts of Aristotle and Aquinas is faced with problems similar to those faced by believers seeking to learn from the Bible. The original texts are lost, other texts were copied by hand, and the copies introduced errors and editorial variations, the Biblical languages of Hebrew and Greek are unknown to many, and we can never be sure what the author meant or (in some cases) who the author was. Nevertheless, the believer recognizes the value of the biblical texts and works from them. And the ethicist can do likewise in a retrieval of older philosophical texts.

It is important to note three things about the older ethics of happiness and prudence retrieved in this book. First, the ethics of prudential reasoning is not a moral relativism. It is a normative ethics, and its norm is a moral absolute. According to its norm, only those feelings, habits, and behaviors constituting a life of happiness and fulfillment for the moral agent understood as a person living in community are morally good. All deliberate feelings and behaviors undermining the agent's flourishing as a good and noble human being living in society are always unreasonable and immoral. Moreover, the ethics of prudential reasoning does allow some absolute moral judgments. Thus, as Aristotle noted, the wrongfulness of murder is absolute. No matter how history develops, murder will never be morally acceptable because murder is, by definition, always the morally unreasonable taking of human life.

Second, the ethics of happiness should not be confused with modern ethical egoisms. In modern versions of egoism the moral agent evaluates behavior only in terms of himself. In the ethics of happiness the moral agent thinks of human existence as interpersonal and social. His happiness and flourishing are inherently entwined with those of others, and thus, their happiness and flourishing matter as well. This is why the predominantly self-centered virtues such as temperance and courage are complemented in an ethics of personal fulfillment by other-centered virtues such as love and justice.

Third, Aristotle did not think the ethics of prudential reasoning was relevant for everyone. In an intriguing but seldom noted remark at the beginning of book VII of the *Nicomachean Ethics*, he acknowledged that certain rare individuals live lives of such heroic virtue that they have no need of prudential reasoning. He also noted that other individuals are so terribly evil—he called them bestial—that they are simply incapable of prudential reasoning. Aristotle was nothing if not a realist. He also thought, with Plato, that many people never grow up morally. They never develop the character virtues or the practical wisdom to make wise decisions about managing their lives. For these people, who unfortunately make up the majority of humankind, the action-guiding laws, principles, and rules developed by others are better than nothing, but their lives are not, according to Aristotle, lives of authentic moral virtue.

The ethics in this book is not written in the language of principles, rules, rights, or duties. It is written in the language of prudential reasoning, the insight and deliberation morally mature people employ to determine how to live fulfilled and happy lives in the situations confronting them. According to Aristotle and Aquinas, prudence is the master virtue for ethical and political decision making. Because prudence is primarily a reasoning attuned to situations and contexts, the study of cases is important for seeing how prudential reasoning works. The cases in this book are therefore presented as an integral part of the chapters describing treatment options. We do not first learn principles and rules and then apply them to cases; we learn about prudential reasoning by working our way through cases involving treatment decisions viewed from the different perspectives of the people involved.

Most cases in this book are not imaginary. They were chosen because they actually happened, and in most instances they were the subject of highly publicized court battles. These public cases were selected because they are morally interesting and instructive and because they give the reader the opportunity to learn something of the history of health care ethics in the United States. As new generations of people interested in health care ethics emerge, they can profit from acquaintance with the widely known cases discussed and debated by those already working in the field.

The book also takes positions in these cases, sometimes agreeing and sometimes disagreeing with what was done. It is important to note that these positions are not intended to be authoritative and dogmatic. Rather, they are invitations for dialogue and discussion. Ethics is not science; we are not studying the physical realities we find around and within our bodies. Ethics is the study of what might become reality as the result of our choices, and an interminable self-correcting process of dialogue and debate is needed to figure out what choices will actually help us live good lives in the ever-changing circumstances of history. As slavery was once seen as ethical and then rejected, what seems ethical today may be rejected in the future as unethical after future discussion and debate.

Each case is presented in an extremely simplified way comprised of two stages. The first stage is called *situational awareness*. Here we attempt to discover and identify the pertinent facts and values in the case. We uncover the facts by asking what is happening here, who are the decision makers, what can be done, and what circumstances are relevant. We become aware of the values involved by asking what features embedded in the situation are good or bad for the people involved and what good and bad outcomes will likely result from our action or inaction.

The second stage is *prudential reasoning*. Here we take the position of each major moral agent in the case—patient, proxy, physician, nurse, attorney, and judge—and ask what each of them could do to live well. The primary goal in life is living well, living a good life, living happily; moral agents behave morally when they behave so as to achieve this goal. This is what we mean by acting according to right reason.

A final word about the cases. The intent in considering these real, and often tragic, cases and in taking a position on what was or was not done is not to attack the personal integrity of the participants in the original story. We simply want to use the stories, which became public when they entered the legal process or were reported in the press, as examples and to learn from them. The analyses of the cases are not intended to make any judgment or to reach any conclusion about the personal or moral character of any person, living or dead, involved in the cases.

This book also differs from many texts in moral philosophy by the place it accords the biblical religious traditions and moral theology. History shows that religion has been a powerful force in shaping ethical attitudes, and it cannot be ignored in ethical analysis. Nonetheless, there are reasons for saying ethics also shapes religion. When it comes to deliberating about how to live well—the major focus of virtue ethics—the moral norm of prudential reasoning embraces all human behaviors, including those proposed in the name of religion and theology. Whether or not to embrace a religious faith is itself an ethical question: will religious commitment enhance or impoverish my flourishing as a human being? The priority of the ethical question that reaches back to Socrates suggests that the eudemonistic ethics of prudential reasoning is relevant, as the texts of Aristotle and Aquinas show so well, both for those who believe in a personal god and for those who do not so believe.

Many people turn to ethics looking for answers. Answers are important, and sometimes we can give them with great confidence. Most of us know the right answer to questions about the morality of slavery, and we also know that, until a few centuries ago, most moral philosophers and theologians (including Aristotle and Aquinas) had the wrong answer.

In addition to moral answers, however, something else is important—moral awareness. The Bible tells a story—and stories are always important in ethics—about moral awareness. King David once spotted a beautiful woman undressed and bathing, and he wanted her. Her husband was a military commander away on a campaign, so they began an affair. When she became pregnant, David recalled the commander from the front lines, hoping that he would sleep with his wife during his home visit so that the king's paternity could be concealed. The commander declined to go home, and stayed in a military camp during his time away from the front. King David then devised a second strategy to cover his tracks—he arranged for the commander to be sent on a useless suicide mission, where he lost his life. David then took the now-widowed Bathsheba as one of his wives, totally oblivious to the immorality of what he and Bathsheba had done—adultery and murder.

A religious man highly respected by King David, Nathan, was not so oblivious to the immorality. One day he told the king how a rich man had taken the young lamb that a poor man had adopted as a pet and loved dearly, and had slaughtered it for a meal. King David was outraged, and ordered the man apprehended and punished. "But," said Nathan, "you are the man." David then realized the terrible thing he had done. He recognized himself as an adulterer and a murderer, and thereby achieved moral awareness, which is the crucial first step in living a good life.

If this book does no more than raise moral awareness about some of the complex ethical issues of health care, it will serve some purpose.

ONE

What Is Ethics?

Iᴛ SHOULD BE NO SURPRISE that ethicists disagree about the answer to this question. The current debates about abortion, nuclear warfare, homosexuality, and euthanasia remind us that ethicists often disagree about ethical matters. We will begin, however, not with the disagreements emerging from the various definitions of ethics, but with the similarities they all share.

DEFINING ETHICS

Despite their differences, most ethical theories include the following features.

Ethics Is about Choices

Here we make but two points, one requiring some explanation, the other needing only a brief statement. First, ethics is concerned with what we choose to do intentionally or on purpose. Ethics is not concerned with what people do accidentally or unintentionally, even if these behaviors cause bad things. If I am getting into a crowded elevator and accidentally step on your foot despite trying to be careful, this is not really an ethical matter. Although I may say "I'm sorry," and thus imply that I did something intentionally, in reality I did not intentionally step on your foot, and nothing unethical or immoral was involved.

The situation becomes more complex if I had stepped on your foot in the process of pushing and shoving my way into the crowded elevator. In this instance I would have to admit some degree of ethical responsibility. True, I did not intend to step on your foot, but I did intend to push my way into the crowded elevator, and thereby I did intentionally choose behavior known to entail a high risk of stepping on someone's foot under these circumstances.

Tremendous debates have existed for centuries in psychology, philosophy, and legal theory about whether human beings are able to choose freely or whether their actions are totally determined by biological, psychological, or sociological factors. These debates need not detain us here. We do know, with the wisdom of everyday experience and of a long criminal justice tradition, that we make choices in life and are therefore responsible in some degree for what we do. To deny this is to deny that a jury could ever find a person guilty of a criminal action. Philosophers and scientists may question our ability to make choices, and some have advanced powerful arguments for explaining our behavior in terms of some form of determinism. But these arguments have not yet convinced us to abandon our experience of choice or to abolish a legal system that holds people responsible, and responsibility implies the person need not have done the deed but indeed chose to do it.

It is important to note that choice embraces what we choose not to do as well as what we choose to do. Choice is about omissions as well as actions. Choosing to do nothing in a situation where we could do something is just as much of a choice as the choice to do something. We are responsible both for what we freely choose to do and for what we freely choose not to do but could do.

Second, although ethics is about choice, not every choice is ethically significant. The only choices of concern in ethics are those giving rise to significant good or bad in the world. Many choices we make in life are too remote from the sphere of good or bad to be of ethical concern. I might very carefully choose what shirt or blouse to wear today, but this choice does not ordinarily give rise to significant good or bad in the world, and so it is not an ethical choice. My choices of what to wear are not usually ethically significant, nor are my choices of what to eat for dinner, of the color of my new car, of computer software, of a television program, and the like.

The recognition that ethical choices are concerned with significant good and bad features in life brings us to the second common theme in ethics—the effort to distinguish what is good from what is bad.

Ethics Is about Evaluation

Ethics inevitably employs determinations and judgments about values. In their simplest form, determinations and judgments about values are differentiations between the good and the bad. Every ethics tells us that certain things are morally good and other things are morally bad and encourages us to choose the good and avoid the bad.

Sometimes the differentiations between good and bad are clear and uncontroversial— nothing bad is involved in the choice of the good, and nothing truly good is involved in the choice of the bad. I take care of my children, for example, or I abuse them. Caring for my children is clearly and simply good; abusing them is clearly and simply bad. Again, I send money to a local charity, or I embezzle money from the local charity. In normal circumstances, contributing to a charity is simply good; stealing from it is simply bad.

Other ethically significant choices, however, are complex in the sense that they involve both good and bad. One and the same action brings about damage and suffering to myself or others but also brings about some good. Euthanasia destroys a human life but brings a quick and peaceful end for a suffering patient dying a slow and painful death. The complex ethical choices, those embracing both good and bad, are the actions and omissions that generate the great controversies in ethics.

Some ethicists distinguish between two types of evaluation: "good or bad" and "right or wrong." They advocate evaluating actions as right or wrong and all other morally significant factors—persons, intentions, motives, character traits, consequences, and the like—as good or bad.

Although there is some merit to distinguishing evaluations of "good or bad" from "right or wrong," this is not the approach we adopt in this text. One reason for not using two types of evaluations (good or bad and right or wrong) is that all ethical evaluations can be expressed in the basic terms of good or bad. Doing the right thing is always good, and doing the wrong thing is always bad.

More important, whenever we distinguish between actions and all other relevant moral aspects in ethics, an unfortunate tendency develops. The distinction inclines us to isolate moral actions from other morally important features, such as feelings, character traits, and the impact of the actions on ourselves and others. The result is an ethics focused on actions considered by themselves and neglectful of the way feelings, intentions, habits, and personal character affect, and are affected by, our actions. As one important contemporary author, William Frankena, put it in two remarks he made in the opening pages of his widely read book titled *Ethics*, (1) "We must not let our decision be affected by our emotions," and (2) "the only question we need answer is whether what is proposed is right or wrong; not what will happen to us, what people will think of us, or how we feel about what has happened."

Frankena is typical of many contemporary ethicists in that he distinguishes the evaluation of actions from the evaluations of other factors. He proposes two kinds of moral judgment: "judgments of moral obligation," which evaluate actions in terms of right and wrong according to principles, and "judgments of moral value," which evaluate motives, intentions, character traits, and consequences in terms of good or bad. He calls this a "double-aspect conception of morality."

Although Frankena proposes that we should regard the morality of principles and the morality of character traits and the other considerations as complementary, he insists that the principles are the basic aspect of morality and that other considerations are secondary. The character traits, for example, are viewed as supporting the principles and are understood in light of them.

Frankena tells us that character traits support moral principles four ways. First, they support us in moments of trial when we are tempted to act contrary to the principles. Second, they sustain us when we have to determine what principle it is our duty to follow when two or more principles conflict. Third, they sustain us when we are trying to revise the working rules of actual duty. Fourth, they allow us to recognize excuses and extenuating circumstances when a person did not act according to the principles but at least tried to do the right thing. In other words, the character traits are considered important only when we need help to carry out the obligations indicated by the principles, or need to resolve conflicts between them, or need to revise rules derived from them, or need to excuse or understand others who have failed to follow the principles. The complementariness of the double-aspect morality is not a complementariness of equals; the principles are basic, and the character traits play a supporting role.

As will become clear in the course of this chapter, the position developed in this book is contrary to that suggested by the two remarks of Frankena. Because virtue pertains to feelings, virtuous feelings will affect our decisions, and rightly so. Second, in an ethics of the good, the most important question in ethics is precisely what will happen to us if we do, or do not, behave in a certain manner. The "only question we need answer" in ethics is not whether our actions are right or wrong but whether our actions, feelings, and character traits are making our lives good lives. Judgments about our actions in an ethics of the good are very much concerned with what happens to us. Actions are good when they help us live well but bad when they undermine our living well.

In an ethics of the good, the virtues and the prudential reasoning needed to establish them in each situation are basic, not the principles. Action-guiding principles enter the picture only when they are helpful, as they often are, in reinforcing the virtues.

Evaluating moral features as good or bad implies, of course, some standard of evaluation. Any ethicist making evaluative judgments about good and bad is employing a criterion or norm. Judgments presuppose standards, and this brings us to our next point—ethical norms.

Ethics Is Normative

Some authors make a distinction between descriptive ethics and normative ethics. This distinction is misleading if it implies that ethics is not normative, that is, if it implies that ethics is a description of what people believe is right or wrong and of how they reason morally. In the long tradition of moral philosophy and ethical theory, ethics has never meant this. Ethics was never understood simply as research into what beliefs people actually hold or how they actually solve moral dilemmas. Ethics was always understood to be normative. It recognized that there were good beliefs, behaviors, and ways of reasoning morally and that there were bad beliefs, behaviors, and ways of reasoning morally.

It would be better to call the important work done in descriptive ethics moral psychology or moral anthropology because it is not ethics in the traditional sense. It is moral psychology and not ethics, for example, when researchers interview people to ascertain how they reason morally or what their values are. A well-known example of moral psychology is the work of Lawrence Kohlberg and his colleagues, who developed first six, and then seven, stages of moral reasoning from their research on children as they grew into adults.

Another example is the work of Carol Gilligan, who pointed out imbalances in Kohlberg's analyses. Other examples of moral psychology or moral anthropology include programs of values clarification and studies of the moralities actually embraced by people of different racial, sexual, cultural, ethnic, and religious backgrounds. In health care, surveys of what nurses or physicians think is ethical regarding certain options—decisions about the withdrawal of feeding tubes, for example—fit into this category of moral psychology.

The key factor in descriptive ethics is that researchers discover, usually by extensive interviews, what people value or what people think is good or bad. The research is important and no good ethicist would want to be without it, but it is not really ethics in the traditional sense because the work is purely descriptive and empirical. Ethics in the traditional sense always included a normative component. Ethicists strove to determine not simply what people thought was good but what was good; not simply what people did in fact value but what was truly valuable; not simply how people reasoned morally but how best to reason morally.

The oldest ethical text we have, the stone tablet recording the Code of Hammurabi (now preserved in the Louvre Museum in Paris), is not simply descriptive of what the Babylonians around 1800 B.C.E. thought was morally good or bad behavior; it is a normative code backed by the authority of the king. Moses did not first interview his people around 1200 B.C.E. to find out what they thought was moral or immoral behavior; he introduced the Ten Commandments as God's laws and made them normative. And Aristotle did not accept what many people of his day (around 350 B.C.E.) thought was the way to live and act but insisted there was a norm for judging the morality of our feelings, habits, and behaviors—and the norm was whether or not these contributed to our living well.

Ethics is not about someone's belief that *x* is good and that *y* is bad. Ethics begins when we ask someone *why* he thinks *x* is good and *why* he thinks *y* is bad. Ethics begins when we begin giving reasons why something is good or bad, and the appeal to the reasons why something is good or bad is an appeal to something normative.

When a person gives reasons why stealing is bad, she is appealing to norms. Perhaps she will say stealing is wrong because it violates God's law, or the natural law, or a person's natural right to his property, or the duty of justice as conceived by Kant, or the greatest happiness principle of Mill. If she is following the older tradition of ethics typified by Aristotle, she may say stealing is ultimately wrong because it threatens to undermine the thief's good life and happiness as both an individual and a social being by violating the virtue of justice, and the virtues are what we need to live well and happily.

Ethicists and moral philosophers disagree on what might serve as the normative basis of moral judgment, but they do not disagree on the need for something normative. The fact that a person believes something is right or wrong is not enough; the moral philosopher insists that those beliefs must be justified by something normative and that the exploration of what is normative for our behavior is the work of ethics. Ethics is not simply about reality—the positions people actually hold as moral—but about norms that enable us to say (to the extent that it can be verbalized) which positions are morally good and which positions are morally bad.

This point about the normative component of ethics is important because some published work in professional journals associated with health care frequently refers to purely descriptive research into what people think is right or wrong as "ethics." Empirical research in ethics, however, is not ethics or moral philosophy in the traditional sense unless it also evaluates the findings in terms of something morally normative, be that norm rights, principles, laws, rules, or human fulfillment and happiness. The important normative component in ethics introduces our next topic—reasoning.

Ethics Includes Reasoning

Faced with the challenges of life, we have to determine what is truly good for ourselves and what is truly bad. The ethical wisdom embedded in our traditions is a rich source for discerning what is good or bad, but it is not enough. Sometimes moral traditions misguide us; our tradition found slavery morally acceptable for centuries but now condemns it. Sometimes, and this is especially true in health care, our moral traditions fail to guide us because our predecessors never experienced or even thought about what we face today.

When responding to the moral questions created by new techniques and technology such as ventilators, artificial hearts, transplantation, cardiopulmonary resuscitation, medical feeding, and medically assisted reproductive interventions, for example, we are very much on our own because we are the first generation to encounter these situations. Following moral traditions, the moral responses given by previous generations, although important, simply will not do. Aristotle correctly identified what we do in ethics—"All people seek the good, not the way of their ancestors." This means we have to think and reason about what will achieve a good life and not simply adopt the ready-made judgments of a moral tradition constituted by our predecessors.

Discerning what is truly good or bad can be difficult for several reasons. First, some things seem good for us but really are not, and some things seem bad but really are good. The pint of ice cream in the freezer looks good to the overweight person with high cholesterol and heart disease but really is not, and fasting from food and fluids for many hours seems bad if we are hungry and thirsty, but it is really good for us if we are about to undergo surgery.

Second, good things are often mixed with bad things. Surgery often brings life-prolonging benefits, yet it also brings the burdens of risk, pain, and physical mutilation. When the good and bad are inextricably entwined, as they often are in health care situations, reasoning can only figure out how best to enhance one's good life and reduce what undermines it.

Third, our ability to figure out what is good and what is bad is always distorted to some extent by psychological and social biases beyond our control. Our view is always a *point* of view, the view of a particular person or persons, in a particular place, at a particular time, with a particular history, and in a particular social, cultural, and (perhaps) religious matrix. This means that the conclusions of our moral reasonings are never absolute but always relative in some degree to our historical and psychological perspectives.

It is also helpful to recognize that the reasoning we encounter in ethics appears on three different levels. The first and most immediate level is the personal level. Here I find myself faced with a situation where I must not only decide what is good but actually do or be affected by what I decide. I am the moral agent. For example I am of advanced years and in declining health, and I need a lung biopsy. I have to decide whether or not it would be better for me to allow physicians to attempt cardiopulmonary resuscitation in the event of a cardiac or pulmonary arrest during the biopsy. As the result of my decision, an order not to attempt resuscitation will, or will not, be written for me.

Another example: I am a physician, and a patient suffering from acquired immune deficiency syndrome (AIDS) has asked for medications I know he intends to use to commit suicide in the future. I have to decide whether it would be better to write the prescription or to refuse a dying man what he considers a reasonable request.

Figuring out what I will actually decide in a particular situation where I am personally engaged is the kind of reasoning the earlier ethics of Aristotle and Aquinas (an ethics we will retrieve in this book) called *prudence*.

The second level of ethical reasoning is judgmental. Here I also find myself considering a particular situation and want to know what will achieve the good in the circumstances, but I am not actually going to do, or be significantly affected by, what I decide. I am not the moral agent. Making ethical judgments on this level is far less personal than practicing prudence because someone else is confronted with the ethical question. In the examples given above I might be a friend of the person wrestling with the decision about cardiopulmonary resuscitation, or I might be a colleague helping the physician decide whether or not he should give the patient with AIDS access to medications that will probably be used for suicide.

Some ethicists do not make a distinction between the *personal* reasoning of the person actually confronted with the ethical challenge and the *judgmental* reasoning of the person considering the case but not so engaged that she will carry out or be significantly impacted by whatever decision is made. They consider both the personal and judgmental levels of reasoning as instances of moral judgment about what should, or should not, be done. In a sense, this is true. There are important similarities between the personal reasoning about what is good or bad when I am faced with doing and being affected by what I decide and the moral judgments I make about what is good or bad for others to do.

Despite the similarities between these two levels of moral reasoning, however, there are reasons for noting the difference between them. The person faced with making a decision about something she will do or be affected by has an important existential perspective not shared by those judging behaviors they will not actually pursue. Her personal reasoning is a part of her life, her story, her future, and these existential and historical factors introduce an important context not shared by anyone else. She is not looking on as a judge; she is the principal involved in the case.

In the last analysis, the final moral decision rests with the moral agent faced with doing or being affected by what she decides, and her position is unique. This uniqueness is better preserved by distinguishing the personal and the judgmental levels of moral reasoning, a distinction reminiscent of that previously made in theological ethics between following one's conscience even when everyone else's ethical judgments might indicate one should do otherwise.

In this book we will not be operating on the personal level of ethical reasoning because you and I are not actually going to carry out, or be affected by, the evaluative decisions we make in the cases we study. When we study the cases we will be operating on the level of judgmental reasoning, not prudence or personal reasoning, just as we do when we try to help friends figure out what is good or bad, or when we review cases in ethics committee meetings at a hospital or nursing home, or when we make moral judgments about particular cases reported in the media, and so forth.

At the same time, since the personal and judgmental levels are similar, experience in reasoning on the judgmental level will ideally help us to make better personal decisions in our lives when we are actually faced with ethical challenges similar to those we study in this book. These challenges are ones that practically nobody can avoid. Most of us will be making morally significant health care decisions for ourselves and for others, most likely our parents, spouse, or our own children.

The third level of ethical reasoning is theoretical. Here we study carefully and critically what others have written and said about ethics, and we attempt to develop some sort of theoretical account that explains the nature of ethics. If I try to show that biomedical ethics is fundamentally a matter of obligations derived from principles and rules, or if I try to show that biomedical ethics is fundamentally not a matter of obligation but of following our natural inclination to achieve a good life and to live well, I am reasoning on the theoretical level. Also on the theoretical level are the attempts to develop an ethics based on divine law (as found in the Hebrew, Christian, and Islamic traditions), and the attempts to base an ethics on natural law, on natural rights, on the greatest happiness principle, and on the respect-for-persons principle that obliges us to treat every person as an end and not merely as a means.

The theoretical study of the nature of ethics, its concepts, and its language is the work of ethicists—the moral philosophers and moral theologians. They try to explain what ethics is all about and to clarify the thoughts and language we use in our judgments and personal decisions. It is very important and very demanding work that requires extensive study. There is a large body of important ethical literature stretching from Plato, Aristotle, the Stoics, and early Hebrew and Christian texts, through Cicero and Augustine, Aquinas, Spinoza, Locke, Hume, Kant, Hegel, Bentham, and Mill, to the seminal authors of our own century. It all must be understood to some extent if one is to enter the conversation about ethics on the theoretical level.

Although the theoretical study of ethics—moral philosophy and moral theology—seems far removed from our personal ethical reasoning about what to do in a particular situation, it is not. Ethical theory does have an impact on our lives, although its role is often unnoticed until we undertake a serious and critical examination of our moral beliefs. Hence, the academic or theoretical work we do in ethics, no less than the cases on which we form judgments, has the same practical goal as does our personal deliberation when we are confronted with a situation where we have to decide what to do. That goal is learning how to live well.

Since this volume is not intended for the specialist, the emphasis is not on the theoretical level. Nonetheless, some theoretical background is necessary, and we will present some theoretical considerations in the early chapters of the book. Most of the time, however, we will work on the judgmental level of ethical reasoning. We will try to make our judgmental reasonings as close as possible to the personal reasoning of a moral agent engaged in an existential situation by looking at actual cases from the different perspectives of the patient, the proxy, the physicians, the nurses, the attorneys, the administrators, and the judges. In this way the ethical analysis of each case will approximate the prudential reasoning each of us practices in life as we strive to live well. The work on the theoretical and judgmental levels will enrich our ability to discern and to do what actually will better achieve the good in our lives. All the work we do in ethics, even the theoretical work, has the same attractive goal of achieving personal happiness in our lives.

We turn next to a description of the two kinds of ethics we find in our cultural tradition.

Two Kinds of Ethics

The major ethical theories in our cultural background fall into two general groups. The theories of the first group are related by the emphasis they place on moral obligation, or duty. Behavior in accord with our moral obligation is considered morally right; behavior not in accord with our moral obligation is considered morally wrong. Underlying these theories is the assumption that people do not naturally tend and desire to live well. If this assumption is embraced, it makes sense to say that people must be obliged to live well and that the morality of behavior is a morality of duty.

Moralities of obligation are moralities of law, where law is understood as a system of precepts or rules people are obliged to follow. Moralities of law appear in different forms. Some rely on divine law, others on natural law, still others (Kant, for example) on the moral law we give to ourselves. Today the morality of law appears most frequently as an ethics based on principles, rules, and rights, where the principles, rules, and rights are understood as action-guides that we have a moral obligation or duty to observe and respect.

The theories of the second group are related by the emphasis they place on the good of the person performing the action. Behavior making our lives good is considered virtuous, and behavior making our lives bad is considered worthless and a vice. These theories of the good assume that most everyone naturally seeks to live well, and they make this desire for a good life the starting point of ethics. The key notion of modern ethics—obligation—is scarcely present in the theories of this group. It makes little sense to say people are obliged to seek what they already want. Instead of obligation, the key notion in an ethics of the good is virtue. Virtues are the feelings, habits, and behaviors that do in fact create a good life.

The two kinds of ethics, of course, are not totally unrelated. After all an ethics encouraging people to live up to their obligations implies it is good for them to do so, and an ethics encouraging people to live well implies living up to their obligations. Yet the differences between an ethics of obligation and an ethics of the good are important, and they result in two significantly distinct approaches to ethics.

An example from a seminal work that has influenced many American ethicists reveals clearly the difference between an ethics rooted in obligation and duty and an ethics rooted in the good and virtue. At the end of his important book *The Right and the Good*, W. D. Ross wonders whether duty or love would be a better motivation for moral actions. In other words, which actions are morally superior—those done for duty or those done for love?

His conclusion is consistent with his preference for what is right over what is good: "The desire to do one's duty is the morally best motive." He acknowledges that many will question this and argue that actions springing from love are morally superior to actions springing from duty, but he argues that they are wrong. When a genuine sense of duty conflicts with any other motive (even love), the sense of duty takes precedence. And if, Ross tells us, both love and duty incline us to one and the same action, our action will be morally better if we act from the motivation of duty rather than from the motivation of love: "We are bound to think the man who acts from sense of duty the better man."

This kind of ethics suggests that parents caring for their children act in a morally superior way when they care for them because it is their duty, rather than because they love them. It suggests that a partner in a marriage behaves in a morally superior way when he supports his wife because it is his duty, rather than because he loves her. It means a physician or nurse acts in a morally superior way when his interaction with patients is motivated by the duties of the clinician-patient relationship rather than by the love of neighbor.

It is precisely this priority of duty over love that separates sharply the moralities of obligation from the moralities of the good. In the ethics of Aristotle and Aquinas retrieved in this text, love is the major virtue whereby we constitute and create our lives as good lives. Aristotle devoted more space to love in the *Nicomachean Ethics* than to any other virtue, and Aquinas made love the crowning virtue of his moral philosophy and theology. There is, then, a kind of fundamental option in health care ethics today—the option between an ethics based on obligation and duty, with its principles, rules, and rights that we must obey and respect, and an ethics based on living well, with its virtues that create a good life.

The ethics of obligation has appeared in many forms in our ethical tradition. We turn next to its major historical manifestations.

HISTORICAL VERSIONS OF THE ETHICS OF OBLIGATION

We can identify five major versions of theories based on obligation. The first two versions originated over two thousand years ago, the remaining three emerged only in the past few centuries.

Divine Law Theories

These influential theories originated in the land recognized today as Iraq but known in ancient times as Babylonia and Mesopotamia. Here a nomadic patriarch named Abraham was born and grew up about four thousand years ago. Consistent with the Semitic cultures in this area of West Asia, Abraham and his people believed that God gives commandments to his people. God's law creates the moral obligations in our lives; human beings are obliged to follow the laws of their Creator.

The divine law theories continue today in the Jewish, Christian, and Islamic religious traditions, for these are the three major world religions tracing their lineage to Abraham and his God. Most people in our culture became familiar with the divine law theory when they first heard of the "Ten Commandments," a set of laws Moses promulgated to his people over three thousand years ago. These commandments, along with hundreds of other divine laws, are preserved in the early books of the Hebrew Bible, which many Christians call the Old Testament.

Natural Law Theories

Plato is widely recognized for his efforts to develop an ethics based on metaphysical norms (that is, on otherworldly, transcendent, eternal, unchanging "Ideas" or normative "Forms") that the wise person must grasp in order to know what is good or bad behavior in the particular situations of this temporal and changing world. At the end of his life, however, after wrestling with numerous difficulties about the famous metaphysical Ideas or Forms, Plato began to speak of physical nature in a morally normative way. He began to argue that actions were virtuous if they were "according to nature" and not virtuous if they were "contrary to nature."

In his last work, *The Laws*, Plato had the "Athenian stranger" (undoubtedly Socrates) say that there is an "unwritten law" against incest recognized by everyone. The Athenian stranger then argues that legislators ought to mold public opinion in such a way that people will recognize that this unwritten law should be extended to all sexual behavior that is not "according to nature" (that is, all sexual behavior not appropriate for reproduction in marriage). Homosexuality, fornication, and masturbation were explicitly condemned by Plato, in addition to incest, as being not according to nature. Homosexuality also received a stronger prohibition: It is not simply not according to nature—it is "contrary to nature," a transgression of nature.

Although "according to nature" is not an exact equivalent of "according to natural law," Plato's use of the phrases "unwritten law," "according to nature," and "contrary to nature" is obviously normative. He believed that sexual actions not in accord with nature are immoral and should become the subject of legal prohibitions.

Early Greek Stoicism (a philosophy inaugurated by Zeno, who had studied at Plato's Academy in Athens more than a half century after Plato's death) also stressed "according to nature" as morally normative. Following Plato, the Greek Stoics did not explicitly speak of natural law, but they did view nature as permeated by a rational order (*logos*) and then concluded that ethics is living and acting "according to rationally ordered nature."

The Stoic influence on ancient thought was immense. Stoicism played a dominant role in the moral thinking of the ancient world until late in the fourth century of the common era, when

Christianity replaced it after the Roman emperor made Christianity the official religion of the vast empire in southern Europe, northern Africa, and the Middle East. Many Stoic ideas continue anonymously in our culture to this day. Most ancient people, for example, believed with Job and Sophocles that bad things happen to good people without reason and that tragedy can destroy a good life. The Stoics were popular because they assured people that this was not so, that "everything happens for the best" in a universe permeated by rational order.

According to some scholars, these two Stoic notions—the *logos* of nature and acting "according to nature"—were independently developed into "acting according to the natural law" by two important figures, Cicero of Rome and Philo of Alexandria. Both of these major figures may have been influenced by a common source, Antiochus of Ascalon (ca. 130–68 B.C.E.), whose doctrine represented a transformation of early Stoicism's "according to nature" to an inchoate notion of "according to the law of nature."

Cicero studied in Greece and wrote extensively on Greek ethics in Latin during the last century before the common era. In his treatments of the Stoics he sometimes freely translated the "*logos* of nature" as the "law of nature," and "according to nature" as "according to the law of nature." Greek philosophy had almost always distinguished nature and law, *physis* and *nomos* (although Plato's remarks in *The Laws* are an exception to this), but Cicero tended to obliterate the distinction. He wrote in his *Laws*: "The highest reason (*logos* in Greek, *ratio* in Latin) implanted in nature is law, which commands what ought to be done, and forbids the opposite" (I, v, 18).

Cicero put the moral law into nature and thus presided at the birth of natural law theories. With him, the transition from "according to nature" to "according to the law of nature" and "according to natural law" became reality. His ideas were later developed at length by Roman jurists looking for a theoretical foundation for civil law, by Christian canonists eager to provide a foundation for Church law, and by medieval theologians and philosophers in the developing universities of the twelfth and thirteenth centuries looking for a basis for ethics in reason to complement the biblical basis rooted in divine revelation.

Philo was of Jewish heritage and wrote from Egypt in the first century of the common era. His language was Greek, and his concept of the law of nature as a source of moral obligation may well have been the result of a desire to reconcile his Jewish tradition of living according to the Law of the Torah with the Stoic philosophy of living according to nature. Philo believed that the universal principles of morality, what he called the "archetypes," are derived from the law of nature and known by all and that the laws formulated in the Torah are more specific statements of these universal principles. His writings influenced a considerable number of his contemporaries, both Jewish and Christian, who were more comfortable thinking and writing in Greek than in Hebrew or Latin.

The natural law concept introduced into Latin ethical thought by Cicero and into Greek ethical thought by Philo exerted a tremendous influence that persists to this day. There are many variations of natural law theory, but they all hold that actions contrary to the natural law are immoral. Natural law, for example, is often cited as a basis for considering homosexual behavior immoral, and Pope Paul VI cited the natural law as the basis for his condemnation of contraception in the 1968 encyclical *Humanae vitae*.

In the past few centuries many ethicists have moved away from the claim that our moral obligations arise either from divine law or from natural law. In place of these older theories, they have created several new approaches. The major ones are natural rights, utilitarianism, and a universal moral law we give to ourselves.

Natural Rights

Some ethicists, following political philosophies developed by Thomas Hobbes and John Locke, say that our moral obligations come from individual rights possessed by all people. People are thought to have natural or *human rights*, chiefly the right to life, the right to choose, and the right to property, and our obligation is to respect these rights. These theories of obligation are called rights-based theories.

Rights-based theories of moral obligation explain the tendencies to justify ethical judgments on the basis of such rights as the right to health care, the right to life, the right to choose, the right to refuse treatment, the right to die, and so forth. If someone has a right to die, a rights-based theory obliges us to respect that right; if a fetus has a right to life, the theory obliges us to let the fetus live; if a woman has a right to choose abortion, the theory obliges us to let her have it; if a person has a right to health care, the theory obliges someone to provide it.

Utilitarianism

Some ethicists, following Jeremy Bentham and John Stuart Mill, say that our moral obligation arises from what will benefit the most people. We are obliged to act on behalf of the greatest happiness for the greatest number. These theories are called *utilitarian* because our obligation is to use whatever means are useful for achieving the greatest happiness. Although it is misleading to say simply that utilitarianism is a philosophy whereby the end, the greatest happiness for the greatest number, justifies the means, this caricature does help us to grasp in a preliminary way the basic dynamic of the moral theory.

Today, most utilitarian theories are rule utilitarianisms; that is, our moral obligation is to follow the rules that will result in the greatest happiness for the greatest number. For example most utilitarians accept the rule stating that it is immoral to kill an innocent person intentionally. They argue that I am always obliged to follow this rule even though, at a particular time, intentionally killing an innocent person might actually result in greater good for a greater number than not killing him.

Autonomous Moral Law

By autonomous moral law we mean a moral law that comes neither from God nor from nature but from ourselves. The Greek roots of "autonomous" are "self" and "law." Each ancient Greek city was autonomous (that is, it made its own laws), and this is why the cities were called city-states. In this moral theory of autonomy, we constitute the moral law for ourselves.

This may sound like pure subjectivism or even anarchy, but it is not. The originator of this powerful moral theory, the eighteenth-century German philosopher Immanuel Kant, insisted that any maxim that we propose as a moral law for ourselves must be universally desirable (that is, the maxim must condone the behavior that we would want everyone to do). Hence, if I find myself in a tight spot and need a lie to escape, I might consider giving myself a moral maxim that permits lying. But no moral maxim can condone lying because no reasonable person would want such a maxim to be universal (that is, to be a maxim that would apply always and everywhere).

And why not? Because a universal moral maxim permitting lying would make life impossible. Such a maxim would make it morally right for the bank to lie about the balance in my account, for the airline to lie about the destination of my flight, for the surgeon to lie about my need for surgery, and for the professor to lie about the quality of my work in the course.

Kant's theory is an example of a *deontological* theory of obligation. Deontological theories oblige us to avoid certain actions without exception. The proscribed actions are always immoral regardless of good intentions, of extenuating circumstances, or of the good consequences resulting from the action. The end never justifies the means. Deontological theories, then, are sharply distinguished from utilitarian theories, yet both are theories of obligation.

All these five theories share a common theme. They view ethics as primarily a matter of obligation. Something—perhaps God's law, perhaps the natural law, perhaps another's rights, perhaps the greatest happiness of the greatest number, perhaps the moral law we give to ourselves—requires us to behave a certain way regardless of whether we want to behave in that way. Morality is a matter of obligation, and obligation connotes doing something we have to do but may not want to do.

MORAL REASONING AND THE THEORIES OF OBLIGATION

The moral reasoning associated with an ethics of obligation tends to manifest two major characteristics: it is both deductive and inductive. We could describe it as *deductive-inductive* reasoning.

Although logically we can clearly distinguish deductive and inductive reasonings, in practice most deductive reasonings have an inductive phase and most inductive reasonings have a deductive phase. It is often said, for example, that ancient science was deductive and modern science is inductive. But this is a gross oversimplification. Aristotle's science was very much inductive, despite his description of science in the *Posterior Analytics* as syllogistic; and modern science is very much deductive once it establishes the hypotheses its experiments are designed to confirm or disprove.

In moral theories of obligation we seldom find purely deductive or purely inductive reasoning. Some theories stress deduction but include induction; some stress induction but include deduction; and some advocate a dialectical balance between deduction and induction whereby the prima facie principles and duties will sometimes dictate a particular judgment and the particular judgments will sometimes modify, revise, or supplement the prima facie principles and duties.

The deductive component begins when we apply one of the general norms—a divine or natural law, or a human right, or an action-guiding moral principle—to a particular situation. By applying the law, right, or principle to the particular situation, we are able to make a moral judgment that reveals our moral obligation in the particular case.

For example if we begin with a human right as a general norm—the right to life, for instance—and apply it to a particular situation involving a feeding tube sustaining the life of a permanently unconscious patient, then we could easily judge that the withdrawal of the tube is unethical because it violates the patient's right to life. This moral judgment would then oblige us to continue the feeding tube.

The inductive component of the deductive-inductive reasoning is what gives rise to the general norms and allows us to modify them. It does this chiefly in two ways. First, from our inherited social practices and rules we can generate general norms and, if necessary, subsequently revise them. The general norms are then applied to future situations. Second, from the judgments we make in particular cases we can develop general principles and rules and then apply them (sometimes in a modified way) to future analogous cases as these occur. This latter form of induction is often called *casuistry*.

The deductive-inductive model of moral reasoning can be sketched as follows.

Moral theory (e.g., theories of divine law, natural law, rights)

↓

General norm (e.g., a natural right, or a principle, rule, or law)

↓

Particular case (e.g., whether or not we should treat this baby)

↓

Particular moral judgment (e.g., we are obliged to treat)

If the moral reasoning makes the theory and norms foundational and then applies the norms to particular cases to determine what we are obliged to do, then it is primarily deductive, and the morality is usually described as applied normative ethics. If the moral reasoning stresses the origin of the norms in particular judgments coalescing over time into a common shared morality giving rise to general rules obliging us in analogous cases, then it is primarily inductive and is sometimes called casuistry. If the moral reasoning moves with ease from the general norm to the particular and from the particular to the general norm, it is thought of as coherentist, and its dynamics is sometimes described as an ongoing reflective equilibrium. *Coherentism* is a term describing the effort to develop a coherence between the general norms and the particular judgments by constantly adjusting each as experience develops. In practice, however, most coherentists tend toward the path staked out by Frankena; that is, the principles are primary.

The deductive reasoning in the deductive-inductive model is analogous to the reasoning we find in geometry. Certain geometrical axioms are given, and from them we can deduce certain truths about particular figures—circles, triangles, rectangles, and so forth. The axioms are true by definition, and if they are applied to a particular figure correctly through deductive reasoning, the conclusions about the particular figure will be true. Moralists disagree on where the analogues to the axioms—the principles or laws—come from. Some say they precede or transcend our experience, as in the theories of divine laws or Kantian moral law; others say they come from a universal common morality. Once established, however, they tend to operate deductively; the principles and laws are norms employed to determine what people are obliged to do.

Sometimes the geometrical flavor of contemporary moral theory emerges explicitly. John Rawls, an advocate of reflective equilibrium, nonetheless wrote in his landmark book *A Theory of Justice*: "The argument aims eventually to be strictly deductive. . . . Clearly arguments from such premises can be fully deductive, as theories in politics and economics attest. We should strive for a kind of moral geometry with all the rigor which this name connotes."

What follows are some extremely simplified examples of deductive moral reasoning in health care ethics using the rights-based and principles-based approaches. When you look at these examples, set aside your opinions; that is, pay no attention to whether or not you agree with the conclusions. Focus instead on the structure of the reasonings. Notice how they employ a general principle or a right that everyone is believed to have, and then apply it to a particular situation in order to generate a conclusion. Remember also that we are leaving aside questions about where the general principles or rights originated; it makes no significant difference in these reasonings whether the principles or rights were derived from a transcendent or transcendental source such as divine law or Kant's pure reason, or from shared moral tradition, a common morality we inherited much as we inherit a language.

1. The general principle is that we must always do what will result in the greatest happiness for the greatest number; this withdrawal of life-sustaining treatment will bring the greatest happiness for the greatest number; therefore, this withdrawal is morally justified.

2. The general principle is that we must always treat another person as an end and never merely as a means; this cesarean section is treating the woman merely as a means because its sole purpose is to let a resident practice the surgery; therefore, this surgery is not morally justified.

3. The most fundamental right is the right to life; withdrawing nutrition and hydration will cause loss of life by starving the person to death; therefore, withdrawing nutrition and hydration is not morally justified.

4. The most fundamental right is the right to choose; terminating my pregnancy is my choice; therefore, terminating my pregnancy is morally justified.

5. The basic moral principle in medicine is beneficence—doing good to others; this surgery will be good for the patient; therefore, this surgery is morally justified.

6. The basic moral principle in health care is patient autonomy or patient self-determination; this competent dying patient wants me to help him commit suicide; therefore, assistance in his suicide is morally justified.

If we could deduce the morally right way to act in any particular case by the deductive-inductive model of reasoning, it would be very comforting. Once general rights and principles are accepted, a person faced with a particular dilemma simply gets the facts straight, recalls the established principles and rights, and then follows the rules of deductive reasoning to find the right answer. Only if more than one principle or right is in play or if the principle or right leads to a highly implausible particular judgment does the person have to engage in some creative and imaginative thinking to balance the conflicting principles or rights, or to revise one of them.

In an ethics of the good, the deductive-inductive kind of moral reasoning is not the primary way we reason. As we will see in chapter two, figuring out how to live well is a matter of prudential deliberation and judgment. Its model is not geometry but figuring out, while actually engaged in a goal-oriented process, how to achieve the goal.

Contrasting the Ethics of Obligation with an Ethics of the Good

The basic idea in an ethics of the good can be expressed in three relatively simple assumptions. First, it is taken as uncontroversial that people do not simply want life, but a good life; that people do not simply want to live, but to live well. Second, it is also taken as uncontroversial that achieving a good life, living well, depends to some extent on the choices we make in life. Finally, it is taken as uncontroversial that intelligent choices, choices that constitute rather than undermine living well, require thought and reasoning. Ethics clarifies the goal we all seek—a good life—and determines, to the extent it can be determined, the choices we need to make to achieve it. Clarifying what truly constitutes a good life and deliberating thoughtfully about how to achieve it in the actual and varied situations confronting us in life constitute the subject matter of ethics in an ethics of the good.

It is important to understand that the good life or living well is not something we should or ought to seek, but something we in fact do seek. A good life is something we all desire—the ultimate and underlying goal of every human being. Nobody in his right mind would strive to live a bad life, to live badly.

It is also important to understand that the good life I seek in this ethics is my own happiness and good. What I seek is my good, a good life for myself. Rightly understood, this is not, as we will see, selfishness. My good is inextricably interwoven with the good of others, especially those who are my family, friends, and members of my communities.

This ethics of the good, no less than the ethics of obligation, is a normative ethics. The norm is a good life, a life of fulfillment and flourishing. The feelings, habits, and behaviors that constitute living well are precisely the feelings, habits, and behaviors that are ethical; those that undermine living well are unethical.

In an ethics of the good, the reasoning is not an effort to deduce moral judgments from rights, principles, or rules. Rather, the person first acknowledges that the overarching goal of life is to live well, and then he figures out what will achieve this goal. The feelings, habits, and actions contributing to a good life are called the virtues; those that undermine a good life are worthless and can be called the vices. The deliberation or practical reasoning called prudence does not lead to a moral judgment that I am obliged to obey whether I want to or not but to a moral decision that I want to execute because the behavior will make my life good.

Retrieving the Ethics of the Good

The ethics of the good has not been fashionable for centuries. One reason why it fell out of favor was the difficulty in clarifying just what constitutes a good life. In this section we need to give a brief account of what we mean by a good life and also to explain why it is important to include a figure such as Aquinas in our retrieval of the ethics of the good from Aristotle.

In chapter six we will develop the notion of what constitutes *one of us*; that is, a notion of what it means to be considered a member of the human population. We will suggest that the notion of "psychic body," what many refer to as sentience, is key for understanding when one of us exists. A human body becomes psychic when it becomes even minimally aware, and a human body ceases to be psychic when it can no longer be even minimally aware. A fetal human body becomes one of us when it begins to feel; and a totally unconscious human body ceases to be one of us when it suffers irreversible loss of all awareness or feeling.

If we consider each one of us a psychic or sentient body, then our question about what constitutes a good life is a question about what is good for a psychic human body. This is, after all, what each of us is, regardless of our age, race, gender, and so forth.

For purposes of analysis we can distinguish several major natural inclinations each one of us—each psychic body—possesses. Although it is somewhat arbitrary to separate the interwoven strands of any existing psychic body, three important sets of inclinations characterize human psychic bodies.

First, some inclinations are markedly biological in nature, and satisfying them contributes to a good life. Living well means we have adequate food, shelter, health, and so forth.

Second, some inclinations are markedly psychological in nature, and satisfying them contributes to a good life. Living well means we have satisfying emotional and cognitive lives and the freedom or liberty to exercise some choice over how we live and what we do.

Third, some inclinations are markedly social in nature, and satisfying them contributes to a good life. Living well means we have healthy interpersonal relationships of love and friendship, contractual agreements with others rooted in justice, and relationships with the political community constituting the society in which we live. Living well means living in supportive political and institutional environments that help people flourish. Human existence is always a coexistence, an existence with others, and this coexistence is sometimes interpersonal, sometimes contractual, sometimes communitarian, and, thought Aristotle, always political.

Each of us has inclinations to forge relations with loved ones and friends, to enter into agreements with others, and to live in just and peaceful communities that we help to build. The political community is not a social contract we establish for the protection of our individual rights; our very existence is fundamentally communal as well as personal. Building community is building a good life for ourselves because living in a well-ordered society working toward peace and justice contributes significantly to living a good life. Satisfying our inclinations for love, friendship, mutual agreements, and a decent society is very much a part of living well.

In recent decades we have begun to realize that our existence is a coexistence in yet another way. Our lives are interwoven with all life on this planet, and we live well when we treat all life well. We are beginning to recognize that the mistreatment of animals and of the environment is something that truly undermines our living well, and thus, it is something we had best avoid.

There are, of course, disagreements about what constitutes a good life, just as there are disagreements among all the various schools of moralities of obligation. The disagreements over what constitutes a truly good life for human beings in particular situations, however, should not blind us to the widespread agreement about many general features of a good human life. We know that health is good and sickness and suffering are bad. We know that adequate nutrition is good and malnutrition is bad. We know that a life with love and friendship is good and a life without love and friendship is bad. We know societies with checks and balances are better in the long run than societies governed by dictators. We know trials by jury are better than the medieval trials by ordeal. We know that a life with adequate resources is good and a life of poverty is bad. We know slavery is not good, nor are torture and political or judicial corruption. We know that education is good, that illiteracy and ignorance are bad. We know that war is terrible and that it is good to make every effort to avoid it. We know reproducing and rearing children in stable and loving relationships are better than other alternatives. We know it is bad when people lie to us, steal from us, break their promises, attack us, and discriminate against us; and we know it is good when people are honest with us, respect our property, keep their promises, support us, and treat us fairly.

In some ways the widespread agreement about what constitutes a good life for humans suggests a universal common morality that many proponents of principle-based and rule-based ethical approaches now advocate, and there are similarities. However there is an important difference: proponents of a universal common morality see it as the foundation of moral obligations expressed in principles and rules, whereas virtue ethics see it as the result of something more fundamental—the common human effort to flourish that we all share.

The shared view of what constitutes a good life manifests itself very clearly when we reflect on what we try to teach children, perhaps as parents, or as relatives, teachers, coaches, and mentors. By word and by example we try to show children how to live a good life, and a great consensus exists on what that good life is. We do not encourage them to lie, steal, or cheat. We do not teach them how to become promiscuous, destructive, or violent. We do try to teach them to be temperate, fair, kind, loving, caring, brave, concerned for others, generous, and so forth. Why do we teach children these virtues? Because we want them to live a good life, and we know living a good life is, in large measure, living virtuously.

The shared ethics of the good actually maintains its identity in a wide variety of different human lives. It is easily adaptable to different cultures and to different eras. The adaptation of

Aristotle by Aquinas is an example of this. The two men lived in two very different worlds— fourth-century B.C.E. Greece and thirteenth-century Europe. Yet Aquinas found Aristotle's ethics relevant, and almost sixteen hundred years after it had been all but forgotten in Europe, Aquinas retrieved Aristotle's ethics of the good.

This is surprising and suggestive given their very different worldviews. Aquinas believed in a God who created the world, conserves it in being, directs it in his providence, loves the people he created, and saves them from the clutches of evil and sin. Aristotle also spoke of god, and sometimes gods, but his god did not create the world, does not conserve it, does not direct it, does not love or even know people, and does not redeem or save anyone. Aristotle's god, at least his god in the *Metaphysics*, is not a deity in any religious sense. The eternal, necessary, first unmoved mover neither knows nor cares about us, and all prayers to this god are unanswered because unheard. In short, Aquinas thought a deep religious faith augmented living well; Aristotle did not so believe.

Moreover, Aquinas accepted the Hebrew Bible as the revealed word of God, a source of truth about the world as well as about God; Aristotle did not. Aquinas believed in a personal life after death, in the immortality of each personal soul destined one day to be rejoined with its resurrected body; Aristotle did not believe in any personal life after death, although his mentor Plato had so believed. Aquinas believed in heaven and hell, states of eternal beatitude and suffering where the good triumph and the bad are punished; Aristotle did not believe in any heaven or hell. Aquinas believed virginity was better than marriage and lived as a religious friar; Aristotle believed that the virtue of temperance indicated a loving sexual relationship was better than the extremes of either promiscuity or virginity and lived as a married man. Aquinas rejected all abortion and suicide; Aristotle accepted abortion and suicide in some situations. Aquinas supported the early Inquisition and thought it was morally good to execute people with heretical ideas; Aristotle fled Athens at the end of his life in fear that he would be executed for his views, a fate that had befallen Socrates earlier in the century.

What is the significance of emphasizing the different worldviews of Aristotle and Aquinas despite their agreement on an ethic of the good? For one thing it shows how their differences did not prevent a deep-seated agreement on what they thought constitutes living well; that is, on what constitutes living virtuously. Aquinas's development of prudence and the moral virtues is very Aristotelian; both men agreed that the goal of ethics is to guide us in living a good life, where living a good life includes living virtuously. What the example of Aquinas and Aristotle shows is that an ethics of the good life can be shared despite great differences in worldviews.

It also presents something that might be relevant for us today. We live in a multicultural society. Some believe in God; others do not. Some are Christian or Jewish; others are not. Some believe in life after death where the good are rewarded and the bad punished; others do not. Some favor libertarian values that emphasize individual rights; others favor communitarian values that emphasize the common good. Some have ethnic and cultural roots in Europe, others in Africa, still others in Asia. What we need in health care is a common ethics that cuts across religious, political, ethnic, cultural, and social backgrounds, an ethics that respects different worldviews but also accommodates what we all share as human beings. Aquinas, despite the vast differences between his religious and cultural worldview and that of Aristotle, saw how Aristotle's ethics of the good had an appeal that could transcend its original cultural matrix. This suggests that an ethics of the good might have important relevance in our multicultural society today.

There are, of course, differences between Aquinas and Aristotle—most notably Aquinas's religious faith—just as there were differences between Aristotle and other ancient Greek theories of the good life developed by the Platonists, Epicureans, and Stoics. These differences, however, should not blind us to the unifying factor these ethical theories of the good share: they are all ethics grounded on our natural desire to live well and are based on the conviction that living and doing well includes living and behaving virtuously.

This book will approach health care ethics from the perspective of an ethics of the good rather than an ethics of obligation. More specifically, it will rely on Aristotle's ethics of the good, an ethics receiving increasing attention by ethicists today. It will also draw on Aquinas's ethics of the good. This approach is somewhat different from the mainstream of current health care ethics. It is presented as an alternative to the more widely known principle-based and rights-based ethics of our culture. Even if you prefer those ethics of obligation and duty, it is still worthwhile knowing about the other major alternative in our cultural tradition—the ethics of the good.

BIOETHICS TODAY

Contemporary health care ethics is currently dominated by the various modern moralities of obligation. The idea that the rights of patients, especially the right to self-determination, the right to life, the right to die, and the right to health care, create obligations binding on others is very strong. Still strong, also, is the idea that both utilitarianism and Kantian deontology, different as these two theories are, somehow generate or at least defend a common set of normative principles (autonomy, beneficence, justice, and nonmalificence) that serve as general guidelines for formulating more specific rules that we are obliged to follow in practice. More recently the idea of a universal "common morality" containing rules of obligation applicable to all people in all places at all times as well as character traits that are universally admired has been gaining attention. Some say that this common morality, and not any moral theory, is what provides the four initial foundational norms or principles for bioethics that develop through a process such as reflective equilibrium into a coherent set of more specific rules for guiding our behavior

If you are at all familiar with the dominant vocabulary of American bioethics, you are undoubtedly aware that it is an ethics based on principles, most notably the principles of autonomy, beneficence, justice, and nonmaleficence. People involved in health care, especially physicians and nurses, are expected to observe rules and rights derived from these general principles to determine what they are morally obliged to do in particular situations. If the principles clash, as they often do, then they must be balanced against each other to determine which one obliges or they must be adjusted to preserve coherence in the system. In the minds of many, making moral decisions and judgments in health care ethics remains a process of guiding our actions in accord with the obligations and rights established by the general principles and the more specific rules derived from them.

In chapter 14, a chapter devoted to medical research, we show how this philosophical approach, now called by some "principlism," received a major boost when Congress set up the National Commission for the Protection of Human Subjects in 1974. Congress asked the Commission to identify basic ethical principles and to develop ethical guidelines derived from these principles that could be applied to biomedical and behavioral research. In 1979 this Commission issued its final report, known as the *Belmont Report*, in which it dutifully identified three basic principles: respect for persons (autonomy), beneficence, and justice. It described a basic ethical principle as a "general judgment that serves as a basic justification for particular prescriptions and evaluations of human actions."

The theoretical background of basing ethics on principles that oblige, however, was established decades before the National Commission. It goes back to several prominent moral philosophers who developed the ethics of duty to a high degree. One such influential philosopher was William Ross, whom we have already mentioned. A brief consideration of ethics of obligation, which has influenced many prominent American bioethicists, will help us to understand something of the background of the National Commission and of American bioethics.

Unlike Kant, who had proposed that some duties deriving from his single basic principle of morality were so strict that no exceptions could be tolerated, Ross suggested a cluster of prima facie duties. For Ross the term "prima facie duty" referred to the characteristic of the kinds of action that we would be obliged to perform if the action in the particular case would not be in conflict with another prima facie duty. For example, the prima facie duty of fidelity requires me to keep my promises, but if I had promised to take my son for ice cream at three o'clock and he breaks his arm at two-thirty, then the prima facie duty of beneficence (taking him for medical treatment) overrides the prima facie duty of fidelity that obliges me to keep my promises.

Ross named six basic prima facie duties: beneficence, justice, not injuring others, self-improvement, gratitude, reparation, and fidelity. Today Ross's prima facie duties, and the exercise of balancing or weighing them when they are in conflict, have reappeared in American bioethics as prima facie principles, most notably the prima facie principles of autonomy, beneficence, nonmaleficence, and justice.

These principles are normative principles, and it is our duty to abide by them. However, and this is what makes them prima facie, whenever these principles conflict, we have to balance them against each other to determine which one prevails in the particular situation. Hence, although these principles are normative (that is, more than rules of thumb), they are not absolute because they can be overruled by other principles.

Most of the textbooks on health care ethics published in the last two decades of the twentieth century—the books designed to help medical and nursing students learn about health care ethics—relied chiefly on a handful of basic principles and rules derived from them as the basis for moral judgment. The ethics of principles is an ethics of obligation; it is never far from the idea that ethics is about our duties and not about the natural desire to live well.

More recently, however, some of the new editions of health care ethics textbooks, largely as a result of the influence of an increasing interest in virtue ethics and in the ethics of care often associated with feminist ethics, now complement their ethics of principles and rules with elements borrowed from virtue ethics. For example, some ethicists who propose a universal "common morality" as the foundation and source of their principles expand the concept of "common morality" so it embraces not only principles and rules of obligation but moral character traits called virtues as well. However, as we will see in the next chapter, the notion of virtue advanced by proponents of common morality in the twenty-first century differs in substantial ways from the virtue ethics adopted in this book and from the virtue ethics found in the tradition, most notably the virtue ethics elaborated by Aristotle and Aquinas.

Despite some similarities, an ethics of the good is not ultimately compatible with an ethics of obligation. An ethics of the good assumes that ethics is primarily about our natural inclination and desire to seek what is good for ourselves, and that we can figure out what is ethical by a practical reasoning called prudence, whereas an ethics of obligation assumes that ethics is primarily about our obligations and duties, and that we can figure out what is ethical by a process of deductive-inductive reasoning based on general principles and tempered by adjustments to achieve coherence or reflective equilibrium. We do have to make a fundamental choice, then, between the two approaches. In this text the choice is to adopt the ethics of the good. Seeking what is good for ourselves is not a matter of obligation but of natural inclination.

SUGGESTED READINGS

Two good introductions to the history of ethics are Lawrence Becker and Charlotte Becker, eds., 1992, *A History of Western Ethics*, New York: Garland; and Robert Cavalier, James Gouinlock, and James Sterba, eds., 1989, *Ethics in the History of Western Philosophy*, New York: St. Martin's. The first volume contains selections from the *Encyclopedia of Ethics*, also published by Garland in 1992. For a history of Christian moral theology, see John Mahoney, 1987, *The Making of Moral Theology: A Study of the Roman Catholic Tradition*, Oxford: Oxford University Press.

For William Frankena's influential position, see his 1963, *Ethics*, Englewood Cliffs: Prentice Hall. The two remarks cited in the text are found on page 2, and his remarks about the basic role of principles in his "double-aspect conception of morality" are found on pages 53–54. For W. D. [William David] Ross's views, see his 1988, *The Right and the Good*, Indianapolis: Hackett, pp. 1–11 and 165–66. The quote from John Rawls is from his 1971, *A Theory of Justice*, Cambridge, MA: Harvard University Press, p. 121.

For a clear description of the difference between the modern and classical approaches to ethics, see Richard Taylor, 1988, "Ancient Wisdom and Modern Folly," in *Midwest Studies in Philosophy*, volume 13 of *Ethical Theory: Character and Virtue*, Peter A. French, Theodore E. Eehling, and Howard K. Wettstein, eds., Notre Dame: University of Notre Dame Press, pp. 54–63; Robert Louden, 1992, *Morality and Moral Theory: A Reappraisal and Reaffirmation*, New York: Oxford University Press, especially chapters 1–5; and G. E. M. Anscombe, 1981, "Modern Moral Philosophy," in *Ethics, Religion and Politics*, volume 3 of *Collected Papers*, Minneapolis: University of Minnesota Press, chapter 4. In the opening lines of this often-reprinted article, which first appeared in 1958, Anscombe states what to many is a startling thesis: namely, "that the concepts of obligation, and duty—*moral* obligation and *moral* duty, that is to say—and of what is *morally* right and wrong, and of the *moral* sense of 'ought,' ought to be jettisoned if this is psychologically possible" (emphasis in the original).

Plato's view on what is not "according to nature" can be found in his *Laws* 636C–D and 838D–839D. For Stoic ethics, see A. A. Long and D. N. Sedley, eds., 1987, *The Hellenistic Philosophers*, volume 1 of *Translation of the Principal Sources with Philosophical Commentary*, Cambridge, UK: Cambridge University Press, sections 56–67.

Unlike the beginnings of divine law moralities in the religions of the Middle East (Judaism, Christianity, and Islam), the beginnings of natural law morality are more indefinite. The traditional view is that it emerged in Greek thought in the fourth century B.C.E., perhaps with Plato but more probably with Stoicism, which began a half-century after Plato's death. However, a careful textual analysis by Helmut Koester suggests the origins of natural law morality should be moved forward several centuries to two sources: Cicero and Philo of Alexander. See Helmut Koester, 1968, "*Nomos Physeos*: The Concept of Natural Law in Greek Thought," in *Religions in Antiquity*, Jacob Neusner, ed., Leiden: Brill, pp. 521–41. In any case, it was the Roman jurists of the first few centuries (especially Gaius in the second century and Ulpian in the third) who made *jus naturale* a foundational concept of jurisprudence. The summation of their work can be found in the first page of Justinian's *Institutes* (sixth century), where natural law is defined as what nature teaches all animals and humans. From the Roman jurists it migrated into Christian and medieval thought. It appears in Aquinas, whose somewhat ambiguous texts on law as an "external source" of human acts along with the devil and God's grace appear in a few passages at the end of his long treatise on the ethics of virtue. See the *Summa Theologiae* I II, Q. 94. For the resurgence of natural law in modern times, see Knud Haakonssen, 1996, *Natural Law and Moral Philosophy: From Grotius to the Scottish Enlightenment*, New York: Cambridge University Press; and Robert George, ed., 1992, *Natural Law Theory: Contemporary Essays*, Oxford: Oxford University Press. It is not difficult to see a strong resemblance between the Roman Stoic concept of natural law that nature teaches to all humans and the recent interest in the "common morality" understood as a set of obligatory norms shared by all persons committed to morality.

A rights-based ethical theory has never been set forth in any comprehensive way despite the widespread popularity of rights claims in moral discourse today, where the rights to life, to choice, to privacy, to die, and so forth are constantly advanced as if they were moral arguments. For the debate about rights in moral theory, see Morton Winston, ed., 1989, *The Philosophy of Human Rights*, Belmont, CA: Wadsworth Publishing; and Jeremy Waldron, ed., 1984, *Theories of Rights*, New York: Oxford University Press.

The best introduction to Kant's moral theory is his *Groundwork of the Metaphysic of Morals* (also translated as the *Fundamental Principles of the Metaphysic of Morals*), available from several publishers. Among the helpful expositions of his theory are two books by Roger Sullivan, 1989, *Immanuel Kant's Moral Theory*, and 1994, *An Introduction to Kant's Ethics*, Cambridge, UK: Cambridge University Press. Lately, some Kantians have been advocating a softer approach to Kant's strict duty-based deontology. See Barbara Herman, 1993, *The Practice of Moral Judgment*, Cambridge, MA: Harvard University Press; and Nancy Sherman, 1997, *Making a Necessity of Virtue: Aristotle and Kant on Virtue*, Cambridge, UK: Cambridge University Press, chapters 1, 4, 5, 7, and 8.

The indispensable source book for utilitarianism is John Stuart Mill's little book published in 1863 titled *Utilitarianism*, available from various publishers. Also important is Book IV of Henry Sidgwick, 1981, *The Methods of Ethics* (first published in 1874), Indianapolis: Hackett Publishing. See also Amartya Sen and Bernard Williams, eds., 1982, *Utilitarianism and Beyond*, Cambridge, UK: Cambridge University Press; and Samuel Scheffler, ed., 1988, *Consequentialism and Its Critics*, Oxford: Oxford University Press.

Examples of typical and thoughtful approaches to developing a health care ethics based on principles include Tom Beauchamp and James Childress, 2009, *Principles of Biomedical Ethics*, 6th ed., New York: Oxford University Press; Thomas Mappes and David DeGrazia, 2001, *Biomedical Ethics*, 5th ed., New York: McGraw-Hill; and Ronald Munson, 2008, *Intervention and Reflection: Basic Issues in Medical Ethics*, 8th ed., Belmont, CA: Wadsworth Publishing. An interesting theological approach to health care ethics based on principles is developed by Benedict Ashley and Kevin O'Rourke, 2006, *Health Care Ethics*, 5th ed., Washington, DC: Georgetown University Press. For an approach based on rights see George Annas, 2004, *The Rights of Patients*, 3rd ed., Carbondale, IL: Southern Illinois University Press. Another very helpful book is Albert Jonsen, Mark Siegler, and William Winslade, 2006, *Clinical Ethics: A Practical Approach to Ethical Decisions in Clinical Medicine*, 6th ed., New York: McGraw-Hill.

For further study of the "common morality" foundation for ethics that is employed by both supporters and critics of principle-based ethics, see Beauchamp and Childress, 2008, especially chapters 1 and 10; and Bernard Gert, 2004 (paperback 2007), *Common Morality: Deciding What to Do*, New York: Oxford University Press. (Gert is a critic of the principle-based approach popularized by Beauchamp and Childress but agrees that a "common morality" is the basis for moral rules.) For a good discussion of the pros and cons of the "common morality" foundation for ethics, see the special issue entitled "Is There a Common Morality?" in the *Kennedy Institute of Ethics Journal* 2003, *13*, 189–274, with articles by Leith Turner, David DeGrazia, Jeffrey Brand-Ballard, and Tom Beauchamp. See also Gene Outka and John Reeder, eds., 1993, *Prospects for a Common Morality*, Princeton: Princeton University Press.

Important sources providing background for the now well-established field of bioethics are Stephen Post, ed., 2003, *Encyclopedia of Bioethics*, 3rd ed., 5 volumes, New York: Macmillan Reference; Peter Singer and A. M Viens, eds., 2008, *Cambridge Textbook of Bioethics*, New York: Cambridge University Press; Jennifer Walter and Eran Klein, eds., 2003, *The Story of Bioethics: From Seminal Works to Contemporary Explorations*, Washington, DC: Georgetown University Press; Albert Jonsen, Robert Veatch, and Leroy Walters, eds., 1998, *Source Book in Bioethics*, Washington, DC: Georgetown University Press; and Albert Jonsen, 1998, *The Birth of Bioethics*, New York: Oxford University Press. Both the *Encyclopedia* (volume 5) and the *Source Book* contain valuable reports and statements issued in the past decades, whereas the *Birth of Bioethics* is a history of the new field from the 1940s through the end of the twentieth century.

TWO

Prudence and Living a Good Life

THIS CHAPTER INTRODUCES the virtue-based ethics that Aristotle first developed in the fourth century B.C.E. and Aquinas retrieved in the thirteenth century. It will explain the starting point and then the three primary ideas of this ethics: happiness, moral virtue, and prudence. The starting point is the deeply rooted desire of human beings to achieve what is truly *good* for themselves; the best good is *happiness*, the best chance of achieving personal happiness is developing authentic *moral virtue*, and the best way to decide what will develop moral virtue is *prudence*. This chapter develops these four topics.

Before we begin we need to make a preliminary remark about terminology. In this book the terms "ethics" and "ethical" will be used interchangeably with "morality" and "moral." Some authors distinguish ethics and morality, but we will not make that distinction. Both words share a common etymology: What the Greek language called "ethics," the Latin language tended to call "morals," and both roots now appear in our English language. Also, it will be helpful to note that what the Greek language called the "character excellences," the Latin language called the "moral virtues," thus showing how the moral virtues pertain to what we often refer to as character integrity or good character. In addition to the moral virtues philosophers writing in both Greek and Latin identified an "intellectual excellence" or a "cognitive virtue" that also plays a major role in virtue ethics.

THE GOOD WE SEEK

Ethics begins, according to the ancient Greeks, when a person wonders how her life should be lived. How should we be living? What should we be trying to achieve? What should we be aiming for in our lives? These questions are the existential and practical questions almost every thoughtful person inevitably asks.

Aristotle's answer begins with the opening sentence of his *Nicomachean Ethics*: "Every skill and every investigation, and likewise every activity and choice, seem to aim at some good; hence the good has been well described as what all things aim at." No reasons can be given to explain why "every activity and choice seem to aim at some good." That they do is simply, for Aristotle, a given of our experience.

Although the immediate aim of our actions and choices is a particular good, we can also think of aiming at an overall good for our lives as a whole. This overall goal is the subject matter of ethics. Ethics clarifies this overall goal and then shows what feelings and behaviors are likely to achieve it in our particular lives.

And what is the overall goal we desire above all for our lives? It it nothing less than making our lives, as a whole, *good* lives. We do not simply desire life—we desire a *good* life. We do not simply want to live—we want to live *well*. We do not simply want to be—we want to *flourish*. Recognizing that the best good we can aim at is making our life as a whole a good life is the starting point of this virtue-based ethics. Aristotle called this starting point the *first principle* of ethics.

Be careful of the word "principle" here. It does not mean what the word "principle" means in modern ethics, in which principles are understood as action-guides deduced from a moral theory or induced from a line of previous moral judgments in similar cases. The *first principle* in the ethics of the good is the absolute beginning, the foundation whence all else is derived.

We cannot prove this first principle; nor can we give any reasons for it. There are no proofs or reasons for first principles. The word "principle" (*principium* in Latin and *arche* in Greek) means beginning, and no reasons can be given to establish the "beginning." If there were reasons for a beginning, the reasons would come logically before the beginning, and then the beginning would then no longer really be the beginning. Both Aristotle and Aquinas agreed that first principles of reasoning are not provable but self-evident. They are self-evident because we soon realize we cannot reason if we do not accept them.

Aristotle was the first philosopher to develop first principles in both *theoretical* reasoning (the reasoning in what he called science—physics, mathematics, and theology) and *practical* reasoning (the reasoning we use when we are making or doing something). The best known first principle of theoretical reasoning is the *principle of noncontradiction*: You cannot think something both is and is not at the same time. You cannot, for example, think something is both a square and not a square; that is, you cannot think something is a square circle. The principle of noncontradiction is so powerful that Christian theologians did not hesitate to say it restricts God. The God of Christian theology is all-powerful, but He cannot create a square circle or a circular square.

The first principle of any practical reasoning is the *principle of the good*—our choices aim at something we perceive as good. The first principle of the practical reasoning known as ethics is that our choices aim at whatever is good for our lives, whatever helps us flourish as human beings. This ethical good is intensely personal. The "good" Aristotle and Aquinas are talking about in ethics is *your* good and *my* good. Aristotle and Aquinas are trying to show their audiences what makes *their* lives good lives. Hence, if you join their audience, it is *your* good, *your* living well, that is meant when they speak of "the good." It is also a shared good, the common good, because both philosophers considered human beings not only personal beings but essentially social beings as well.

People do, of course, disagree on what above all makes a life good. Some say the overall good in life is money and property, others say it is pleasure, some say it is power, and still others say it is honors and recognition. Certainly money, property, pleasure, power, honors, and recognition are good, but are they the best goods we can aim at or desire for our lives as a whole?

To answer that question ask yourself whether a person could achieve these goods and still not be living a life you would consider good overall. Certainly money, pleasure, power, honors, and recognition are desirable goods, but they are at least arguably not the most desirable goods achievable in a human life.

The first moral philosophers thought that the most desirable overall good was something else, and, despite variations in their accounts, they generally agreed on what it was. They called the best good we can desire for our lives *eudaimonia*. The word has no exact equivalent in English—literally it means something like "good fate," but "happiness," or perhaps "flourishing," is probably the best translation. The Greek ethicists began with the idea that the overall good any thoughtful person would desire for his life is his happiness. A human life is successful if it is a happy life.

HAPPINESS

Happiness, of course, is a very general and vague term that can be understood in many different ways. Hence the challenge now is to explain what is meant by happiness. And the challenge is a demanding one for two reasons. First, human life is complex and supports many different ways of achieving happiness. And second, happiness is somewhat paradoxical in this sense: We achieve happiness not by aiming at it directly as if it were a concrete objective but by pursuing the concrete feelings, behaviors, and habits that make a life happy. We begin our explanation of happiness by saying what it is not.

What Happiness Is Not

First, we do not equate happiness with feelings of pleasure and the absence of pain. Pleasure may well accompany happiness, but this is not necessary, and as is well known pleasure can mislead us about what is truly good and thus undermine our happiness. And the presence of pain, although unpleasant, does not necessarily indicate that we are doing something bad.

The identification of happiness with feeling pleasure and avoiding pain has a long history going back at least to Epicurus (342?–270 B.C.E.) and his famous cloistered garden outside the walls of Athens. In modern times Thomas Hobbes and Jeremy Bentham, both important political philosophers, were leading proponents of reviving this notion. But feelings of pleasure cannot be equated with happiness understood as what is truly good for ourselves, because pleasure often distracts us and sometimes leads us toward what is not truly good.

Second, we do not equate happiness with the satisfaction of whatever desires a person might have. Happiness is not getting what we happen to want at the moment but achieving a good life. Sometimes a particular thing we want is not good for us, and getting it will not bring us happiness despite our thinking that it will.

Third, we do not equate happiness with whatever a particular person believes it to be. A person might believe happiness is living promiscuously and so live this way, but his belief that he is happy does not provide the happiness of which we speak because such a life is not truly good for human beings. The word happiness designates what is truly good for a person, not what the person believes is good or brings happiness. In an ethics of happiness, the simple fact that someone declares he is happy is not enough for us to say he has achieved happiness; it must also be shown that he has achieved what will truly bring happiness—that is, a good life. It is always possible for people to think that they are living fulfilling lives when in fact they are not. People afflicted with Down syndrome, for example, often seem more happy and content in life than many other people, but no Greek moralist would have said such a life was a good life, something any rational person would deliberately seek.

Happiness Is Agent-Centered

Making personal happiness the starting point and goal of ethics could easily suggest something close to narcissism, egoism, individualism, or a crass "looking out for number one," but it should not. Any understanding of personal happiness implying selfishness is incompatible with a credible morality.

Sensitivity to this threat of egoism or selfishness is at least partly the reason why many modern moral philosophers and theologians have proposed something other than personal happiness as the foundation of ethics—perhaps rights, or principles, or an altruistic Christian life of self-sacrifice. These modern theories are so influential that many people have forgotten the blunt appeal to personal happiness in earlier philosophical and religious ethics.

Although the ethics of Aristotle is typical and perhaps the best-known ancient morality grounded in personal happiness, his understanding of ethics was not unique in the earlier centuries. Just about every philosopher and religious leader of the time proposed personal happiness as the goal of morality. Consider two examples, one from Plato (427?–347 B.C.E.) and one from the Christian scriptures (ca. 60–ca. 100).

In the beginning of Plato's *The Republic*, a man named Thrasymachus insists that there is no good reason for being ethical or just: "The just man is always a loser, my naive Socrates. He always loses out to the unjust" (343D). Socrates disagrees and insists that the just and ethical person is a winner. He tells the mythical story of Er, a good man killed in battle. On the twelfth day Er rose from the dead and reported what he had witnessed in the life after death: Evil people were being punished tenfold and good people were being rewarded tenfold. Socrates drew the obvious conclusion—the wise person will choose the ethical life, "for this is how a man will find his greatest happiness" (619B). If we live justly, "we shall be friends to the gods and to ourselves both in this life and when we go to claim our rewards, like the victors in the games go forth to gather their prizes" (621C–D). Socrates' point is clear: Ethical living is what achieves the best for ourselves—our greatest happiness.

The Christian tradition also insists that living morally is in our best interest. It never tires of reminding us that bad people "will go away to eternal punishment, and the virtuous to eternal life" (Matt. 25:46). Christ's teachings were demanding, and his followers often wondered what was in it for them. Sometimes they spoke in blunt terms: "What about us?" he (Peter) said to him. "We have left everything and followed you. What are we to have then?" The response was equally blunt: Jesus told Peter he will "be repaid a hundred times over, and also inherit eternal life" (Matt. 19:27–29; cf. Luke 18:28–30). It is undoubtedly difficult for a man to give up home, land, and loved ones to follow Jesus, but he has the assurance that the loss will be balanced by compensation a hundred times greater in this life and then, after death, by eternal life as well. Christian living is constantly presented in the Christian scriptures as the way to gain great happiness for yourself both before and after death.

Socrates willingly gave up his life for the sake of what he saw as the good, and Peter left all to follow Jesus and was eventually killed for his choice. These actions are complex. On the one hand they represent the ultimate self-sacrifice, the greatest act of altruism a human being can make—sacrificing one's life for a good and noble cause. On the other hand Socrates and Peter performed these actions of great sacrifice convinced that they would in the end gain ten or a hundred times more than they gave up.

The dynamic is clear: invest now, profit later; sow now, reap later; give up a lot, gain much more. Socrates and Peter sacrificed much, but the sacrifices were investments in a far greater happiness. Does this make them selfish and narcissistic? Not according to the ancient philosophical and religious traditions. In these traditions, paradoxical as it seems to us today, living rightly is in our self-interest because it results in the greatest possible personal happiness; yet this self-interest is neither narcissistic nor selfish.

It is well to remember that most people who existed before the past few modern centuries did not have as individualized a notion of each person as we do today. People did not think of themselves as isolated individuals joining together in some sort of social contract to protect their individual rights and freedoms. It was Descartes, the father of modern philosophy, who said in the seventeenth century, "I think, therefore I am"; most people before him said "I belong to a community, therefore I am." Personal human existence was always a social human existence, an existence intricately integrated with the existence of others in personal and political relationships.

Some philosophers of the twentieth century have tried to recapture this older notion of social existence and to redress the excessive individualism of modern philosophies and liberal political theories that stress individual rights. Our existence, they tell us, is never singular but always a coexistence. Being human is not the same as being a rock or any other thing. Take away all the rocks in a pile but one, and that remaining rock is every bit the rock it was before the others were removed. Take away all the people in a community but one, and that remaining person is no longer the human being she was before the others were removed. Since human existence is a coexistence, if the existences of others are undermined, so is mine. Human being is social being; my being is a being-with-others.

Once we understand ourselves not as discrete atomic entities related to others by some kind of social contract we decide to embrace, but as existentially interconnected with others in the very being we call human being, then the tendency to understand an ethics advocating personal fulfillment and happiness as selfishness is derailed. If my life is always a life-with-others, then my happiness and flourishing is always entwined with the happiness and flourishing of others. If my existence is a coexistence, then it is impossible for me to flourish at the expense of others. Treating them unjustly or insensitively undermines my good as well as their good.

Understood in the framework of its origination, where human beings were thought of as essentially social beings, an ethics of personal happiness is anything but an ethics of selfishness. The happiness of any human being is the happiness of a social being, not of a discrete individual. This is why, for Aristotle, the study of ethics—how I go about making moral decisions—is only a phase in a larger study, a study he called politics.

This can be difficult for the modern mind to understand because the modern approach (whether influenced by the liberal political philosophies extolling individual rights and liberty but neglecting community or by the more conservative political philosophies extolling family and communitarian values but neglecting the important modern values of liberty and self-determination) assumes the dichotomy of self and others, of individual and community, and then opts for one over the other. But it is anachronistic to place the ethics of personal happiness developed by Aquinas or

Aristotle in the modern conceptual framework that dichotomizes the individual and her societies and then to criticize it.

The familiar dichotomies of egoism and altruism and of self and community were, in the forms we experience them, unknown to earlier moralists. They never hesitated to claim that acting for the sake of virtue was acting in our own best interest. Nor did they hesitate to claim that acting for the good of others was also acting in our own best interest. They simply assumed that human beings are political beings, that human existence is always a coexistence with others in communities.

Hence an ethics of the good retrieved from Aristotle and Aquinas is not an ethics of the liberal self striving primarily for his happiness, nor is it an ethics of the communitarian self striving primarily for the common good; it is both. Living well has both individual and communal dimensions. Speaking of my good is also speaking of the common good; speaking of my happiness is also speaking of the happiness of others; speaking of my flourishing is also speaking of the flourishing of my communities.

Happiness Is a Collective Term

We have said that the happiness we speak of in ethics is not simply pleasure, nor is it the satisfaction of whatever desire we happen to have, nor is it whatever we happen to think it is, nor is it anything selfish. What, then, is this personal happiness? What can we say about it?

We can begin by saying that happiness in ethics is a collective term describing the right balance and coordination of all the important goods in a person's life. That is why it was described by Aristotle as the "complete" good.

An analogy may help us to understand how a collective term is used. A rope is composed of, let us say, a thousand strands twisted together. The rope is not something added to the strands. We do not have a thousand and one things—the thousand strands and one rope—but the strands themselves constitute the rope. In a similar way, our happiness is not some additional good that comes as the result of achieving other good things in life. It is, rather, the life we call good because it combines successfully all the important elements and strands that constitute the human good. Happiness is not the reward gained after a life has been lived well but the good life itself.

The good things in our lives come from two sources: luck and choice. Under luck we include any good thing we receive apart from our own effort. Some people prefer to speak of "blessings" instead of luck. By luck or blessings we may have inherited good health or happen to live in peaceful times with an abundance of friends and wealth, for example. Good luck and many blessings will certainly contribute to our personal happiness, but they are not the crucial factors. Luck will not by itself bring us the personal happiness envisioned in ethics, and its absence will not preclude this happiness. Something else is much more important.

The second and more important source of our happiness is the particular goods we choose to pursue as we live our lives. Aristotle noted but never organized, at least in the texts we have, the various good elements composing a happy life. Some later commentators did attempt some organization, however, and their schema is helpful. They identified three categories of goods according to the importance of their contribution to happiness. The categories are clear enough, although translating the ancient terms into English is somewhat awkward. The categories of goods constituting happiness, beginning with the most valuable, are these:

- Noble goods
- Potential goods
- Useful goods

Noble Goods

These are the essential feelings, behaviors, and habits creating a happy life. By "behaviors" we mean *actions* as well as *omissions* (things you could do but choose not to do). By "behaviors" we also mean both *private* actions and omissions as well as a whole range of *social* actions and omissions with other people, interactions ranging from intimate love and friendship to all forms of social, political, and commercial relationships. Finally, by "habits" we mean acquired *dispositions* for feeling and behaving in certain ways. We develop these habits through constant repetition of the feelings and behaviors.

The feelings, behaviors, and habits called the *noble goods* are the principal ingredients of happiness. We choose them for the sake of our happiness and, since they are also valuable in themselves, for their own sake as well. The Greeks called these feelings, behaviors, and habits "excellent." The subsequent Latin word for them was *virtutes*, the etymological origin of the English word "virtues." The essential noble goods are the *virtues*. The ethics of happiness is a *virtue ethics*.

Potential Goods

These are goods providing us with opportunities to pursue the all-important virtues. They were called *potential goods* because they have the potential for contributing to the virtues and to happiness. Some examples of potential goods are health, financial resources, pleasure, religion, art, music, science, charitable work, and almost any legitimate occupation. These are all goods that foster opportunities for virtue and happiness. These potential goods share one similarity with the virtues—we seek them for their own sake as well as for the sake of higher goods. They differ from the noble goods or virtues because, according to Aristotle, you need all the virtues for happiness but you do not need all the potential goods.

Useful Goods

These are goods sought not for their own sake but only for the sake of other goods, either the noble goods (the virtues) or the potential goods. An example of a useful good is an antibiotic: We do not take an antibiotic for its own sake but for the sake of a more valuable good—our health. Tools are another example: We do not buy a lawn mower for its own sake but for the sake of cutting grass. *Useful goods* are like tools that we need to accomplish something valuable. We do not seek them for their intrinsic value but for some other good we desire.

Once we distinguish the major kinds of good, we can see how happiness, the most desirable good in a human life, is actually composed of several different categories of goods. Of these the most important are the *noble* goods (the virtues); then come the *potential* goods and finally the *useful* goods. The virtues play the major role in our happiness, but they need support from some *potential* and *useful* goods.

Today the word "goods" seems a little awkward for the ideas just presented. It might make things more clear if we use the word "value" and recast the schema in terms of a hierarchy of values. The goal of life is happiness—making our lives truly good lives. The highest values are the virtues, and they are valuable both because they are the principal elements in happiness and because they have intrinsic value as well. Next in line after the virtues are things humans value for their potential to contribute to happiness and virtue as well as for their intrinsic value. Finally, at the lowest level, are the utilitarian values valuable only for their contribution to the higher values.

Ancient commentators on this schema of goods and values all agreed that the best good we could pursue in a human life was happiness, and most agreed on what feelings, behaviors, and habits should be counted as virtues. They debated interminably, however, about what goods or values are "potential" and what goods or values are merely "useful." Their disputes about this issue need not detain us. All we need to know is that happiness, the good we desire most, is a collective noun embracing virtues and some other goods or values as well.

Another ancient dispute however is of some interest. Do the virtues guarantee happiness? If our feelings, activities, and habits are virtuous, does that mean we will certainly be happy and have a good life? Or is it possible to be virtuous and not have happiness and a good life? In other words, can tragedy destroy the happiness of a virtuous person? This question was the subject of an extensive debate in ancient ethics.

Happiness and Tragedy

A serious challenge to the idea that living virtuously guarantees happiness comes from all too frequent examples of good people whose lives are haunted by tragedy. Bad things do happen to good people. Ancient ethics proposed three major responses to this challenge of tragedy to virtue. Socrates and Plato thought that virtue guarantees happiness but admitted that the happiness might not come until life after death. Aristotle, rejecting personal existence after death, thought that virtue makes happiness likely in this life but does not guarantee it. The Stoics, coming after Plato and Aristotle, thought that virtue could actually guarantee happiness in this life. However, their view on this matter was never widely accepted because most people could not see how any virtuous human being's happiness could be unaffected by tragedy in one's own life or the life of a loved one. Even the Stoics admitted that only a few "sages" could ever muster enough stoical detachment to remain unaffected by significant personal losses and tragedies. Hence we are left with two plausible answers to the question of whether virtue guarantees happiness. One assertion denies that tragedy can ultimately destroy happiness because no matter how tragic an earthly life, there is a life after death, and one assertion admits that tragedy could destroy happiness.

There is no way to resolve this difference of opinion about happiness—whether it can occur only in this life and can be undermined by bad luck or whether it can also occur in a life after death where all bad luck can be neutralized. Each person is left with a fundamental option on the question of whether or not there is personal survival after death. One will opt for the view of Aristotle, which was also the view of Abraham, Moses, and Job; another will opt for the view of Socrates and Plato, which is also the view of Christians and Muslims.

For our purposes it makes no difference which option is embraced, for both are compatible with the ethics we develop in this book. Aquinas has shown us the way here. His ethics is very much a revival of Aristotle's approach, yet he embraced the Christian belief in life after death. The lack of consensus about whether happiness is confined to this life or extends beyond death does not undermine the central thesis in this ethics of the good: Ethics is about our personal happiness, what it is, and how we achieve it.

There is, however, one very important and generally ignored question facing those who believe with Aristotle that this life is all there is. Sometimes people find themselves in a situation where nothing they can choose will result in happiness. None of the options will promote a good life; no chance for any significant happiness exists. If happiness is the goal of life and the criterion for what is ethical and unethical, what happens when nothing the person can do will promote her happiness? If she believes in life after death, of course, there is no problem because the impossibility of happiness in this life is not final; happiness is always possible in the life after death.

But Aristotle did not believe in life after death. What, then, can be said about an ethics of seeking our good when none of the available choices promotes a good life? Does the ethics of the good go on a holiday when this tragic situation arises? Suppose, for example, a person is dying of widespread and painful cancer. Realistically, these are his choices: (1) he may choose to remain alert as long as possible and thus experience great pain; (2) he may choose heavy pain medication and thus spend his last days so drugged that he loses all meaningful contact with reality; or (3) he may choose euthanasia or suicide and thus give up his life. None of these options leads to happiness. Living in pain or in a drugged state is not living a good life, nor is euthanasia or suicide, for that ends life. What, then, could an ethics of the good and personal happiness offer in tragic situations when achieving a good life and happiness is no longer possible?

The answer to this question in Aristotle is important. In tragic situations where no choice will lead to happiness, an ethics of the good acknowledges an important corollary: When we can no longer achieve a good life, the best we can do is avoid what is contrary to a good life. In other words when none of our choices will promote our happiness, when all options are undesirable and unwanted, then we are reduced to choosing the less worse option. The ethical aim of our life is to live well and be happy; if living well and happiness are not possible, then all we can do is reduce the bad features in the situation as far as possible. Not choosing the less worse is immoral because it undermines an ethics of the good by promoting more bad than is necessary.

The ethics of the good, then, is understood this way: Behavior is moral when we choose what promotes living well or, in tragic situations where living well is no longer possible, when we choose the less worse. Thus Aristotle, in his discussion of battlefield courage, argued that in some situations a soldier has but two choices, and neither promotes his living well. He can stand, fight, and be killed, or he can desert his post and be a coward. Neither choice brings happiness; there is no happiness in being killed or in living as a deserter and a coward. The soldier is caught in a tragic situation and can only choose the less worse. Aristotle argued that fighting unto death will in most circumstances be less worse than fleeing and hence deserves to be recognized as a virtue, the virtue of courage.

In the rare and tragic situations when living well is not an option, when the only choices are the choices promoting a life no one would desire, all the good person can do is to choose the less bad. The first principle of an ethics of the good, then, was fully stated by Aquinas as: "Happiness or living well is to be sought and promoted, and the bad is to be avoided." Virtuous action is action done for the sake of living well and happily or, when happiness is no longer a realistic option, for the sake of avoiding as far as possible whatever undermines living well and happiness.

The full statement of the first principle of an ethics of the good is especially important for ethics dealing with areas of human life haunted by tragic situations in which no available option can really be considered a contribution to the agent's happiness. Military ethics focuses on one such area; health care ethics focuses on another. Sometimes in health care ethics no option available to a patient, proxy, physician, or nurse promotes to any significant degree what Aristotle called happiness.

The hypothetical situation of the dying cancer patient is an example of such a case. Nothing he can choose will bring him happiness, but he behaves morally by choosing the least bad option. His moral reasoning might well unfold as follows. Retaining alertness despite the pain may at first be less worse than masking the pain but losing awareness. Then, if the pain intensifies, the reverse may be true, and masking the pain despite the loss of awareness may be less worse than retaining awareness with the pain. At this stage he then has two choices: live his last days without pain but heavily drugged, or ask his physician to kill him. It is at least arguable, as we will see in the chapter on euthanasia, that medicating patients even to the point of unawareness if necessary is a less worse way of controlling suffering than killing them, even if they ask to be killed.

Happiness and Moral Obligation

It is important to remember that any ethics of the good also contains an ethics of obligation in two ways. First, there is a sense in which we can say that, given the natural inclination to seek happiness in life, then we ought to seek happiness; that is, we ought to seek a fulfilled and flourishing life, a good life. The language of "ought" is a language of obligation. In an ethics of the good, however, the "ought" denotes obligation in a weak sense because happiness is what each of us already desires anyway.

Second, an ethics of the good may well include laws, principles, and rights. In fact whenever promulgating laws, principles, and rights will help us to live a good life, they are reasonable. Proponents of an ethics of the good can agree with Kant that a moral law requiring us to keep our promises is helpful in most situations; with Bentham that our social welfare programs should do the most good for the greatest number; and with Locke that people have rights to life, liberty, and property. And we can agree with the prevailing principles of American bioethics that capture important values: Patient self-determination, beneficence, and justice are very important considerations, and behaving in accord with them preserves the human good in most cases.

The important point, however, is that human well-being or flourishing is the foundation for what is good, not the laws, principles, and rights. What constitutes a good life determines what the laws, principles, and rights will be and when they will be relevant; the laws, principles, and rights derived from moral theories or from a common morality, no matter how important, do not determine a priori what constitutes a good life.

Happiness and Virtue

A key notion in any ethics of the good is virtue. Virtue meant "excellence" in ancient Greek, and the word was used for both living and nonliving things: A machine can be excellent, or a horse, or a human being. Something is excellent when it is well formed *and* performs well. A machine is excellent if it is well made and works well; a horse is excellent if it is well formed and functions well. A flutist is excellent if she is an outstanding flutist and actually plays exceptionally well. A flutist is not excellent if she has mastered the instrument but does not play; nor is she excellent if she has not mastered the instrument but happens to play well in a particular concert. In the *Iliad* Homer called a soldier excellent only when the man was a courageous fighter and actually did fight courageously. A courageous soldier who does not fight is not excellent; nor is a cowardly soldier excellent who fights courageously only when stimulated by the wine he drank out of fear.

From these examples we can see that excellence is related to a goal. If a thing is so formed and so functions that the goal is achieved, then it is an excellent thing. If the machine, the horse, and the flutist are so formed and so function as to achieve the goals appropriate to that machine, horses, and flutists, we call them and their performances excellent. The goal is the norm for excellence. Only when we know what the machine, horse, and flutist are expected to accomplish can we judge whether their structures and functions are excellent.

As we have explained, the goal of any human life considered as a whole is personal happiness. We say "considered as a whole" because the subsidiary goals are not those that concern us here. These are many and worthwhile and include, for example, graduation from school, earning a good living, developing loving relationships, having a family, being a good clinician, and so forth. But in ethics it is the overall goal of every human life that concerns us, and this, as we saw in the last section, is personal happiness.

We can now define an excellent or virtuous human being as a person so formed and so functioning as to achieve personal happiness. Simply put, whenever our habits, feelings, and behavior are in fact achieving personal happiness, we call them excellent or virtuous. The virtues are those human qualities that promote personal happiness. Virtues are the feelings, habits, and behaviors constitutive of living well.

Two kinds of virtue play major roles in the morality of happiness: *moral* virtue and *intellectual* virtue. The inclusion of an intellectual virtue in virtue ethics is absolutely crucial; in fact it is the intellectual virtue, what Aristotle called *phronesis* and Aquinas called *prudentia*, that is the action-guiding norm in virtue ethics. We cannot stress the intellectual decision-making virtue in virtue ethics enough because many contemporary accounts of virtue ethics either ignore the intellectual virtue or reduce it to a secondary role. Although we will explain them separately, they always work together in practice. A degree of moral virtue is necessary for the relevant intellectual virtue, prudence, to function well, and a degree of prudence is necessary for morally virtuous decision making in each particular situation. Every moral virtue presupposes prudential reasoning, and sound prudential reasoning presupposes the person has already developed some level of moral virtue.

Moral Virtue

The moral virtues are the excellences of a person's character—the feelings, behaviors, and habits that contribute to character integrity and thus contribute to his living well, living a good life. As previously noted, "moral virtue" is synonymous with "character virtue" or "character excellence." This section will explain five moral virtues that play a major role in traditional virtue ethics: temperance, courage, justice, love, and pride. The section that follows it will explain the intellectual virtue that plays the normative role in virtue ethics: prudence.

Emergence of the Moral Virtues

The different moral virtues originate in various natural inclinations or tendencies that have evolved in human beings over time. We will live well by embracing these natural inclinations and cultivating them so that they will enrich rather than impoverish our lives. In other words the different moral virtues are nothing more than our natural inclinations shaped by intelligence so they will likely enhance rather than undermine our happiness.

Aristotle's writings suggest five major natural inclinations in human life and give a name to the moral virtue appropriate for each:

- Our inclinations to satisfy our appetites for eating, drinking, and sex
- Our inclinations to act despite fears and risks
- Our inclinations to seek close personal relationships
- Our inclinations to seek working relationships with others
- Our inclinations to seek honors and recognition

First, we have natural inclinations to seek food and fluids when we are hungry and thirsty. We may also seek mood-enhancing substances such as alcohol, nicotine, and so forth. And we seek some form of sexual gratification.

Second, we have a natural inclination to engage in activities despite the fears that accompany them. Sensing that we could never live a rich and fulfilled life unless we are willing to take some risks, we are inclined to take them.

Third, we have a natural inclination to bond closely with others. We were born into a network of relationships, some kind of family. And as we mature we naturally pursue personal relationships as we come to realize a life lived without intimate connections is a life not well lived.

Fourth, we also have a natural inclination to encounter others in less personal ways. We relate to other people every day, sometimes for the first and last time, sometimes over extended periods of time. All human lives are interwoven with various social, political, commercial, and professional encounters.

Finally, we have a natural inclination for honors and praise, especially when we do well or bear up well under great challenges, adversity, sickness, or tragedy. We naturally seek recognition for our achievements. We want our success to be recognized and acknowledged.

You can easily see how these major natural inclinations can hurt as well as help us live well. We know that not all eating, drinking, and sex; not all risky behaviors; not all relationships; and not all honors and praise contribute to our living well and flourishing as human beings. Of course, other natural inclinations exist as well—inclinations to anger and to aggression, for example—and these too can hurt as well as help us live well.

When these natural inclinations spontaneously give rise to good feelings and behaviors—those contributing to a good life—Aristotle called them natural virtues. We often see natural virtues in children when they share cookies or perform an act of kindness or carefully try something risky. Moral training can shape and strengthen these natural virtues.

Spontaneous natural virtue and early moral training provide an orientation toward living well, but they are woefully inadequate for the complexities of adult life. For a mature moral life we need more than natural virtues and moral training—we need what Aristotle called the *authentic* moral virtues. Whereas natural virtues arise spontaneously and are shaped by training, the *authentic* moral virtues arise from intelligent choices guided by prudence. Whenever we deliberately and intelligently guide the feelings and behaviors arising from our natural inclinations, we are forming authentic moral virtues.

Looking at the five major domains of life we singled out earlier, we can name five major *authentic* moral virtues:

- Good management of eating, drinking, and sex is *temperance*.
- Good management of risk taking is *courage*.
- Good management of personal relationships is *love* or *friendship*.
- Good management of general encounters with others is *justice*.
- Good management of honors and recognition is *pride*.

Aristotle's claim is that developing the *authentic* moral virtues gives us the best chance of achieving happiness in life. You probably recognize the first four moral virtues—temperance, courage, love, and justice—and have some idea of what they are. However, you are probably not familiar with the fifth moral virtue, pride. Yet Aristotle actually considered pride to be the most important moral virtue. Since his views on pride have often been neglected in the virtue theory tradition, we need to say something about it.

Pride—The Forgotten Virtue

By "pride" Aristotle meant managing intelligently our natural inclination to seek honor and recognition for our accomplishments in life. It is natural to want our achievements to be honored and recognized. But honor and recognition bestowed by others can be tricky. They may not recognize our achievements or they may misunderstand them or find them politically unattractive. Hence we cannot reliably depend on others to satisfy our natural desires for honor and the recognition of our achievements.

The greatest accomplishment in life is to make the choices that will form our characters in an excellent way and thus be living a good and noble life. If we are making significant progress toward this goal, we would do well to recognize it and be proud of it and to accept recognition given by others if they honor us properly for our moral nobility. Actually truthful self-recognition is more accurate than recognition by others for two reasons. First, the bestowal of honors by others is unreliable—people bestow honors on others for many reasons other than honest evaluation of significant achievement. Second, those truly deserving of honor and recognition are often neglected because they lack political connections or clever public relations.

The Greek word we are translating here as pride is *megalopsychia*, which literally means "greatness of soul." There is no exact English equivalent. Magnanimity is also a literal translation but does not tell us much. Some translate *megalopsychia* as dignity, which is fairly accurate. In any event, Aristotle tells us that this virtue is the capstone of a life well lived and that the person living a noble life should recognize the achievement because it is difficult to do and not many people actually succeed in living morally noble lives. A person with virtuous pride so esteems herself that she will not compromise her character for other goods no matter how enticing they may be. Pride is the virtuous self-respect and self-esteem that has been earned over time and tested by adversity and temptation. A person with this virtue has great moral dignity.

Making pride a virtue is somewhat unsettling for many in the Christian tradition. This tradition, after all, suggested that pride was the first of the seven capital sins and encouraged people to seek the virtue of humility. But Aristotle's idea is this. If people have work to do—painting a picture, building a house, practicing as a nurse or a physician, writing a term paper, or whatever—experience suggests that they will do a better job if they take pride in what they do. Now the most important work in life according to traditional virtue ethics is becoming a noble human being, and we will do a better job at succeeding in this if we take pride in how we live our lives. Aquinas seems to have recognized the value of Aristotle's virtue in his *Commentary on the Nicomachean Ethics*, for he declined to oppose *megalopsychia* to humility and suggested that Christians could legitimately take pride in their moral achievement as long as they acknowledge God's help.

Lists of Moral Virtues

No canonical list of the moral virtues exists. The traditional moral virtues of temperance, courage, love, and justice appear in some form on just about every ancient list of moral virtues, but other virtues are often mentioned as well. Lists often vary with the same author. Aristotle, for example, gives various lists. His *Rhetoric* names seven moral virtues: justice, courage, temperance, magnificence, dignity, generosity, and gentleness. The moral virtue of love is noticeably absent here, but he does define and discuss it at some length in book II of the same work. The *Eudemian Ethics* lists the seven moral virtues of the *Rhetoric* and adds love, respect for self and others, righteous indignation, truthfulness, solemnity, and patience. The *Nicomachean Ethics* also lists the seven moral virtues of the *Rhetoric* and adds love, truthfulness, and several other virtues for which Aristotle says there are no names.

The lack of a definitive list of moral virtues is not a problem because the moral virtues in a morality of happiness do not play the role moral principles play in the various moralities of obligation. Unlike action-guiding principles and rules, the moral virtues are not a stock of maxims that we apply to particular situations to determine what we ought to do. They are simply the ways of feeling and behaving that make up a good life, that is, a life of personal happiness. Any feeling, behavior, or habit contributing to a truly good life is an ethical virtue. In the health care field caring, empathy, sympathy, kindness, and so forth are important moral virtues.

According to Aristotle, philosophical reflection shows that a life will likely be happy if it is composed of feelings, behaviors, and habits known as temperance, courage, love, justice, dignity, and so forth. In other words, the moral virtues give us the best chance of flourishing as human beings.

You may disagree with Aristotle, but if you do, you will need to show that the chances of living a good and happy life will be better if a person feels and behaves in nonvirtuous ways. You will need to show how happiness will be more likely in a life lived without the moral virtues of temperance, courage, love, justice, and dignity. It is not easy to find intelligent arguments that support the position that a good life is a life constituted by the lack of moral virtue or by the vices contrary to them.

The notion of *authentic* moral virtue is now beginning to emerge. Authentic moral virtue is rooted in our good management of our natural inclinations. Our natural dispositions become morally virtuous when we go beyond the formation we received in our youth and from our secular and religious culture and begin to deliberate personally about what we might do to live well and then choose this course. Only when we choose our behavior—choose to be kind, just, loving, courageous, and so forth—for the sake of virtue and not simply because it is a duty or obligation are we achieving *authentic* moral virtue and living a truly good human life. These chosen actions of virtue gradually build up our moral character, and the stronger our moral character, the more easily and often we will continue to choose truly virtuous behaviors. A reciprocal dynamic occurs whereby our good choices and our virtuous character mutually reinforce each other. Unfortunately the converse is also true: The more we choose contrary to virtue the more our character becomes bad, and the worse our character becomes the more we tend to make bad choices.

Making good choices—choices that make our lives good and happy lives—about the feelings and behaviors arising from our natural inclinations is accomplished by the other virtue that we mentioned: *prudence*. This indispensable intellectual virtue guides every decision that results in *authentic* moral virtue. Prudence plays the crucial management role in traditional virtue-based ethics, and without the personal practice of prudential reasoning, there is no *authentic* moral virtue. As Aquinas puts it: "And thus the whole matter of the moral virtues falls under the single reasoning of prudence."

Prudence

Two kinds of intelligence play major roles in the philosophy of Aristotle and Aquinas: *theoretical intelligence* and *practical intelligence*. Theoretical intelligence strives to know about the realities that exist independently of us. These independent realities comprise two domains. One domain embraces the beings our senses encounter, and the other embraces the beings our senses cannot encounter, such as human souls and the God or gods functioning as sources of motion. Knowledge about the sensible beings is of two kinds; it is either physics (natural philosophy) or, if it focuses only on the quantitative aspect of sensible beings, mathematics. (The Aristotelian separation of physics and mathematics lasted until Isaac Newton, building on the work of Copernicus, Kepler, and Galileo, showed in his revolutionary book of 1687, *The Mathematical Principles of Natural Philosophy*, that physics is actually mathematical.) Knowledge about the nonsensible beings—souls and gods—Aristotle called *first philosophy* and *theology*; others later termed it *metaphysics*.

The ideal of theoretical knowledge—the knowledge of given realities—exhibits several important characteristics. It is consistent—its major first principle is the principle of noncontradiction. It is deductive—once its general principles are discovered by induction or set forth in theory, we can understand all the particulars covered by the principles and rules. It is universal—its truths hold everywhere and always. And it is necessary—if achieved, it allows its possessors to claim the certitude that comes only with knowing their truth is necessarily so.

Practical intelligence, on the other hand, is not ultimately about realities that exist independently of us. It is about knowing what voluntary human activities will work in the world. These voluntary activities fall into two domains: We make things and we do things. Building a good structure or writing a good play calls for practical intelligence in making things, whereas directing a military operation well or treating a patient well calls for practical intelligence in doing things. The most important thing we can do is to make our lives good lives, and the practical intelligence for doing this is the intelligence we need in what Aristotle and Aquinas call ethics.

This practical knowledge does not, indeed cannot, reflect the rigidity of theoretical knowledge. The knowledge for knowing how to make and do successful things is not the same as knowledge about what is already made and done. Since ongoing situations are always changing and developing, practical knowledge is not so much consistent, deductive, necessary, and universal as it is variable, experiential, provisional, and situation specific.

The moral virtues are the chief elements of a good and happy life, but they alone are not capable of directing us in ever-changing circumstances. They require on-the-spot intelligent management. Aristotle called this intellectual aspect of every moral virtue *phronesis*, Cicero and Aquinas called it *prudentia*, and we are translating it as *prudence*. Prudence is the intellectual virtue that clarifies the overall good we are aiming at for our lives, and it manages our feelings, behaviors, and habits in each situation so that we will likely achieve a measure of this happiness.

For many reasons that we cannot go into here, later modern European languages lost the ability to express the rich notion of *phronesis* and *prudentia* that we find in the ethics of Aristotle and Aquinas. The words *prudence* in English and French, and *klugheit* in German, simply do not convey what *phronesis* and *prudentia* meant in the older ethics. In fact the "prudent" person today is often not the morally noble person characterized by the *phronesis* and *prudentia* of the earlier ethics but rather an overly careful person bent on avoiding difficulties in his life. Such prudence, however, may in fact be unethical. In health care for example, some physicians, possibly influenced by legal counsel, think it prudent to avoid any behavior that might result in litigation. They never see that such prudence could be highly immoral in some circumstances—when it leads to medically unnecessary tests, for example.

Modern authors discussing Aristotle's *phronesis* and Aquinas's *prudentia* therefore shy away from using the misleading English word "prudence." They employ instead phrases such as "practical wisdom," "practical reason," "practical rationality," "moral insight," "intelligence," and "non-scientific deliberation."

There are good reasons for using these phrases, but there are also drawbacks. One drawback is the confusion caused by the use of different English words to translate one Greek or one Latin word with a very definite meaning in ethics. Another is the fact that, in his *Ethics*, Aristotle takes great care to show that *phronesis* is not associated with wisdom, and thus the frequent translation of *phronesis* as "practical wisdom" is misleading. Moreover, Greek has common words for practical and wisdom (*pratike* and *sophia*), and this suggests that we should translate *phronesis* by another English word.

Despite the problems associated with the word prudence in English, we will use the word to translate what Aristotle called *phronesis* and Aquinas called *prudentia*. The complex and rich meaning these authors gave prudence will, I hope, emerge in what follows. Prudence or prudential reasoning is, quite simply, how we figure out what choices are most likely conducive to our goal in any given situation. In ethics prudence is the deliberation we use to determine what will give us the best chance to achieve happiness (that is, to determine what is ethical or morally good). It tells us what to do in order to achieve a good life.

What Prudence Is Not

We begin by saying what prudence is not. It is not, as we explained earlier, a moral judgment deduced from general norms such as principles, rules, or rights. Prudence never reasons this way. It is much more imaginative, narrative, and creative.

This does not mean, however, that any of the conclusions deduced from principles and rules are necessarily wrong or incompatible with those of prudence. In many cases the conclusions deduced from the ethics of principles and rights are compatible with those generated by an ethics of prudence. But the contrast we are making here between prudential reasoning and principle-based reasoning centers not on conclusions but on the process of arriving at conclusions.

Prudence does not make general principles or rights central and then proceed by deductive logic to a particular judgment. Recognizing this may leave some people uncomfortable because the logical certitude available with deductive reasoning is not available. Prudence simply does not provide us with the logical comfort we expect in deductive geometry, or in science, or with religious dogma. An ethics of prudence accepts this discomfort and, with Aristotle and Aquinas, acknowledges that in matters of concrete human behavior our knowledge is, at best, valid "only for the most part."

Morality is simply not science. Galileo and Newton taught us how to measure physical bodies and how to predict a high tide or an eclipse or a sunrise a thousand years from now, but no historian or psychologist or sociologist or ethicist can measure human choice and predict future human action with such precision. What should make us uneasy in ethics is not that we do not have the certitude we think we have in modern science or thought we had in ancient metaphysics and theology but that so many people think we have, or should have, such certitude in the field of deliberate and free human conduct.

This does not mean prudence is some form of guessing or little more than a matter of personal beliefs and opinions. We can certainly guess or sincerely believe or have a strong opinion that something is good or bad, and our guess, belief, or opinion might well be correct, but this is not prudence. The judgments of prudence are always supported by reasons. Feelings play an important role, as we shall see, but they do not replace the need for reasons. What we always have to show in an ethics of prudence is *why* we think something will indeed contribute to what is truly good. This is why, in the second part of this book in which we consider concrete ethical issues, we will always insist on reasons to support the ethical judgments we suggest. And the reasons are valid when they show that an action or omission truly contributes to living well.

Adopting an ethics of the good employing prudence as the reasoning that directs our conduct means that we can never say a behavior is morally good or morally bad "because I believe it with all my heart" or "because that is the way I was brought up" or "because this is what civil or religious authorities say." Prudence, the intellectual virtue at the heart of morality, always supports its judgments with reasons why the behavior in question will, or will not, actually contribute to my human good. Aristotle and Aquinas always insisted that acting prudently is, in the last analysis, acting not according to mere beliefs, nor according to how I was brought up, nor according to the dictates of authority, but "according to right reason."

Finally, we should not confuse prudence with a purely instrumental kind of reasoning, a reasoning concerned exclusively with the means needed to achieve a goal and not with the goal itself. In instrumental reasoning the end and the means are distinguished. Vacationing in the Caribbean is one thing; buying the ticket weeks ahead of time is quite another. The distinction between ends and means in instrumental reasoning becomes very clear when we have a good end and a bad means—we desire money, so we steal it.

In prudence there is no sharp distinction between means and end. The behavior is not simply the means to happiness but happiness itself. The end, happiness, is embedded in the means. Happiness is not distinct from the virtuous activity that achieves it; happiness is living virtuously. Prudence is therefore a reasoning about the end as well as about the means. Prudence grasps the complete good of human life as well as the means to achieve it. We totally misunderstand Aristotle and Aquinas if we think their ethics is an instrumental reasoning wherein "the end justifies any means." In every case, prudence must grasp the end—living well—and show how the means will promote it.

What Prudence Is

Prudence is the deliberation and reasoning in any particular situation that determines what feelings and behaviors will truly promote my good or at least avoid the worse bad. But how does prudence determine what behavior is virtuous and reasonable? How do I decide what behavior makes my life a good life?

Outside of tragic situations and excluding situations in which what I am contemplating is clearly contrary to a good life by definition (murder, for example), Aristotle suggests that prudence begins by recognizing that a good life is enhanced by striking a balance between feelings and behaviors that are neither excessive nor deficient.

Some behaviors, for example, contribute in a significant way to the biological aspects of the human good. The primary examples are eating, drinking, exercise, and sex. But if we eat too much or too little, we undermine living well. Just how much and what to eat will vary from person to person and from circumstance to circumstance, and prudence is needed to determine how much we should eat in any given situation. I know too much is not good for me, and obviously too little is not good. I also know circumstances play a role—I should not eat anything before major surgery. So I cannot simply say eating is good for me.

What is good for me is eating reasonably, that is, eating well or virtuously. Eating is reasonable when, given the circumstances, it is neither too much nor too little for me. The knowledge I need to figure out how much I should eat is primarily practical, not scientific, and it is circumstantial. This example of practical knowledge in the matter of eating—which Aristotle and Aquinas considered a matter of the moral virtue known as temperance—gives us a preliminary idea of how prudence works. Prudence, recognizing that good behavior is undermined by excess or by defect, endeavors to determine just where on the spectrum between those extremes the behavior promoting my good will fall in the particular circumstances facing me at any given time.

Prudence not only determines what achieves my good, it is also decisive. It directs me to behave in a certain way. This is what distinguishes prudence from what we called judgment. The processes of reasoning in prudence and in judgment are similar, but unlike judgment, prudence directs the person doing the reasoning to do, or not to do, something.

The controlling role of prudence is clearly seen when it overrides what would normally be morally virtuous. Consider the following situation adapted from an ancient example in virtue ethics. A person borrowed a friend's rifle last week and promised to return it today. The friend comes to the house to retrieve his gun. Justice and promise keeping indicate the borrower should return it as promised.

But now think of this. The owner is going after someone who has wronged him. You know he can be violent and may use the gun to threaten or even shoot at the other person, so you hesitate to return his gun. But he reminds you that the gun is his property and that you promised to return it today. He argues that keeping his property without his consent violates the moral principle of justice. He also points out that the great moralist Immanuel Kant insisted that everybody is bound by a strict moral duty never to break a promise.

Obviously you cannot simply think of justice and promise keeping in this situation and then return his property. What more do you need to do? You need to figure out what would really be a good choice for you in these circumstances. Once you realize that giving a weapon to someone on the way to threaten and maybe shoot at another person is not the kind of action that is likely to make your life a good life, you know what decision is intelligent—the decision to keep his property without his consent despite your promise. By so doing you reveal how prudential reasoning is the controlling factor in virtuous decision making.

The actual practice of prudential reasoning can be difficult at first. There is no clear methodology similar to the deductive method of deducing particular moral judgments from ethical principles. Indeed some think that method is the enemy of the prudential reasoning needed in ethics.

Fortunately, the person practicing prudence in any moral situation does not start from scratch. Before trying to determine what is right in a particular case, she has the benefit of three things. First, every person has a preliminary natural orientation toward a good life. Living things, including human beings, strive not only to live but to live well. Second, she has received some moral education from parents, from schools, from society, and frequently from religious organizations. This moral education provides a preliminary apprehension of how to go about living a good life. Third, if she is reasonably mature, she has complemented her natural orientation and moral education toward a good life with a personal awareness that living well is the overall goal of life.

When the practitioner of prudence is faced with a challenging concrete situation, these three background features have already provided a preliminary orientation. Now she must determine what behavior will achieve her personal happiness in the situation. Prudence will provide the answer to the extent it can be provided, so we must examine its features more closely.

The Features of Prudence

Aquinas lists eight features of prudence and three additional secondary virtues associated with it. His list is a compilation of features drawn mostly from Aristotle but from others as well. It is not intended to be exhaustive. It is a convenient way to organize the chief characteristics of prudence, as long as we do not mistake the list for any kind of highly organized methodology or for any kind of sequence such as we find in manuals telling us how to operate equipment or build something. Prudence is not like that. It is a way of thinking that cannot be considered a science, or a craft, or a technique, but only as a unique and somewhat disorganized process.

The list that follows is, therefore, not to be taken as steps of a method to be followed every time we make a moral decision. It is simply a compilation of features embedded in prudence and largely unnoticed by the prudent person in the process of exercising prudence. Only through analytical reflection on prudential activity does the list emerge. Not every feature on the list is of equal importance. Some features are rather obvious and simple, whereas others will require some explanation. And some features are debatable. With these remarks in mind, we now take up the eight features of prudence and the three secondary intellectual virtues associated with it.

Memory

We learn from experience, sometimes the hard way, what contributes to our fulfillment and what does not. What happened to us in the past can serve as plausible grounds or "quasiarguments," as Aquinas calls them, for figuring out what we should do in the present.

Understanding

This term requires some comment for a correct appreciation of its meaning. "Apprehension" might be a better translation of the Greek *nous* and the Latin *intellectus* but, since "understanding" is so often used, we will retain it. We shall have to be careful, however, how we understand this word, understanding. It is a highly technical term with a precise meaning for Aristotle and Aquinas. It refers to the ability to know something directly (that is, without a reasoning process). Aquinas says things known this way are "known per se." They are self-evident and obvious. They need no proof, no arguments, no reasons. Aristotle and Aquinas thought this understanding of the self-evident was the way we came to know two kinds of things: (1) the first principle of theoretical reasoning (the principle of noncontradiction) and the first principle of practical reasoning (our choices always seek what is thought to be good) and (2) the moral issues in the concrete situations we face in the course of a life.

We have already seen how this understanding of the self-evident grasps the first principle of practical reasoning, but now we need to note the second area where we have to rely on this direct apprehension called understanding—the immediate grasping of moral issues, what is significantly good or bad, in each concrete situation that we face in life. Understanding grasps directly the particular situation with its salient moral features. Prudential reasoning thus begins with two starting points grasped by understanding: the first principle (people seek their good) and the moral nuances embedded in the unique particular situation facing us.

Learning from the Prudent

In *The Republic* Plato advanced a famous theory: our communities should be run by philosopher-kings who master philosophy and ethics and then direct the moral lives of the citizens. The philosopher-kings were the ethical experts. In some religious traditions a similar theory exists: the community should be run by theologian-authorities who master theology and ethics and then direct the moral lives of the believers.

Aristotle and Aquinas proposed a fundamental revision to this model. They still embraced the idea that a special group provided moral direction, but membership in the group is not confined to philosopher-kings or theologian-authorities. Rather, the group is composed of experienced people who have actually achieved a high degree of moral success in their personal lives. The group comprises people who are in fact prudent or were prudent when they were alive. They are the people who actually live, or did live, good lives. These people are the ethically successful people; we recognize them as noble human beings.

Aristotle called these people the *phronimoi*, the people who had mastered *phronesis*; Aquinas called them the "experts," the "elders," and the "prudent." We have all met these people in life. They are the people we recognize as being of high moral integrity; they are good, decent, and noble people. Some are rich, but many are poor; some are powerful, but many are weak or even exploited. Some are political or religious leaders, but many are not. We trust and admire these people of high moral integrity, and both Aristotle and Aquinas insisted we should learn from them.

And how do they teach us? Not in a scientific or theoretical way and not by statements backed by whatever authority they might have. They do not give us principles, rules, laws, and regulations to follow. Nor are the particular behaviors they chose in their lives necessarily the model for what we should choose in our lives. We do not simply imitate their lives and do what they did. Rather, we learn from their ability to deliberate prudently. In the different situations of their lives they were able to figure out the behavior constitutive of a good life. They did this by prudence. So we want to learn from their example, from how they practiced prudence and went about perceiving the right thing to do in their lives.

These good and noble people do not tell me what behavior is right in my situation; they teach me how to perceive the moral dimensions in particular situations and how to figure out what behavior is best suited to achieve happiness. The prudent people who serve as role models do not dictate what is the right thing to do; they offer advice and show us how to figure out for ourselves what is the right thing for us. They serve as examples. We want to study how they made virtuous choices in their concrete situations so we can make them in our own.

Shrewdness

This is the ability to grasp very quickly what is the right thing to do. The shrewd person has the ability to hit the mark, to get right to the point, to cut through all the irrelevant factors and see, while on the spot, what is really necessary to achieve the end. Shrewdness quickly grasps what we should start doing now, in this situation, to achieve our goal—a good life.

Reasoning

Reasoning consists of showing how certain feelings and behavior will truly achieve my good in the particular situation. My reasons will, or should, show how the behavior is better suited to my good than the other options available in the circumstances. And if my action causes bad things to happen to me or to others, then I must produce convincing reasons for the bad I cause.

Consideration of Consequences

We can call this foresight. Aquinas calls it "providence" because it is a foreseeing or seeing ahead. We know our actions have consequences, and so we look to these consequences and try to discern how they fit into our personal happiness. Prudence acknowledges that we must always consider the consequences of our actions and whether they will bring good things or bad things for ourselves and others.

Consideration of Circumstances

Prudence is about individual actions in particular situations, and hence many circumstantial factors are involved. Some of the circumstances are morally significant and should be a part of prudential consideration. Circumstances can sometimes make all the difference in the world. Something considered good in one situation might not be good in other circumstances. Thus, to use Aquinas's example, it is good to treat another person kindly—unless she happens to be a suspicious and cynical person, for then the kindness may very well make her more suspicious and eventually disturb and upset her.

The ethical person not only does the good thing but does it in the right way and at the right time. Virtue is living well and doing well, and this depends in large measure on circumstances. We have to look at all the circumstances to make a good moral decision because the virtuous mean always depends on the circumstances in which the moral agent finds herself.

The major circumstantial factors affecting morality were well known in Greek, Roman, and medieval ethics. They revolve around who is performing the action, what kind of action it is, where it is being done, by what means it is being done, why it is being done, how it is being done, and when it is being done. Cicero and the medieval moralists often summarized these factors as follows: "who, what, where, by what means, why, how, when." Except for the "what," which refers to the action itself, and the "why," which refers to intention and purpose, all these factors are circumstances.

Caution

Moral situations are often not clear-cut. The good is often mixed with the bad. Therefore, we have to be very careful as we make our way through the jungle of moral dilemmas. Caution rules out any kind of dogmatic or fundamentalist approach in ethics. Prudence always tiptoes along, for it recognizes the complexity and contradictory nature of many situations and knows that no simple answer is possible in difficult and complex cases.

Listing these eight factors characterizing the intellectual virtue of prudence helps us to understand the virtue better. Prudence is a complex intellectual virtue embracing memory, understanding the first principle and concrete situations, learning from the truly prudent, shrewdness, reasoning ability, the consideration both of consequences and of circumstances, and an element of caution.

Prudence and Feelings

It has been noted with some reason that Aquinas's description of prudence is overly intellectual and neglects an important aspect of good prudential decision making—feeling. Traditional wisdom has long warned us about letting emotions and feelings disrupt our thinking. What we now realize more and more, however, is the disruption in moral reasoning that occurs when emotions and feelings are not part of thinking, especially thinking about living well and how to achieve it. Studies in psychology have shown how some people with normal cognitive abilities but who lack emotions because of brain damage consistently fail to make good decisions about living.

Undoubtedly emotions and feelings can inhibit or overwhelm thinking and lead to poor decisions. But the lack of emotion also leads to poor decisions. Emotions and feelings can lead us in the right direction as surely as they can lead us astray, and they can help us create a happy life as surely as they can create unhappiness. Living without emotion and feeling is not living well, and choices without emotion and feeling are not morally mature.

Emotion plays a major role in figuring out what it takes to live life well. Our longing for happiness—our primary goal—is primarily emotional although rational reflection certainly clarifies this goal. Emotions shape our deliberations and choices chiefly by conveying more rapidly than unemotional, detached reasoning the good and bad features of a situation.

In some situations emotions and feelings give immediate and clear moral direction. If you see a child tormenting an animal for example, the unpleasant feeling you experience at seeing the animal being tortured will be the major factor prompting you to stop the child's cruel behavior. Emotions enable us to respond correctly to some situations without the slower processes of deliberation. Emotions and feelings often apprehend the ethical features in a situation more quickly and sometimes more accurately than deliberation.

Emotions and feelings obviously play a larger role in some areas of life than they do in others. They are significant features of decision making in matters of love, friendship, courage, and being unjustly victimized, for example, but they are less significant when it comes to matters of what we owe in justice.

A major emotional attitude of great importance to prudence is *caring*. Caring about a person or a project is feeling a concern for that person or project to flourish and be successful. In the virtue-based morality of personal happiness outlined here, we care for ourselves by helping ourselves grow toward a good and flourishing life. We care for other people—lovers, family, friends, communities, and so forth—and for projects by helping them flourish. And we care for animals and the environment by helping them flourish.

Caring plays a major role in living well. If we care about ourselves, we will choose what is good for ourselves; if we care about our work, we will do it well; if we care about others, we will treat them well; and if we care about our political and social institutions, we will help make them good. Care is truly an integral component of prudential reasoning.

Feelings, then, are an integral part of prudence. They shape its cognitive descriptions and evaluations and in turn are shaped by them. Prudence, as Aristotle observed, can be thought of either as *desiring reason* or as *reasoning desire*.

Next we turn to the final stage of prudence—making and implementing a decision to feel or behave in a certain way.

Prudential Decision Making

Prudence not only perceives our moral goal (happiness) and the feelings and behaviors likely to achieve it but actually directs our feelings and behaviors. Prudence culminates in decisions to do whatever will likely make our lives truly good lives.

Practical decision making has been the object of intense study in recent decades. Two major paradigms have emerged: one is generally known as *rational choice*, and the other is often described as *naturalistic decision making*. Rational choice strategies emerged from psychological studies of problem solving in controlled laboratory situations. Naturalistic decision making, on the other hand, emerged from observations of how experienced people actually make good decisions in real-life situations.

The defining feature of the rational choice strategy is that it is a comparative strategy—it lays out as many alternatives as possible and then compares the favorable and unfavorable consequences of each. Some authors suggest laying out all the alternatives together in what they call a decisional balance sheet. Others suggest that we compare only two alternatives at a time, pick the better one, and then compare that one with a third, pick the better one, continuing until the best alternative is found.

Do these comparative rational choice strategies work? To a point, yes. Comparing alternatives can play an important role in some decisions, especially when the decision maker wants or needs to justify the decision to others or when he is expected to seek maximization in his decision making, that is, the best that can possibly be achieved. But is rational choice strategy the best way to make practical decisions in ambiguous moral situations? Probably not.

Naturalistic decision making is more promising and supports Aristotle's ancient idea of prudence and choice. When researchers watched experienced people make decisions in real life rather than as subjects of controlled research in problem solving, they realized that they did not compare the many possible alternatives with each other to identify the best one. Rather, after assessing the overall situation, they perceived a possible solution and decided to try it. Instead of laying out all the alternatives and comparing them by weighing the advantages and disadvantages of each, they recognized key patterns as well as anomalies in the unfolding situation, imagined a solution compatible with their goal, and then evaluated it as they implemented it. They developed a situation awareness highlighting both familiar and novel features and then saw a promising response they could pursue. Instead of comparing the advantages and disadvantages of many alternatives with each other, they considered only one or a few options in light of their goal and then recognized what would likely achieve that goal.

How do experienced people size up a situation and perceive a promising response so readily? They do so by what researchers call *expertise*. What happens is this: Experience provides the expertise that primes the decision-making process by enabling the experienced decision maker to recognize quickly what is going on and what to do about it. Hence, one important version of naturalistic decision making is aptly called the *recognition-primed decision* model. This model emerged from decades of studying how people actually made good decisions in their area of expertise. As researchers watched firefighters, nurses, pilots, engineers, nuclear plant operators, and military commanders make good decisions and then discussed with them how they did this, they found that experienced people arrived at their decisions not by rational choice strategies but by a recognition-primed decision strategy. Only beginners with little or no experience, or people whose decisions would be carefully analyzed by others, employed the laborious comparative analysis suggested by rational choice theory.

One way to grasp the difference between a rational choice strategy and a recognition-primed decision strategy is to think of how a computer plays a game of chess. The computer uses a rational choice strategy. It considers all the possible moves, then the opponent's possible counter moves to these moves, then its possible moves after these counter moves, and so on. After comparing thousands of alternatives, it picks the best move. This artificial intelligence is so powerful that good computer programs can now beat the best chess players. The beginning chess player, by the way, also relies on rational choice strategy. He compares the advantages and disadvantages of possible moves to find the best one. Of course his ability to compare moves and counter moves is far less than that of a computer.

The expert player, on the other hand, relies chiefly on a recognition-primed decision approach. He perceives key patterns on the board, considers them rather briefly, and then makes his moves. He has neither the time nor the cognitive ability to calculate the huge number of possibilities implied by each move he could make. The computer, of course, can do all the calculations quickly, and that is why computers can now beat the best human players.

You might think that this shows that a rational choice strategy is better than a recognition-primed approach for making decisions, but this is not so for at least three reasons. First, although computers with rational choice software can now beat chess experts, players using rational choice strategy cannot beat them. An expert chess player will inevitably defeat any human player using rational choice strategy. A rational choice strategy gains the advantage only when coupled with the incredible calculating power of computers. No human brain, not even the brains of expert chess players, can compare the advantages and disadvantages of the available moves as quickly and as accurately as the computer. When human chess players try to imitate the decision-making strategies of machines, they actually degrade their decision-making ability.

Second, rational choice strategy works well when the environment is rule governed, as it is with games. When preexisting rules determine what moves can and cannot be made, a comparative analysis of options is feasible even when the options are numerous as they are in chess. But preexisting rules do not ultimately determine human choices in life. Humans make the rules as they go along, and important areas of life—relationships of love, for example—are never well managed by rules.

Third, rational choice strategy is rather detached and unemotional. The comparisons tend toward calculation and quantification, and personal feelings do not play a major role. Making ethical decisions, however, is a very personal and often emotional affair, and the practical reasoning that we need to make them well is not primarily that of rational calculations.

The recognition-primed decision model of recent naturalistic decision theory is very similar to prudence. Aristotle insisted that prudence only works well when the decision maker has already developed some level of expertise in the moral virtues. Virtuous habits provide the moral expertise that permits a person confronting a new situation to recognize the morally salient features and then to perceive rather quickly an appropriate response. A virtuous person seldom compares all the alternatives with each other and then calculates their relative advantages and disadvantages. Rather, she recognizes the morally significant features in the situation and then perceives a move likely to achieve her overall goal in life—happiness.

Only beginners in ethics rely on a rational choice strategy. Without the expertise to size up a situation and readily see a promising course of action, beginners have to rely on comparing the advantages and disadvantages of all the alternatives. As people develop virtue in ethics, however, they rely less on comparative analysis and more on recognizing patterns and perceiving directly the choices in any developing situations likely to accomplish their overall aim in life—happiness.

Modern psychological research thus suggests that Aristotle was on the right track centuries ago when he distinguished practical reason from rule-based deductive reason and insisted that practical reasoning is what we need for human affairs such as ethics, politics, military tactics, medical practice, and so forth. Practical decision making in ethics is prudence—a naturalistic decision-making process distinctly different from rational choice strategies.

Prudence and Deliberation

Aquinas makes a distinction between prudence and another virtue closely allied to it, *deliberation*. The difference seems to be this. A person well advanced in having acquired the moral virtues generally makes moral decisions more by experience, insight, and intuition than by deliberation, as we have just noted. However, when faced with the radically new situations that we so often encounter in bioethics today, even the person with a high level of moral virtue and decision-making expertise needs to deliberate carefully and dialogue widely. Strictly speaking, however, prudence is not deliberate; but deliberation is a virtue closely allied to it.

Prudence and Formal Reasoning

Understanding prudence as a natural decision-making process requiring virtue and practical expertise does not do away with all formal reasoning in ethical decision making. Prudence is not science or geometry, nor is it calculating the advantages and disadvantages of as many options as possible, but it often benefits from some formal reasoning. Usually this formal reasoning occurs after the decision maker has identified a tentative decision. To show how this is so, it will be helpful to note how formal reasoning plays a role in another form of practical reasoning—legal reasoning.

Imagine a civil dispute for which both sides present documentation and testimony to the court. As the judge reads the evidence and listens to the testimony, her intelligence probably begins to formulate a decision in her mind. Her developing decision is shaped by her experience with the law and her expertise with cases as well as by her consideration of the evidence and testimony. Gradually a tentative decision takes shape. Only then does she begin formally gathering the legal reasons to support it from relevant legislation, regulations, and previous court decisions.

When the judge writes her decision, however, she will cite these legal reasons as premises leading to her conclusion. Logically, this is correct. Existing laws, regulations, and precedents are important reasons that support judicial decisions. In actuality, however, the judge finally organized her legal reasons for the decision only after she made it. Her perception and reflection on the case, along with her experience with the law, first led to her decision. The formal legal premises appearing in her written decision as steps that led to her decision were actually developed formally only after she had reached a decision.

In some cases the judge may formulate a decision and then be unable to support it with adequate legal reasons. If this occurs, she will reconsider the case, revise her conclusion, and then look for legal reasons in support of her revised decision. More probably, however, her experience and review of the testimony in the case will have led her to a conclusion supported by legal reasons, and she will write her decision accordingly.

It is somewhat the same in ethical reasoning in difficult and complex situations. We perceive the situation in its complexity and see a good response. Only then, if we have the time, might we explicitly formulate the reasons for our decision. When we explain the decision, we undoubtedly present the reasons as coming before the conclusion, although in fact we developed them after it.

Does this make the formal reasoning in prudence no more than rationalization? Are we simply making up reasons to give a veneer of respectability to our preferences? Not really, if the prudential reasoning is authentic. The reasons we develop after we make a tentative decision do play a role. Formulating the reasons serves as a check. When we are able to develop good reasons that show that our decision is likely to help achieve what we are aiming at above all—a good and happy life—we can go forward with added confidence. On the other hand when we are not able to develop good reasons for our decisions, we can abandon our conclusion and take another long look at the situation so that we can make a more reasonable choice.

Prudence and Bad Moral Decisions

Most people tend to call a bad decision one that results in a bad outcome and, conversely, a good decision one that results in a good outcome. This, however, is not the case. Some bad decisions have good outcomes; for example, we may make a decision inconsistent with temperance or courage and actually things may nonetheless turn out well for us. And some good decisions may have bad outcomes; for example, we may make a decision consistent with temperance or courage and actually things may not work out well for us. A truly good decision might bring tragedy, and a truly bad decision might not. There are no guarantees. All we can say is that over the long run, moral decisions made with intelligence and prudence are more likely to contribute to our happiness and living well than decisions not so made.

What then is a bad practical decision? It is not one that happens to have a poor outcome but one that was poorly made. And what is a poorly made decision? In the practical decision making guided by prudence, a poorly made decision is one made by someone who lacks situational awareness and the virtuous experience needed to cope well with the situation. In other words the major causes of a poorly made practical decision are not, as rational choice theorists suggest, faulty comparative analysis of all the alternatives or psychological biases preventing us from thinking clearly. The major causes of bad ethical decisions are an inadequate awareness of what is going on and insufficient experience to handle it well so that the decision maker can achieve what he desires most—a good life.

Prudence and Religion

Religion is a complex and difficult topic. It is complex because so many religions exist in the world, and most of them encompass internal factions ranging from "fundamentalist" to "liberal." Also it is a difficult topic because many believers consider matters of religious faith to be inappropriate subjects for rational discussion and critical thinking. Moreover, the religions that trace their roots back to the God of Abraham—Judaism, Christianity, and Islam—present a unique challenge to the ethics of happiness and prudential reasoning. These religions teach that morality originates with God and obligates the religious faithful to obey the divine law as presented and interpreted by religious authorities.

A conflict thus exists between these religious ethics and the virtue-based ethics pioneered by Aristotle. A religious believer will be torn between two fundamental questions: Does ethics originate from his religion or from his humanity? Does the guide for living well come ultimately from divine law or from human intelligence? Does religious faith or human reason provide the primary insights about how one should live one's life?

Religious believers do not agree on how to answer these questions. Some believers say that religious faith provides the norm for moral decision making. Others say that religious faith is important but does not provide the norm for moral decision making. Still others say that religious faith and virtue combine in complementary ways and together provide the norms for making moral decisions. Often, however, proponents of this last view tend not to consider religion and reason truly complementary—in controversial issues of human behavior, they give the last word to religious faith, not reason.

The debate over whether morality and ethics ultimately come "from above" in some kind of religious revelation of commandments presented and interpreted by religious authorities or "from below" in some kind of rational or intelligent modification of the desires and inclinations inherent in our nature has existed for centuries and will likely continue for a long time to come. We cannot hope to solve it here. However, one way to look at the relation of the virtue-based ethics and religious faith is to encourage each person to ask whether religious faith is valuable in achieving his aim of living a good life. If he finds that religious faith is valuable for living virtuously, then it is one of the potential goods, which are, you may remember, goods that are valuable in themselves and valuable also because of their contributions to the virtues.

Might religious faith be more than a potential good? Might it be what the virtue-based tradition called a *noble* good, that is, a moral virtue? Probably not. The moral virtues are the necessary components of a morally good life. If religious faith is a moral virtue, we would have to say it is necessary for a morally good life, which seems clearly false because it is not hard to find people who live truly virtuous lives without embracing any organized faith or religion.

If religious faith is considered a virtue, and some theologians do so consider it, then it is best thought of as a theological virtue granted as a gift from God and not a moral virtue gained by intentionally and repeatedly choosing morally virtuous feelings and behaviors for their own sake and for the sake of personal happiness in life. This was the general position Aquinas adopted. He argued in the *Summa Theologiae* (I II Q. 62) that the theological virtues (faith, hope, and charity) are specifically distinct from the moral and intellectual virtues for three reasons: They have a super-human aim (God); they come as gifts from God (and not from our decisions and behavior); and knowledge of them comes from biblical revelation (not human reason).

In evaluating whether and to what extent religious faith might be a value that contributes to living well, it is important to remember that religion is much more than a moral code. Religions point to something sacred; provide rituals of celebration, mourning, conversion, and forgiveness; offer faith in something transcendent, hope in times of despair, and love in the midst of obligations. Religions also preserve important traditions and practices and provide communities where morality is taken seriously and endlessly debated. All these religious elements may help people achieve their primary aim—living a good and happy life. To the extent that they do, it makes sense in a virtue-based ethics to embrace them. In other words, the virtue-based morality of happiness can, but need not, include religion as a potential good in a well-lived life.

It is not without interest to note that Aristotle, the architect of the morality of happiness presented here, acknowledged the importance of religion for good living. This is somewhat surprising because in his theoretical philosophy he described God as an unmoved mover who neither knew of nor cared about humanity. On the political level, however, he felt it important to acknowledge recognition of Greek religion. Apparently he thought that religious practices conducted by the priests contributed something valuable to the social and political well-being of the community.

Aristotle also spoke of "the divine element" in us as the ultimate source of our desire for happiness and of our natural tendencies to seek the goods that compose it. Finally, he claimed that contemplation of "god" is the best of human activities and thus an integral part of human happiness. The exact meaning of these remarks at the end of the *Nicomachean Ethics* is a matter of much dispute, so it would not be wise to make too much of them. Still, the passages exist and are suggestive. It is important to note, however, that Aristotle never felt that the divine element in us or the god we contemplate would tell us how to live a good life. That is the job of prudence rooted in moral virtue.

This concludes our sketch of prudential decision making in the virtue-based ethics of happiness initiated by Aristotle and retrieved by Aquinas. The cases in this book will bring you as close to prudential reasoning and ethical decision making as possible by examining dilemmas in health care from the various perspectives of the moral agents involved—the people who had to decide to do something, or to do nothing. Only after their perspectives have been considered will a general ethical reflection be introduced. The purpose is not to judge others but to consider what they faced so we can better make the practical decisions in our lives that will likely make our lives good lives and bring us the happiness we desire. Before looking at particular cases, however, we need to consider some preliminary notions. The next chapter looks at the language we use and often misuse in health care ethics.

SUGGESTED READINGS

For a splendid account of the beginning of the moralities of happiness in ancient Greece, see Julia Annas, 1993, *The Morality of Happiness*, New York: Oxford University Press. Helpful comments on this book by noted Aristotelian scholars Nancy Sherman, John Cooper, and Richard Kraut, with a response by Annas, appear as a symposium on the book in *Philosophy and Phenomenological Research* 1995, *55*, 909–37.

Although the assumption that happiness is the overriding good in life was widespread in ancient Greece, it was not universal. A notable exception was the Cyrenaic school. Influenced by Aristippus, one of Socrates' followers, its members claimed our ultimate good was pleasure, and if we seek happiness, it is only because it gives us pleasure. Unlike the Epicureans, who claimed happiness is pleasure, the Cyrenaics taught that happiness is a means to pleasure. See Terence Irwin, "Aristippus against Happiness," *Monist* 1991, *74*, 55–82.

We rely on Aristotle and Aquinas for the development of personal good or happiness as the central theme of ethics. The classical texts are Aristotle's *Nicomachean Ethics*, especially books 1 and 10; the *Eudemian Ethics*, books 1 and 2; the *Rhetoric*, book 1, chapters 6 and 7; and the *Topics*, book 3, chapters 1 and 2. In the past decade a major movement in psychology inaugurated by Martin Seligman and known as positive psychology has reintroduced the ancient notions of *eudaimonia* and a set of virtues or "strengths of character" that enable people to achieve this happiness in their lives. Positive psychology's focus on happiness (rather than mental illness) and the core character virtues needed to attain it reawakens the work of the original virtue ethicists, especially when we read that the six core virtues positive psychology proposes are the familiar ones we find in ancient virtue ethics: temperance, courage, justice, love, spirituality (which the Greeks called piety), and wisdom. See Martin Seligman, 2002, *Authentic Happiness*, New York: Free Press; Christopher Peterson and Martin Seligman, 2004, *Character Strengths and Virtues*, New York: Oxford University Press; and Jonathan Haidt, 2006, *The Happiness Hypothesis: Finding Modern Truth in Ancient Wisdom*, New York: Basic Books. Also helpful are the online site positivepsychology.org and numerous articles in the *Journal of Positive Psychology*. The emphasis of positive psychology is on subjective well-being and happiness, whereas virtue ethics focuses on objective well-being as well; that is, virtue ethics focuses on what truly makes a human life good. It is not enough simply to experience happiness; the ethical inquiry seeks in addition what is in fact a good and noble human life for a human being.

See also Stephen White, 1992, *Sovereign Virtue: Aristotle on the Relation between Happiness and Prosperity*, Stanford: Stanford University Press, especially parts 1 and 2; Richard Kraut, 1989, *Aristotle on the Human Good*, Princeton: Princeton University Press, especially chapters 1, 4, and 5; John M. Cooper, 1977, *Reason and Human Good in Aristotle*, Cambridge: Harvard University Press, especially chapters 2 and 3; and Sarah Broadie, 1991, *Ethics with Aristotle*, New York: Oxford University Press, chapters 1 and 7. Three papers in Amelie Oksenberg Rorty, ed., 1980, *Essays on Aristotle's Ethics*, Berkeley: University of California Press, are also helpful: Thomas Nagel's "Aristotle on *Eudaimonia*," J. L. Ackrill's paper with the same title, and John McDowell's "The Role of *Eudaimonia* in Aristotle's Ethics." See also Julia Annas, "Aristotle on Virtue and Happiness," and J. L. Ackrill, "Aristotle on *Eudaimonia*," in *Aristotle's Ethics: Critical Essays*, Nancy Sherman, ed., New York: Rowman & Littlefield; and Mary Hayden, "Rediscovering Eudaimonistic Teleology," *Monist* 1992, *75*, 71–83.

See also Julia Annas, "Self-love in Aristotle" *The Southern Journal of Philosophy* 1988, *27* (Suppl), 1–18; John Cooper, "Aristotle on Friendship," in Rorty, *Essays on Aristotle's Ethics*, pp. 301–40; Nancy Sherman, 1989, *The Fabric of Character: Aristotle's Theory of Virtue*, New York: Oxford University Press, chapter 4; Bernard Williams, 1985, *Ethics and the Limits of Philosophy*, Cambridge, MA: Harvard University Press, chapter 3; A. W. Price, 1989, *Love and Friendship in Plato and Aristotle*, New York: Oxford University Press, chapters 4–7; J. O. Urmson, 1988, *Aristotle's Ethics*, New York: Basil Blackwell, chapters 9 and 10; and Carlo Natali, 2001, *The Wisdom of Aristotle*, Albany: State University of New York Press. For a thoughtful article explaining how Aristotle's morality of happiness leads us to choose the less bad when no available option leads to happiness, see Robert Heinaman, "Rationality, *Eudaimonia* and *Kakodaimonia* in Aristotle," *Phronesis* 1993, *38*, 31–56.

The major texts in Aquinas supporting the Aristotelian view are the *Summa Theologiae*, I II, questions 1–5; the *Summa Contra Gentiles*, book 3; the *Sententia Libri Ethicorum* (Commentary on the Book of Ethics); and his detailed analysis of Aristotle's *Nicomachean Ethics*, revised, titled *Commentary on Aristotle's Nicomachean Ethics*, C. I. Litzinger, trans., Notre Dame: Dumb Ox Books, 1993.

Aquinas's treatment of the parallel between the self-evident first principle of theoretical reasoning (the principle of noncontradiction) and the self-evident first principle of moral reasoning (people seek their good) is found in the *Summa Theologiae*, I II, q. 91, a. 3 and q. 94, a. 3. In q. 94, a. 2, he wrote: "The first principle (*primum principium*) is all seek their good, and this leads to the first precept (*primum praeceptum*), which is: do and seek the good, and avoid the bad." For a provocative, and controversial, reading of Aquinas on the first principle of practical reasoning, see Germain Grisez, "The First Principle of Practical Reason," *Natural Law Forum* 1965, *10*, 168–96, reprinted in an abridged form in Anthony Kenny, ed., 1976, *Aquinas: A Collection of Critical Essays*, South Bend: University of Notre Dame Press, pp. 340–82. Aquinas also states that the first principle of human action is reason: "Reason is the *principium primum* of all human actions" (*Summa Theologiae*, I II, q. 58, a. 2). This is merely another way of making his point. Reason apprehends what is good for us and directs us in achieving it.

Both Aristotle and Aquinas insist that an ethics of seeking our good (that is, our personal happiness) is an ethics advocating an abiding and sincere concern for others. Both insist that we cannot be happy without justice and love. See books 4, 5, 8, and 9 in the *Nicomachean Ethics* and *Summa Theologiae* I II, qq. 26–29 and II II, qq. 23–27 and 57–63. See also Arthur Madigan, 1991, "Eth. Nic, 9:8: Beyond Egoism and Altruism," in *Aristotle's Ethics*, John P. Anton and Anthony Preus, eds., 1991, Albany: State University of New York Press, pp. 73–94; and Mary Hayden, "The Paradox of Aquinas's Altruism: From Self-Love to Love of Others," *Proceedings of the American Catholic Philosophical Association* 1990, *63*, 72–83.

The classic texts in Aristotle elaborating his doctrine of the intellectual and moral virtues are the *Nicomachean Ethics*, books 2–7, and the *Eudemian Ethics*, books 2 and 3. See also Sherman, *The Fabric of Character*, chapters 1–3; and Broadie, *Ethics with Aristotle*, chapter 4. The major text for the capstone moral virtue *megalopsychia*, which we are now translating as pride, is book 4 of the *Nicomachean Ethics*, section 3. For a thoughtful explanation of Aristotle's moral virtue of pride, see Daniel Russell, 2005, "Aristotle on the Moral Relevance of Self-Respect," in *Virtue Ethics, Old and New*, Stephen Gardiner, ed., Ithaca, NY: Cornell University Press, pp. 101–21.

The central texts on the virtues in Aquinas are the *Summa Theologiae* I II, q. 49–67, and II II, q. 47–170. Also important is his more technical analysis titled *De Virtutibus in Communi* (The Virtues in General), one of the *Questiones Disputatae* (Disputed Questions). See *Questiones Disputatae*, volume 2, Turin: Marietti, 1949, pp. 707–51. Aquinas claims virtuous habits are necessary for three reasons: (1) they give a certain uniformity to our actions, so that we respond habitually in just or loving or courageous ways to individual situations; (2) they enable us to respond promptly by relieving us of the necessity of an elaborate inquiry to figure out what is right every time we are faced with a moral decision; and (3) they enable us to act more easily and with enjoyment, since such actions become second nature thanks to the virtuous habits (*De Virtutibus in Communi*, a. 1).

Aristotle's development of prudence (*phronesis*) is set forth in book 6 of the *Nicomachean Ethics*. See also Pierre Aubenque, 1986, *La prudence chez Aristote*, Paris: Presses Universitaires de France, pp. 33–152; Norman O. Dahl, 1984, *Practical Reason, Aristotle, and Weakness of the Will*, Minneapolis: University of Minnesota Press, pp. 3–135; Paul Schuchman, 1980, *Aristotle and the Problem of Moral Discernment*, Frankfort am Main: Peter D. Lang, chapters 1, 4, and 5; David Wiggins, "Deliberation and Practical Reason," in Rorty, *Essays on Aristotle's Ethics*, pp. 221–40; Hans-Georg Gadamer, 1991, *Truth and Method*, 2nd revised ed., New York: Crossroad, pp. 312–24; Martha C. Nussbaum, 1986, "Non-scientific Deliberation," in *The Fragility of Goodness*, Cambridge, UK: Cambridge University Press, chapter 10; Charles Larmore, 1987, "Moral Judgment—an Aristotelian Insight," in *Patterns of Moral Complexity*, Cambridge, UK: Cambridge University Press, chapter 1.

For more recent work see Nancy Sherman, 1997, "Aristotelian Particularism," in *Making a Necessity of Virtue: Aristotle and Kant on Virtue*, Cambridge, UK: Cambridge University Press, chapter 6; John McDowell, 1996, "Deliberation and Moral Development in Aristotle's Ethics," in *Aristotle, Kant, and the Stoics*, Stephen Engstrom and Jennifer Whiting, eds., Cambridge, UK: Cambridge University Press, chapter 1; Dominique Panzani, "La *phronesis*: disposition paradoxale," pp. 23–43, and Jean-Yves Chateau, "L'object de la *phronesis* et la vérité pratique," pp. 185–261, in Jean-Yves Chateau, ed., 1997, *La Vérité Pratique: Aristote, Ethique a Nicomaque*, Paris: Librarie Philosophique; J. Vrin and Danielle Lories, 1998, *Le Sens Commun et le Jugment du Phronimos*, Louvain: Editions Peeters, especially chapter 2, "*Phronesis*"; Gerard Hughes, 2001, *Aristotle on Ethics*, New York: Routledge; and Sarah Broadie, 2002, "Philosophical Introduction," in *Aristotle: Nicomachean Ethics*, Christopher Rowe, trans., New York: Oxford University Press, pp. 9–91. Rowe's translation and extensive commentary provide a valuable guide for those interested in the serious study of Aristotle, as does the translation with extensive notes by Terence Irwin, 1999, *Aristotle: Nicomachean Ethics*, 2nd ed., Indianapolis: Hackett Publishing Company. In the second edition Irwin begins translating *phronesis* as "prudence."

Aquinas's development of prudence (*prudentia*) is set forth in the *Summa Theologiae*, I II, q. 57, a. 4–6, q. 58, and II II, q. 47–56. His statement that "the whole matter of the moral virtues falls under the single reasoning of prudence" is from I II, q. 65, a.1, ad 3 and reads in Latin "*Et ideo tota materia moralium virtutum sub una ratione prudentiae cadit.*" His discussion of deliberation, a virtue allied to prudence, is in the *Summa Theologiae*, II II, q. 51 and follows closely book 6, chapters 9–11 of the *Nicomachean Ethics*. See also Josef Pieper, 1966, *The Four Cardinal Virtues*, Notre Dame: University of Notre Dame Press, pp. 3–40. For an overview of Aquinas's doctrine of prudence showing that it, and not the natural law or the moral virtues, provides the ethical directions for the activities of our lives, see Daniel Nelson, 1992, *The Priority of Prudence*, University Park, PA: Pennsylvania State University Press, especially chapters 2, 3, and 5. For an excellent collection of articles on the ethics of Aquinas, see Stephen Pope, ed., 2002, *The Ethics of Aquinas*, Washington, DC: Georgetown University Press, especially James Keenan, "The Virtue of Prudence," pp. 259–71.

After being overshadowed so long by moralities of obligation with their action-guiding moral laws, maxims, principles, and rules, moralities of happiness and virtue are now receiving enormous attention in the literature. Some important early work in English was done by Alasdair Macintyre, Philippa Foot, Iris Murdoch, Bernard Williams, and G. E. M. Anscombe. For more recent literature see Michael Slote, 1992, *From Morality to Virtue*, New York: Oxford University Press, especially parts II and IV. Collections of essays on virtue theory include Roger Crisp, ed., 1996, *How Should One Live? Essays on the Virtues*, New York: Oxford University Press, especially chapter 1 by Crisp titled "Modern Moral Philosophy and the Virtues" and chapter 2 by Rosalind Hursthouse titled "Normative Virtue Ethics"; Roger Crisp and Michael Slote, eds., 1997, *Virtue Ethics*, New York: Oxford University Press; Ellen F. Paul, Jefferey Miller, and Fred Paul, eds., 1997, *Self-Interest*, Cambridge University Press; and Ellen F. Paul, Jefferey Miller, and Fred Paul, eds., 1998, *Virtue and Vice*, Cambridge, UK: Cambridge University Press; Rosalind Hursthouse, 1999, *On Virtue Ethics*, New York: Oxford University Press; Raymond J. Devettere, 2002, *Introduction to Virtue Ethics: Insights of the Ancient Greeks*, Washington, DC: Georgetown University Press; Stephen Darwell, ed., 2003, *Virtue Ethics*, Oxford: Blackwell Publishing; Timothy Chappell, ed., 2006, *Values and Virtues: Aristotelianism in Contemporary Ethics*, New York: Oxford University Press; and Stephen Gardiner, ed., 2005, *Virtue Ethics, Old and New*, Ithaca, NY: Cornell University Press. For thirteen articles relevant to a virtue-based ethics of happiness, see the issue of *Social Philosophy and Policy* 1999, *16*, which is devoted to the theme "Human Flourishing." For an excellent overview see Rosalind Hursthouse's 2007 article "Virtue Ethics" with a good bibliography in the online *Stanford Encyclopedia of Philosophy* at plato.stanford.edu.

Examples of virtue-based ethics in health care include Candace Gauthier, "Teaching the Virtues: Justifications and Recommendations"; Eric Loewy, "Developing Habits and Knowing What Habits to Develop: A Look at the Role of Virtue in Ethics," *Cambridge Quarterly of Healthcare Ethics* 1997, *6*, 339–46 and 347–55; and Edmund Pellegrino and David Thomasma, 1996, *The Christian Virtues in Medical Practice*, Washington, DC: Georgetown University Press. For an example of practical moral reasoning similar to Aristotle but based on the pragmatism of John Dewey, see Joseph Fins, "Approximation and Negotiation: Clinical Pragmaticism and Difference," *Cambridge Quarterly of Healthcare Ethics* 1998, *7*, 68–76; and Joseph Fins, Matthew D. Bacchetta, and Franklin G. Miller, "Clinical Pragmaticism: A Method of Moral Problem Solving," *Kennedy Institute of Ethics Journal* 1997, 7, 129–45.

For a classic text on rational choice decision making, see Irving Janis and Leon Mann, 1977, *Decision Making: A Psychological Analysis of Conflict, Choice, and Commitment*, New York: Free Press. A seminal text in the rational choice tradition that attributes poor decisions to biases infecting our reasoning is Jay Russo and Paul Shoemaker, 1989, *Decision Traps: Ten Barriers to Brilliant Decision Making and How to Overcome Them*, Garden City, NY: Doubleday. See also John Hammond, 1998, *Small Choices: A Practical Guide to Making Better Decisions*, Boston: Harvard Business School Press.

A good collection of decision-making scenarios showing that experienced people do not rely on rational choice theory is Caroline Zsambok and Gary Klein, 1997, *Naturalistic Decision Making*, Mahwah, NJ: Lawrence Erlbaum. The naturalistic decision model that so closely resembles prudence is explained with numerous examples in an important book by Gary Klein, 1998, *Sources of Power: How People Make Decisions*, Cambridge, MA: MIT Press. For some of the philosophical theory behind the psychology of naturalistic decision making, see Hurbert Dreyfus, 1972, *What Computers Can't Do: A Critique of Artificial Intelligence*, New York: Harper & Row; and Hurbert Dreyfus and Stuart Dreyfus, 1986, *Mind over Machine: The Power of Human Intuitive Expertise in the Era of the Computer*, New York: Free Press. For more recent literature see David Myers, 2002, *Intuition: Its Powers and Perils*, New Haven: Yale University Press; Gerd Gigerenzer, 2007, *Gut Feelings: The Intelligence of the Unconscious*, New York: Viking

Penguin; and Gary Klein, 2004, *The Power of Intuition* (originally titled *Intuition at Work* in 2003), New York: Doubleday.

For a consideration of the role religion and spirituality might well play in health care ethics, see David Thomasma and Erich Loewy, "Exploring the Role of Religion in Medical Ethics," *Cambridge Quarterly of Healthcare Ethics* 1996, *5*, 257–68; Joseph Tham, "The Secularization of Bioethics," *National Catholic Bioethics Quarterly* 2008, *8*, 443–53; and Bernard Lo et al., "Discussing Religious and Spiritual Issues at the End of Life: A Practical Guide for Physicians," *JAMA* 2002, *287*, 749–54. For an excellent book on spirituality and health care by a Catholic physician and ethicist who is also a Franciscan friar, see Daniel Sulmasy, 2006, *The Rebirth of the Clinic: An Introduction to Spirituality in Health Care*, Washington, DC: Georgetown University Press. See also Carol Taylor and Roberto Dell'Oro, eds., 2006, *Health and Human Flourishing: Religion, Medicine, and Moral Anthropology*, Washington, DC: Georgetown University Press; and David Kelly, 2004, *Contemporary Catholic Health Care Ethics*, Washington, DC: Georgetown University Press. Several journals are also helpful, among them *Christian Bioethics* and the *National Catholic Bioethics Quarterly*.

For a helpful confirmation from contemporary cognitive science of the inadequacy of the rule-based ethics inherited from ancient theories of divine and natural law, as well as from the modern Enlightenment theories of principles, rules, and duties, see Mark Johnson, 1993, *Moral Imagination: Implications of Cognitive Science for Ethics*, Chicago: University of Chicago Press. Johnson describes the "extremely narrow definition" of morality characterizing our culture as follows: "Morality is a set of restrictive rules that are supposed to tell you which acts you may and may not perform, which you have an obligation to perform, and when you can be blamed for what you have done. It is not fundamentally about how to live a good life or how to live well. Instead, it is only a matter of 'doing the right thing'—*the* one thing required of you in a given situation" (p. 246). This narrow definition of morality neglects what he calls prudential reasoning, which is "the practical use of reason to determine the most efficient means of attaining the comprehensive human end of happiness or well-being" (p. 247). Johnson's emphasis on imagination, metaphor, and narrative in moral reasoning is comfortably compatible with the older notions of prudence.

THREE

The Language of Health Care Ethics

WE USE LANGUAGE in many different ways. Some sentences state facts, others ask questions, and still others give commands. Our words may be simple descriptions, or they may change our lives. The man who says "I do" when someone asks him whether he likes ice cream is simply reporting a preference, but the man who says "I do" when asked whether he takes a woman as his wife is, if the consent is mutual, making a marriage.

The meaning of language depends to a great extent on what is going on when the language is used. We have to know the "language game," as the philosopher Ludwig Wittgenstein put it, to know what words and sentences mean. For example, normally we think stealing is immoral and shameful, yet we are delighted when a member of our team steals second base.

One important use of language is classifying and distinguishing the realities we encounter. When classifications and distinctions bring order and clarity to the expression of our thoughts, they can be very helpful. Yet classifications and distinctions can become a source of mischief and sometimes mislead us. In health care ethics, this can happen in two ways.

First, some well-established classifications and distinctions are not always suitable for newly developed techniques and technologies, yet we continue to use them. Instead of recognizing the newness and originality of recent developments, we force or shoehorn them into traditional classifications and distinctions. This distorts our descriptions of them, and the distortions undermine our moral deliberations and judgments.

The confusion that results from using traditional classifications for new procedures can be seen readily in the following example. When long-term nourishment by feeding tubes became a reality not so long ago, there were two ways people could classify it. They could say feeding tubes were (1) a way of feeding people or (2) a medical treatment. Neither classification is really fitting. Inserting nutrition and fluids through a tube running into the stomach through the nasal passages or surgically inserted through the abdominal wall is not what we call feeding in any ordinary meaning of the term. Nor is it a typical medical treatment, because it does not provide medicine or medication but what everyone, sick or healthy, needs for life—nutrition and fluids. These techniques are too much like treatment to be classified as feeding, but too much like feeding to be classified as treatment. For purposes of moral deliberation, nourishing people by feeding tubes is better understood and classified as a new category of action.

Worse than the misleading classification of new techniques and technologies is the tendency to substitute distinctions for moral reasoning. For example, some use the distinction between ordinary treatment and extraordinary treatment to justify a moral judgment. They claim that (1) the refusal of an ordinary treatment such as an antibiotic for an infection is never morally justified, whereas (2) the refusal of an extraordinary treatment such as an artificial heart is morally justified. This looks like moral reasoning, but it really is not. Proponents have simply made a distinction between *ordinary* treatment and *extraordinary* treatment and then claimed that the former is always morally obligatory but not the latter.

Sometimes poorly classifying a new technique or technology, or substituting a distinction for authentic moral reasoning, is unintentional and harmless. The process looks like legitimate reasoning and is carelessly accepted as such, but no great harm is done because the conclusion happens to be morally sound.

Sometimes, however, poorly classifying things or substituting distinctions for reasoning is not unintentional and harmless. People may deliberately employ poor classifications and substitute distinctions for reasoning in order to avoid authentic discussion about issues on which they have already taken a firm position. They do not use classifications and distinctions to clarify a subject but, rather, to convince an audience.

People tend to do this when their minds are already made up. Ideologues have nothing to gain from careful classifications and thoughtful distinctions in controversial moral matters. Ideologues are not about to change their minds for any reason. They believe there is nothing to figure out—they already have the right answer. If withdrawing a feeding tube undermines their commitment to the right to life, they will classify it as feeding and insist that patients must always be fed. If withholding antibiotics undermines their conception of the value of human life, they will make a distinction between ordinary and extraordinary treatment, call antibiotics "ordinary treatment," and conclude that they cannot be withheld.

All attempts to show these people that using feeding tubes to keep permanently unconscious patients alive for decades is not reasonable and therefore not morally obligatory fall on deaf ears. A classification has become an ideology: "Feeding tubes feed, and if we do not feed those who cannot feed themselves, they starve to death, and that is wrong." Similarly, attempts to show that using antibiotics to reverse the pneumonia of a ninety-year-old man dying in discomfort of metastasized cancer is not reasonable, and therefore not morally obligatory, fail. A distinction has become an ideology: "Antibiotics are simple, inexpensive, painless, and ordinary treatment, and we are not according human life its proper value if we fail to use ordinary means to preserve it."

This chapter will first call attention to several distinctions that often cause confusion in the reasoning and debates about health care ethics and then will note several other distinctions that can be helpful in our prudential reasoning.

DISTINCTIONS THAT CAN MISLEAD

The following distinctions need to be used with exceptional care or not at all because their use so often hinders good prudential reasoning.

Actions and Omissions

The distinction between action and omission, doing something and not doing something, is certainly valid. I can take my medicine or not take it; I can treat or not treat a patient.

The distinction between action and omission, however, can easily mislead us in ethics. A major problem arises when the distinction is used in situations in which the foreseen outcome is not wanted or desired, and a distinction is made between actions and omissions giving rise to the unwanted outcome. For example, the unwanted outcome of removing life-support equipment is the patient's death. Since many people believe that it is immoral to perform an action leading to the patient's death, they think of what will be done as an omission, the omission of technology needed to support life. This enables them to claim that they are not performing an action leading to death; they are simply omitting inappropriate treatment.

Using the action-omission distinction this way obviously twists language in an unacceptable manner. The action of removing life-support equipment is just that—an action. It is not an omission. Twisting language this way is objectionable because it undermines moral reasoning. We cannot reason well if our language is distorted.

Using the action-omission distinction this way also camouflages an important moral consideration. The unspoken assumption behind using the action-omission distinction is often the belief that omissions contributing to a death are easier to justify morally than actions contributing to a death. Sometimes this is true, but not always. Omissions can be as immoral as actions. Not doing something we should do is as morally significant as doing something we should not do. Some actions are ethical, and some are not; some omissions are ethical, and some are not. The danger is that making a distinction between action and omission can blind us to the fact that omissions can be as immoral as actions. Unless we see this, we will not properly consider ourselves morally responsible for the foreseen bad outcomes that follow our omissions.

In health care ethics the basic action-omission distinction appears in two widespread formulations: the distinction between withdrawing and withholding treatment, and the distinction between intentionally causing death and letting die (or permitting a person to die). We need to say a few words about each.

Withdrawing and Withholding Treatment

There are two major problems associated with this distinction. First, the distinction between withdrawing and withholding treatment is not always clear. It is not clear, for example, in situations in which we stop treatment by withholding the next step. If we interrupt a series of discrete chemotherapy treatments (one today, one tomorrow, and so on), we could say either that we are withdrawing the chemotherapy treatment or that we are withholding the remaining treatments. The same can be said of discrete dialysis treatments. And some have claimed we do not really withdraw medical nutrition—we simply withhold the next drop in the tube or line.

At other times of course, the distinction between withholding and withdrawing treatment is clear. One example is the distinction between not connecting a patient to a ventilator and disconnecting the ventilator. Even when the distinction is clear, however, it is not really relevant for making a moral judgment. Both withdrawal and withholding are moral in some situations and immoral in others.

Second, the distinction between withholding and withdrawing treatment can distort our moral judgment. A widespread conviction, for example, holds that it is more difficult to justify withdrawing treatment than withholding it. Psychologically of course, it is more difficult to withdraw than to withhold life-sustaining treatment from a patient, especially when he will die moments after the withdrawal. But this does not mean that it is more difficult to establish the moral justification of withdrawal than to establish the moral justification of withholding.

Actually, withdrawal of treatment is often easier to justify morally than withholding it in the first place. This is so because in questions of withdrawal we have important information that we do not have in cases of withholding, namely, we know how the therapy actually affects the patient's condition. Moral judgments require the best possible information, and we have better information when we are actually using the treatment than when we have not yet tried it. The added information we have from using a treatment puts us in a better position to make a good moral decision about its benefits and burdens.

Failure to acknowledge the advantage we have in making decisions about treatment withdrawal can lead to unfortunate consequences. For example, if providers think it is morally more difficult to justify withdrawing a ventilator than withholding it, they may not begin the ventilation when they are unsure of its medical value for fear that once they start it, they can not stop it. This means a patient who could have benefited from the ventilator will not have the chance to benefit from it. Again, if providers think it is morally more difficult to justify withdrawing a ventilator than withholding it, they may not withdraw a ventilator that they never would have started in the first place if they had known it would be so burdensome. This means a patient who is unreasonably burdened by a ventilator will be left on it.

Intentionally Causing Death and Letting Die

This is the most sensitive variation of the distinction between action and omission. From childhood we are taught "Do not kill." Later most of us learn to accept the morality of exceptions, most notably killing as a last resort in self-defense or killing enemy soldiers in what is traditionally called just warfare. And many people also make an exception for the killing in legal executions. But a long tradition of medical ethics going back to the Hippocratic writings condemns the killing of patients by physicians.

There were always challenges to this tradition, and today, as we will see in chapter 13 on euthanasia and assisted suicide, these challenges are stronger than ever in recent history. Nonetheless, the American Medical Association's (AMA) ethical guidelines continue to say that "the physician should not intentionally cause death." What the guidelines mean is clear—the AMA is opposed to physicians giving lethal injections—but the language is misleading. It forces physicians to think of behaviors with a causal impact on a patient's death as if they were not causal in any way. Thus, some describe the action of removing life-support equipment as "letting die" and maintain that the disease, not the life-support removal, is the only cause of death.

Sometimes the distinction between intentionally causing death and letting die (or, to put it another way, between causing death and letting the disease cause death) is clear. If I intentionally give a lethal injection, I cause death, and if I do not attempt CPR, I am letting the person in cardiac arrest die. But frequently the distinction between intentionally causing death and letting die is not clear because the providers' actions play a definite causal role in patients' deaths. Consider the following behaviors.

1. Physician gives a lethal injection to the patient.
2. Physician assists a patient with suicide.
3. Physician gives a dying patient medication needed for pain relief although the drugs will hasten death.
4. Physician withdraws nutrition and hydration through tubes or lines.
5. Physician withdraws needed life-sustaining equipment.
6. Physician withholds nutrition or life-sustaining treatment.

The first five behaviors all involve causal impact on the death of the patient. The causal impact is strongest in the first behavior and weakest in the fourth and fifth. Only the sixth behavior makes no causal contribution to death. Withholding nutrition and treatment is the only real case of letting die on the list. In every other situation the provider's actions have a causal impact on the patient's death.

The distinction between intentionally causing death and letting die is too simplified to serve as a substitute for moral reasoning. It is disingenuous to ignore the causal impact, for example, of withdrawing a ventilator from someone who will die without it. We would have no trouble acknowledging that a stranger walking into an ICU and withdrawing a ventilator causes the patient's death. Yet if a physician withdraws the same ventilator, some want to pretend that the action plays no causal role in the patient's death. They claim that the physician is only "letting the patient die."

What is really happening when a ventilator is removed from a person needing it, of course, is that both the disease *and* the withdrawal are causes of death, but neither alone is a *sufficient* cause of death. For death to occur at this time, the disease must be making it impossible for the patient to live without the ventilator *and* someone must remove or shut off the ventilator. Sound moral analysis will admit that the physician's action has a causal impact on the patient's death at this time and then go on to ask whether the withdrawal of the ventilator is morally reasonable in the circumstances.

Paternalism and Autonomy

The distinction between paternalism and autonomy rests on where we place the power of authorizing medical treatment and on how we perceive the relationship between what the physician thinks is good for the patient and what the patient wants. In general the older medical tradition made physicians the authorities and made the paramount moral value doing good for, or at least no harm to, patients. This tradition argued that the physician knows more than the patient and has more experience and that the patient's ability to think clearly and to choose rationally is often undermined by the illness. Hence, it made sense to say that the physician should do what he thought was best for the patient.

The relationship between physician and patient thus resembled the relationship between a wise and caring father and his child. When the physician acts like a caring father toward a patient, who is a beginner or a child in the world of medicine, we call it paternalism. The physician-father knows best, and the patient-child is expected to follow doctor's orders.

Some claim that the Hippocratic Oath, a cornerstone of medical ethics for centuries, is one of the sources of this medical paternalism. This oath is thought to have originated around the fourth century B.C.E. among a group of Greek-speaking people, the Pythagoreans, who flourished for a time in southern Italy, then a part of the Greek world. These followers of Pythagoras (known to every high school student as the discoverer of the geometric theorem that bears his name) formed a distinct social group with shared religious, philosophical, and moral beliefs. Most people of that era did not share those beliefs, and thus the Hippocratic Oath represents the views of a small and somewhat idiosyncratic group in the classical world.

The physician taking the oath says he will take measures "for the benefit of the sick according to my ability and judgment." This does suggest medical paternalism, especially since there is no mention of any judgment by the patient. The oath also says that the physician will not provide lethal drugs to patients requesting them or give an abortifacient to a woman, but these prohibitions were probably not so much paternalistic as important moral values for the Pythagorean physician, who would have accepted the strong belief of his group in the interconnection and value of all life, human as well as animal.

Perhaps an even stronger source of medical paternalism in the tradition was the realization that the power of medical knowledge should be used for good and not for harm. Many people were horrified by the thought that physicians would use their expertise for evil—to devise more exquisite techniques of torture, for example. So the tradition insisted that the physician should always act for the patient's good and do what he thought was best for the patient.

In most cases the physician knew better than the patient what was good for the patient. From this the tradition concluded that, if he really cared about his patient, he should simply do what was best for the patient. If this meant doing things without the patient's knowledge and consent, so be it. The important thing was to do what was good for the patient, and the physician was the authority in determining this. The physician was like a parent, responsible for the well-being of the patient, and must act accordingly. This commitment to paternal beneficence, to the good of the patient, was one of the great moral values of traditional medicine.

Recently, however, all forms of paternalism in our culture have been widely criticized. In the past few centuries various philosophies have arisen that locate the source of decision making more and more in the individual rather than in political or religious authority.

Examples of this trend are many and well known. The Lutheran Reformation in Christianity, for example, encouraged vernacular translations of the Bible so each individual could read and interpret it rather than have church authorities interpret the Latin text. The powerful political theory of John Locke made the right to liberty one of the three basic natural rights, and his theory is a major source of the right to choose and the right to privacy that we hear so much about today. The influential moral philosophy of Immanuel Kant held that the moral law comes not from God, nor from the law of nature, but from ourselves—we are morally autonomous in that we give the universal moral law to ourselves. The popular philosophy called utilitarianism, developed extensively in the nineteenth century by John Stuart Mill, stressed liberty and placed minimal limitations on human freedom: we are not free to do things that will harm others or undermine the greatest good for the greatest number. Finally, various existentialist philosophies beginning with Kierkegaard and Nietzsche in the nineteenth century held that choosing and willing, rather than thinking and knowing, are the hallmarks of human existence. Kierkegaard urged individuals to move beyond ethics to what he called a "religious" stage; Nietzsche saw only decadence in existing European morality and encouraged individuals to exercise a will-to-power that would inaugurate a transvaluation of all values.

Major trends such as these, different as they are from each other, all reinforce a central notion, namely the important value of self-determination and personal choice.

Medical paternalism was bound to run into difficulties with the many modern philosophies and theologies of individual choice. The major value is no longer what someone else, even a caring physician, thinks is good but what the patient thinks is good and what the patient chooses. Beneficence remains an important value—no patient in his right mind wants anything bad done to him—but the autonomy of the patient has become a crucial value as well. In the language of those who conceive of ethics as a matter of principles, the principle of autonomy has emerged and in some cases has come to dominate the principle of beneficence in health care ethics.

The beneficence supporting traditional medical paternalism meant doing good for the patient in a medical sense; that is, it meant trying to achieve a good clinical outcome. It did not really take into account the patient's personal commitments that might conflict with good clinical care. A classic example of this is the treatment of a Jehovah's Witness when blood is needed. The physician may know the unconscious patient in the operating room will die without a transfusion and is thus driven by beneficence to give it, but the patient may have insisted for religious reasons that blood not be given. In this case most ethicists, and several important legal decisions, say that respect for the autonomy of the patient should take priority over the beneficence of the physician trying to save the patient's life.

Autonomy, self-determination, and respect for persons are important notions in medical ethics. Sometimes as in the above example they can clash with the older idea that the doctor should do what is good for her patient. This leads some to think that we must make a choice between medical paternalism and beneficence on the one hand and patient autonomy and self-determination on the other. Almost always when the choice is presented this way, it is the paternalism that is rejected.

Now things are changing again. In the past few years ethicists have been moving away from the language of autonomy as they recognize that patients, especially very sick or elderly patients, are really not that autonomous. Moreover, some patients and proxies have misused autonomy and self-determination to demand medically inappropriate treatments. This places physicians in a difficult position. No physician wants to order inappropriate medical treatments simply because his patient or the patient's proxy wants them.

The choice forced by the distinction between paternalism and autonomy, however, is not helpful, and that is why the distinction is best avoided. Both paternalism and patient self-determination reflect important values in a rich ethic of health care. The driving force of paternalism is doing good for the patient, and the driving force of self-determination is the recognition that patients remain persons who cannot be disenfranchised of the responsibility and freedom to make important personal choices in life.

There is no need to distinguish between paternalism and autonomy and to prefer one over the other. Given the physician's experience and knowledge, and a lack of the same in most patients, and given the way in which disease makes it difficult for patients to remain in control of their lives, a paternal (or maternal) attitude has its place in medicine and health care. And given the importance of respecting the personal commitments of patients who see the world differently from the physician, autonomy or self-determination also has its place.

The ideal will be to maintain the best of both paternalism and self-determination, and the most promising way to do this is to have the physician and the patient share the decision making. This avoids having the physician behave like a parent with his child. It also avoids reducing the physician to a hired hand ordered around by a patient autonomously authorizing his or her medical treatment in such a way that the physician no longer exercises professional judgment but simply carries out the patient's decisions.

It is important to avoid considering the physician's paternalism morally suspect and the patient's autonomous decisions morally acceptable. It is not this simple. In some situations paternalism can be justified, and in some situations the decision of the patient is simply immoral. The fact that a patient exercises her right to choose what will be done to her body does not thereby justify the morality of what she chooses. It is not enough to say, "This is what the patient wants; therefore, this is the right thing to do." The test of the right thing to do is whether what is done achieves the truly good, not whether the patient autonomously chooses it. Important as autonomy or self-determination is, it is not a criterion of what is morally right.

Ordinary and Extraordinary Means of Preserving Life

This distinction has been losing the popularity it once enjoyed. It originated several centuries ago in Roman Catholic moral theology, and, when medical treatments were much simpler, it served a useful purpose. It has been kept alive by a number of landmark court cases where judges described respirators and tubal feeding as extraordinary and then used that description in justifying withdrawal. The New Jersey Supreme Court, for example, described Karen Quinlan's respirator as extraordinary treatment, and the Massachusetts Supreme Judicial Court found that Joseph Saikewicz's chemotherapy and Paul Brophy's tubal feeding were extraordinary. These courts then allowed medical personnel to honor requests of proxies for the patients to forgo the life-sustaining treatments.

The fundamental idea behind the distinction between ordinary and extraordinary treatment is this: Although human life is an important value, ethics does not require people to use extraordinary means to preserve it. Hence, if a patient chooses to forgo extraordinary treatment, providers withholding or withdrawing that treatment are acting morally even if death follows. On the other hand, the patient's decision to forgo so-called ordinary treatment is not morally justified.

There are several problems with this approach. The first is now familiar—the temptation to rely on a distinction instead of moral deliberation and reasoning to determine what is morally good behavior.

The second problem centers on just what we are to consider extraordinary life-sustaining treatment. Those supporting the value of the distinction speak of treatment that is very expensive, or unusual, or very painful, or very risky, or highly technological. Sometimes it is easy to use these notions. Most everyone would agree that a heart transplant is, at least at the present time, extraordinary. But in many other situations the distinction is simply not clear. The courts have considered respirators extraordinary, but many people would consider a respirator in an operating room or in an intensive care unit quite ordinary. And the courts have considered long-term use of a feeding tube for an unconscious person not expected to recover an extraordinary treatment, but many people consider nutrition supplied by a simple tube an ordinary means of nutritional support.

Because there is no way to provide a satisfactory definition of extraordinary treatment in modern medicine, the distinction is not helpful and, in fact, can be misleading. If used instead of moral reasoning, for example, it would require us to give ordinary antibiotics to fight the pneumonia of an elderly dialysis patient on a ventilator and dying of painful cancer. The distinction between ordinary and extraordinary means of preserving life, no less than the others we have considered, is no substitute for the prudential reasoning and moral reflection we need to determine what achieves the human good in any situation.

Futile Treatment and Effective Treatment

Futile treatment was not a problem until recently. When physicians were the sole decision makers, there was no futile treatment—if the physician thought a treatment was futile, he would never provide it. The recent upsurge of patient autonomy and self-determination has created the problem of futile treatment. At first this trend toward patient autonomy and self-determination centered on the patient's right to refuse treatments, but now the other side is beginning to show itself. Patients or their proxies are demanding treatment, and sometimes the providers are convinced the treatment they demand is futile or useless.

This presents a problem for providers. If they honor the patient's request for treatment they believe is inappropriate, they act contrary to their professional judgment. Sometimes they can transfer the patient to other providers, but sometimes they cannot, and this leaves them in a difficult position. Parents, for example, have demanded painful treatments for their children that providers believed were medically useless. This is upsetting for providers because they are being asked to do something that causes suffering for their patient but which they perceive as providing no benefit.

To resolve this difficulty, some now propose a new distinction: futile treatment and effective treatment. They would like to use the distinction to justify morally a physician's refusal to supply inappropriate medical treatments demanded by a patient or a proxy. The idea is simple: once the treatment is deemed futile, providers have no obligation to provide it even if the patient or proxy wants it. In fact, some argue that there is a moral obligation not to provide treatment defined as futile. The main effect of the judgment of futility, then, is to limit the autonomy of patients by allowing them to authorize only effective treatment. Once physicians determine a treatment is futile, they no longer have the obligation to provide or continue it, and they do not need the consent of the patient to withdraw or withhold it.

One example of this thinking can be seen in some recent policies about providing cardiopulmonary resuscitation (CPR) in hospitals. Some new policies allow writing a do-not-resuscitate (DNR) order without the patient's consent if the physician believes resuscitation efforts would be futile. This is a new development; hitherto, most hospital policies required consent from the patient or proxy before the DNR order could be written. This development reflects the new idea that providers can define futile treatment and then unilaterally withhold or withdraw it. Another example is the 1999 Texas Advance Directives Act (ADA) that was extended to cover children in 2003. It provides legal protection for physicians to stop treatments they consider futile despite what the patient or family wants. We will consider the pros and cons of this legislation in chapter 17.

At first glance this approach seems reasonable because, at least in some cases, the distinction between effective and futile treatment is clear and does suggest a basis for moral judgment. Treatment of people on life support who have suffered whole brain death, for example, is obviously futile. So is periodontal surgery to prevent the loss of teeth ten years from now when the patient is dying. But these are the easy cases, where the futility is clear.

In most cases the distinction between futile and effective treatment is not so clear. This is primarily because the notion of futility is so complex it is useless, much as the confusing notion of extraordinary rendered the ordinary-extraordinary distinction useless. Suppose, for example, the probability of a painful treatment's success is one in a thousand. Providers may consider it futile to provide such a treatment, but a desperate mother may think that one in a thousand is a worthwhile chance for her baby. Again, suppose the respirator is merely preserving an irreversible vegetative state. Providers may consider the treatment futile, but the proxy may consider the treatment effective because it is still preserving human life. We will consider such a case—the Wanglie story—in chapter 7.

We can see from this that the judgment of futility is often not a clear and objective judgment and that many factors other than medical effectiveness are involved. The distinction between effective and futile treatment is too controversial to serve as the basis of ethical judgments. The distinction should not become a substitute for thoughtful moral deliberation, no more than should the other distinctions we have considered. Providers may well conclude a treatment is futile, but that alone is not enough to justify its removal. Other relevant values and circumstances must be considered.

The futility debate intensified in the 1990s for at least two reasons: the increasing number of cases where families demanded unreasonable CPR efforts and life-sustaining treatments and the upsurge of managed care. We will consider some of the better-known cases—Helga Wanglie, Baby K, Baby L, Catherine Gilgunn, and Barbara Howe—in later chapters. In response to these conflicts some institutions developed policies on futility, but the difficulty in finding an acceptable objective definition of futility remains a weakness in policies trying to identify any treatment that might prolong life as futile. One state, Texas, has an Advance Directives Act that does allow hospitals to define treatment as futile and stop treatment unilaterally, but as we will see in chapter 17, it has produced some unfortunate situations that may do more harm then good. The AMA has taken a different approach. In March 1999 its Council on Ethical and Judicial Affairs issued a helpful report that recommended that institutions avoid policies that try to define futility and develop instead a fair and open multistep process to resolve conflicts about treatments at the end of life. The process can help but unfortunately does not always resolve the dispute.

A major reason why the "futility" debates can be so intractable in the United States emerged in an article published in the *Archives of Surgery* in 2008 that suggested many Americans are basing their demand for treatment on their belief in miracles. Even in cases where there is no reasonable hope of reversing the condition or preventing death, some people believe treatments should be continued to allow for the possibility of a miracle. Researchers found, for example, that 61 percent of the public believe, despite the impossibility of medical reversal, in the real possibility of a miraculous reversal of persistent vegetative state (PVS) and that 27 percent of the public believe life-sustaining treatments should be continued even when it is obvious there is no hope of medical recovery since there is always the real possibility of miracles. However, only 20 percent of health care professionals think it makes sense to believe a miracle might reverse PVS, and very few think advanced life support should be continued when there is clearly no hope of medical recovery. The disparity between what the public believes and what health care providers believe obviously sets up an environment where disagreements about what is and what is not "futile" will easily emerge.

Belief in miracles is indigenous to many major religions—both the Hebrew and Christian biblical books recount numerous stories of miracles, and both Jesus and his followers reversed many physical and mental illnesses, even death itself, thanks to miracles—and it does not usually give way to reason. However, belief in the possibility of a miracle does not necessarily mean that medical nutrition and other life-sustaining treatments should be continued indefinitely. One can believe in miracles and also decide that feeding tubes and ventilators should be withdrawn. The following examples look like good reasoning but are not.

- A miracle could restore awareness and cognitive ability for a patient in PVS.
- Mother was diagnosed as being in PVS two years ago.
- Therefore, we should continue the feeding tube.

There is no logical connection between believing in the possibility of a miracle and concluding that life support treatments should be continued. When Jesus raised Lazarus from the dead, he had been dead for days, and the Gospel tells us, the tomb smelled from the corruption of the body when it was opened. If a miracle is going to occur, no help from feeding tubes or life support is needed. There is no contradiction between believing in miracles and also thinking there are times when it is reasonable to withdraw life-support interventions. Unfortunately, as long as many people think that belief in the possibility of a miracle cure entails keeping feeding tubes and ventilators going no matter how grim the prognosis, the stage is set for conflicts over futile treatment.

Finally we should note that the distinction between futile treatment and effective treatment is especially dangerous in the current era of intensive cost control. Under the rapidly disappearing system known as fee-for-service where providers were paid for their services, the financial incentive was to provide them. Now in many payment systems the financial incentive is reversed—hospitals and physicians often have financial inducements to limit their services. This is especially true if the patient is one of the more than 45 million Americans who have no health insurance and the hospital has no way of collecting payment for the expensive care they provide the uninsured. In some cases then, hospitals have a financial interest in defining expensive treatments as futile so they need not provide them. And this makes patients and families wonder about the motives of their physicians and hospitals whenever they define treatment as futile and then take steps to avoid providing it. It is not a scenario that builds trust between providers and the families of needy patients.

Direct and Indirect Results

Our actions invariably have many results that we might call consequences, outcomes, or effects. Some of these consequences are unforeseen and unexpected, and these are not morally relevant. The foreseen consequences, however, are morally relevant. We recognize that some of these effects are good and thus desirable, whereas others are not good and thus undesirable. When a provider gives chemotherapy, for example, the desired effect is the shrinkage of the tumor, and the undesirable effects include hair loss and nausea. One and the same action causes both good and bad effects.

In the language of medicine, we sometimes speak of the secondary effects as side effects. Thus, hair loss is a side effect of chemotherapy, an effect alongside the main effect. In the language of some moral philosophies and theologies, we find the term *double effect* used to describe situations where our action gives rise to two effects, one good and the other bad. The desired good effect is considered the direct result of our behavior, whereas the undesired bad effect is considered the indirect result of our behavior.

The distinction between two results (one called direct because it is desired and good; the other called indirect because it is undesired and not good) has given rise to what is called the *principle of the double effect.* However, although this principle is clear and helpful in some scenarios, it is currently the source of great debate both within and beyond the Roman Catholic moral theology that originally generated it. Its fundamental intuition is laudable; it recognizes that the moral world is sometimes an ambiguous place and that we can morally justify some behaviors despite the bad effects they cause. The use of the principle of double effect, however, often undermines, as does the employment of any moral principle, sound moral deliberation and reasoning.

The classic moral example behind the principle of the double effect is found in Aquinas's analysis of killing in self-defense. As a Christian, he accepted the biblical injunction: Thou shalt not kill. But, he argued, if a criminal makes a life-threatening attack on me, I may use force, even lethal force if necessary, to save my life. My action will have two effects: the direct and good effect of saving my life and the indirect and bad effect of killing a human being. I can justify the killing, however, because it was not directly intended. I intended to save my life, not to kill someone. The death is an unfortunate, unwanted, and unavoidable bad effect of the same action that saved my life.

Actions with double—perhaps it would be better to say multiple—effects abound in health care. The surgeon removing an appendix, the endodontist doing a root canal, and the nurse starting an intravenous (IV) treatment are all performing actions with multiple results, some good and some bad. The direct effect of the surgery is the removal of an infected appendix; the indirect effects are the pain and trauma to the body. The medical goals are good; but other results—pain, scarring, trauma, and the like—are bad.

From this we can see that the notions of direct and indirect results are grounded on intention. The direct results are the effects we intend; the indirect effects are those we know will occur but do not intend and regret. In self-defense, for example, what we intend is saving our lives, not the death of the attacker, although we know very well when we resort to lethal force to stop him that he will die. And in doing surgery, we intend the removal of the infected gall bladder, not the attendant pain and trauma, although we know very well when we operate that we will cause pain and trauma to the body.

It is important to realize, of course, that we are responsible for all the known effects, indirect as well as direct, of our actions. We are responsible for the attacker's death, and the surgeon is responsible for the bad things such as pain and trauma that accompany any surgery. Just because they are side effects or indirect effects does not mean they fall outside the moral sphere.

In moral evaluation, then, the effort to describe something as a direct rather than indirect effect, as something I intend rather than as something I foresaw but did not intend, is not ultimately crucial. Rather, what we have to determine is whether what we are going to do is reasonable, and reasonableness will depend to a great extent on all the expected consequences, both intended and unintended, of our behavior. Aquinas seems to have realized this. Apart from mentioning two effects in his example of self-defense, he never developed what was to be known later as the principle of double effect.

Prudential reasoning considers all the significant effects of our actions and gains little by dividing them into direct and indirect. In practice this means prudence looks at the whole picture, considers the complex mixture of good and bad that is involved in the process, and then determines the most reasonable thing to do given the circumstances and the consequences we think will follow our behavior.

There is, however, a valuable insight captured in the famous principle of the double effect. It recognizes that our actions often have bad as well as good effects, and it justifies our performing such actions when the reasons for acting override the bad we cause. This famous principle, although not really helpful in an ethics of prudence and not used by Aristotle and Aquinas, is a principle of moral realism. It reminds us that if we are not prepared to do bad things for good reasons, then ever more terrible bad things will multiply in life. And it reminds us we need good reasons to compensate for the bad we know will follow from the good we are trying to do.

Immoral and Intrinsically Immoral

Some ethicists advocate a distinction between what we might call the simply immoral and the intrinsically immoral or the intrinsically evil. They argue that some actions are immoral by their very nature. To understand their point, it is helpful to analyze moral behavior into several components.

1. The actual physical action that is performed
2. The intention of the agent in performing the action
3. The circumstances in which the action is performed
4. The consequences resulting from the action

The idea behind the notion of intrinsically immoral actions is that some physical actions are immoral regardless of the agent's intention, the circumstances, or the consequences. Other actions may also be immoral, but their immorality depends on the intention, the circumstances, or the consequences. In other words, intrinsically immoral actions are always and everywhere immoral—there are no exceptions.

Once the notion of intrinsically immoral actions is accepted, the ethicist invariably proposes a set of moral laws or rules forbidding these actions always and everywhere. The laws or rules allow no exceptions, no matter what the intentions, circumstances, or consequences. Actions that are not intrinsically immoral, on the other hand, may or may not be immoral, depending on the circumstances and consequences, and no moral laws or rules forbidding them can be absolute—exceptions are always possible.

What actions do ethicists propose as intrinsically evil? The list, as you might expect, varies, but many ethicists who promote the notion of intrinsically immoral actions include lying, suicide, contraception, sterilization, abortion, extramarital sex, and masturbation. Killing another human being is not proposed as intrinsically immoral because it is morally justified in some situations—war and self-defense, for example. However, some ethicists consider killing the innocent intrinsically immoral, and its prohibition a moral absolute.

Those ethicists who hold certain actions always and everywhere immoral and who promulgate moral rules that never allow exceptions are known today as *deontologists*. Deontologists are convinced that there must be some concrete moral absolutes, otherwise morality will quickly degenerate into a situation ethics in which the appeal to extenuating circumstances or to consequences, as the utilitarians advocate, will soon be used to justify the worst evils.

The current idea that some actions are intrinsically immoral developed from two major sources. The first is a movement that began in the fourteenth century within Roman Catholic moral theology, and the second is the influential moral philosophy developed by Immanuel Kant in the eighteenth century.

Catholic Theology

As ancient writings from the early church fathers and Augustine attest, a strain of moral rigor was present in Catholic moral theology from the beginning. The doctrine of intrinsically immoral or intrinsically evil actions, however, was not formally developed until the fourteenth century. It grew out of a moral problem that fascinated the medieval theologians—the status of the Ten Commandments. They wondered whether there could be exceptions to God's laws prohibiting killing, adultery, and stealing. If killing is against God's law, how could God tell Abraham to kill his son Isaac? If adultery is against God's law, how could God tell Hosea to sleep with a prostitute? And if stealing is against God's law, how could God condone the theft of Egyptian property as the Hebrews left Egypt in the Exodus?

The creative efforts employed by theologians to explain actions in violation of the Ten Commandments, but which had been commanded or at least approved by God, need not detain us here. The solution of one relatively unknown fourteenth-century theologian, however, is of interest. Durand of Saint Pourcain (Durandus in Latin) claimed that God could not dispense from the commandments forbidding adultery and stealing because the "matter" forbidden by these commandments has the character of evil or immorality *intrinsically*. Adultery and stealing are intrinsically immoral.

According to Durand, killing is not intrinsically immoral, and therefore God could order Abraham to kill Isaac. But he could not have ordered Hosea to have intercourse with a prostitute nor the Hebrews to steal from the Egyptians, because these actions are intrinsically immoral. How, then, did Durand resolve the biblical accounts of Hosea's sexual liaison with the prostitute and the Hebrews' theft of Egyptian property? By what critics consider a weak argument. He claimed God, the Lord of all, gave the prostitute to Hosea as his wife, so he was not really ordering him to commit adultery or to fornicate with her; and he claimed that God gave the Egyptian property to the Hebrews, so they really were not stealing it when they took it. If you accept this explanation, then you can say that God was not making exceptions to his commandments forbidding the intrinsically immoral actions of adultery and stealing.

It is important to remark, however, that Aquinas, who lived the century before Durand, never held that any physical actions, considered by themselves without any reference to circumstances, could be intrinsically immoral. He did hold, as did Aristotle, that some actions are immoral *secundum se*; that is, they are immoral "by definition" in that the words used to describe them denote a moral judgment as well as a simple description. Actions so defined are actions described in such a way that a moral judgment is embedded in the description. Aquinas and Aristotle both claimed, for example, that deliberate homicide was always immoral, and Aquinas would agree that God could never command anyone to commit homicide. But homicide is not an action defined in simple physical terms; a judgment is embedded in the word homicide. Homicide means a killing that should not happen. God could never command people to commit a homicide but he could and, according to the Hebrew Bible, did command people to kill.

As the Middle Ages ended, theologians tended to lose interest in reconciling the biblical accounts approving killing, adultery, and stealing with God's commandments, but the idea of intrinsically immoral physical actions remained, and the list began to grow. Although later theologians tended to exclude stealing from the list of intrinsically immoral actions—if you were starving you could steal food as a last resort—they added other actions, among them lying, suicide, and various sexual sins.

By the nineteenth century many of the manuals used to train seminarians had adopted a list of intrinsically immoral actions, and by the twentieth century the moral theology of intrinsically immoral actions had found its way into important papal documents. In *Casti Connubii*, the 1930 encyclical forbidding contraception, for example, Pope Pius XI wrote: "The conjugal act is of its very nature designed for the procreation of offspring; and therefore those who in performing it deliberately deprive it of its natural power and efficacy, act against nature and do something which is shameful and *intrinsically immoral*" (no. 54, emphasis added).

Since then, several important official documents of the Roman Catholic Church have insisted that a number of other physical actions, most notably abortion, sterilization, homosexual behavior, and masturbation, are also intrinsically immoral. The theology of intrinsically immoral actions continued in the encyclicals of Pope John Paul II titled *Veritatis splendor* (*The Splendor of Truth*, 1993) and *Evangelium vitae* (*The Gospel of Life*, 1995).

In November 2007 the United States Conference of Catholic Bishops (USCCB) continued the trend in its guide for Catholic voters titled *The Challenge of Forming Consciences for Faithful Citizenship*. The guide reminds Catholics of seven themes of Catholic social teaching that provide a moral framework for decisions in public life. One theme is that human life is sacred and direct attacks on innocent human life are never morally acceptable, and among the "direct attacks" are the "intrinsic evils" of "abortion, euthanasia, human cloning, and destruction of human embryos for research." Curiously, another section of the document summary states that, although Catholics are not single-issue voters, "a candidate's position on a single issue that involves an intrinsic evil, such as support for legal abortion or the promotion of racism, may legitimately lead a voter to disqualify a candidate from receiving support." It is one thing to call abortion intrinsically evil but another thing to call advocating limited legal support for it in a pluralistic society also intrinsically evil. And the "promotion of racism" is a new arrival not found on the centuries-old lists of intrinsic evils.

In December 2008 the Vatican's Congregation for the Doctrine of the Faith released a new Instruction titled *Dignitas personae* (The Dignity of the Person), which concerns "certain bioethical questions." The Instruction continues the Vatican's theology of intrinsically evil actions, specifically mentioning in vitro fertilization and intracytoplasmic sperm injection, pregnancy reduction, as well as other kinds of abortion including any research that destroys a human embryo, "artificial fertilization," and human cloning even if confined to research.

The adoption of this ethics of intrinsically immoral actions by the leaders of the Catholic Church has had a major impact on health care ethics in the United States, where many hospitals are under Catholic auspices. It explains why the *Ethical and Religious Directives for Catholic Health Care Services* (fourth edition, 2001) imposed by the American bishops on these facilities forbid all abortions, even for ectopic pregnancies; all vasectomies, tubal ligations, and medical interventions for contraception, regardless of the circumstances; and all masturbation, even to obtain sperm for fertility diagnosis or for reproductive assistance within marriage by procedures considered acceptable, e.g., husbands and wives using artificial insemination or the transfer of gametes (sperm and ova) to the fallopian tubes.

Immanuel Kant

The second major source of the current idea that some actions are intrinsically immoral (that is, always and everywhere immoral regardless of the agent's motive, the circumstances, or the consequences) is the extremely influential moral philosophy of Immanuel Kant. Kant's basic moral principle was a general imperative that reason imposes on all of us. He called this principle the *categorical imperative*. It is an imperative because it commands and obliges us; it is categorical because it is absolute and generates absolute moral norms.

Kant almost always described the categorical imperative in terms of the moral obligations or duties that it generates. Some of these moral duties are positive, some negative. Some of the negative duties are *strict* or *perfect*, and these are the ones that interest us. According to Kant, the strict negative duties oblige us to avoid certain actions always and everywhere. Strict negative duties define a class of actions that are always wrong. They can never be morally justified under any circumstances because every attempt to consider any violation of a strict negative duty as moral results in a contradiction. Since the rational aspect of Kantian morality does not admit contradictions, violations of strict negative duties are *necessarily* immoral.

Suicide is the paradigm example. The categorical imperative generates moral duties toward myself, among them a strict negative duty never to harm myself. Any moral maxim allowing suicide obviously contradicts the duty never to harm myself. Hence, no moral maxim permitting suicide is possible. Suicide is always immoral.

Kant did not describe violations of strict negative duties as intrinsically immoral, but his doctrine of strict negative duties, duties whose every violation would constitute a contradiction at the heart of morality, was certainly analogous to the medieval doctrine. The doctrine generates a list of actions that are universally and necessarily immoral. No good intention, no circumstances or consequences, could ever morally justify performing one of these actions.

What physical actions were necessarily immoral for Kant? His list included, in addition to suicide, mutilation of the body, drunkenness, gluttony, contraception, homosexual behavior, extramarital sex, masturbation, bestiality, and lying. Kant's list bears an uncanny resemblance to the list of intrinsically immoral actions developed by the Catholic theologians, but Kant was not a Catholic, and he was not arguing from a theological position. His moral absolutes, he claimed, are deduced from what he called "pure practical reason." By pure practical reason Kant meant a reasoning concerned with behavior (the practical) based on necessary and universal principles unaffected by circumstances, history, or change (the pure).

Kant's inclusion of so many sexual actions in his list of necessarily immoral actions is based on the view expressed in his *Metaphysics of Morals* (Part II, section 7) that sexual actions are intended by nature for the preservation of the species. Our duty, if we choose to engage in sex, is to preserve the race, and corresponding to this is a strict negative duty not to act contrary to this purpose. Any moral maxim permitting masturbation, contraception, homosexuality, and bestiality would contradict this strict negative duty, and hence these actions are necessarily immoral. Even extramarital reproductive sex was necessarily immoral for Kant since he believed that reproduction should occur only in marriage.

Kant's insistence that certain actions such as contraception, lying, homosexuality, and masturbation are necessarily immoral did not, any more than did the theological and papal proposals that these actions are intrinsically immoral, go without challenge. One critic of Kant brought up a disturbing example involving lying. If lying is necessarily immoral, if the maxim forbidding lies always holds regardless of the circumstances, then we run into strange situations where behaving morally promotes immorality. Suppose, the critic said, someone is pursuing my friend with the intent to kill him, and he is hiding in my house. If the would-be murderer asks me if my friend is hiding in my house, what reasonable person would think it immoral if, unable to avoid answering the question, I lied to save my friend's life?

In his *Lectures on Ethics* (1780), Kant had toyed with the idea of distinguishing falsehood from lying and had suggested that deceiving a person who had no right to know the truth was a falsehood and not a lie. However, in the essay titled *On the Supposed Right to Lie from Altruistic Motives*, published in 1797 to answer this very critic, Kant made no such distinction and insisted on the absolute prohibition against lying. Regardless of the circumstances and the terrible consequences that follow when the murderer tracks down my friend after I tell the truth, Kant held that I must tell the truth if I cannot avoid answering the question. The moral law simply forbids all lying; there are no exceptions. Lying is always immoral.

Today many ethicists claiming allegiance to moral principles and rules grounded in Kant's moral philosophy simply ignore many of the strict negative duties his theory generates. It is not unusual to see those who consider themselves Kantians in theory accepting, in some situations, the morality of contraception, organ donation from the living (which involves mutilation), abortion, masturbation (for in vitro fertilization and artificial insemination, for example), and even physician-assisted suicide, yet Kant condemned all these actions as *necessarily* immoral because they contradict the strict negative duties generated by the supreme moral principle of the Kantian moral theory—the categorical imperative.

One might be tempted to say that this is not important and that, after all, those retrieving Aristotle also reject some of his moral positions. This is certainly true—nobody retrieving the ethics of Aristotle would agree with his positions on any number of issues. Aquinas did not accept Aristotle's approval of infanticide, and no one retrieving Aristotle today accepts his position on slavery. But there is a major difference between the moral theories of Aristotle and those of Kant. Aristotle's theory allows a self-correcting process of reevaluation for all actions; Kant's theory does not allow any reevaluation of necessarily immoral actions deduced from the categorical imperative.

Aristotle's theory is based on right reason and the human good, and the rejection of slavery is a question of learning to see how slavery is morally unreasonable because it is contrary to the human good. New moral evaluations occur easily within a moral theory founded on the human good. They do not undermine the foundation of the theory. The prudential reasoning and judgments in Aristotle's theory do not give us necessary conclusions valid for always and everywhere. They produce only our best efforts at the time and in the circumstances to say what will promote our good. Prudential judgments in future times and other circumstances may produce other conclusions. Circumstances are always a factor in prudential judgments about good and bad, and circumstances can vary from time to time as well as from place to place. Hence Aristotle's theory allows the historical development of moral evaluations. Aristotle thought infanticide did not undermine the human good, but prudence could easily move him to hold the opposite belief today.

Kant's doctrine of strict negative moral duties, however, allows no such development. Any theory which holds that certain physical actions are necessarily immoral cannot allow any of these actions ever to become morally acceptable. Once actions such as killing oneself, sterilization, or homosexual behavior are defined as contrary to strict negative duties, no circumstances now or in the future can reverse their immorality. Kant's moral theory is rooted in a categorical imperative that transcends history, and allowing exceptions to a strict negative duty as history unfolds would undermine the theory itself.

Kant seemed aware of this problem and did raise questions about some of the strict negative duties. He asked, for example, whether it would really be suicide if a person going mad killed himself lest, in his madness, he harm others. But he did not show how such a suicide could be morally justified as an exception to the strict duties we owe ourselves. He raised the question of possible exceptions to the universal maxim against suicide, but he did not elaborate on how any exceptions to the universal moral maxim proscribing suicide could be possible.

Moral philosophers studying Kant are also aware of the problem created by defining violations of strict negative duties as always immoral. They have proposed various solutions to it, solutions sometimes reminiscent of the creative efforts employed by medieval theologians to reconcile God's commandments with God's commands directing certain biblical heroes to kill the innocent, to fornicate, and to steal. Many health care ethicists who appeal to Kant for support of their positions, however, seem unaware of the philosophical problem. It is truly curious to see some ethical writings on health care justify abortion, contraception, sterilization, and physician-assisted suicide by an appeal to the Kantian principle of autonomy, when what Kant called the Law of Autonomy condemns these actions as always and everywhere immoral.

Many Kantians clearly have difficulty with Kant's notion of strict negative duties and the necessarily immoral actions these duties denote, just as many theologians within the Catholic tradition have difficulty with the notions of intrinsically evil and intrinsically immoral actions. These difficulties alone suggest that the distinction between the simply immoral and intrinsically immoral is problematic. A more important reason for not using the distinction, however, is its incompatibility with an ethics of prudential deliberation and judgment. And, of course, the whole idea of intrinsically or necessarily immoral actions is foreign to the prudential reasoning of Aristotle and Aquinas.

HELPFUL DISTINCTIONS

We turn now to a set of distinctions that can help us. These distinctions are not faultless, but they can nonetheless serve a useful purpose in moral reasoning about health care issues.

Reasonable and Unreasonable

This will be a key distinction in our analysis. In moral matters the reasonable thing to do or not do will be the ethical thing to do or not do. The norm in the ethics of the good is reason. What is according to reason is ethical. What is unreasonable is unethical. There is never a situation in which the ethical thing to do is unreasonable or the reasonable thing to do is unethical. As Aquinas put it: "Reason is the first principle (*primum principium*) of all human actions." Of course, we have to explain what according to reason means in this context. What, indeed, is reasonable in moral matters?

Put simply, the reasonable is whatever achieves what is truly good for us in the circumstances. If we are deliberately doing something that truly promotes living well, then we are acting reasonably. If we deliberately pursue a course of action opposed to our good, then we are not acting reasonably. Since our good is personal happiness, we can also say that the reasonable is whatever achieves our happiness in the circumstances, and the unreasonable is what undermines it. In practical matters what is reasonable is determined, to the extent we can determine it, by the reasoning we have been calling prudence.

As we have already pointed out, it is not always easy to determine what is the reasonable or ethical thing to do in a particular situation. We have to acknowledge this and admit that ethics is not a science with definitive answers for every particular case. Moreover, health care ethics usually involves an added complexity, namely, most decisions involve at least two major moral agents: (1) the patient (or her proxy or proxies) and (2) the primary physician (and often several other providers as well).

In a time when the physician made the treatment choices on the basis of what he thought was good for the patient, he was the major (and often the only) moral agent. Today we recognize the patient (or proxy) as a major moral agent along with the physician. This plurality of moral agents adds a tremendous complication to many ethical situations in health care. Physician and patient may not reach the same conclusions about what is good.

In health care, therefore, moral agents not only have to figure out what to do about treatment, but, since treatment is a joint effort involving a patient and a number of providers, they must determine what to do when there is disagreement on ethical matters among the several moral agents involved. What is the most ethical way to proceed when the physician and patient (or proxy) do not agree on what is the ethical way to proceed? This is an especially difficult problem for providers when they think that patients or proxies are not making reasonable and right decisions about life-sustaining treatment.

Nonetheless, despite the practical difficulties, the norm of ethics remains what is according to reason, where what is according to reason is understood as what will truly achieve the good, or at least avoid the worse, in the situation. If there is a moral conflict between patient and providers, it can only be resolved by figuring out what is reasonable in the circumstances. Hence, the distinction between reasonable and unreasonable is crucial and universal; it is no less than the distinction between the ethical and the unethical, the moral and the immoral.

Prudence and Moral Judgment

Much of the literature on ethics fails to recognize the difference between prudence and moral judgment. As we saw in chapters 1 and 2, prudence is the moral reasoning employed by a moral agent, that is, a person actually enmeshed in a situation and faced with deciding what to do or not do. It is the moral reasoning you and I employ when we are faced with a decision that we will have to carry out. Prudence tells us what to do in the actual situation in order to achieve our good.

Moral judgment, on the other hand, is the moral reasoning we employ when we are reviewing situations in which we are not actually involved. Here we are not the moral agent. We are not going to do what we decide is the right thing to do, but we are making judgments about how we think the people actually involved will promote living well.

As was already noted this means that the work we do in this book is not, strictly speaking, the work of prudence. We will be making moral judgments. However, the way we will go about making moral judgments about particular cases and the way we practice personal prudence are very similar, and thus, what we said about prudence in the first chapters will apply also to the moral judgments we will make in later chapters. The two are so related that work in making moral judgments will enhance prudence, just as a highly developed prudence in our personal lives will enhance our ability to make good moral judgments about the situations confronting others.

In the later chapters as we examine particular cases, we will strengthen the similarity between prudence and moral judgment by considering each case from the perspectives of the various moral agents—patients, proxies, physicians, nurses, attorneys, administrators, judges, and others. This will make our moral judgments as close to prudence as possible, for we will ask what we would do if we were the patient, the proxy, the physician, and so forth, in the particular situation.

Descriptive Language and Evaluative Language

People often confuse description and evaluation when they speak and write about ethical matters. This is understandable because a purely descriptive natural language simply does not exist. The language we speak in life is always biased in some degree. Words, phrases, and sentences are always colored by social, historical, and personal perspectives.

Early in the twentieth century some philosophers tried to escape the bias inherent in natural languages by developing a purely formal language using letters of the alphabet to stand for propositions. If you wanted to develop a logical argument, you would first make your language a series of propositions, and then use the letter "p" for the first proposition, "q" for the second, and so forth. Then you would join the propositions together in one of several clearly defined ways indicated by symbols. The idea was to develop a language of logical elegance and clarity and to encourage people to "watch their *p*'s and *q*'s," that is, to think and speak in a clearly defined and logical way. The result was a language that was mathematical in its precision and logic but so narrow and impoverished that it was of little use in life. For this and other reasons the project was abandoned by everyone except specialists interested in its mathematical and logical features.

The desire for a purely descriptive language also arose in the modern philosophy of science. Philosophers tried mightily to speak of pure facts in science. They attempted to show how the scientists' belief in the facts meant science was objective and represented things as they truly are, not as what we think they are.

Today most philosophers of science acknowledge that there are no pure facts, that everything we perceive as fact is theory-laden, that facts cannot be perceived without a theoretical background that will, among other things, indicate what will be counted as a fact. Galileo saw moons circling Jupiter in 1610 and considered it a fact; his adversaries, whose biblical and Ptolemaic conceptions of the universe did not allow such facts, did not consider what he saw to be a fact. And the fact that the shortest distance between two stars is not a straight line is not a fact for someone convinced that the axioms of Euclidean geometry apply to vast distances in real space. And the fact that minutes and hours pass more slowly on stars moving faster relative to our solar system is not a fact for someone convinced that the Newtonian concept of absolute time holds for all velocities, even velocities approaching the speed of light.

A purely descriptive or purely factual language is not really possible in the natural languages used in science, nor in the language of ethics. Nonetheless, we do need to strive in ethical reflection for language that is not overloaded with conceptual and evaluative biases. If we are going to talk intelligently about ethical issues, we need to use language that, while admittedly not completely descriptive and factual, is essentially so. In ethics we need to contrast this essentially descriptive language with language that is significantly evaluative. To do this we have to learn how to recognize language that looks descriptive but actually smuggles in moral judgments. Consider the following sentences.

1. John killed Jack.
2. John murdered Jack.

The structures of the two sentences are similar. They have the same "A did something to B" format, and both subjects and objects are identical. The verbs also share the same meaning—they indicate lethal actions. But from an ethical point of view, the sentences are very dissimilar. The first is fundamentally descriptive. It describes an action—an action that causes death—but it does not evaluate that action. It does not tell us whether the killing was legal or illegal, moral or immoral. Perhaps Jack stumbled drunk onto a busy high-speed road on a rainy night, and John, despite driving carefully, struck and killed him. Perhaps John and Jack were soldiers fighting opposite each other in a war, and John fired the weapon that killed Jack. The first sentence tells us something bad happened but does not tell us whether that something was moral or immoral. "John killed Jack" is an essentially descriptive sentence.

The second sentence is more than descriptive; it makes a moral judgment. Murder is a particular kind of killing. In law it is illegal killing, and in morality it is immoral killing. The second sentence is essentially an evaluation, although it retains a descriptive component. It speaks not just of a killing, but of a killing that is illegal and immoral. When I say "John murdered Jack," I am saying (1) John killed Jack and (2) the killing was immoral and illegal. Unlike the first sentence, which describes an action without making a moral or legal judgment, the second sentence both describes an action and makes a moral and legal judgment. "John murdered Jack" is essentially a moral and legal evaluation; it is not a simple description.

The distinction between description and moral evaluation is important in discourse about controversial moral issues. Descriptive language enables people to deliberate and to discuss the issue and then to move toward a thoughtful moral judgment. Evaluative language subverts moral deliberation and discussion about controversial issues by introducing moral judgments prematurely. True deliberation and discussion become impossible when the moral judgments are already made—we are not really deliberating when we have already made up our minds. When there are moral dilemmas or disagreements about what is moral, then people, regardless of their personal commitments, must step back from their evaluative language and use descriptive language to talk about the issue. Otherwise they are preaching to each other or shouting at each other.

The importance of the distinction between descriptive and evaluative language is relatively easy to see in the example we gave, yet it is often confused in practice. In discussions about abortion, for example, opponents of it sometimes use the language of "murder" and "killing babies." In effect this ends the moral discussion before it begins, because everyone considers murder and deliberately killing babies immoral. The language of murder and killing babies is not a language of description—it is a language of moral evaluation.

On the other hand, advocates of choice in abortion sometimes describe abortion in terms of rights—the right to reproductive freedom, the right to privacy, the right to choose, and so forth. This also ends the moral discussion before it begins because most everyone favors personal rights and freedom for themselves. The language of rights and freedom is not a language of description but a language of moral evaluation.

Another example in which evaluative language occurs prematurely is in discussions about withdrawing life-sustaining treatments from seriously defective newborns with poor prognoses. On one side are people so dedicated to the infant's right to life that they view withdrawing life-sustaining treatment as killing babies. On the other side are people so sensitive to the burdens of invasive treatment with little benefit for the infant that they view providing it as child abuse. Both descriptions are loaded with moral evaluations and thus hinder sound moral deliberation and judgment.

When we talk about controversial subjects such as abortion and treatment withdrawals from infants, we need a clear and morally neutral description of what happens. We need a language describing abortion as the termination of a pregnancy or, more exactly, as the destruction of a fetus. And we need to discuss what treatments are promoting what is truly good for the infant and what treatments are not. Only then can we reason morally to determine whether or not we have adequate reasons for destroying a human fetus or withdrawing life-sustaining treatments from the child.

Intelligent discourse about the morality of any action subject to sincere and serious disagreement has to begin with relatively neutral descriptive language. Reflections on health care issues in the following chapters attempt to avoid heavily loaded evaluative language in favor of essentially descriptive language. Providing a good description, however, is not an easy task. As we pointed out, no description is completely neutral or clean from an evaluative standpoint. But some expressions are more prejudicial than others, and these we must try to avoid. Keeping the distinction between description and evaluation in mind can help us do this.

Bad and Immoral

Some theologians have recently introduced a distinction between what they call "premoral evil" (or nonmoral evil, or ontic evil) and moral evil. Premoral evil is anything harmful and damaging to life, especially human life. Moral evil is anything harmful and damaging to life arising from morally unreasonable human choice. Instead of using the language of premoral and moral evil, we will distinguish the bad and the immoral. We will call premoral evil (or nonmoral evil or ontic evil) bad, and we will call moral evil immoral or unethical.

The bad is not, of itself, immoral. It is simply bad, something we prefer not to happen. Sometimes these bad things arise from the dynamics of nature: perhaps a violent storm causes death or a virus makes me sick. Sometimes these bad things result from human behavior: perhaps someone accidently steps on my foot or perhaps someone intentionally does something causing me pain but has a good reason for having done it. The bad things caused (1) by nature or (2) by unintentional human behavior or (3) by intentional human behavior with adequate reasons are not immoral. They are simply bad, and it is unfortunate that we have to deal with them in life.

Only the bad caused by *intentional* human behavior without adequate reasons is immoral. The immoral embraces only the bad things done (1) intentionally and (2) without a sufficient reason. Intentional actions or omissions giving rise to bad things without good reasons are what we mean by immoral or unethical behavior.

An obstetrician performing a cesarean section causes pain and damage to the woman's body, and these are bad things. If the surgery is done for a good reason—to prevent injury to the baby, for example—the action is morally reasonable. But if the surgery is not done for a good reason—if it is done chiefly for the convenience of the obstetrician, for example—then the surgery is not reasonable, the pain and damage are immoral, and the obstetrician behaves in an unethical way.

We are constantly doing things intentionally that cause bad things in our own lives as well as in the lives of others. We cannot live in the world without hurting people: Sometimes the soldier has to fight the enemy, sometimes the judge has to sentence a criminal, sometimes the dentist has to drill a tooth, sometimes a person has to break off a relationship, sometimes a parent has to say no, sometimes an employer has to fire an employee, and so forth. These actions all cause other people grief, but they are not immoral or unethical if the agents have sufficient reasons balancing the bad things they cause.

Only if we do not have sufficient reasons for causing bad things is our behavior unreasonable and immoral. Intentional behavior giving rise to bad things without sufficient reason is immoral because I can never achieve a truly good life by causing needless pain and suffering or by damaging or destroying life unnecessarily.

The distinction between the bad and the immoral is a useful distinction. There are times when doing good things will cause bad things—injury, pain, and even death. The distinction between the bad and the immoral allows us to recognize that intentionally engaging in behavior that gives rise to bad things such as suffering and even death is not necessarily immoral. Morality centers on whether or not the suffering and death we cause are reasonable; that is, whether or not there are adequate reasons for doing or not doing whatever brings about the suffering or the death.

The ultimate moral issue is not whether someone suffers or even dies, because suffering and dying, although bad, are not immoral. The ultimate moral issue arising from deliberate behavior that gives rise to bad things is whether or not there are overriding reasons for allowing or causing the bad outcomes to occur. If we have overriding reasons for the suffering, injury, or death we cause, then we are acting according to reason and in a moral way; if not, we are acting unreasonably and in an immoral way.

Put simply, doing bad things to ourselves, to others, or to the environmental web of life we share with all the living becomes immoral if (1) done deliberately and (2) without a sufficient reason.

Removing nutrition, withholding life-sustaining treatment, destroying fetuses, and the like all involve insults to life. The ethical person will not bring them about unless she concludes from her moral deliberation that she has substantial overriding reasons to do so. Morally good people strive never to cause any bad things; in fact, they try to prevent them whenever possible, but sometimes they cannot achieve a good life without damaging or even destroying life.

This suggests a practical guideline: Whenever what we are going to do, or not going to do but could do, will result in the bad (that is, will give rise to suffering or damage to life), then we will avoid the behavior unless there are overriding reasons not to avoid it. And the greater the bad, the stronger the overriding reasons have to be.

Although ethics is primarily a positive endeavor—it shows us the feelings, habits, and behaviors that promote happiness in our lives—a great deal of effort in ethics is devoted to becoming aware of the bad things arising from our intentional behavior and to figuring out whether we have sufficient reasons for causing or allowing them to happen. This aspect of ethics is especially important in health care ethics, where much of what providers might do, or not do, causes pain, suffering, and even the risk of death in patients.

It is well to remember, however, that an ethics devoted only to avoiding the bad would be an impoverished ethics. An adequate health care ethics encourages us to promote the good whenever possible. It encourages us to behave with kindness, compassion, caring, justice, love, honesty, and the like, for this is how we live well and happily.

Research and Treatment

This is a good distinction to keep in mind. The failure to distinguish scientific research and medical treatment causes great mischief in moral reasoning and undermines the ability of people to think clearly about difficult personal decisions and develop wise policies for the regulation of drugs by the FDA. Most of us have a pretty good idea of what we mean by medical treatment. We go to a doctor, and he or she provides approved treatments that often include giving us drugs directly or giving us prescriptions for drugs. The physician's primary intention is to benefit us by curing our problem, or by extending our lives, or at least by reducing our discomfort.

An understandable confusion can arise in several analogous situations. For example, as we will see in chapter 14, persons enrolled in clinical trials often go to a doctor who also provides them with drugs, and thus they can easily think of themselves as patients and of the doctor as providing medical treatment intended to benefit them. What the doctor in a clinical trial is providing, however, is neither treatment nor something primarily for the benefit of the persons receiving the drug. Rather, the doctor is performing a clinical experiment, and the primary intention is to find out whether the drug or device being tested will qualify as a treatment. Persons enrolled in clinical research are no longer "patients" but "human subjects" or "participants in research." Yet many people receiving drugs or devices in clinical trials fail to make the distinction between research and treatment. Often, in what is called the "therapeutic misconception," they assume falsely that they are receiving treatments designed to benefit them. Studies show, for example, that people in clinical trials with a placebo arm frequently do not understand that there is a good chance that what they will receive will be something deliberately designed not to have any medicinal value for them.

Another example where people fail to distinguish treatment and research occurs, as we will see in chapter 17, in the ongoing debate about allowing seriously ill and dying people access to unapproved drugs and devices if they cannot get into clinical trials. Advocates of giving people greater access to unapproved drugs—drugs not currently approved by the FDA—almost invariably speak of desperately ill people being denied "life-saving treatments." In fact, however, these people are not being denied "treatments." It would be more accurate to say they are being denied "risky experimental drugs" because the drugs are not yet accepted as treatments and probably, on the basis of our experience with testing unapproved drugs, never will be accepted because researchers will discover that they are not safe or not effective, or both. Unapproved drugs, whether given by doctors to people in clinical trials or outside of clinical trials, may look like medical treatments, but they really should be thought of as experiments likely to fail.

The purpose of this chapter is to simplify our work later on when we consider various topics in health care ethics. By taking these steps to clarify language and to set aside some popular but potentially misleading distinctions, we sidestep a number of confusions haunting many recent discussions of ethical issues in health care.

We turn next to a topic of primary importance in health care ethics. Who decides what to do, and how do they go about making their decisions?

Suggested Readings

Deciding to Forego Life-Sustaining Treatment, 1983, a report of the President's Commission for the Study of Ethical Problems in Medicine and Biomedical and Behavioral Research (hereafter the "President's Commission"), noted that four distinctions (actions versus omissions leading to death, withholding versus withdrawing treatment, intended versus unintended but foreseeable consequences, and ordinary versus extraordinary treatment) are "inherently unclear" and that using them "is often so mechanical that it neither illuminates an actual case nor provides an ethically persuasive argument" (pp. 60–90).

The report also states, however, that variations of the distinction "intentionally cause death—let die," although often "conceptually unclear and of dubious moral importance," are useful in persuading people to accept sound decisions that would otherwise meet unwarranted resistance" (p. 71). There are strong reasons for disagreeing with this position. Good ethics is undermined by the use of unclear distinctions, and convincing someone to accept a sound decision by deliberately using unclear distinctions suggests manipulation, if not deception. See Raymond J. Devettere, "Reconceptualizing the Euthanasia Debate," *Law, Medicine & Health Care* 1989, *17*, 145–55.

The moral value of the "ordinary-extraordinary" and "withhold-withdraw" distinctions is also challenged in the report of the Hastings Center titled *Guidelines on the Termination of Life-Sustaining Treatment and the Care of the Dying*, pp. 5ff. The 1980 Declaration on Euthanasia issued by the Roman Catholic Church acknowledged that the "ordinary-extraordinary" distinction is "perhaps less clear" than it once was because it is imprecise and because of the rapid progress in treatment interventions. This document is printed as Appendix C in *Deciding to Forego Life-Sustaining Treatment* (1983).

Early legal decisions accepted the "ordinary-extraordinary" distinction (cf. *Matter of Quinlan*, 70 NJ 10 [1976] and *Superintendent of Belchertown State School v. Saikewicz*, 373 Mass 728, 738, 743–44 [1977]), but some more recent decisions either reject it or relegate it to a very minor place in the decision-making process. See, for example, *Matter of Conroy*, 98 NJ 371–72 (1985).

The distinction between "futility" and what could be called "utility" (that is, what would be effective treatment) is now the subject of intense debate. Daniel Callahan, "Medical Futility, Medical Necessity: The Problem without a Name," *Hastings Center Report* 1991, *21* (July), 30–35, frames the issue well. See also Robert Truog, A. S. Brett, and J. Frader, "The Problem with Futility," *New England Journal of Medicine* 1992, *326*, 1560–64; Robert Truog, "Beyond Futility," *Journal of Clinical Ethics* 1992, *3*, 143–45; and Stuart Youngner, "Who Defines Futility?" *JAMA* 1988, *260*, 2094–95. Also helpful is a collection of seven articles on medical futility in *Law, Medicine & Health Care* 1992, *20*, 307–39, and another collection of articles on futility in a special section of the *Cambridge Quarterly of Healthcare Ethics* 1993, *2*, 142–227.

For later developments in the debate on futility, see Marjorie Zucker and Howard Zucker, eds., 1997, *Medical Futility and the Evaluation of Life-Sustaining Interventions*, Cambridge: Cambridge University Press; Lawrence Schneiderman and Nancy Jecker, 1997, *Wrong Medicine: Doctors, Patients, and Futile Medicine*, Baltimore: Johns Hopkins University Press; Amir Halevy and Baruch Brody, "A Multi-Institution Collaborative Policy on Medical Futility," *JAMA* 1996, *276*, 571–74; Howard Brody, "Bringing Clarity to the Futility Debate: Don't Use the Wrong Cases," *Cambridge Quarterly of Health-care Ethics* 1998, *7*, 269–73 with a commentary by Lawrence Schneiderman on 273–78; S. Van McCrary et al., "Physicians' Quantitative Assessments of Medical Futility," *Journal of Clinical Ethics* 1994, *5*, 100–03 with commentaries by Nancy Jecker, Howard Brody, Clarence Braddock, Janicemarie Vinicky, and James Orlowski on pp. 138–49. For the AMA report suggesting that institutions should develop a fair process approach rather than a policy with substantive definitions, see "Medical Futility in End-of-Life Care: Report of the Council on Ethical and Judicial Affairs," *JAMA* 1999, *281*, 937–41. The article reporting how belief in miracles is a factor that complicates some disputes about futile treatment is Lenworth Jacobs, K. Burns, and B. Bennett Jacobs, "Trauma Death: Views of the Public and Trauma Professionals on Death and Dying from Injuries," *Archives of Surgery* 2008, *143*, 730–35. See also Paul Helft, M. Siegler, and J. Lantos, "The Rise and Fall of the Futility Movement," *New England Journal of Medicine* 2000, *343*, 293–96.

The direct-indirect distinction has been well known in moral theology for centuries. Thomas Aquinas distinguished direct and indirect voluntary behavior in the *Summa Theologiae* I II, q. 6, a. 3 and q. 77, a. 7, but his distinction is not the same as that used today. According to Aquinas, if I choose to steer the ship against the rocks, I *directly* cause the shipwreck, but if I decline to steer the drifting ship away from the rocks when I could and should have done so, then I *indirectly* cause the shipwreck. Later theologians, however, used the direct-indirect distinction in a different sense, usually in conjunction with the principle of double effect. Here, "direct" referred to the intended effect of the action, and "indirect" to the unintended but foreseen effect. See Bruno Schuller, "Direct Killing/Indirect Killing" and Albert Di Ianni, "The Direct/Indirect Distinction in Morals," both in Charles Curran and Richard McCormick, eds., 1979, *Readings in Moral Theology No. 1*, New York: Paulist Press, pp. 138–57 and 215–43; and Richard McCormick, "Searching for the Consistent Ethic of Life," in Joseph Selling, ed., 1988, *Personalist Morals*, Leuven: Leuven University Press, pp. 135–46. A version of this essay also appeared as a symposium paper titled "The Consistent Ethic of Life: Is There an Historical Soft Underbelly?" in Thomas Fuechtmann, ed., 1988, *Consistent Ethic of Life*, Kansas City: Sheed & Ward, pp. 96–122.

John Dedek has provided a good introduction to the development of the doctrine of intrinsically immoral actions in several articles. See his "Moral Absolutes in the Predecessors of St. Thomas," *Theological Studies* 1977, *38*, 654–80; "Intrinsically Evil Acts: An Historical Study of the Mind of St. Thomas,"

68 — *The Language of Health Care Ethics*

Thomist 1979, *43*, 385–413; and "Intrinsically Evil Acts: The Emergence of a Doctrine," *Recherches de Theologie Ancienne et Medievale* 1983, *50*, 191–226. See also Josef Fuchs, 1984, "An Ongoing Discussion in Christian Ethics: Intrinsically Evil Acts?" in *Christian Ethics in a Secular Arena*, trans. Bernard Hoose and Brian McNeil, Washington, DC: Georgetown University Press, chapter 5; and Charles Curran, ed., 1968, *Absolutes in Moral Theology?* Washington, DC: Corpus, especially Curran's own essay, "Absolute Norms and Medical Ethics," pp. 108–53. A summary of the 2007 United States Conference of Catholic Bishops' *Challenge of Forming Consciences for Faith Citizenship* can be found at usccb.org. The full text is at faithfulcitizenship.org. The 2008 Instruction *Dignitas Personae* is also available at usccb.org.

Aristotle's examples of feelings and actions that are immoral by definition and therefore beyond the scope of prudential reasoning in particular situations are the feelings of spite, shamelessness, and envy and the actions of adultery, theft, and murder. See the *Nicomachean Ethics* 1107a9–26. It is important to note the importance of feelings in an ethics of the good life. Feelings of spite, shamelessness, and envy do not promote my well-being; they do not make me happy. They are, therefore, always immoral by definition.

One of the best recent introductions to Kant's complex and seminal ethical theory is Roger Sullivan, 1989, *Immanuel Kant's Moral Theory*, Cambridge, UK: Cambridge University Press. As Sullivan points out, Kant had a very dim view of human sexuality. The sexually sensual and the erotic were simply lust in his mind, a manifestation of our animal appetites. Only the preservation of the race in marriage justified engaging in sexual behavior. Kant is not even clear on whether married couples could have intercourse when pregnancy is impossible, but he does suggest that sex in such circumstances, something "certainly unallowed," might be allowed "to prevent some greater transgression (as an indulgence)." See Kant, *The Metaphysics of Morals*, in Kant, 1983, *Ethical Philosophy*, trans. James Ellington, Indianapolis: Hackett, p. 87. Kant's ethic of duty runs throughout this work.

Kant is especially vehement in his condemnation of homosexuality and masturbation, which he considers both contrary to reason (the moral law) and contrary to nature as well, and contraception, which is contrary to the purpose of our sexual organs. According to him, these actions degrade us below the level of animals, which, he said, avoid any of these behaviors. He thought masturbation, homosexuality, and contraception were actually worse than suicide. At least suicide, he says, requires courage, and where there is courage there can be some respect. But in masturbation, homosexuality, and contraception there is no courage, merely a "weak surrender to animal pleasure." See *The Metaphysics of Morals*, pp. 85–88, and 1963, *Lectures on Ethics*, trans. Louis Infield, New York: Harper Torchbooks, pp. 162–71. After reading Kant's dim view of sexual behavior and of marriage ("It is by marriage that woman becomes free; man loses his freedom in it," cited by Sullivan, Kant's *Moral Theory*, p. 355), learning he was a lifelong bachelor comes as no surprise.

The idea that ethics is doing what is reasonable recalls Aquinas's remark that "reason is the first principle of all human action," found in the *Summa Theologiae* I II, q. 58, a. 2. For both Aquinas and Aristotle, the ethical is what they repeatedly claim is according to right reason, and it is clear from the contexts that the right reason is prudential reasoning or prudence. This does not contradict the idea that my personal good is the first principle of ethics because my good and reason are understood in terms of each other. The morally reasonable is what achieves my good, and whatever achieves my good is the morally reasonable. Hence, to say my good or happiness is the first principle of ethics, or to say behaving according to reason is the first principle of ethics, is to say the same thing in two different ways.

It should again be noted that some translations of Aristotle and Aquinas present their respective phrases *kata ton orthon logon* and *secundum rectam rationem* in a misleading way as "according to the right principle" or "according to the right rule," thus suggesting (incorrectly) that Aristotle and Aquinas advocated a principle-based or rule-based morality much as we find in an ethics of obligation today. These phrases should be translated as "according to right reason," and the context makes it clear that the right reason for ethics is prudential reason, not deductive reason relying on laws, principles, or rules.

The distinction between description and evaluation in natural language is actually much more complicated than it appears, as J. L. Austin, 1975, *How to Do Things with Words*, 2nd ed., Cambridge, MA: Harvard University Press, reminds us. See especially lectures XI and XII.

For background to the distinction between the bad and the immoral, see Louis Janssens, "Ontic Evil and Moral Evil," *Louvain Studies* 1972, *4*, 115–56, reprinted in Curran and McCormick, 1979, *Readings in Moral Theology*, No. 1, New York: Paulist Press, pp. 40–93. Josef Fuchs speaks of "premoral evil" in his 1983, *Personal Responsibility and Christian Morality*, Washington, DC: Georgetown University Press, pp. 136–39; whereas Richard McCormick prefers "nonmoral evil" in "Notes on Moral Theology," *Theological Studies* 1976, *37*, 76–78. See also Bernard Hoose, 1987, *Proportionalism*, Washington, DC: Georgetown University Press, especially chapter 2.

For an explanation of "therapeutic misconception" see Paul Applebaum et al., "False Hopes and Best Data: Consent to Research and the Therapeutic Misconception," *Hastings Center Report* 1987, *17* (March-April), 20–24; and Paul Applebaum and Charles Lidz, "Re-evaluating the Therapeutic Misconception: Response to Miller and Joffe," *Kennedy Institute of Ethics Journal* 2006, *16*, 367–73.

FOUR

Making Health Care Decisions

Decision making in clinical settings can be very complicated. Various parties have legitimate interests, and one of the parties, the patient, may be so affected by medical problems that for him or her to make good decisions is unlikely or impossible. In this chapter we focus on the decision making of the patient and the physician. In chapter 5 we will describe what happens when a patient has lost decision-making capacity and a proxy or surrogate, usually from his family, speaks for the patient with the physician.

The first section of this chapter discusses the complexity inherent in making health care decisions. The second section considers the capacity of a patient to make decisions, what constitutes capacity, and how it is determined. The third section explains informed consent, the most distinctive feature of patient decision making in clinical settings. The fourth section covers the advance directives people can put in place to retain some decision-making authority if they should ever lose the capacity to make decisions. The final section discusses the Patient Self-Determination Act and shows, by looking at the research project known as SUPPORT and a case study, how difficult it has been to change the clinical culture in hospitals so that patients and their families can carry out their reasonable wishes at the end of life.

Complexity of Health Care Decisions

The complexity arises from three main sources: (1) both the physician and the patient are actively involved in making decisions, and they may disagree about what is proper medical treatment; (2) the patient's ability to make decisions may be undermined by his illness—it is hard to make good decisions about anything when we are sick or limited by external factors; (3) health care decisions often involve important moral issues, and good moral decisions are not always good clinical decisions.

Disagreements between Physician and Patient

As was noted in chapter 3, for a long time it was taken for granted that the physician should make the decisions about treatment. This is known as medical paternalism. When it was operative, there were seldom disagreements between physician and patient because the physician made the decisions unilaterally. More recently some have reacted to this paternalism by proposing the principle of patient autonomy or patient self-determination and by encouraging patients' rights. This movement makes the patient the primary decision maker. It also sets the stage for conflict; physicians cannot abdicate their responsibility for the medical treatment they provide, or can provide, for their patient.

We now recognize that neither medical paternalism nor patient autonomy provides the best in health care decisions. Medical paternalism, however well motivated, disenfranchises the patient. On the other hand, patient autonomy, however well grounded in a person's right to choose what happens to him, disenfranchises the physician.

Today a new conception of health care decision making is gaining credence—one that avoids the extremes of both paternalism and autonomy. This new conception, supported by the President's Commission reports titled *Making Health Care Decisions* and *Deciding to Forego Life-Sustaining Treatment*, is called "shared decision making." It envisions the patient and the physician deciding together how care can be managed best. It tries to combine the best of both worlds—the physician's expertise and the patient's values. The process of making the decision becomes a shared process, a partnership between the patient and the physician. In shared decision making, the answer to the question "who decides?" is "the patient *and* the physician."

Shared decision making in any field, however, is a complex phenomenon. Sometimes it runs smoothly, but the potential for conflict is always present. The physician may want something done, but the patient refuses. And the patient may want something done, but the physician refuses, perhaps because it is not good medical practice, or illegal, or unethical. Even in shared decision making, then, each participant retains autonomy. Patients can always refuse the proposed medical intervention, and physicians can always refuse to practice bad medicine or to behave immorally.

Although the center of the shared decision-making process is the patient-physician relationship, the sharing in the decisions often extends to a wider circle, and this complicates matters even more. On the patient's side, family members frequently play a major role in the health care decisions. On the physician's side, other providers are frequently consulted and may share directly in the decisions.

Limitations Affecting the Patient's Ability to Make Health Care Decisions

There are four major ways a patient's role in making effective health care decisions can be limited or lost. First, the patient's capacity to make, or to make known, her decisions may be lost or diminished. She may become unconscious, or be conscious but so overwhelmed by medication, disease, pain, or confusion that she is not really capable of making decisions or, if she can make them, of communicating them to the physicians. If a patient loses the capacity to make or to communicate decisions, a proxy or surrogate will normally step in and try to speak for the patient. We will consider decision making by proxies or surrogates in the next chapter. If a patient retains decision-making capacity, but it has been diminished by age or illness, enabling him to play an appropriate role in the decision making can become very challenging for the physicians, nurses, and family.

Second, when a person becomes a patient he enters an environment in which other people are also making decisions about his care. Not only physicians but nurses, other providers, and the institution itself have a say in what they do for the patient because they are responsible for their actions. At times their disagreement will limit the patient's ability to make an effective decision.

Sometimes this conflict can be resolved by communication and negotiation, but occasionally the disagreement persists. For example, a patient imminently dying from widespread cancer may insist on cardiopulmonary resuscitation when he suffers the expected arrest, but the physicians and nurses responsible for performing the CPR may be convinced that attempting resuscitation is medically inappropriate and not want to do it. If they are convinced that it would be medically and morally wrong for them to attempt resuscitation, they cannot do it in good conscience. If the patient insists on resuscitation efforts, their only alternative is to transfer the patient to other providers. In practice, however, this may not be possible at the moment. Thus, it is not inconceivable that providers will have to tell the patient that they will not attempt resuscitation if the arrest occurs while he is under their care. The providers' refusal of treatment limits the patient's ability to make an effective decision about his treatment.

Third, as we will see, the law sometimes restricts a patient's ability to make effective decisions about health care. By law we mean both legislation and the court decisions constituting the tradition of case law. Thus, a patient may want a physician to kill her by a lethal overdose, but the law forbids it, so the physician refuses. And the single mother of young children may want to refuse a blood transfusion for religious reasons, but a court may overrule her decision lest the children lose their only parent.

Finally, much of health care in the United States is not paid for by the patient but by third-party payers, most notably Medicare, the Veterans Administration, the military health care system, Medicaid welfare programs, and various private health insurance plans and health maintenance organizations (HMOs). Any of these payers can effectively restrict the patient's ability to make effective decisions about a particular treatment by refusing to fund it when the patient has no other way to pay for it. If an insurance company declines to pay for the surgery a patient wants, this will override the patient's decision and the physician's decision as well, if the patient cannot afford to pay for the surgery himself or is unable to find another funding source.

Potential Conflict between Clinical and Ethical Goals

Almost every health care decision has two goals. One goal is to decide what will be good health care for the patient. This is often an enormously complicated question—it is not always easy to know what constitutes good patient care. We are tempted to say that good patient care is treating to cure disease and preserve life, and this is true is most cases, but not always. Sometimes good care consists in declining or discontinuing treatment because the interventions cause more burdens than any possible benefits they could provide. When this happens the goal is not cure but comfort, not mindless preservation of life but recognition of medicine's inherent limitations.

The second goal is to decide what will be morally good for the patient and for the providers. Health care decisions are seldom simply about treatment; morality almost always intrudes. This is so because most treatments have risks and harmful side effects, and the need for reasons to justify causing these bad events is a main concern of ethics. Patients and physicians have to decide not only what is good medical care but what is ethical care, given the circumstances.

The clinical and moral goals sometimes conflict because clinical practice is not identical with clinical ethics. The goal of clinical practice is the good considered as good clinical outcome; the goal of clinical ethics is the good considered as good ethical outcome. The right clinical decision is often the right moral decision, but not always. Transplanting black-market kidneys bought from desperate and impoverished people, for example, might be the best clinical outcome for patients needing the kidneys, but from an ethical point of view, good reasons exist for saying that the implantation of black-market kidneys is immoral. The potential clash between clinical and ethical goals is one more reason why making health care decisions can become so complex.

These, then, are some of the factors that give rise to the complexity inherent in decisions about health care. Next, we turn to an examination of the most essential condition that must be present before a patient can make a health care decision—capacity. By decision-making capacity we mean the ability to make thoughtful and voluntary decisions about health care. Decision-making capacity is a major issue when patients participate in decision making because the dysfunction that makes them patients may very well also limit or undermine their ability to make important decisions. Determining whether or not a patient has decision-making capacity is one of the more important, and difficult, challenges facing physicians and nurses.

DECISION-MAKING CAPACITY

Decision-making capacity in health care is the ability to make reasonable decisions about what to do when confronted with disease, injury, and pain. In a general sense providers as well as patients need to have decision-making capacity, but we will consider this capacity only in patients. We presume the physicians and other providers have the capacity to make decisions.

Many authors use the words "competence" or "competent" to describe what we are calling decision-making capacity. Using competence to indicate decision-making capacity could be misleading because competence has long been used in a precise legal sense. Our legal system normally assumes an adult is competent unless a court has ruled otherwise. Obviously then, the legal meaning of competence and what we mean by decision-making capacity are not the same. Many adult patients not declared incompetent by a court do not have the capacity to make decisions about their health care.

Clear examples of patients without the capacity to make informed and voluntary decisions include children, the unconscious, many with mental illness, and the like. In many cases, however, the lack of capacity is not so clear. Although it is wise to begin by presuming that conscious adults have decision-making capacity, we know that some of them do not have it and that others will have to make decisions for them. Physicians have the difficult task of determining whether or not their patients have decision-making capacity. This determination is a serious matter because once a physician determines a patient is incapable of making decisions about his health care, she in effect disenfranchises him of his prerogative to make what could be very important decisions about his life. We need, therefore, a clear understanding of this decision-making capacity.

Capacity is the ability to do something specific; it is related to a particular task. A blind person lacks the capacity to drive a car but does not lack capacity to hear a symphony. In health care, our interest is chiefly in the capacity or ability of patients to perform a particular task—to make their health care decisions. This capacity for making health care decisions is very specific. Some patients may have the capacity for making health care decisions but not for making other decisions—decisions about their finances, for example. Some patients may retain the capacity to make health care decisions despite psychiatric disorders or organic mental disabilities that leave them confused about other things. And some patients may have the capacity to make some treatment decisions but not others, or they may have the capacity to make treatment decisions at some times but not all the time.

The capacity for making health care decisions has three aspects, and all three must be present for us to say that the patient has decision-making capacity.

1. *Understanding.* Decision-making capacity means a patient can understand relevant information about the disease, the treatment options, and the recommendations of the physician. It also means he is able to communicate with providers.

2. *Evaluation.* Decision-making capacity means a patient has some framework of values that will enable him to judge whether a particular health care decision will accomplish what he considers good for himself.

3. *Reasoning.* Decision-making capacity means that a patient can deliberate and reason about how all available courses of action will likely affect him. This implies that he can grasp cause-effect relationships, notions of probability and percentages, and the basic form of "if X, then Y" reasonings.

A question that frequently arises is whether or not a patient can be partially capable of making a health care decision; that is, whether or not there are degrees of capacity. Experience certainly suggests that there are degrees of capacity. A person's capacity for decision making could diminish for any number of reasons and yet not be totally lost. This suggests that we could say some people have a partial capacity for making health care decisions.

This may seem like a wise move, but in practice, it is not. For practical reasons, it is important to draw a sharp line between decision-making capacity and incapacity. Capacity is an either-or situation: either the patient has decision-making capacity for this situation or she does not have it.

If we did not draw a sharp line between capacity and incapacity, we could never determine just who has the final responsibility for making the decision about the patient's care—the patient or the proxy. If the patient is capable, the patient has final responsibility for decisions; if the patient is not capable, the proxy has the final responsibility. If we embrace the notion of partial capacity, the physician would be placed in an untenable position. She would not know whether to accept the decisions of the patient with partial capacity or those of the proxy. Only by making a sharp dividing line between capacity and incapacity can we determine who ultimately decides—the patient or the patient's proxy.

Capacity is thus a threshold notion, and a patient is on one side or the other. We cannot think of someone as straddling the threshold between capacity and incapacity. The physician determines whether a particular patient has, or does not have, the capacity to make a particular decision at a particular time.

The major question emerging from considering capacity a threshold notion is just how diminished any of the three aspects of capacity (understanding, evaluating, and reasoning) must be before a patient has crossed the threshold from capacity to incapacity. Ultimately this determination is, as the President's Commission noted, a matter of personal judgment based on common sense. And as we will see in the next chapter, the physician has the responsibility of making this judgment about his or her patient.

However, physicians should not judge patients incapable of making decisions simply because they make a decision that is idiosyncratic or at variance with what the physician thinks is best. For example, a few people routinely refuse blood for religious reasons. Their decision to refuse a treatment almost everyone else considers reasonable is not a reason for their physicians to conclude that they have lost the capacity for making health care decisions. In other words, a decision most would consider unreasonable does not automatically mean the person making it lacks capacity. People with capacity can make unreasonable decisions, and they can make mistakes. Conversely, people can make reasonable decisions, yet not have decision-making capacity. We cannot use the outcome of the decision process, the decision itself, as evidence that the person has, or does not have, decision-making capacity.

On the other hand, when a patient decides on something that physicians and other providers think is unnecessarily dangerous or obviously unreasonable given the circumstances, it certainly raises a warning flag. Physicians concerned about their patient's well-being will be moved to probe deeper into the decision-making process and to question the person's capacity. The more harmful the decision, the more carefully the physician will investigate the issue of capacity when the decision appears unreasonable. An unreasonable decision is not a reason for saying the person does not have capacity, but it is a reason for investigating more carefully the presumption of capacity.

Perhaps the easiest case in which providers can accept what they consider an unreasonable decision is when the decision is based on tenets of a sincerely held religious faith. Nearly everyone considers a patient's commitment to a recognized religious faith an appeal that outweighs all other reasons for using life-saving treatment. Thus, many physicians and nurses would consider the refusal of blood in the face of death by a practicing Jehovah's Witness an unreasonable decision from a medical perspective but not something that they should question because it is based on a sincerely held religious faith.

It is more difficult for physicians and nurses to accept other appeals that patients might use to justify their refusal of reasonable treatment necessary to preserve life. Sometimes paternalistic intervention may be appropriate, sometimes not, and usually only those on the scene can make the right decision. Imagine, for example, a man with a history of heart attacks suddenly having symptoms of another attack as he plays golf. His golfing partners are concerned and want to call an ambulance, but he refuses because he wants to finish the hole. He has not lost the capacity to make a health care decision, although he is certainly making a stupid one. Imagine also that a physician is playing with him, and he knows that a serious situation is developing. One would hope the physician would act in a paternalistic way, ignore the man's refusal to summon paramedics, and take the necessary steps to save his life. Refusing medical help for a life-threatening heart attack in order to finish playing a hole in golf simply does not carry the same weight as refusing life-saving treatment for religious reasons.

When a patient with decision-making capacity makes an unusual decision for reasons the providers believe are trivial, they must respond with a great deal of what we have called prudence. If the patient persists in his position, they must decide whether it is ethical for them to respect the decision, to override it, or to withdraw from the case. Withdrawing from the case is preferable to overriding a patient's request, but withdrawal is not always possible. When no other physician is available and willing to accept responsibility for the care of the patient, an attending physician cannot abandon a patient. This presents, as we saw in the example of the patient dying with cancer who wants resuscitation attempted, a difficult situation for the providers.

In summary, then, we want to remember the following key points about capacity:

1. We begin by presuming conscious adult patients have the capacity to make health care decisions. This assumption ceases when there is evidence that the capacity does not exist, and the physician determines that it is indeed lacking.

2. The capacity for making health care decisions has three aspects: the ability to understand and communicate; the ability to deliberate and reason about alternative courses of action; and the ability to evaluate what is good.

3. Capacity is a threshold notion. It must be determined that a patient either has or does not have decision-making capacity for a particular option at a particular time. However, capacity may come and go, and capacity may exist for some decisions but not for others.

4. An unreasonable decision does not by itself indicate decision-making incapacity; nor does a reasonable decision indicate capacity. However, an obviously unreasonable decision, especially when serious harm will result, should trigger a more extensive probing into the question of the patient's capacity.

One of the most important things a patient with decision-making capacity does is to give informed consent for medical interventions. We turn now to an examination of this important concept.

INFORMED CONSENT

Informed consent is a major feature of twentieth-century health care. Most of us encounter it for the first time when we need some kind of surgical or medical intervention. A health care provider, usually the physician, explains the medical problem to us, the various options we have, a recommended treatment to correct the problem, and the risks involved in the interventions. We then sign a form indicating our consent for the procedure.

Many patients and providers alike confuse the signing of this form with the reality of giving informed consent. Patients often think they are giving consent by signing the form, and providers often think they are getting informed consent by having it signed. Actually, informed consent has little to do with the signing of a form. We should think of the signed form as the documentation of informed consent, something we need for the records, but not the informed consent itself.

Informed consent is a personal exchange between physician and patient. The physician provides information so the patient becomes "informed," and the patient then "consents" to the proposed treatment. This interaction between physician and patient constitutes the reality of informed consent. The signed form is the record that this interaction did indeed occur, but it is not the informed consent itself.

Where did the notion of informed consent originate? Undoubtedly its origins are as old as medicine. People got sick, knew that physicians might be able to alleviate the illness, and turned to them for help. This seeking of medical aid implied that the afflicted person was somewhat informed about what physicians do and was willing to have this done to him. Moreover, we can easily suppose that many physicians said something to their patients about what they thought was the problem and what they were going to do about it before they intervened. We have no historical evidence to suggest that physicians routinely invaded people's lives and forced treatment on them every time they became sick. People knew something about treatments and sought out persons skilled in providing them. This is a long way from the doctrine of informed consent as we now know it, but it does remind us that many patients were getting some information and giving something of consent long before informed consent became the popular doctrine it is today.

The modern doctrine of informed consent emerged from several developments over the past few centuries. The modern liberal philosophy of personal rights and liberties certainly provided an important philosophical background. More recently there has been an understandable reaction to the institutionalization of medicine in hospitals. Informed consent was not as necessary when physicians visited homes. Patients had more control in their homes than they do in hospitals, and they knew more about the traditional remedies than they know about the advanced life-prolonging techniques and technologies associated with modern hospitals.

The most important source of today's doctrine of informed consent, however, is not philosophical or sociological but legal. Informed consent as we know it today originated in the courts. Several landmark decisions played a key role in making informed consent a fact of life in health care, and reviewing these decisions will help us to understand more clearly the meaning of informed consent.

The Legal History of Informed Consent

We will consider four of the landmark legal decisions that shaped the doctrine of informed consent as we know it today.

The *Schloendorff* Decision (New York, 1914)

Mrs. Schloendorff had steadfastly insisted, despite her physician's recommendation, that she did not want surgery to remove a fibroid tumor. She did agree that he could administer ether and perform an abdominal examination to determine whether or not it was malignant. The physician was so concerned about the tumor that he removed it while she was under the anesthesia.

She sued for damages but did not prevail because no serious harm ensued. However, Justice Cardozo's decision contains one of the most quoted sentences in the legal history of informed consent: "Every human being of adult years and sound mind has a right to determine what shall be done with his own body; and a surgeon who performs an operation without his patient's consent commits an assault, for which he is liable in damages."

This was not the first time the key word "consent" appeared in court decisions about medical treatment. Almost a decade earlier, decisions in two cases (*Mohr v. Williams*, 1905, and *Pratt v. Davis*, 1905, affirmed 1906) stated that a citizen's first right, the right to himself, forbids physicians and surgeons from violating his bodily integrity without his consent. But the *Schloendorff* decision attracted considerable attention. Justice Cardozo was a well-known jurist, and his language was clear, even eloquent. Most of all, it was ominous: it spoke of an operation without consent as an "assault" and said the surgeon was liable for damages.

The *Schloendorff* decision made people more aware of the legal requirement for consent, but this was still a long way from *informed* consent. Although the decision called for consent, it said nothing about informed consent. Consent can be uninformed or misinformed (perhaps we could say "disinformed," as in "disinformation"). Consent is uninformed when the patient consents to a procedure without receiving enough information to know what will happen to him, or, if he did receive information, did not understand it. Consent is misinformed when the patient has been misled about what will happen. The notion of informed consent did not appear until a California case more than forty years after the *Schloendorff* decision.

The *Salgo* Decision (California, 1957)

Mr. Salgo had consented to a translumbar aortography, a diagnostic procedure intended to locate the cause of the chronic pain in his leg. The procedure involved the injection of a dye to give the pictures greater clarity. Unfortunately, the procedure caused paralysis in his legs. He sued the Stanford University hospital. His attorneys initially argued that the physicians were negligent in doing the procedure. Later, they added the argument that the physicians had failed to provide their client with information about the risks of the diagnostic procedure.

The trial court ruled in favor of Stanford University, and Mr. Salgo's attorneys appealed. The California Court of Appeals reversed the lower court's decision. In the ruling favoring the patient, the court used, for the first time in a major legal decision, the now well-known phrase "informed consent."

The story of how these famous words "informed consent" appeared in the decision is of interest. The judge writing the decision was struggling with two important values. He wanted to protect the right of patients to know what might happen to them in medical procedures. He also wanted to respect the discretion of physicians and enable them to use their best judgment when they discuss the risks of a procedure with patients. Obviously, if the physicians describe in great detail every possible bad outcome or side effect or risk associated with a procedure, some patients will be so frightened they will decline truly beneficial interventions.

One organization very interested in protecting the right of physicians to use discretion in telling patients about risks associated with surgery was the American College of Surgeons. It submitted an *amicus curiae* (friend of the court) brief to the judge in which it argued that, although physicians did need to disclose all the facts, they also needed to use discretion when discussing risks. The College of Surgeons, of course, was hoping the judge would not find the physicians had acted improperly when they failed to tell Martin Salgo about the risk of paralysis.

The Court of Appeals did not agree—it decided in favor of Mr. Salgo. And in an ironic twist, the judge writing the opinion in favor of the patient used the language of the *amicus curiae* brief that had been submitted to support the physicians. In so doing the judge precipitated the jump of the phrase "informed consent" into the everyday language of health care. The famous words in the *Salgo* decision, words first found in the brief submitted to the court by the College of Surgeons, are: "In discussing the element of risk a certain amount of discretion must be employed consistent with the full disclosure of facts necessary to an informed consent."

The decision recognized that physicians must use discretion in telling patients about risks lest they frighten them, but it said this discretion cannot undermine the patient's need to know the facts. If patients do not know the facts, including facts about risks, they cannot give *informed* consent to the procedure. Mr. Salgo's consent was not truly informed because he had not received all the facts about the risks. The court found the patient's need to know outweighed the physician's effort to be discreet.

This decision made it clear that consent to a medical procedure is not enough. The consent must be informed; that is, physicians must fully disclose the facts. Any recourse by the physician to discretion is strictly limited to what will not undermine this disclosure of the facts necessary to give an informed consent. It is not an exaggeration to say that informed consent for medical treatment, as we know it today, was born in California in 1957.

Of course, like any neonate, the legal doctrine of informed consent was not yet mature. Other cases would follow, and their findings would contribute to its development. We will mention two of these cases. The first one is considered by many to be almost as important as the *Schloendorff* and *Salgo* cases.

The *Canterbury* Decision (District of Columbia, 1972)

In 1959 nineteen-year-old Jerry Canterbury was suffering from back pain. After he had a diagnostic myelogram, his surgeon told him he would need surgery to correct a suspected ruptured disk. On the day after the surgery Mr. Canterbury slipped off the bed while trying to urinate. He became paralyzed from the waist down.

Emergency surgery that night reversed some of the paralysis but left him dependent on crutches and with chronic urologic problems. The patient sued the hospital and the surgeon, but the judge in the district court ordered a directed verdict: He told the jury it must find in favor of the hospital and physician. Attorneys for Canterbury appealed. The U.S. Court of Appeals sent the case back to district court and ordered a full trial in which a jury could hear the evidence and make its own decision. In an ironic twist, the subsequent jury trial also resulted in a decision exonerating the hospital and the surgeon.

What is important for the legal history of informed consent, however, was the position taken by the Court of Appeals when it sent the case back to the lower court for trial. One of the charges against the surgeon was that he had failed to inform the patient of the risk of paralysis The court had to acknowledge that it was not clear whether the surgery or the fall had caused the paralysis, but it insisted that this uncertainty did not change the fact that the surgeon might have failed in his duty to disclose the risk. The court then set forth some first principles to guide physicians in telling patients about available treatments and their associated risks. Four of those principles provide a richer understanding of informed consent.

1. The "root premise" that every human being has a right to determine what shall be done with his or her body means the person needs whatever information is necessary to make an intelligent decision. The physician has a duty to disclose the information a patient needs for an intelligent decision, even if the patient does not ask for it.

2. The physician's duty to disclose information about all the options and their risks is not something the medical profession itself determines. There is a difference between treatment and disclosure. The standards of the medical profession determine what is appropriate treatment. But the medical profession does not determine what is the appropriate disclosure about medical treatment. This is determined by the more general standard of what is "reasonable under the circumstances."

3. The question of what is "reasonable under the circumstances" is itself a tricky one. Ideally the physician must disclose whatever the particular patient would find relevant to his decision. In practice, however, this is a difficult standard because it is impossible for physicians to know what each individual patient would consider relevant to his decision. Hence, the standard of disclosure is more general; it is what a "reasonable person" in the patient's position would consider relevant in deciding whether to give or to withhold consent for treatment.

4. There are two exceptions to the duty to disclose: first, emergencies where treatment is needed and circumstances do not allow disclosure; second, rare situations in which disclosure would present a threat to the patient's well-being because of the adverse reactions it would cause.

The *Canterbury* decision clearly set forth what we now recognize as the two crucial aspects of informed consent. It insisted on *consent* because the patients have the right to control what providers do to their bodies, and it insisted on *information* because patients cannot make intelligent decisions unless they know all the options and the associated risks. If patients are going to consent intelligently, they require information, and it is the responsibility of physicians to provide that information. And the standard of how much information has to be disclosed is not determined by what the physician thinks is relevant but, rather, by the "reasonable person" standard, that is, by what a reasonable person in the patient's position would consider relevant.

All this seems so simple today, but the philosophy supporting informed consent is not the philosophy we find in the influential Hippocratic Oath. The Hippocratic tradition encouraged the physician to do whatever he thought was best for the patient. Informed consent, on the other hand, empowers a patient to accept what she thinks is best, and this may not be what the physician, a nurse, or even a judge thinks is best. Informed consent can therefore sometimes collide with the medical beneficence advocated in the Hippocratic tradition.

Before we leave the legal history of informed consent, we give as an example a case in which a court acknowledged the prerogative of a patient with decision-making capacity to decide against life-saving surgery when her daughter, her physicians, and the court all thought her decision was irrational.

The *Candura* Decision (Massachusetts, 1978)

Mrs. Candura had gangrene in her leg, and her physicians recommended amputation without delay. She was properly informed and consented to the surgery, but then she changed her mind. Her daughter went to probate court, asking to be appointed her mother's guardian with the authority to give consent for the surgery. The probate court judge granted the daughter's request; however, the Massachusetts Appeals Court reversed the decision. It ruled that the daughter could not be the guardian and give consent for this surgery because there was no evidence that her mother was incompetent. The Appeals Court acknowledged that most people would regard Mrs. Candura's refusal of the life-sustaining surgery as unfortunate, but nonetheless, it was an informed decision, and physicians could not force treatment on her without her consent. In short, the "law protects her right to make her own decision to accept or reject treatment, whether that decision is wise or unwise."

This case, which we will consider more in detail in chapter 7, shows the important reverse side of informed consent. The legal doctrine means patients must be informed so they can refuse treatment as well as consent to it. When people have decision-making capacity, their decisions generally should be respected. Family members may consider the decision unwise and irrational, but that is not grounds for overriding the wishes of a person with decision-making capacity. As the Appeals Court wisely stated, "the irrationality of her decision does not justify a conclusion that Mrs. Candura is incompetent in the legal sense." Nor, we might add, does an irrational decision necessarily mean a person is without decision-making capacity in the ethical sense.

The Ethics of Informed Consent

The legal background of informed consent sets forth the two major elements of the informed consent doctrine: information and consent. We now consider these elements in a wider moral context.

Information

What information must the physician disclose and discuss, and what information must the patient be able to understand and discuss, for the consent to treatment to be an informed consent?

    1. Physicians will tell patients their medical diagnosis and the prognosis if nothing is done. In other words, physicians must be sure their patients understand what is wrong and what will happen if the condition is not treated.

    2. Physicians will tell patients about all the medically accepted treatment options for their condition, as well as the risks, burdens, and benefits associated with each. There is a temptation for physicians to neglect disclosure of the burdens because they are naturally reluctant to discuss comprehensively the burdens and possible side effects of interventions that they feel the patient really needs. Yet the patient needs this information if her consent is going to be truly informed. The requirement that physicians disclose all medically accepted treatments also means that the physician may have to provide information about treatments he does not favor or cannot provide.

    3. Physicians will also recommend a treatment plan and give the reasons why they think it is best for the patient. One of the physician's roles is giving professional advice, and patients rightly expect this. Often a patient will ask, "What would you do in my situation?" or "What do you think is best?" The responses to these kinds of questions allow an important conversation to take place and provide the basis for a truly shared decision. It is not really adequate for a physician to do no more than lay out the options and let the patient decide; she must participate with the patient in the decision, and this means informing him of her opinion if she has one.

Consent

Consent requires a certain degree of freedom. If you point a gun at a cashier and tell him to hand over the money in the cash register, most likely he will give you the money. Obviously we would not say he truly consented to giving you the money; he decided to give it to you because he was threatened by the gun and fearful of getting shot. We can truly consent to something only when we have significant freedom to accept or reject it. This means consent in health care must not be forced, coerced, or manipulated.

    Treatment is *forced* when it is given without consent to a patient capable of giving informed consent. In this day and age of informed consent, it might seem that forced treatment is a thing of the past, and to a great extent this is true. But subtle forms of forced treatment can still occur. Suppose a hospice patient wants his do-not-resuscitate order followed in the operating room. During the subsequent operation, he suffers cardiopulmonary arrest. If the physicians attempt resuscitation, they are forcing treatment on him against his will, and this is unethical. If the surgeons had operated on Mrs. Candura against her wishes, that would have been another example of forced treatment.

    Treatment is *coerced* when it is given to a patient who gives consent but not freely. The person is under so much pressure to give consent that the consent is not freely given. Usually the coercion is accomplished by some kind of threat, as when the cashier was threatened by the gun. Coercion is rare in health care, but it sometimes occurs. A husband might threaten to leave his wife unless she has an abortion, for example. She may consent to the procedure, and the providers may think her consent is voluntary, but if the threats are what make her seek the abortion, then she is not truly consenting to it. Her consent is coerced. Again, nursing home personnel may threaten to discharge an elderly welfare patient who needs time-consuming spoon feeding unless he consents to a gastrostomy tube for nutrition. He may agree to the surgery, but his consent is coerced, not voluntary.

A rare kind of coercion occurs when civil authorities put pressure on people to accept medical interventions. Thus, a judge may tell a woman who irresponsibly reproduces every year and so neglects and abuses her babies that a state agency must find foster homes for them that she has a choice between a prison sentence or sterilization. If she gives consent for medical procedures to sterilize her in order to stay out of prison, her consent is not voluntary but coerced. This does not mean, however, that this coercion is necessarily immoral. Some ethicists would argue that it is not immoral to give a woman with a history of frequent pregnancies and convictions of child abuse a choice between serving time or sterilization; others would disagree.

It is important to distinguish between threats and information about adverse consequences. Providers may certainly tell, indeed many times must tell, patients about unpleasant things that will happen if they don't accept treatment. But this is providing information, not threatening patients, as long as no effort is made to coerce the patient to give consent to a procedure.

Treatment is the result of *manipulation* when some technique is used to get the patient to give consent. There are many ways to manipulate people. Some are trivial and can be ignored, but some methods are not trivial and are clearly immoral. Giving a little encouragement to a person hesitating to have a needed but difficult procedure is not the kind of manipulation that causes ethical concerns. But there are less savory ways of manipulating people.

Suppose the physician really thinks the patient ought to have the risky procedure and tries to get consent by saying "Don't worry, most people come through this with no problem" when 40 percent of the people suffer serious consequences or die as the result of the intervention. Strictly speaking what the physician said was true (60 percent is indeed "most" people), but presenting the information this way can be manipulative. If the patient knew 40 percent of the people had serious problems or died as a result of the intervention, he might have withheld consent.

Again, suppose the resident in anesthesia has administered numerous spinal block anesthesias in recent months but has had no opportunity to administer general anesthesia. She understandably wants more experience with general anesthesia and tries to get her patients to accept it. She spends extra time telling them how safe general anesthesia is for healthy people and tells them in great detail of the risks associated with spinal blocks. This can easily become a form of manipulation. She is slanting the preoperative conference in an effort to have patients accept general anesthesia; she is trying to manipulate them, and this is unethical.

Psychological manipulation is also possible. There are ways to make people feel bad, or guilty, or upset if they do not follow what you want them to do. Consider the following: A person has given informed consent for surgery. All the preparations are made. He is prepped, the operating room is ready, and the anesthesiologists, nurses, and surgeon are standing by. It is a busy hospital, and the schedules are always tight. Moreover, the administration is making every effort to achieve maximum utilization of the facilities. Then, on the way to the operating room, the patient says he has changed his mind.

The nurses and residents immediately tell him what a terrible disruption this will cause in everybody's schedule and how his decision will waste valuable operating room time. They do everything they can to make him feel guilty for waiting so long to have changed his mind, for not living up to his agreement when he gave informed consent, and so on. In brief, they are trying to manipulate him so he will agree to the surgery. Without question his action has caused a major problem, and if there is no good reason for it, they have legitimate reason for being upset. But this does not justify the manipulation.

Ethical Significance of Informed Consent

Informed consent fits very well into the ethical framework advanced in the earlier chapters. This framework views ethics as the way each person seeks his or her good. Each moral agent desires a good life, and whatever behavior contributes to a truly good life is morally reasonable. This ethics places a great premium on the individual's figuring out what is truly good in her situation. The ethical person engages in what may be described as either "deliberative reason" or "rational deliberation," to use Aristotle's phrases, and then does what she has decided is good, that is, what she has concluded will achieve her good. Prudence is the intellectual virtue whereby a person "orders" herself to behave in a certain way because that behavior is seen as what will result in good.

All this obviously points to the values underlying informed consent. The ethics of personal responsibility requires the moral agent to deliberate, to figure out how best to achieve happiness in what is often a very confusing situation. This stress on personal deliberation, on practical rather than pure reasoning, on the existential rather than the metaphysical, on the prudence of each moral agent rather than principles, on personal decision rather than authoritarian direction is strongly reinforced by the doctrine of informed consent.

Documentation of Informed Consent

Informed consent is a process involving two major players, the patient and the physician. Normally the patient does not have all the necessary information, so the physician must disclose it. The patient must understand the information, evaluate the impact of the treatment options on his life, deliberate about those options, and then decide to consent or not consent to a course of action. From a moral point of view, we have informed consent when this process occurs. Thus, informed consent may exist even though the informed consent form itself is not signed. And, conversely, informed consent may not exist even though the form is signed. This happens when information was not adequately disclosed or when it was adequately disclosed but not sufficiently understood or when the consent was forced, coerced, or manipulated.

In our society, however, it is extremely important that the process of informed consent be properly documented. It is important to have a record of the informed consent process. Moreover, the documentation requirement can actually encourage the important shared decision-making process and remind everyone of its seriousness.

Informed Consent and Medical Education

Although informed consent is now widely accepted in principle as an integral part of medical and surgical care, there are still areas where this key doctrine is neglected. One of these areas occurs in teaching hospitals where medical students have direct contact with patients and where residents actually provide much of patient care. Here two important values collide: Medical students and residents need to learn how to practice medicine; and to practice medicine they need to practice on the patients. On the other hand, patients deserve the opportunity to make decisions about what happens to them when they are patients in hospitals. Patients need to know what is going on and to have an opportunity to accept or reject the role of becoming a participant in medical education. Sometimes, however, the worthy goal of medical education has overshadowed the need to keep patients well informed and to allow them to be able to make choices about what happens to them.

Part of the problem is that many people are not familiar with the culture of teaching hospitals—hospitals where clinical professors, residents, and medical students play key roles in their care. Briefly stated, a teaching hospital is where people learn how to be doctors. American medical education puts great stress on practical experience, so after the first two years in the classroom medical students spend the next two years at various health care facilities where they learn first hand how to practice medicine by "rotating" through the different services: obstetrics, psychiatry, internal medicine, surgery, and so forth. They usually dress in "scrubs" and perform simple tasks like taking patient histories and actually practice some procedures. Many patients do not understand the system and are not well informed that medical students may be practicing procedures on them. Patients have a right to refuse procedures performed by medical students who are not doctors and should not be practicing on patients without their permission.

Another integral part of teaching hospitals is the presence of newly minted doctors called interns or residents who are not licensed to practice on their own and who are spending three or more years actually practicing on patients under the close supervision of instructors. Thus, for example, when a person in a teaching hospital receives anesthesia, is intubated, undergoes surgery, delivers a baby, or needs some kind of physical examination, it could well be a resident and not an anesthesiologist, surgeon, obstetrician, or physician who provides the intervention. Patients also need to know that medical students may be present before and during the procedures and may actually be practicing some procedures on them. Procedures performed by medical students, of course, are not necessary for patient care. Such procedures benefit the student, not the patient.

What happens in teaching hospitals seldom causes physical harm to patients. They actually receive good care because the supervision is strict and the supervisors are most often among the best in the field. The ethical issue of harm in this instance emerges from two other sources. First, it is not good to disenfranchise patients by not disclosing adequate information and giving patients the opportunity to decide about participating in medical education. Second, it is not good to undermine the trust people have in the medical profession by not disclosing in some detail that goes beyond the general statement that "medical students and residents may be involved in your care." The general practice of resorting to generalities instead of concrete information lest some patients reject the intervention of medical students and residents provides students with more learning opportunities but at the expense of the important moral value of informed consent and personal decision making about what will be done to one's body and by whom.

Adequate disclosure is often lacking because there is a fear, largely unfounded as we will see, that so many people will refuse the interventions of medical students that medical education will be compromised. It is true that patients in teaching hospitals have signed a form on admission or before surgery that says something like "medical students and residents may be involved in my care." But the crucial question is whether this is enough information for truly informed consent that allows medical students to engage in many procedures. Several studies suggest that it is not. These studies show that a significant percentage of patients would decline procedures performed by medical students if they knew about them.

What kind of procedures are we talking about? Two of the most controversial are rectal examinations and pelvic examinations. Sometimes clinical instructors allow medical students to perform these procedures, and often the patient may be under anesthesia at the time and not be aware of them.

In one study published in 2000 two physicians, Peter Ubel and Ari Silver-Isenstadt, reported that about 25 percent of patients definitely would not allow medical students to perform rectal or pelvic exams (the number grows to about 39 percent if the exams occur while patients are under anesthesia). In another study at an OB/GYN clinic in England, 54 percent of women would refuse to let a medical student perform a pelvic exam, and 21 percent would refuse to let a medical student take their medical history. Because patients have a right to decline making themselves available so medical students can learn, these studies suggest that clinical instructors should first explain exactly who medical students are (they are not "student doctors") and obtain permission from patients before they allow medical students to practice these procedures.

In a study reported in the *British Medical Journal* whose chief author was a medical student, a survey reporting the experiences of 386 undergraduate medical students showed that among 702 sedated patients who underwent "practice" rectal or pelvic exams by medical students under anesthesia, written permission existed in only 24 percent of the cases, oral permission in about 50 percent, and students reported that no permission had been given in 24 percent of the cases. And often, more than one medical student practiced these exams on a sedated patient. The survey showed that medical students were often uneasy about doing this without full informed consent, but they felt unable to voice their hesitations.

The problem also exists with residents. In a teaching hospital every anesthesia resident will give general anesthesia, a spinal, or an epidural for the first time to someone, and every surgical resident will perform a first surgery. Because patients can choose to have a fully qualified physician perform these procedures, good ethics suggests that they be made aware of what is happening and be given the opportunity to consent or decline. There is something ethically suspect when a patient is thinking a fully qualified anesthesiologist is going to be administering anesthesia when, in fact, it is a resident who will administer it, or when a patient is thinking her surgeon is going to be performing the surgery when, in fact, it is a resident who will be doing much of the operation and perhaps a medical student who will be suturing the incision.

What might a reasonable approach to this area of conflicted interests be? Perhaps, as so often happens in virtue ethics, the best course is something of a middle path that protects both values—medical education and respect for patients who deserve the opportunity to accept or decline procedures performed by medical students or residents. A key to resolving the dilemma is approaching patients diplomatically and explaining to them the importance of medical education and how they can help. The studies show that, although a significant percentage of patients would decline interventions by medical students, enough will consent to their participation to ensure opportunities for educational practice. This is the approach taken by the AMA in Opinion 8.087 of its Code of Medical Ethics, which includes the following statements:

- Patients are free to choose from whom they receive treatment. When medical students are involved in the care of patients, health care professionals should relate the benefits of medical student participation to patients and *should ensure that they are willing to permit such participation.*
- In instances where the patient will be temporarily incapacitated (e.g., anesthetized) and where students' involvement is anticipated, involvement should be discussed before the procedure is undertaken whenever possible. Similarly, in instances where a patient may not have the capacity to make decisions, student involvement should be discussed with the surrogate decision-maker involved in the care of the patient whenever possible.

Exceptions to Informed Consent

There are times when medical interventions without the patient's informed consent are ethical. One obvious instance occurs when the patient does not have the capacity to give informed consent. In these situations a proxy will be making the decisions and giving the informed consent. Proxy decision making on behalf of patients without decision-making capacity is the subject of the next chapter.

For patients with decision-making capacity, there are four major exceptions to the legal and ethical requirement for informed consent before medical interventions are begun.

Legal Requirements

Sometimes laws or military directives require health care interventions. Examples here include the law of a country requiring immunizations for public health reasons, or a military order requiring immunizations or drugs to protect the health of military personnel and to maintain an effective fighting force.

Emergencies

In most emergencies there is no time to disclose the necessary information for an informed consent. Here the providers simply act according to what they think will be in the best interests of the patient. These situations frequently happen in hospital emergency rooms and when emergency medical personnel arrive on the scene of an accident or sudden illness.

The emergency exception to informed consent is often quite obvious, but this is not always so. It does not apply, for example, when personnel taking care of somebody in an emergency happen to know what the patient wants. In such a situation they would not do what they think is best for the patient but what they know the patient wants.

Consider the following situation. A hospitalized dying patient, with an order not to be resuscitated if respiratory or cardiac arrest occurs, is being transported by ambulance to a nearby facility for a treatment the hospital cannot provide. The patient has not been discharged from the hospital, and he is to be returned in a few hours. During the transport a cardiac arrest occurs. The ambulance crew are trained in CPR and instructed to begin emergency CPR whenever they are called to the scene of a cardiac arrest. Despite knowing the patient has given informed consent for the do-not-resuscitate order, the ambulance crew attempts resuscitation. In effect they are forcing treatment on a patient who knew an arrest was a real possibility and who had made it clear that he did not want resuscitation attempted.

Ambulance personnel will sometimes claim it is ethical for them to attempt resuscitation in such circumstances. They claim emergency personnel must always treat in an emergency and that a cardiac arrest is an emergency. Moreover, their employer's protocols probably require them to treat all people having arrests. This is excellent general advice—the primary response of emergency personnel is to treat if they can.

But attempting resuscitation in these circumstances raises several questions. First, is this really an emergency? The fact that a patient has an order to withhold resuscitation indicates, in most cases, that an arrest is not unexpected. The patient is in the ambulance for routine transportation and not because of an emergency. Second, how can it be plausibly argued that attempting resuscitation for a patient who has declined it is morally reasonable? If the arrest had occurred at the hospital an hour earlier, no attempt to resuscitate the patient would have been made, and everyone would have thought that not attempting resuscitation was the morally right response for this patient. It is difficult to say withholding CPR is no longer the morally right thing to do simply because the patient is being transported in an ambulance for treatment elsewhere.

This example suggests that some interventions made without informed consent under the heading of an emergency are arguably morally suspect, perhaps because it is not really an emergency or perhaps because providers know it is not what the patient wants. A few states have begun to recognize the problems inherent in this kind of emergency resuscitation performed by emergency medical technicians (EMTs) and paramedics, and they are taking steps to introduce legal measures to protect patients from unwanted CPR by EMTs and paramedics. Some emergency department personnel, however, seem to cling to the idea that in an emergency it is up to them to determine what should be done regardless of the known wishes of the patient.

It is important to note that the emergency exception that allows physicians to do what they think is best for the patient without obtaining informed consent from the patient or proxy has one major restriction; namely, they cannot do what they think is best if it is otherwise than what they know the patient or proxy wants. Sometimes, for example, emergency department personnel might know from previous admissions that a particular patient from a local nursing home desires only palliative care. If that patient arrives by ambulance at the same emergency department, it is hard to see how it would be morally reasonable for physicians to take aggressive measures to keep the patient alive when, even though there is no time to obtain consent for orders not to attempt resuscitation or not to intubate, they know he or she or a proxy has decided not to have aggressive life-sustaining measures performed.

An interesting incident some years ago at Massachusetts General Hospital (MGH) resulted in a clear judicial statement limiting the authority of physicians to decide unilaterally what is best for their patients in an emergency. Early on a Sunday morning in March 1990 a young woman named Catherine Shine, who had a long history of asthma, had a serious attack at her sister Anna's apartment. She was improving but let her sister take her to MGH, where she agreed to accept treatment but made it clear that she did not want to be intubated. At first she was given a nebulizer, but after an arterial blood gas test and an examination Dr. Jose Vega decided she had to be intubated. She objected, and a few minutes later she left the cubicle and ran to the exit doors where a security guard, aided by another physician, forcibly escorted her back to the cubicle. Dr. Vega ordered her placed in four-point restraints and then intubated her against her wishes. She recovered and was released from the hospital the next day. Her family later testified that she had been traumatized by the experience.

In July 1992 the same patient suffered another serious asthma attack while at home with her fiancé and brother. She refused to go a hospital, but when she became unconscious, they called an ambulance. She died two days later at the hospital (not MGH).

Her father, also a physician, then sued Dr. Vega and MGH alleging that her experience at MGH in 1990 left her fearful of hospitals and thus caused her to decline hospitalization in 1992, a delay that led to her death. His central claim was that Dr. Vega and MGH had wrongfully restrained and intubated Catherine, which so traumatized her that she later refused transport to a hospital, a situation that led to her death. Lawyers for Dr. Vega and MGH argued that Dr. Vega was faced with a life-threatening emergency and that he acted properly in the emergency situation.

The Superior Court jury decided that the intubation of Catherine against her wishes in 1990 was not wrongful because it was a life-threatening emergency. The judge's instructions to the jury left them little choice. She instructed them to ask first whether Catherine's life was threatened and, if it was, then they should go no further because the life-threatening emergency would absolve the defendants of all liability. The jury decided, correctly, that it had been a life-threatening situation and then, following the judge's instructions, exonerated the doctor and hospital.

Lawyers for Catherine's father appealed the jury verdict and the Massachusetts Supreme Judicial Court (SJC) accepted the case. The basis of the appeal was the prejudicial nature of the judge's instructions despite a long history of informed consent cases that prevent physicians from forcing treatment on patients. The SJC vacated the Superior Court judgment and sent the case back for trial. The case never went to trial, however, because the defendants decided to settle after they read the SJC decision.

In its decision to vacate the lower court decision, the SJC cited the 1972 *Canterbury v. Spence* case that said the emergency exception to informed consent comes into play only when the patient is incapable of giving informed consent, something obviously not true in this case, and even then consent from a relative should be sought. And relatives acting as proxies should, as we will see in the next chapter, choose what the patient would want if they know this. In emergencies doctors can treat unilaterally only if neither the patient nor the family is able to give consent or explain the patient's wishes. The SJC also ruled that the judge should have instructed the jury to consider first whether Catherine was capable of informed consent. If she was, then they should conclude that it was wrong to restrain and intubate her against her wishes.

The case law about informed consent in emergencies is consistent with a virtue-based ethical approach which insists that ethical maturity occurs when we take responsibility for managing our lives, something Catherine was trying to do. For her the reasonable thing was to reject intubation, which had never been necessary before and, since she was actually improving when it was ordered, may not have been necessary that morning. The morally reasonable thing for the doctor to do would have been to respect her wishes rather than put her in restraints and force the intubation on her.

An interesting and seldom discussed aspect of this case is the decision the patient's fiancé and brother made in 1992. At her second major attack she refused hospitalization, and they delayed until she became unconscious and then called for help. Was this a morally reasonable response, or were they forcing hospitalization on her against her wishes? In defense of their actions, one could argue that she may not have expected to lapse into unconsciousness, and thus her refusal was no longer clearly what she would have wanted in these circumstances. Moreover, if she regained consciousness in the hospital, she could always decline any treatment and leave any time she chose. Hence their actions, which showed that they were erring on the side of caution, can be supported by plausible moral reasons. Yet if she had lapsed into unconsciousness at MGH two years earlier, would it have been reasonable to intubate her then? Perhaps it would have been because she could always have requested withdrawal if she recovered decision-making capacity; yet intubation is an emergency intervention that the patient clearly said she did not want. There seems to be no clear morally reasonable response in this kind of situation. It is generally not reasonable for physicians or family to let someone die from an asthma attack that could be reversed by temporary intubation; nor is it generally reasonable to force intubation on someone against her clearly stated wishes.

Waivers

Sometimes patients with decision-making capacity waive their prerogative to give informed consent. They might choose not to be informed of the diagnosis, or of the prognosis, or of the risks. They may even not want to make any decisions about treatment, preferring to leave that in the hands of the physician or another person, perhaps a family member. From a moral point of view there is no problem with patients' waiving their option to give informed consent.

If the patient waives informed consent and expects the physician to make the decisions, however, a difficult situation ensues. In the present cultural climate many physicians will hesitate to accept a patient's wish that the physician make treatment decisions without obtaining informed consent. So strong is the legal and social climate in favor of informed consent that many physicians are uncomfortable working without it, and they will often seek an appropriate proxy to give informed consent and to sign the form.

A patient's waiver is a complex phenomenon. The patient certainly is morally justified in choosing to waive the rights of receiving information and of giving consent, but it is less certain that he can waive the physician's responsibility to disclose information and obtain consent before providing treatment. In effect the patient's waiver is requesting the physician not to disclose information and not to obtain consent before treatment, and the physician may well be unhappy with this arrangement. Moreover the waiver undermines the ideal of shared decision making by putting the whole burden on the physician.

There are times, however, the waiver allowing a physician to treat without informed consent may be morally appropriate. A physician who has known her patient for many years might accept a waiver as the patient, declining with age, becomes less and less able to understand what is going on. Accepting the patient's waiver in these circumstances is more likely to be appropriate when the patient has no immediate family and when the appropriate treatment remains straightforward. Even in these cases, however, a prudent physician may be more comfortable designating a proxy to share the health care decisions.

If a person other than the physician is to make the decisions under the waiver, then the situation is not quite so problematic. It is easy to imagine, for example, an elderly person asking the physician to discuss treatments with a son or daughter and to accept whatever this person decides. Once the physician is certain her patient wants to proceed this way, there is no moral objection to following the patient's wishes. The major responsibility of the physician will then be to supply the family member with all the information needed for informed consent to the interventions.

Therapeutic Privilege

This is a rather controversial exception to obtaining informed consent from a patient with decision-making capacity. The idea is that giving people the truth about their unfortunate diagnosis and expecting them to make an agonizing choice to give or withhold consent for burdensome treatment with an uncertain outcome might devastate them. Physicians and family sometimes fear that the disturbing information and the need for a decision in a tragic situation will cause the patient to become upset, depressed, or emotionally unresponsive, and these negative reactions will make his condition worse. As a result, withholding the bad news might seem to be the right thing to do.

When patients are never told of their unfortunate diagnoses, however, an intolerable situation often develops. Treatments are given, and providers and friends have to perform a dance of pretending—pretending that the illness is only temporary, pretending that the patient "will soon be fine."

Although it may seem that this is the merciful thing to do, most often it is not. There is no evidence that informing patients of their situation when the diagnosis and prognosis are not good is more dangerous to them than pretending everything is fine. Moreover, there are several good reasons for avoiding the dance of pretending. First, it often does not work. People soon begin to sense they are seriously ill and getting worse. And people also sense that others are not being honest with them.

Second, it forces the physicians and nurses to live a lie. They know the truth, but they are expected to conceal it from the patient. This is especially difficult when patients ask pointed questions about their status and when the providers do not agree with the concealment in the first place. Sometimes nurses have to deal with the pointed questions of a patient whom the physician had declined to inform about the serious nature of the illness. Sometimes physicians have to care for patients whose families insist that the patient could not cope with the diagnosis. This undermines the relationship of trust that should exist between providers and patients.

Third, it denies the patient the opportunity to tidy up relations with loved ones and friends and to prepare for death. For many patients this is an important process.

For these reasons the appeal to therapeutic privilege is rarely justified. One situation in which we might be inclined to invoke it involves the medical care of people from other cultures without a strong tradition of individual rights, autonomy, and personal freedom, and with a strong tradition of medical paternalism. People from these cultures might even become hopelessly confused, especially if they are older, when they fall ill in this country and are confronted with the unfamiliar process of informed consent.

Another situation in which therapeutic privilege might be justified centers on patients with a history of psychiatric problems. These cases require very delicate judgment calls, and great sensitivity is required lest the physician prematurely disenfranchise patients of a say in what happens to them.

In general there is widespread agreement that therapeutic privilege should be an extremely rare exception to informed consent and that sufficient information, no matter how terrible, ought to be provided so the patient can participate meaningfully in the decision-making process. The disclosure may be difficult for the physician and upsetting for the patient, but this is often less harmful than the efforts at concealment. Concealing the truth disenfranchises patients by preventing them from making their own decisions. Taking this power away from people is a serious step indeed, and it is the major reason why therapeutic privilege should be so rarely invoked.

ADVANCE DIRECTIVES

Many of us will one day lose our capacity to make health care decisions. When that happens our primary physician will turn to a proxy for decisions about our treatment. Someone else will be giving informed consent for our surgery or ventilator or feeding tube.

If the proxy does not know what treatments we would have wanted, then he may be inclined to give consent for anything that might help to keep us alive. And once life-sustaining therapies are being used, the proxy may find it difficult to request their withdrawal if they become unreasonable. It is not easy to request treatment withdrawals when the result is death.

And if the proxy does request withdrawal of life-sustaining treatment, providers may hesitate to remove it from us unless they have strong evidence that we had previously indicated we did not want the particular therapies. This is so because some state courts, most notably those in Missouri and New York, have insisted that life-sustaining treatment cannot be withdrawn from unconscious patients unless clear and convincing evidence exists that the patient had previously indicated he did not want the specific intervention.

In other words, when we lose our capacity to make decisions, we lose a great deal of control over what happens to us. And it is quite possible that things will be done to us that we would not want done to us.

We can keep some control over what will happen to us in the event we lose our decision-making capacity by making advance directives. Advance directives are our instructions for health care that will become effective if we ever lose our decision-making capacity.

We can set up advance directives two ways: (1) We can prepare written directions about how we want to be treated if certain conditions afflict us, and (2) we can designate someone to report our instructions or, if we didn't give instructions, to make decisions for us. In other words we can write out how we want to be treated, and we can choose someone to speak for us. We will call the instructions for treatment *treatment directives* and the instructions designating who is to speak for us *proxy designations*.

Treatment Directives

There are two kinds of written treatment directives, living wills and medical care directives. Many people call all written directives living wills, but they are not. The major differences between the living will and the more generic medical care directive are that (1) the living will is a formal legal document, and the medical care directive is not; and (2) the living will usually designates only unwanted treatments, whereas the medical care directive almost always includes treatments the person wants. It is helpful, then, to think of a living will as a special type of medical care directive.

Living Wills

Strictly speaking a living will is a legal document similar to the legal will that directs the disposal of our property after death. In the 1960s two groups, the Euthanasia Society of America and Concern for Dying, advocated legal recognition of a will that would allow people to set forth their wishes to have life-support systems withheld or removed in certain situations. For a few years all attempts to pass legislation recognizing such a will failed.

Then the great publicity surrounding the efforts of a New Jersey father to have the respirator removed from his severely brain-damaged and permanently unconscious daughter attracted national attention. The patient was Karen Quinlan, and her landmark case will be considered later. The well-known story of Karen Quinlan, more than anything else in the 1970s, made people aware of the new life-support systems being developed and how they could keep the vital functions of a human body going long after there was any hope of significant recovery.

Legalization of living wills followed soon after the Quinlan case. In 1976 California became the first state to recognize them by what it called the Natural Death Act. In the next year efforts to introduce legal living wills were made in forty-two states and were successful in seven. Today over forty states have some form of legal living will. The laws vary from state to state. Most states insist on some strict conditions that must be met before the living will can be accepted as valid and then executed. Some states, for example, allow only terminally ill people to make them and may require a waiting period after the patient has been informed of such a diagnosis. Other states nullify the will if the person becomes pregnant. The conditions are designed to prevent abuse. Unfortunately they also severely limit the value of the document as an advance directive.

Without question, living will laws represented an important first step in respecting a person's desires not to be treated in ways he would consider unreasonable. But they were only a first step, and today we can see their inadequacies.

1. Many living will laws allow only terminally ill patients, or people whose death is expected within a short time, to make these wills. This leaves everyone else without a means of making advance decisions about treatment.

2. The directives are narrow in that they apply only to treatments people do not want and ignore what treatments they might desire.

3. The language is often vague, using such hard-to-define terms as "heroic measures" or "meaningful quality of life."

4. Most laws providing for living wills do not legislate any penalties if providers choose to ignore them.

5. Providers, especially those working in an emergency situation, have to worry about whether the document really was the person's legal living will. It is always possible that the person had executed it but was thinking of canceling it or that the person had executed a more recent living will or that the document is a forgery.

Efforts are being made, with some success, to overcome the deficiencies of living will laws. At the same time there has been a movement toward a better type of advance directive, the medical care directive.

Medical Care Directives

A medical care directive is a written instruction indicating the care people want if they should ever become incapacitated. The directive is more broad than a living will because (1) anyone capable of informed consent can make one—the person does not have to be terminally or seriously ill, as the laws governing living wills often require; (2) the directions are for providing treatment as well as forgoing it; and (3) the language describing the medical problems that might develop, and the treatments that might be employed, is more concrete and complete than the language found in most living wills.

A typical medical care directive will consider three things: what medical problems might occur, what treatments are available, and what treatments I, as patient, want. The section on what I want can be further nuanced; perhaps I want some care no matter what, or the same care on a trial basis with the understanding it will be withdrawn if it becomes unreasonable. And in some cases I might be undecided about what I would want and state this, leaving the decision up to a proxy.

The kinds of medical problems most often included in a medical care directive are these:

1. Being in a vegetative state or in a coma with little or no hope of regaining awareness
2. Suffering brain damage or any disease that leaves the person totally and permanently incoherent and confused all the time
3. Having any condition, especially a painful one, that is expected to bring death in the next year or so regardless of whether treatments are provided

The major types of treatment most often mentioned in a medical care directive are major surgery, dialysis, providing air by mechanical devices (ventilators and respirators), providing nourishment by tubes or lines, blood transfusions, antibiotics, and cardiopulmonary resuscitation.

Medical care directives are especially important in states such as Massachusetts where living wills are not legally recognized. At the very least they help the physician and proxy decision maker to know what the now incapacitated person would have wanted in the circumstances. As we will see in the next chapter, this puts the proxy in a better position to make good decisions.

Medical care directives have two major advantages for patients. First, they extend the patient's prerogative of informed consent beyond the loss of capacity. Second, they protect the patient from treatments that make little or no sense and that practically no person really wants but that might be given if no advance directives exist.

Some patients, for example, lost all awareness years ago and live on in a persistent vegetative state. They will never again recover any awareness. Most people do not want to be kept alive this way, yet thousands of people are because they left no advance directives. Without evidence that they explicitly said they would not want the life-sustaining interventions, some state courts and some physicians will not honor a proxy's decision to withdraw the life-sustaining treatment.

Although medical care directives are an improvement over legal living wills, they also have their weaknesses. First, it is impossible to anticipate every medical problem that might happen, so the instructions we leave may not be helpful, and they may even mislead those caring for us. Second, people often change their minds as time goes on, and the directives of last year might not reflect the desires of this year. The person functioning as our proxy might be aware of our latest wishes and thus be trapped between honoring our written directives and doing what is more consistent with our later wishes. Third, many people attempting to compose advance directives become bewildered as they think about all the different kinds of medical situations and treatment options available for each. The task overwhelms them, and if they manage to produce a document at all, it is poorly done.

There is a more serious practical problem as well. The medical care directive is really an extensive and extended informed consent document. It usually covers a whole series of hypothetical medical problems and a host of possible treatments. The average patient will need hours of instruction to understand adequately the various diagnoses, prognoses, risks, benefits, costs, alternative treatments, and so forth that are involved in informed consent. Someone has to provide the information leading to advance directives. Normally the physician would be explaining the treatments, risks, side effects, and expected benefits, but few physicians have the time to provide all the necessary information and to discuss the many possible situations covered in a medical care directive. And if they had the time, few physicians would be inclined to do it, knowing that almost all the time would be wasted because so many of the problems and treatment options—unfortunately, we cannot be sure which ones—would never be a real issue for that particular patient.

This has led many to suggest a second kind of advance directive—the designation of a proxy or surrogate who will make decisions for us if ever we cannot.

Proxy Designations

The second type of advance directive, the proxy designation, allows us to designate a person who will make the decisions about withholding and withdrawing our treatments or who will give informed consent for treatment if we ever become incapacitated. We can distinguish two general kinds of proxy designations: the durable power of attorney and the more general health care proxy designation.

Durable Power of Attorney

The law allows us to give another person the power of attorney. This power allows the designated person to carry out certain functions on our behalf. If we are going to be away for an extended time, for example, we can give someone the power of attorney to sign checks to pay our bills. Although the power of attorney usually applies to our property, it could also apply to our person; that is, we could designate a person to make certain decisions about our personal matters as well as about our property. This would seem to make the power of attorney procedure a natural basis for appointing someone to make health care decisions on our behalf if we should ever become incapacitated. Paradoxically, however, this is not the case; the ordinary power of attorney lapses when the person granting the power becomes incapacitated, and this is precisely when we would need the designated attorney to make health care decisions.

One way to prevent the power of attorney from lapsing when the person granting it becomes incapacitated is to authorize a durable power of attorney. The durable power of attorney retains its power when the person granting it loses capacity. All states recognize the durable power of attorney, and most allow it or a similar procedure for the purpose of designating someone to make personal health care decisions for us if we should be unable to make the decisions ourselves. Some states have even instituted a durable power of attorney law designed explicitly for health care matters.

Health Care Proxy Designation

The durable power of attorney is not the only way to designate a proxy decision maker for health care. A simple written directive designating a person to make health care decisions is most often all that is needed. This is because the physician is the person who will have to find the appropriate proxy, and except for extraordinary circumstances, the physician will obviously be relieved to know that the patient has already designated the person he should consult when the patient can no longer make decisions.

Some states, however, have formalized the designation of a proxy or surrogate decision maker by passing laws designed to strengthen the power of such a proxy idea. In July 1990 New York enacted a health care proxy law, and Massachusetts followed in December 1990. A brief review of the Massachusetts law will give us a good idea of recent developments in the trend to formalize the designation of a proxy or surrogate in a legal way.

The Massachusetts Health Care Proxy Act (HCPA) allows an adult with decision-making capacity to designate another adult as his agent to make health care decisions on his behalf in the future. The authority of the agent does not become effective until the attending physician determines that the patient has lost the capacity to make decisions and to give informed consent. The physician must notify the patient orally and in writing of this determination (unless the patient is unconscious or otherwise unable to comprehend) and must enter the determination of incapacity in the patient's medical record.

The designation of the health care agent must be in writing, but there is no required legal form. To be legally recognized, however, the form must clearly identify the agent and indicate that the person intends to have the agent make health care decisions on his behalf. The form must be signed by the person designating the agent and by two witnesses other than the designated agent or any alternate agents who might be named. The witnesses verify that the person was over eighteen, had the capacity to designate an agent, and did it voluntarily.

The form must be dated, and it is revoked automatically if the person makes another proxy designation at a later date. It is also automatically revoked by divorce or legal separation if the agent is the person's spouse. And the person may choose to revoke it at any time orally or in writing or by some action such as crossing it out or tearing it up.

Once the physician has formally determined that the patient has lost the capacity to make health care decisions, the designated proxy in Massachusetts can make any decisions, including decisions to withhold or withdraw life-sustaining treatment, unless the person had restricted the agent's authority on the proxy designation form.

However, the patient, despite being considered incapable of making decisions by the physician, may always veto any of his agent's decisions, unless a court has ruled that the patient is incompetent.

If the physician later determines the person has regained capacity, the proxy loses the authority to make the decisions but regains it if the physician subsequently determines the patient is again incapable of making the decisions. Physicians may, for ethical or religious reasons, choose not to comply with the agent's decisions, but they will then arrange to transfer the care of the patient to another physician or, if this fails, to seek relief in court. Physicians also enjoy immunity from criminal and civil liability if they carry out in good faith the decisions made by the agents properly designated by the Massachusetts HCPA. And, if there is good cause, a physician can always challenge the agent's decisions in court.

This kind of law can be a big help in reinforcing the moral responsibility we have to help others take care of us if we ever lose the capacity to make decisions. In effect the laws extend our powers of decision making and of informed consent into a time when we may be incapable of making decisions. We may expect these laws to become more refined as time goes on and to be accepted in more and more states. New York, for example, has an excellent health care proxy law similar to that of Massachusetts, although there is one notable difference. Although the designated agents in Massachusetts can decide to withhold or withdraw any life-sustaining treatment including medical nutrition and hydration based on the patient's best interests, the proxies in New York can withhold or withdraw all such treatments *except* medical nutrition and hydration; for that they need to have "reasonable knowledge of the patient's wishes" before authorizing the withdrawal. And a family member who is not a designated proxy in New York cannot authorize the withholding or withdrawal of any life-sustaining treatments including CPR unless there is "clear and convincing evidence" that the patient wished not to have those treatments.

We can expect new developments in this direction. Some states, for example, are fashioning laws that would designate an agent for incapacitated patients who did not make such a designation themselves and do not have a court-appointed guardian. The proposed laws would empower a spouse, adult children, parents, siblings, even close friends, to act as designated proxies for those who failed to designate a proxy before they lost capacity.

Since December 1991, there has been a federal law supporting advance directives. It is called the Patient Self-Determination Act (PSDA), and we conclude this chapter with a brief consideration of it.

THE PATIENT SELF-DETERMINATION ACT

In December 1991 the first federal statute on treatment directives and proxy designations went into effect. The law applies to all hospitals, nursing homes, hospices, health maintenance organizations, and home health agencies receiving Medicare or Medicaid funds. Since almost all these institutions do receive these federal funds, the law is almost universal in scope.

The act requires these institutions to provide written information to each adult patient about the right to make health care decisions, to refuse treatment, and to write advance directives for use if the person should ever become incapacitated. The law encourages, but does not require, adults to make both treatment directives and proxy designations.

This statute provides an excellent opportunity for people to think about advance directives and to make some provision for them. Only if people make some kind of advance directives can we avoid the guessing game that often transpires when providers, family, and friends do not know what a patient would want, and it is too late to ask. To this end the statute encourages community education programs to increase the general public's awareness of advance directives and to urge people to formulate them. This is one of the more important aspects of the act because it helps to create a general social attitude encouraging advance directives.

Only time will tell how successful the PSDA will be. One weakness lies in the process itself. The information about the right to make decisions and formulate advance directives is provided on admission to the hospital or nursing home or on enrollment in the health maintenance organization. As we all know, clerical personnel, not physicians or other health care providers, take care of the formalities of admission to a clinic or of enrollment in an HMO. The danger is that the very important matter of treatment directives may become separated from dialogue with the physician and become lost in the admissions or enrollment processes.

Formulating advance directives is really a kind of informed consent for future treatment as well as a decision to forgo certain treatments. These consents and treatment refusals are serious matters, and the decisions are best shared with the attending physician. If the act encourages people to discuss with their physicians their wishes about the more common forms of medical treatments available for serious problems that may arise, then it will be a great success.

Not everybody is happy with the PSDA legislation. Some pro-life groups have opposed it, perhaps fearing it would lead to euthanasia. Some people agreed with the idea of treatment directives but felt it was not a good idea to have a federal law intruding into the area of personal health care decisions. Others felt the legislation should have made physicians rather than institutions responsible for providing the information because physicians are the people primarily responsible for treating patients according to their wishes.

How successful have the PSDA legislation and other efforts been in encouraging patients to express their wishes and in having physicians follow them? Many feel the progress has been less than satisfactory. Too many people still become patients without indicating how they want to be treated or who they want to make decisions for them if they should ever lose decision-making capacity. More important, a major study published four years after the PSDA showed that the preferences of many patients at the end of life are being ignored. The study is known as SUPPORT (Study to Understand Prognosis and Preferences for Outcomes and Risks of Treatment) and deserves our attention.

The first phase of SUPPORT was a two-year project to determine how physicians in five teaching hospitals were treating people at the end of life. At the conclusion of the two years a review of nine thousand cases revealed some serious problems. Nearly 40 percent of the dying patients spent the last days of their lives receiving aggressive life-support treatments in intensive care units, and families reported that about one-half of them were in serious pain. In 80 percent of the cases physicians did not understand their patients' wishes about resuscitation efforts. And physicians declined to write orders to withhold resuscitation efforts for one-half of the patients who indicated they did not want any resuscitation efforts. The overuse of aggressive life support, the failure to provide comfort care, and the disregard of patients' wishes at the end of life are disturbing.

The second two-year phase of SUPPORT covered 1991–1993, a time when the PSDA became effective. Researchers set up a control group of about twenty-five hundred patients whose physicians became the subjects of intense efforts to make them more responsive to their patients' pain and preferences at the end of life. Despite expectations that the situation would improve, the results were a shocking surprise. The efforts to have patients treated the way they wanted to be treated in the hospitals had practically no impact on the way physicians actually treated them. The culture of medicine with its emphasis on intervention clearly overwhelmed the wishes of very sick hospital patients.

Why were so many physicians in teaching hospitals ignoring their patients' wishes? Undoubtedly many factors are at work but a significant one is the tendency of some physicians to let their desire to save lives override moral values. The culture of medicine has long taught physicians to do what they think is best for their patients regardless of what the patient wants, and cultures change slowly.

The following true story shows how this can happen. It is taken from *How We Die*, a best-selling book in the 1990s written by a professor of surgery at Yale–New Haven Hospital who was also a member of the institution's Bioethics Committee. The brief case will help explain the dismal results of the SUPPORT study by showing how clinical decisions sometimes override ethical values.

As noted in the Introduction, the cases are presented as an integral part of the discussions describing decision making about treatment options. Each case is presented in two stages: the first stage provides situational awareness, and the second suggests how each major agent might engage in prudential reasoning as each faces the various available options.

Our consideration of cases in this and subsequent chapters illustrates the prudential reasoning described in chapter 2. The format in which the cases are presented might suggest a rigorous method, but this is not the case. The format is, rather, simply an illustration of one way prudential deliberation and moral judgment might unfold in situations suggested by the cases. Practical moral reasoning—deciding what to do when we do not have all the facts, are faced with much uncertainty, and cannot predict exactly how our decision will turn out—is not a logical exercise that lends itself to a rigorous method. Rather, we work our way through life and the dilemmas it presents by relying on our moral character, experience, insight, intuition, and feeling to perceive a promising move that will enhance virtuous personal human flourishing, be consistent with the common good, and reduce what undermines these goods.

The Case of Hazel Welch

The Story

Hazel was a ninety-two-year-old resident in a convalescent unit of a senior citizen residence. She could no longer walk because of her advanced arthritis. Her circulation problems would soon require amputation of a toe. She also suffered from leukemia, but it was in remission. Her mental abilities were intact.

After collapsing in her room she was rushed to the hospital where doctors diagnosed a perforated digestive tract. After receiving IV fluids she regained awareness and became completely lucid. The surgeon explained that food and fluid leaking into her abdominal cavity were causing infection. He said immediate surgery was needed to close the perforation and sought her consent. To his surprise she refused, saying she had been on this planet "quite long enough, young man." He then used every argument he could muster to persuade her to have the surgery. He admitted the surgery would give her only a one in three chance of survival but pointed out that those odds were certainly better than certain death without the surgery. And he downplayed negative aspects such as a difficult postoperative recovery because of her age and circulatory problems.

Hazel adamantly refused to consent, so he gave her some time to think it over. When he returned fifteen minutes later she looked directly into his eyes and said "I'll do it but only because I trust you." She signed the consent form, and the surgery was performed.

Ethical Analysis

Situational awareness. Here we pause and consider the main facts and ethical features, both good and bad, in the story. We are aware of the following facts.

1. Hazel was ninety-two and unable to walk. She suffered from a gangrenous toe that would require amputation in the near future, leukemia that was in remission, severe arthritis, and serious

circulation problems. Then her digestive tract became perforated, which is a life-threatening situation.

  2. Hazel was also cognitively intact; she had the capacity to make decisions about her treatments. When she learned that the surgery on her intestines would probably fail, she decided against it.

  3. The surgeon, knowing that the surgery was the only thing that might save her life, persuaded her to change her mind to have the surgery.

We are also aware of the following good and bad features in Hazel's story.

  1. Hazel will die without surgery, and the loss of life is bad.

  2. The surgery might save her life, and this would be good.

  3. The surgeon is experiencing distress from two sources. He does not want his patient to die, and he does not want his colleagues at the weekly surgical conference to criticize him for poor judgment and negligence if he lets Hazel have her way. He wrote: "I would almost certainly be castigated over my failure to overrule such a seemingly senseless wish." His distress over losing a patient and over future criticism is a bad experience for him.

  4. The surgeon truthfully pointed out that Hazel had only a one-in-three chance of survival with the surgery, and this is good. However, in an effort to get her consent, he admitted that he "played down what she could realistically be expected to experience" during her postoperative recovery, and this is bad.

Prudential Reasoning in the Hazel Welch Story

Patient's perspective.   Hazel's perspective is most important here because she is cognitively intact. She is in the best position to weigh the benefits and burdens of major surgery at this point in her life. At ninety-two, she has already lost much of what makes a human life good. She has no family, is confined to a bed and chair in a convalescent wing of a senior citizen home, suffers from arthritis and circulatory problems, will likely soon need surgery to remove a toe because of her circulation problems, and has other health problems. In her mind, the abdominal surgery is not a reasonable choice for her. It will probably fail, and if it does succeed it will add additional discomfort to her life while at best only restoring her to a very limited life.

  It would be difficult to say her decision is unreasonable. She knows the surgery will probably fail, and if it does succeed, she doesn't think the benefits to her at this stage in her life outweigh the burdens. It is possible that another person in a similar situation would find it reasonable to accept surgery. In other words, when ethics comes down to its bottom line—the personal decision by a particular person—it sometimes happens that what one person will see as a good choice another will see as a bad one.

  A virtue-based ethic of the good, unlike a rule-based ethics of obligation, allows this discrepancy because prudence puts the ultimate moral decision in the hands of the person trying to live well. It does not ask what would be the patient's moral obligation in a situation such as this; it asks what would be good, and in a situation such as this, the good is something the person herself can best determine.

Surgeon's perspective.   The surgeon was naturally upset when Hazel declined the surgery. He sincerely wanted her to live and knew she needed the surgery for that. He also admitted that he dreaded the criticisms of his colleagues at a distinguished medical school if he let her have her way and refuse the surgery. So he decided to persuade her to give consent for the surgery. Efforts at persuasion are not normally morally problematic. Persuasion is not coercion, and it can be helpful when people need encouragement to undergo something difficult that might be good for them. But the physician also acknowledged that he decided not to inform her fully of what she could expect with the surgery and during recovery. His intentions were good, but, as we saw in this chapter, his decision to downplay the side effects was morally problematic because it misled the patient. In effect, the surgeon did not really receive a fully informed consent for the surgery.

Ethical Reflection

The surgeon in this case was Dr. Sherwin Nuland, author of the best-selling book *How We Die*. His comments on the case show how clinical concerns can unfortunately override ethical values in some cases. On the one hand he acknowledged that he had not made a good ethical decision: "For Miss Welch, the effort was not justified, no matter what success might have resulted, and I was not wise enough to recognize it. I see things differently now." He went on to say that "paternalism was precisely the source of my error in treating Miss Welch."

Yet, on the other hand, Dr. Nuland wrote that it would be a "lie" for him to imply that he would have acted differently even if he had recognized his error. He admitted that he probably would have done the same thing again, partly because "the code of the profession of surgery demands that no patient as salvageable as Miss Welch be allowed to die if a straightforward operation can save her." His clinical concerns trumped ethics: "Viewed by a surgeon, mine was strictly a clinical decision, and ethics should not have been a consideration." He concluded that "ethicists and moralists run aground when they try to judge the actions of bedside doctors."

The view that clinical decisions override ethics is incoherent in an ethics of the good. If ethics is about seeking the bottom-line goal in one's life; that is, making one's life a good life, then ethical decisions trump all others. Once a moral agent allows professional goals to override the greatest goal of any human life—happiness, living a good life, living virtuously—he misses what Aristotle called the "target."

The actual outcome of the case is of interest even though it has no bearing on the ethics of the surgeon's decision to ignore his patient's reasonable wishes. The surgery repaired Hazel's digestive tract but left her in a confused state and kept alive by a ventilator. A week later her mind cleared, and two days after that she improved enough so the ventilator could be removed. As soon as she could talk she began criticizing Dr. Nuland. "She lost no time in letting me know what a dirty trick I had pulled, [and] she didn't hesitate to let me know I betrayed her by minimizing the difficulties of the postoperative period." Hazel had trusted the physician but felt that he had betrayed that trust. This is unfortunate because trust is a crucial moral ingredient in any productive physician-patient relationship.

When Hazel returned to her room in the senior citizen residence, she wrote out advance directives with emphatic directions indicating that she wanted nothing but nursing care if anything else happened to her. Two weeks later she suffered a massive stroke. The staff at the home, unlike those in the hospital, respected her wishes and did not transfer her to the hospital. She died the next day. Her story is a vivid example of what the SUPPORT study uncovered—how the culture of medicine in teaching hospitals tends to ignore people's wishes at the end of life by forgetting ethical considerations at the bedside.

FINAL REFLECTIONS

Informed consent, advance directives, state health care proxy laws, and the federal PSDA fit very well with the ethical perspective outlined earlier. This ethics is a morality of the good understood as the good we achieve for ourselves by the moral choices we make in life. Advance directives are an expansion of this ethics into future situations that might happen to us. We imagine what could happen to us, and we indicate what we think our moral response in these situations would be. Our advance directives extend our decision making into a future when we might no longer be able to make prudential decisions in our lives.

Treatment directives are important for another reason—making them is a virtuous thing to do. They prevent our physician, other providers, and our loved ones from being left in the predicament of trying to figure out how we would want to be treated if we ever lose the capacity to decide. Doing something good for others for their sake is what we call the virtue of love.

Making advance directives also manifests the virtues of courage and justice. It takes courage to deal with our disintegration and death, and arranging to forgo unreasonable treatment exhibits justice. Spending money for treatments a person would not want is a terrible waste of resources.

In an ethics where the goal is the good life, rightly understood, of the persons behaving as moral agents, the personal responsibility of persons for their own well-being is obvious. In an ethics whose norm is "according to right reason," treatment directives make a lot of sense. The morally good behavior is always the reasonable behavior designed to achieve the good. Without advance directives, the unreasonable is often done, and the good is not achieved.

Good ethics encourages people to make advance directives carefully. Perhaps the best way to do this is by making an advance directive that combines treatment directives with a proxy designation. We might call this the *combined advance directive*.

The combined advance directive has two parts. In one part we consider what might happen in the future and how we want to be treated and then indicate this in writing to help others know our wishes if it should happen that we are no longer able to communicate them. In the other part we appoint a proxy (and, if possible, an alternate in case the proxy is not available) and grant the proxy the general authority to decide whether to provide, withhold, or withdraw treatment and medical nutrition subject to whatever limitations, if any, we indicate on the form designating the proxy.

The key to any advance directive is clarity. The underlying assumption is that providing all possible treatment all the time is, in this era of modern technology and medical technique, simply not reasonable or moral. So advance directives are decisions about treatment—what to provide and what to forgo, and who is to make decisions when I no longer can. But these directives need to be concrete. It is not enough to appoint a proxy; I have to make sure my proxy knows my thoughts about life, suffering, and death and about treatments I would find reasonable.

The combined advance directive brings together the best of treatment directives and of proxy appointments. It gives my directions in some degree of detail, but it also designates a person for making decisions. This is important because I cannot anticipate every possible aspect of future events in my written directives, and a proxy is very helpful in resolving difficulties of interpretation and in dealing with complications unforeseen by me. The proxy is also someone with whom the physician and other providers can communicate when communication with me is impossible.

The combined advance directive, of course, is not a perfect solution to this difficult problem of extending informed consent and patient decision making beyond the loss of capacity. Many of the problems associated with treatment directives and proxy designations still haunt the combined directive. Moreover, a conflict may develop between my written directives and what my appointed proxy thinks I would want in a particular set of circumstances. For example, my proxy may conclude that I did not really intend my directive to be followed in the unanticipated situation that actually developed. The proxy may also have reasons for thinking I was changing my mind about some of the treatment directives.

It is not easy to sort things out when my treatment directives and the proxy's opinion of what I would now want are in conflict. I can reduce the problem somewhat if I include in my combined directive some instructions on how I would want such a conflict resolved. I could say that my proxy has the final say, or I could say that the treatment directives should prevail in the event of a conflict. Without such a provision in the combined directive, providers and others will be in a real quandary when these conflicts occur. Seeking relief in the courts is a last resort in health care because the adversarial atmosphere of the courts is not really the place for personal health care decisions, but sometimes there is no alternative.

Advance directives and the 1991 Patient Self-Determination Act remind us of the important role proxies play in health care decision making. The next chapter considers the matter of proxy decision making and explains how a proxy makes health care decisions for others.

Suggested Readings

A valuable online source of thoughtful articles on bioethics and suggested readings that has been appearing monthly is the AMA Journal of Ethics at virtualmentor.org. The August 2008 issue (virtual mentor.ama-assn.org/2008/08) was devoted to decision-making capacity and informed consent. A good introduction to the notion of decision-making capacity is found in two reports of the President's Commission, 1982, *Making Health Care Decisions*, volume I, Washington, DC: U.S. Government Printing Office, pp. 55–62; and 1983, *Deciding to Forego Life-Sustaining Treatment*, Washington, DC: U.S. Government Printing Office, p. 45. Also helpful is the 1985 American Hospital Association report titled *Values in Conflict: Resolving Ethical Issues in Hospital Care*, Chicago: AHA, pp. 9–12. See also Paul Appelbaum and Thomas Grisso, "Assessing Patients' Capacities to Consent to Treatment," *New England Journal of Medicine* 1988, *319*, 1635–38; Bernard Lo, "Assessing Decision-Making Capacity," *Law, Medicine & Health Care* 1990, *18*, 193–201; James Drane, "Competency to Give an Informed Consent: A Model for Making Clinical Assessments," *JAMA* 1984, *252*,925–27; Mary Cutter and Earl Shelp, eds., l991, *Competency: A Study of Informal Competency Determinations in Primary Care*, Dordrecht: Kluwer Academic Publishers; E. Haavi Morreim, "Impairments and Impediments in Patients' Decision Making: Reframing the Competence Question," *Journal of Clinical Ethics* 1993, *4*, 294–307; Paul Appelbaum, "Assessment of Patients' Competence to Consent for Treatment," *New England Journal of Medicine* 2007, *357*, 1834–40.

An excellent source for the history of informed consent is Ruth Faden and Tom Beauchamp, 1986, *A History and Theory of Informed Consent*, New York: Oxford University Press. For a complete overview of informed consent from the important legal perspective, see Fay Rozovsky, 2007, *Consent to Treatment: A Practical Guide*, 4th ed., New York: Aspen Publishers. See also Franz Ingelfinger, "Informed (But Uneducated) Consent," *New England Journal of Medicine* 1972, *287*, 466; Eugene Laforet, "The Fiction of Informed Consent," *JAMA* 1976, *235*, 1579–85; Charles Lidz and Allen Meisel, "What We Do and Do Not Know about Informed Consent," *JAMA* 1981, *246*, 2473–77; Charles Lidz et al., "Informed Consent and the Structure of Medical Care," in *Making Health Care Decisions*, volume II, pp. 317–410; Gerald Dworkin, "Autonomy and Informed Consent," in *Making Health Care Decisions*, volume III, pp. 63–81; and the series of articles in the special section titled "Informed Consent in Medical Practice," *Journal of Clinical Ethics* 1994, *5*, 189–223 and 243–266.

For a very comprehensive bibliography (377 entries, each with a brief summary) on informed consent conveniently indexed according to main topics such as decision-making capacity, disclosure of information, understanding, and voluntariness, see the Special Supplement by Jeremy Sugarman et al., "Empirical Research on Informed Consent," *Hastings Center Report* 1999, *29* (January–February), S1–S42. The literature on informed consent is vast. Some notable texts include Jessica Berg et al., 2001, *Informed Consent: Legal Theory and Clinical Practice*, 2nd ed. New York: Oxford University Press; and Neil Manson and Onora O'Beill, 2007, *Rethinking Informed Consent in Bioethics*, New York: Cambridge University Press.

There is a growing awareness that not all people consider patient self-determination and informed consent as valuable as does traditional American bioethics with its emphasis on the principle of (patient) autonomy. Many people from other cultures and some from Western culture, especially if they are elderly or severely ill, often prefer to rely on family members for decision making even when they have decision-making capacity. For background on this see the special section "Difference and the Delivery of Healthcare," *Cambridge Quarterly of Healthcare Ethics* 1998, *7*, 1–87; and another special section, "Cultural Difference," *Journal of Clinical Ethics* 1998, *9*, 99–193. A prudent physician could ask his patients how much they want to be involved in decision making and, if they wish to defer to proxies, ask them to waive their prerogative and note the waiver in the medical record.

The citations for the landmark legal decisions shaping informed consent are *Schloendorff v. Society of New York Hospital*, 211 N.Y. 125 (1914); *Salgo v. Leland Stanford Jr. University Board of Trustees*, 317 P.2d 170 (1957); *Canterbury v. Spence*, 464 F.2d 772 (1972); and *Lane v. Candura*, 376 N.E.2d 1232 (1978). The Catherine Shine case is *Shine v. Vega*, 709 N.E.2d 58 (1999). For a summary of the Shine case see George Annas, "The Last Resort—Use of Physical Restraints in Medical Emergencies," *New England Journal of Medicine* 1999, *341*, 1408–12.

For the importance of informed consent in medical education see Adam Wolfberg, "The Patient as Ally—Learning the Pelvic Examination," *New England Journal of Medicine* 2007, *356*, 889–90; Yvette Coldicott et al., "The Ethics of Intimate Examinations—Teaching Tomorrow's Doctors," *British Medical Journal* 2003, *326*, 97–101; and Peter Ubel et al., "Don't Ask, Don't Tell: A Change in Medical Student Attitudes after Obstetrics/Gynecology Clerkships toward Seeking Informed Consent for Pelvic Examinations on an Anesthetized Patient," *American Journal of Obstetrics and Gynecology* 2003, *88*, 575–79 (Ubel discovered that students are *less* likely to seek informed consent for pelvic exams after their ob/gyn rotations). See also the Case Study titled "Moral Priorities in a Teaching Hospital," *Hastings Center*

Report 2006, *36* (November–December), 13–14; and Peter Ubel and Ari Silver-Isenstadt, "Are Patients Willing to Participate in Medical Education?" *Journal of Clinical Ethics* 2000, *11*, 230–35.

For advance directives, see chapter 3 of the President's Council on Bioethics 2005 report titled "The Limited Wisdom of Advance Directives," available at bioethics.gov; George Annas, "The Health Care Proxy and the Living Will," *New England Journal of Medicine* 1991, *324*, 1210–13; Linda Emanuel et al. "Advance Directives for Medical Care—a Case for Greater Use," *New England Journal of Medicine* 1991, *324*, 889–95; Nancy King, 1991, *Making Sense of Advance Directives*, Boston: Kluwer Academic Publishers; Linda Emanuel and Ezekiel Emanuel, "The Medical Directive: A New Comprehensive Advance Care Document," *JAMA* 1989, *261*, 3288–93; Ezekiel Emanuel and Linda Emanuel, "Living Wills: Past, Present, and Future," *Journal of Clinical Ethics* 1990, *1*, 9–19; Judith Areen, "Advance Directives under State Law and Judicial Decisions," *Law, Medicine & Health Care* 1991, *19*, 91–100; and Linda Emanuel, "Advance Directives: What Have We Learned So Far?" *Journal of Clinical Ethics* 1993, *4*, 8–16.

Commentaries on the Patient Self-Determination Act include John La Puma, "Advance Directives on Admission: Clinical Implications and Analysis of the Patient Self-Determination Act of 1990," *JAMA* 1991, *266*, 402–405; Susan Wolf et al., "Sources of Concern about the Patient Self-Determination Act," *New England Journal of Medicine* 1991, *325*, 1666–71; Elizabeth McCloskey, "The Patient Self-Determination Act," *Kennedy Institute of Ethics Journal* 1991, *1*, 163–69; Charles Sabatino, "Surely the Wizard Will Help Us, Toto? Implementing the Patient Self-Determination Act," *Hastings Center Report* 1993, *23* (January–February), 12–16; Mathy Mezey and Beth Latimer, "The Patient Self-Determination Act: An Early Look at Implementation," *Hastings Center Report* 1993, *23* (January–February), 16–20; Joanne Lynn and Joan Teno, "After the Patient Self-Determination Act: The Need for Empirical Research on Formal Advance Directives," *Hastings Center Report* 1993, *23* (January–February), 20–24; Elizabeth McClosky, "Between Isolation and Intrusion: The Patient Self-Determination Act," *Law, Medicine & Health Care* 1991, *19*, 80–82; and Jeremy Sugarman et al., "The Cost of Ethics Legislation: A Look at the Patient Self-Determination Act," *Kennedy Institute of Ethics Journal* 1993, *3*, 387–399. See also the special supplement titled "Practicing the PSDA," *Hastings Center Report* 1991, *21* (September–October), S1–S16; and Lawrence Ulrich, 1999, *The Patient Self-Determination Act: Meeting the Challenge in Patient Care*, Washington, DC: Georgetown University Press.

The results of SUPPORT were published as "A Controlled Trial to Improve Care for Seriously Ill Hospitalized Patients," *JAMA* 1995, *274*, 1591–98. For thoughtful commentaries see the special supplement "Dying Well in the Hospital: The Lessons of SUPPORT," *Hastings Center Report* 1995, *25* (November–December), S1–S36. The Robert Wood Johnson Foundation funded SUPPORT, and after it was finished the Foundation provided additional grants to improve care at the end of life. One such initiative funded a project called EPEC (Education of Physicians on End-of-life Care) to develop a standardized core curriculum to train physicians about ethics, communication, palliative care, and pain control at the end of life. See also Andrew Skolnick, "End-of-Life Care Movement Growing," *JAMA* 1997, *278*, 967–69. The story of Hazel Welch is taken from Sherwin Nuland, 1995, *How We Die*, New York: Random House, pp. 250–58.

For two important articles underlining what constitutes good end-of-life care from the patients' point of view, see Peter Singer et al., "Quality End-of-Life Care: Patients' Perspectives," *JAMA* 1999, *281*, 163–68; and Peter Singer et al., "Reconceptualizing Advance Care Planning from the Patient's Perspective," *Archives of Internal Medicine* 1998, *158*, 879–84. The American Board of Hospice and Palliative Medicine began board certifications in 1996. See Mary Bretscher and Edward Creagan, "Understanding Suffering: What Palliative Medicine Teaches Us," *Mayo Clinic Proceedings* 1997, *72*, 785–87; Sean Morrison et al., "The Growth of Palliative Care Programs in United States Hospitals," *Journal of Palliative Medicine* 2005, *8*, 1127–34; and Benjamin Goldsmith et al., "Variability in Access to Hospital Palliative Care in the United States," *Journal of Palliative Medicine* 2008, *11*, 1094–1102. See also nineteen articles relevant to palliative care in the ICU in a supplement to *Critical Care Medicine* 2006, *34*, S301–420; and a Hastings Center special report: Bruce Jennings et al., eds., 2007, *Improving End of Life Care*, Garrison, NY: The Hastings Center. The Center's earlier special supplement, Bruce Jennings et al., eds., 2003, *Access to Hospice Care: Expanding Boundaries*, Garrison, NY: The Hastings Center, is also helpful.

FIVE

Deciding for Others

MANY PATIENTS do not have the capacity to make health care decisions. Some, children and those with congenital mental impairments, never had decision-making capacity. Others had it once but have lost the capacity because of various medical or psychological problems. Because patients without decision-making capacity can no longer make decisions to receive or to refuse treatment, other people will make these treatment decisions and give consent on their behalf. The person making these decisions is called a *proxy* or a *surrogate*.

In the previous chapter we defined the three essential elements of decision-making capacity. They were (1) the ability to understand and communicate relevant information, (2) the possession of a framework of values providing a context for particular value judgments, and (3) the ability to reason about different outcomes, risks, and chances of success. If any one of these three elements is absent to a significant degree, then the person does not have decision-making capacity.

The responsibility of determining the absence of the capacity to make health care decisions rests with the physician. This is so because apart from exceptional circumstances such as emergencies, a physician cannot treat a patient without voluntary and informed consent, and consent is valid only if the person has the capacity to give it.

Although the physician determines when a patient lacks decision-making capacity, the determination is not normally based on medical criteria or on a psychiatric consultation. The determination of incapacity is a practical judgment that any mature person who knows the patient can make. It is a judgment made by a medical professional, but it is not a medical or professional judgment. The exception to this is mental illness. When mental illness has been diagnosed, medical expertise and psychiatric consultations are often needed to determine whether or not the patient has decision-making capacity.

Sometimes a person lacks all decision-making capacity. This is the case, for example, with unconscious patients or young children. Sometimes, however, a person lacks decision-making capacity in a more limited sense. A patient may have the capacity to make decisions about some treatments but not about others, or she may have the capacity to make decisions at this time but not at another time. Hence, what the physician must determine is whether or not the patient has the capacity to decide about a particular treatment at a particular time.

It is also the responsibility of the physician to identify the appropriate proxy when his patient lacks decision-making capacity. Sometimes this is a simple matter. The patient may have already designated a proxy, or supportive family members may be available. When a patient has not designated a proxy or when family members are not available, the physician's task of identifying the appropriate proxy can be difficult.

When the physician is working with a proxy, he must be aware of any conflict of interest or of any emotional baggage that could distort the proxy's decisions. For example, some children anxious to preserve an inheritance might decline life-sustaining treatment for an elderly parent suffering from a stroke because they know it can lead to years of expensive care in a nursing home. Again, some children, feeling guilty about neglecting a parent for years, might insist on "doing everything" when the treatment is burdensome and of no real benefit to their parent. The physician's primary clinical responsibility is always the care of the patient, and he will reject the unreasonable requests of proxies.

BECOMING A PROXY

A person can become a proxy and make health care decisions for an incapacitated patient in several ways.

Patient-Designated Proxy

The best way of becoming a proxy is to be designated by the patient before decision-making capacity has been lost. When patients have chosen their proxies, it makes everything much easier for the physician as well as for everyone else. If the patient loses capacity, the physician simply turns to the designated proxy for treatment decisions and informed consent.

In many cases, however, patients have not selected a proxy, and the physician of an incapacitated patient must find the person or persons with whom the shared decision making will occur and who will give informed consent whenever it is required for treatment interventions.

Family Members as Proxies

If the patient has supportive and capable family members, identifying a proxy is normally a relatively simple matter for the physician. A spouse is usually the proxy for a mate, a child or children are usually appropriate for a widowed parent, and parents are the proxies of first choice for their minor children.

There is growing recognition, however, that in many families, even loving families, people often do not really have a good idea of their loved one's treatment preferences. Caring about someone and living with her for years does not guarantee that we would know what she would want if she became incapacitated. Many people in families retain a significant degree of privacy about certain areas of their lives, including how they might want to be treated when ill. Adult children may not really know what their aging parents want, and some spouses may not really know what their partner wants.

We cannot, therefore, always assume that members of a family know the wishes of an incapacitated family member. Perhaps they do know; perhaps they do not. This is why physicians cannot simply accept a family member's decisions for a loved one who once had decision-making capacity. Physicians need to ask family members *why* they believe an intervention is something their loved one would, or would not, want. When family members say "She would not want a feeding tube" or "He did not want to be kept alive by machines," physicians do well to ask such questions as: "What did your mother or your father ever say or do that makes you think she or he would, or would not, want the feeding tube or the life-support equipment?"

Significant Others as Proxies

It is always possible that someone outside the family has a better idea of what the patient wants. If this is so, then this person would be in a better position to act as proxy for the patient. Of course this could easily generate a very volatile situation if the family members object. Unfortunately, if their objections are successful, it could mean a patient will be denied the proxy best suited to report what he wanted.

The typical situation where a significant other would make a better proxy than a family member occurs when the patient no longer lives with family and has established a close and enduring relationship with another person but never married him or her. No simple formula exists for determining when this significant other is a better proxy than a family member. It is yet another area where prudence is a valuable resource.

People from the pastoral care and social work support systems and other members of the health care team can sometimes provide information of great help to the physician in identifying a significant other as the appropriate proxy. The idea is to designate as proxy a person who knows and cares about the patient, is aware of the patient's desires, is available, and is willing to become informed about the diagnosis, the prognosis, the available treatments, and the side effects and risks of treatments. If a patient has had no meaningful contact with his family for decades, it makes no sense to think a family member is the most suitable proxy.

Court-Appointed Proxies

Problems can arise over the designation of a proxy for any number of reasons. Perhaps there is no family or significant other available, or the family is available but hopelessly divided over what should be done. Perhaps a proxy is requesting something clearly inappropriate for a patient.

Sometimes the physician and social workers can resolve the difficulty, but at other times they must fall back on the last resort and seek a court-appointed guardian. If a court does appoint a guardian to make health care decisions, the guardian's decisions have priority over those of any other proxy. If the physician or the family disagrees with the court-appointed guardian's decisions, they cannot overrule him, but they can challenge the decision in court.

Once the matter of designating a proxy lands in the courts, the process often becomes complicated, especially if the decision involves withholding or withdrawing life-sustaining treatment. Courts rely on an adversarial process—that is, people present arguments both pro and con. And instead of a simple procedure to appoint a guardian with the power of making a decision, the legal process often extends to the treatment issue itself and thereby turns the case into a whole new question that sometimes involves judges making decisions either for treatment or for its withdrawal.

STANDARDS FOR MAKING PROXY DECISIONS

When proxies make health care decisions for other people, they need to rely on some kind of standards to guide their judgments. The two widely recognized standards in health care ethics are called *substituted judgment* and *best interests*. Both these standards are patient centered. In cases of substituted judgment, the wishes of the patient prevail; in cases of best interests, the benefit to the patient prevails.

Sometimes, however, neither of these standards applies, and the proxy will have to rely on a third standard, what we will call the *reasonable treatment* standard. This standard is provider-centered; the proxy determines what is reasonable treatment in the circumstances.

Substituted judgment is the preferred standard, and the proxy will rely on it whenever possible. Only if the proxy cannot use substituted judgment will she turn to the best interests standard. And only if neither substituted judgment nor the best interests standard is appropriate will the proxy turn to the reasonable treatment standard.

The Substituted Judgment Standard

Substituted judgment is a rather awkward term, but its meaning is simple. The "judgment" in substituted judgment is the judgment of the patient. All the proxy does is step in as a substitute for the patient and report the patient's wishes to the physician. When using the substituted judgment standard, the proxy is like a substitute teacher who steps in and uses the lesson plan the assigned teacher had already developed. The substitute teacher does not really make the plan for the day, nor does the proxy using substituted judgment really make the treatment decisions. Just as the substitute teacher carries out the lesson plan chosen earlier by the regular teacher, so the proxy using substituted judgment carries out the treatment plan chosen earlier by the patient.

This means the proxy must know how the person wants to be treated if she becomes an incapacitated patient. There are three ways a proxy can know this:

1. The patient could have explicitly told the proxy, orally or in written advance directives, what she wants done.

2. The patient could have implicitly made clear what she wants, perhaps by offhand comments about how silly it is to keep unconscious people alive on machines for months, and so forth.

3. The patient could have revealed enough about her thinking and values so the proxy knows what she wants, even though the matter was never discussed or even mentioned. This is an extremely weak basis for substituted judgment but may be valid in some cases. The spouse in a happy marriage where the couple was open and communicated well with each other, for example, may be in a position to rely on it.

The proxy's role in substituted judgment is, therefore, a limited one. The proxy does not really make the decision; he communicates the decision of the patient. In substituted judgment, the proxy reports to the physician what the patient wants. Substituted judgment works very well when patients have discussed in a clear and explicit way their wishes about future treatment with their proxies. Proxies find it more difficult to use substituted judgment when they have to rely on a patient's comments and on their familiarity with the person and the person's attitude toward life, sickness, and death. This is why treatment directives and communication with the person who will act as proxy are so vital.

Proxies can use substituted judgment only when they know what the patient would have wanted. The substituted judgment standard cannot be used when proxies have to make decisions for babies or young children, or for adults who never had capacity, or, if these individuals once did have it, never revealed enough for the proxy to know what they wanted.

Although this explanation of substituted judgment reflects the standard use of the term in health care ethics, we should note that the phrase is sometimes used differently by the courts. Some legal decisions—and this includes a long history of decisions in Massachusetts—use the phrase "substituted judgment" for decisions to withhold or withdraw treatment from incapacitated people who never had capacity (babies or adults with severe congenital mental deficiencies) or who had it but never indicated what they wanted before they lost it. These courts claim that declining treatment is something that these people would have chosen if they were capable of choosing, and they call this hypothetical construct "substituted judgment." For example, there is a Massachusetts case involving a young child named Beth who was diagnosed as being in a persistent vegetative state (PVS) after a tragic automobile accident. The state had legal custody of the child, and the director of a pediatric intensive care unit asked the court to authorize a DNR order years after Beth had lost consciousness. The judge relied on the legal interpretation of substituted judgment and found that Beth, given the situation, would, if she could, want a DNR order, and he issued an order to withhold CPR. Beth's guardian *ad litem* appealed, but the state Supreme Judicial Court upheld the judge's decision.

This is not really the substituted judgment standard we use in ethics, where substituted judgment means we have some evidence of what the person actually wants. Some judges are aware that the legal doctrine allowing judges to claim they know what a never-competent person would have decided if she were able to decide is not a solid legal approach. In the case of Beth, for example, a dissenting justice wrote a strong objection:

> The court again has approved application of the doctrine of substituted judgment when there is not a *soupçon* of evidence to support it. The trial judge did not have a smidgen of evidence on which to conclude that if this child who is now about five and one half years old were competent to decide, she would elect certain death to a life with no cognitive ability. The route by which the court arrives at its conclusion is a cruel charade which is being perpetuated whenever we are faced with a life and death decision of an incompetent person.

Why do some court decisions allowing the withdrawal or withholding of life-sustaining treatment insist that substituted judgment is the standard for making the decision, even when the patient never had the capacity to make health care decisions? Two reasons come to mind.

First, the courts recognize a serious obligation to preserve human life, especially vulnerable human life, and thus some judges are uncomfortable with decisions to stop treatments that are preserving life. It is difficult for these judges to give up the obligation to preserve life, and if they do, they want the patient, and not anyone else, to make the decision. If the patient never had decision-making capacity, the best these judges can do is claim that the patient would have decided to forgo treatment if he could have decided to forgo treatment.

Second, the law supports rights of self-determination and privacy, including, as we saw in our discussion of informed consent, the right of people to refuse treatment. The courts do not think these rights are lost just because a person is not able to assert them. The courts are careful about rights, and some judges can accept the withholding or withdrawal of life-sustaining treatment only if they can construe the case as one in which the patient would, if he could, exercise his right to refuse treatment.

Although the efforts of these courts to justify the withholding or withdrawal of inappropriate treatment are laudable, their use of substituted judgment to conjecture what patients who never had capacity would have wanted if they did have capacity is not helpful. In fact, it causes unnecessary confusion. It would be better if these courts could refrain from viewing every decision to withdraw treatment from an incapacitated patient as a form of substituted judgment and acknowledge that the second criterion of proxy decision making, best interests, is legally relevant.

The Best Interests Standard

The best interests standard is what the proxy falls back on when the patient's wishes are not known and the substituted judgment standard cannot be used. The interests in best interests are the interests of the patient, what will best benefit the patient. Often the patient will derive benefit from treatment, but sometimes treatment is more of a burden than a benefit. In such cases, the treatment would not be in the best interests of the patient.

The benefit in question is a net benefit—that is, what will be in the best interests of the patient, all things considered. Best interests does not refer to the benefit of a specific treatment. Suppose a proxy were making a decision for a terminally ill person with periodontal disease. Gum surgery, an uncomfortable procedure, will obviously be a benefit by curing the gum disease, but, when everything is considered, it is not in the patient's best interests. The gum disease will not cause distress or tooth loss for another decade, and the person is not expected to live more than a year. We have a similar case when people in pain are clearly dying and then contract pneumonia. Using antibiotics will produce a benefit—the curing of pneumonia—but this treatment may not be in the best interests of these dying patients, all things considered.

The word "best" in best interests is somewhat misleading and could be confusing. It does not mean that the proxy must provide the absolutely best treatment for the patient. If the patient needs surgery, for example, the proxy need not seek the best surgeon in the world for the operation, or seek to place the person in the best medical center in the country. The word "best" in best interests simply means that the proxy should decide on the basis of what he thinks is good for the particular patient—that is, what he thinks will truly benefit him.

Both the substituted judgment and the best interests standards can be overridden in some rare situations. In an emergency triage situation, for example, a provider may decide to withhold or remove treatment in order to provide such treatment for another with a better chance of survival even though the first patient wanted the treatment or it is in her best interests to have it. And a national health service may put limits on certain treatments that will place them beyond the reach of most citizens despite the fact that some patients would want the treatment or that it would be in their best interests to receive it.

The Reasonable Treatment Standard

Sometimes neither the substituted judgment nor the best interests standard is applicable. We cannot use substituted judgment if the patient never gave any indication of what was wanted. And we cannot use best interests if the patient has no interests, and sometimes we do not use it when the patient has interests. Two examples where a proxy cannot rely either on substituted judgment (the patients never expressed their wishes) or on best interests are (1) some permanently unconscious patients and (2) some incapacitated dying patients kept on life support to preserve organs for transplantation. In the first case, the proxy may decide to withdraw life-sustaining treatment; in the second, she may decide to continue it. In neither case can the proxy's decision be based on substituted judgment (the patients never indicated what was wanted) or, as we will see, on best interests. Hence, we need a third standard, the reasonable treatment standard. To see why this is so, we will look at these situations more closely.

Permanently Unconscious Patients

Patients in a permanent coma or in a PVS no longer have any interests in the usual sense of the word. They are beyond experiencing anything, and therefore beyond all burdens and benefits. It truly makes no difference to them whether they live or die. Their family, friends, and their society may still have interests in what happens to them, but these patients have no interests. Nothing we do to or for them is a burden or a benefit. Life-support systems and surgeries are neither benefits nor burdens for them because they do not, and never again will, feel anything.

Some ethicists argue that the permanently unaware patient does have interests, or at least has one interest, the interest in living. They say that we can speak of the interests of a permanently unconscious person just as we speak of the interests of a deceased person who left instructions in a will about the disposition of personal property. The executor of the estate respects those wishes and, as we say, looks out for the interests of the deceased.

The interests we speak of in reference to the deceased, however, are not the same as the interests designated in the best interests standard. The interests in reference to the deceased refer to their earlier wishes and thus relate to the substituted judgment standard, not to the best interests standard. The interests in the best interests standard refer not to what the patient wanted but to what is beneficial for the patient now that we do not really know what she would have wanted.

Imagine this situation: A ventilator-dependent patient has been in a PVS for years, and the proxy now wants to withdraw the life-support systems. Since the patient never gave any indication of how he wanted to be treated if he ever permanently lost consciousness, the proxy cannot use substituted judgment. Nor can she use the best interests standard because permanently unconscious patients have no interests. Nothing matters to them. Yet it is at least arguable, and more likely reasonably certain, that the proxy is morally justified in seeking withdrawal of life-sustaining treatment from a PVS patient.

But what standard guides the proxy's decision? In such a case, the proxy falls back on what we are calling the reasonable treatment standard. The proxy requests the withdrawal of life-sustaining treatment because there is no cogent reason to treat, and many reasons not to treat, permanently unconscious patients year after year. Treatment of a PVS patient is not reasonable because it is of no possible benefit to the patient, withdrawing it is of no burden to the patient, and providing the treatment is a considerable burden for others.

Sometimes the reasonable treatment standard is appropriate even when we do know what the patient would have wanted. Imagine this situation: A person once told his proxy that he wanted major heart surgery if he ever needed it. Many years ago, he lapsed into a PVS. Now he needs the heart surgery. Should the proxy, using the substituted judgment standard, try to arrange for the heart surgery? Or could the proxy ignore the patient's wishes and decline to seek the surgery? It is at least arguable, and more likely reasonably certain, that we should not perform major heart surgery (or kidney dialysis or organ transplantation) on a person in a PVS even though the patient may have wanted "everything done" to preserve life.

But what is the basis of this judgment? It is not substituted judgment—the patient said he wanted the intervention. And it is not best interests—the permanently unconscious patient has no interests. The standard guiding the proxy's decision can only be what we are calling the reasonable treatment standard. And in this kind of case, the reasonable treatment standard of proxy decision making actually overrules the substituted judgment standard.

Incapacitated Organ Donors

The reasonable treatment standard may also be invoked in a second kind of situation involving conscious but incapacitated patients. Consider the following. A young child on life-support systems is dying, and the parents and providers have reached the conclusion that withdrawing the life support is in the best interests of the child.

The parents are also ardent supporters of organ transplantation and would now like to donate the organs of their child after death. It may be that the best chance for successful transplantation will be to keep the child alive on life-support equipment for several days until the recipients of the organs can be located, brought to the hospital of the dying child, and prepared for the surgery. Suppose also that the child can be medicated to prevent suffering while kept alive on the life-support equipment.

If we do decide to continue the life support to preserve the organs, the decision is not based on substituted judgment—a proxy cannot use this standard for a baby. Nor is it based on best interests—we have already said that withdrawal of the treatment is now in the best interests of the child. Hence, neither substituted judgment nor best interests can justify the parents' decision to continue the life support keeping the child's organs healthy for transplantation. Quite simply, the baby's life is not being preserved for her own benefit, but for the benefit of the organ recipients. Is this ethical?

Once again, the appropriate standard guiding the proxies' decision is the reasonable treatment standard. If it is reasonable, the proxies may decide to continue treatment even when it is no longer in the child's best interests. Given the shortage of infant organs, it is at least arguably reasonable to continue the life-sustaining treatment for a short time provided we have reason to believe that the prolonged treatment is not causing the baby any suffering.

In summary, then, when patients do not have decision-making capacity, a proxy will decide for them. The proxy normally bases his decision on one of three standards. First, the proxy tries to use the substituted judgment standard and report what the patient wants. If this is not possible, the proxy turns to the second standard—best interests—and tries to decide what is in the best interests of this particular patient. If the patient has left no indication of her wishes and has no interests because of the permanent loss of all awareness, the proxy can only decide on the basis of the third standard—what is reasonable treatment in the circumstances.

The substituted judgment and best interests standards are now widely understood and accepted in health care ethics, and they are easily compatible with the ethics of right reason that we are developing. Our third standard, reasonable treatment, normally used only when the other two are not applicable, is not so widely recognized, although there is growing awareness that neither substituted judgment nor best interests are relevant in all cases of deciding for others, as our examples have shown.

In most cases of deciding for others, the standards just outlined can be applied in a straightforward way. Deciding for some classes of patients, however, can be a real challenge. We will now look at three such groups: older children, the mentally ill, and patients from other cultures.

DECIDING FOR OLDER CHILDREN

The task of making health care decisions for neonates and young children, while often difficult because it is so hard to know what is the right thing to do, is fairly straightforward. Since the young children never had decision-making capacity and do not have it now, the decisions made on their behalf are usually based on the best interests standard.

Deciding for children becomes much more complicated when the children are older and have some grasp of the information and some ability to give consent yet still lack the maturity of an adult. These children are not yet fully capable of making mature decisions but are not far from it and may actually have the capacity to make some decisions. The situation is further complicated because the medical needs and the problems they face after puberty are often the kind of problems many children might not want their parents to know of—pregnancy, sexually transmitted diseases, drug abuse, and the like. The desire of some minors to prevent their parents from knowing about their problems makes it impossible for physicians to consider their parents as appropriate proxies.

In trying to sort out the conflicting issues surrounding the medical treatment of older children, a brief historical comment may be helpful. Until recently our common law tradition, along with our ethical heritage, viewed parents as having almost total control over their minor children. Children were not thought to have rights of their own. Parents made all the decisions affecting the children, including health care decisions, until the minor became an adult or established an independent life. For a long time the age of becoming an adult in the United States was twenty-one, but since the federal voting age was lowered to eighteen in 1971, most legislatures now consider eighteen the age at which a child becomes an adult.

The idea that parents have almost total control over their children slowly broke down in recent centuries. One major factor in the breakdown occurred in the nineteenth century when a heightened awareness of the exploitation of children emerged. Parents had always used their children as laborers to work long hours tilling the land and tending the animals. With the rise of industrialization, however, the sight of children working long hours in the miserable nineteenth-century factories led to laws designed to protect and promote children's welfare. In some cases these laws prevented parents from doing what they wanted to do with their children—send them off to work in factories.

The movement to protect children and improve their welfare did not, of course, immediately enhance their self-determination. The laws restricted what their parents could demand of them, but they did not give children more power in decision making. This came much later and not without considerable social upheaval and family stress. At the present time, however, our society has arrived at the point where most people agree that older minors should play a major role in significant decisions affecting their lives, including decisions about their medical treatment.

On the other hand parents still retain a considerable interest in providing for their children, especially those not yet eighteen years of age. And most children under eighteen can still benefit from parental guidance, especially when they are ill and major medical decisions need to be made. The tricky question with a teenage minor, then, is how the real but limited capacity for self-determination in the not-yet-mature child can be harmonized with legitimate parental concerns and important parental guidance. This is the kind of question not susceptible to a definitive answer; all we can hope to do is grope toward some kind of response.

We will first show how studies on the cognitive development of children suggest strongly that the absolute minimum age necessary for a child to have the capacity to make health care decisions is about twelve years. Before this age, parents or another proxy must make the decisions because the child lacks the cognitive development to do it. Then we will examine how parents or a proxy should be involved in making decisions for minors twelve years and older. We will see how in some cases it may be morally appropriate for the parents or proxy to have nothing to do with the decision, whereas in other cases it is morally appropriate that they share in, and perhaps actually make, the health care decision.

The Minimum Age for Minors to Make Health Care Decisions

The first thing to determine is when an older minor has developed sufficient capacity to understand, to evaluate, to reason about the medical realities confronting her, and to consent freely to proposed interventions. In other words, when does a child develop the capacity to make health care decisions?

The answer of course will vary from child to child. Some mature very quickly; others take a slower route. Yet developmental studies of normal children show definite stages of advancing toward maturity in understanding, evaluating, reasoning, and consenting. These studies indicate that most children younger than twelve years of age have not yet developed decision-making capacity, that children between twelve and fourteen years are in a kind of transition period, and that children fifteen and older may well have enough capacity to make major health care decisions on their own. This is not to say that making such decisions on their own is the ideal; obviously, most children under eighteen could benefit from the assistance of loving and caring parents.

Some suggest that minors suffering from chronic illness for many years achieve an understanding and an ability to make decisions about their treatment long before other children. This seems to be so for older minors, but the reverse may be true for younger children, in whom the illness may retard mental and moral development.

It is important to determine when minors achieve the capacity to make their health care decisions because we want to avoid two situations: We do not want to ignore their decisions if they truly have the capacity to make them, and we do not want to accept their decisions if they really do not have the capacity to make them. In other words we do not want to disenfranchise a child capable of deciding, and we do not want to force decision making on a child not yet ready for it.

To determine when the health care decisions of a minor are valid, we must examine his capacity to make such decisions. In the previous chapter we identified three elements of capacity: understanding, evaluation, and reasoning.

Understanding

Studies of normal children suggest that a child's understanding of illness is closely related to the developmental stages of cognitive development first outlined in some detail by Jean Piaget decades ago. In this developmental schema children do not really begin to understand illness, let alone prognoses and the impact of various treatments that might cure or mitigate the illness, until some time after the age of eleven. Then this realistic understanding of illness grows over the next few years.

Evaluation

A child's appreciation of what is good and bad also grows in developmental stages. Here the basic work was done by Lawrence Kohlberg, who continued Piaget's work in the relationship between cognitive and moral development. The developmental studies of Piaget, Kohlberg, and others elaborating on their work strongly suggest that mature moral judgments cannot be made until about the age of twelve. Although Kohlberg's work has been criticized, with some reason, because it emphasized the moral development of boys as they grew into men and thus slighted the moral development of girls as they grew into women and because his stages of moral development presuppose a Kantian moral framework, his conclusions about when children begin to make moral judgments remain widely accepted.

This does not mean mature moral judgments *are* made at this age—only that the minor has the capacity to make them. Both Piaget and Kohlberg insisted on what we all know: Achieving a mature cognitive development does not mean moral maturity necessarily follows. People cannot make moral decisions without advanced cognitive development, but this cognitive development does not guarantee that they will make morally mature decisions.

Reasoning

In Piaget's schema formal reasoning also begins around the age of twelve, when the advanced level of cognitive development that enables adolescents to reason abstractly occurs. At this stage the child can consider various possibilities, form hypotheses and deduce conclusions from them, and then test these conclusions against experience. Moreover, a child at this stage of cognitive development can reason simultaneously about the alternative treatments and about the risks associated with each. As was pointed out in the last chapter, this is the level of reasoning a person must achieve, at least in rudimentary form, before we can say that he has the capacity to make health care decisions and to give informed consent.

From the developmental studies pioneered by Piaget and Kohlberg then, it seems clear that children below the age of twelve simply do not have the capacity to make heath care decisions and to give informed consent. Their parents or some other proxy must do it for them.

This leaves us with the problems associated with minors aged twelve to eighteen years. It is the difficult, gray area, because children this age are achieving the cognitive development that allows them to understand, evaluate, and reason in a mature way, but this maturity is obviously not fully developed, and it will vary significantly from child to child. The difficult question now is what role parents play in the health care decisions of this group of children?

Limitations on the Parental Role in Decisions Affecting Older Minors

Children from twelve to eighteen years are still considered minors, and therefore the assumption is that they are still subject to their parents' decisions. As the following examples show, however, there are many situations in which parents no longer have the authority to make health care decisions for their older minor children, and the children decide for themselves.

Emancipated Minors

Emancipated minors have been recognized in law for years, and the recognition seems morally sound. Emancipated minors are no longer subject to parental control. In general an emancipated minor can make her own health care decisions and give informed consent for medical interventions. Emancipated minors are usually no longer living at home and are supporting themselves. Marriage is an action that emancipates a minor, even if the marriage is followed by divorce and the minor returns to the parental home. Entry into military service also emancipates a minor. A college student under eighteen living at college is in an ambiguous situation if the parents are still supporting him financially, but there is a general tendency to consider a college student not living at home emancipated and capable of giving informed consent. A high school student at a boarding school, however, is generally not considered emancipated, and thus parents are the ones to give consent for his medical treatment.

A minor child who has run away from home presents another ambiguous situation, but it seems reasonable to consider him sufficiently emancipated to give informed consent, especially if the runaway teenager does not want the parents involved in the situation, which is often the case. It would also seem appropriate to consider a minor who has become a parent as emancipated. Since parents give consent for the treatment of their child, they should be able to give consent for their own treatment even if they are still minors.

Minor Treatment Statutes

Many states have laws allowing minors above a certain age—which varies from state to state—to give consent for some medical treatment without notifying their parents. The need to treat venereal disease was the problem behind many of these laws. Obviously, many minors would not want their parents to know that they had contracted a sexually transmitted disease, and they would not be inclined to seek treatment if the physicians had to contact their parents to obtain consent for treatment. Without treatment, however, not only would the infected minors suffer, but very likely some of them might spread the disease and create a public health problem. Hence, accepting consent from minors for treatment of sexually transmitted diseases became legally acceptable in many states.

A second situation often covered by these minor treatment statutes is drug abuse. It is easy to understand why many minors would not want their parents to know they have a drug problem, so accepting consent for treatment from the minors themselves also makes sense.

A third situation often covered by these statutes is prenatal care. Many states have laws permitting pregnant minors to give consent for appropriate health care during pregnancy without parental approval or notification.

Contraception

As we will note in the chapter on reproduction, a series of Supreme Court cases has found that restrictions on contraception violate the constitutional right to privacy. In 1965 *Griswold v. Connecticut* allowed access to contraception for married couples. In 1972 *Eisenstadt v. Baird*, a case originating in Massachusetts, allowed access to contraception for unmarried adults; and in 1977 *Carey v. Population Serivces International*, a case originating in New York, allowed access to contraception for unmarried minors. These interpretations of the Constitution allow sexually active unmarried minors to give consent for contraceptive medical interventions such as anovulant pills, diaphragms, and Norplant implants without parental notification.

Allowing minors access to contraceptive medical interventions is, of course, a highly charged controversy in our society at this time. On one side people argue that such access is for the good of the sexually active minor and of society because it prevents unwanted pregnancy. On the other side people argue that such access encourages immature sexual relationships, undermines the legitimate concern parents have for their children, and weakens society in general by seeming to encourage widespread sexual activity outside the social structure of marriage and the family. There are thoughtful and caring people on both sides of this debate.

There is not much debate, however, about contraceptive sterilization. These surgeries raise a host of more serious questions because they are very difficult to reverse, and the sterilized minor might well want children at a later date. Many, if not most, people consider the surgical sterilization of minors at their request morally objectionable. Most physicians, of course, would refuse to perform these surgeries on teenagers, and with good reason, since there is no justification for these radical contraceptive interventions at an early age.

Abortion

In 1973 the Supreme Court extended the notion of privacy to abortion in the first two trimesters of pregnancy in *Roe v. Wade* and *Doe v. Bolton*. The women in these cases were adults, so the question of whether a pregnant minor could give informed consent for an abortion was not specifically addressed by the Court at that time.

Massachusetts then passed a law requiring both parents, if they were available, to give consent before their daughter under the age of eighteen could have an abortion. In *Bellotti v. Baird* (1979) the Supreme Court struck down this law, thereby allowing minors to give consent for their abortions. The opinion required states that considered pregnant minors too immature to give authentic informed consent for abortion to arrange an alternative procedure that would not force the minor girl to seek parental consent for her abortion.

One such alternative procedure exists in Massachusetts and in some other states. A minor seeking an abortion without parental consent must appear before a judge. He or she then determines whether the minor has the capacity to give informed consent for the abortion. If the judge finds the minor has the capacity, then she can give consent for her abortion. If the judge finds she does not have the capacity, then the court must decide whether the abortion is in her best interests. If the court so finds, it can issue an order allowing the abortion. In practice, judges in Massachusetts almost invariably find the pregnant minor has the capacity to give consent for the abortion.

The legal developments allowing minors to give consent for treatment of sexually transmitted diseases and drug problems, and for medical interventions to prevent or terminate pregnancy, have encouraged a trend whereby older minors are considered to have the capacity to make health care decisions for other medical problems as well. This trend implies that they also have the capacity to withhold consent for treatment that their parents may want them to have. The assumption that parents make all the decisions for their minor children has given way to the recognition that older minors are able to make many of their health care decisions.

From an ethical point of view, there are both good and bad features in this trend that allows minors to make their own decisions. The major good feature centers on recognizing the increasing capacity of a maturing minor to assume responsibility for his life. The maturing minor has to form some kind of life plan and make decisions that will determine what kind of adult he will become. It is impossible to do this if parents make all the important decisions until age eighteen, and then the minor suddenly assumes decision-making responsibility. Rather, the process of maturity requires a more gradual transition from a child subject to parental control to a young adult responsible for his decisions. Older minors naturally desire to assume more and more control over their lives and are actually able to do so successfully to a considerable degree.

Yet the value of self-determination for minors is less than it is for adults, primarily because the decisions teenagers make are limited by their lack of experience and maturity. Good decision making comes only with time, practice, and experience, and the minor simply has not had enough of these. Hence the notions of autonomy and self-determination that are so popular in contemporary health care ethics are of limited value when the patient is a minor.

There are good reasons for allowing minors to give consent for treatment involving health problems associated with sexuality and drugs if they do not want their parents to know of their problems. But this does not mean it is a good idea for them to make all their health care decisions.

In many other cases it is in the self-interest of the minor to have parental consultation and guidance in making health care decisions. And if teenagers have a trusting and open relation with their parents, they might well benefit from parental help in making decisions about the medical issues surrounding sexuality and drugs as well.

A major bad feature of the trend to accept health care decisions from minors without parental consent is the seldom noticed impact it has on the legitimate interests of parents to care for their children. Most parents care about their children and often know them and their needs better than the children know themselves. This parental caring and interest in the child's welfare does not end as soon as the child develops a minimally adequate decision-making capacity but continues long afterward. The fact that this parental interest can be distorted, and that some parents try to run their children's lives, should not blind us to the legitimate parental interest and caring that continues through the teenage years and often beyond.

Once this is acknowledged, the determination that a minor has developed decision-making capacity does not imply that he should exercise it without parental involvement. In some situations—venereal disease, for example—it may be reasonable not to confide in parents, but in many other health care situations the minor will benefit greatly from the involvement of caring parents. Hence, there are many situations where good ethics suggests the participation of parents in the medical decision making affecting their minor children even though these children may have achieved sufficient decision-making capacity to be able to make the decisions on their own.

There is an additional reason for encouraging parental involvement in the health care decisions of minors whenever possible: the legitimate interest of parents in their family. Parents and other children in the family as well may be affected by the health care decision of a minor, and therefore, the parents should have some say in what goes on. The parents, for example, may be paying for the treatment, or the proposed treatment may adversely affect the other children in the family, whom the parents have a responsibility to protect. Whenever the minor's treatment impacts on important family interests, the parents have a legitimate interest in participating actively in the decision making.

Making decisions for children when they are between the ages of twelve and eighteen, then, is a very complicated matter if these minors are not emancipated or if they are seeking one of the special forms of treatment where parental notification would create more burdens than benefits. It calls for a great deal of prudential insight. The following comments may provide a general moral orientation.

First, parents are the usual proxies for children who lack the capacity to make health care decisions. Sometimes, however, it may be necessary for the courts to appoint a guardian or proxy because the parents' behavior disqualifies them from making medical decisions for their children.

Second, when parents make decisions for older minors, they use the familiar standards of substituted judgment and best interests, but in a qualified way. Substituted judgment cannot be used unless the child is an older minor and has indicated some preferences about how he wants to be treated; even then his immaturity has to be taken into consideration. And the best interests standard has to be qualified because parents must consider the decision in light of the best interests of others in the family, especially other children.

Third, when children begin to achieve some capacity to understand and to consent voluntarily to medical treatment, parents should include them in the decision-making process to the extent it is possible. Parents and physicians treat children with respect by sharing information with them and by letting them participate in the decision-making process to the extent they are able to do so. Before children are sufficiently mature to give true consent for treatment, they are able to assent to the decisions being made in their best interests, and physicians and parents should seek this assent.

Fourth, when minors have achieved decision-making capacity, parents should still play a role in the decision making, unless it would not be helpful as may be the case with medical problems caused by sexual activity or drug abuse. Just how strong this parental role should be will depend on the circumstances and the maturity of the minor. The ideal situation will be a shared decision making among the parents, the minor, and the physician, but this is often not feasible.

Fifth, it sometimes happens that responsible parents want to make an informed refusal of routine treatment for their children. The classic example of this involves families who are practicing Jehovah's Witnesses. This religious group believes that the Bible forbids blood transfusions. Parents, however, may not refuse consent for normal life-saving treatments for their children. If they do, providers may appeal to the state child protective agencies or directly to the courts. The courts tend to respond in one of two ways: Either they issue an order for the treatment, or they temporarily remove the child from the parents' custody and appoint a guardian to give consent for it. The basis of the courts' reactions are state child abuse laws, which consider the withholding of necessary medical treatment from a child a form of child abuse and neglect. A state supreme court decision known as *Prince v. Massachusetts* made the important point that a parent may become a martyr for his religious beliefs, but "he is not free to make a martyr of his child."

Deciding for the Mentally Ill

Mental illness can be a terrible tragedy affecting not only the patient but the family and society as well. Many mentally ill people cannot care for themselves, and they may be a danger to themselves or others. Frequently, proxies must make health care decisions for them.

Making health care decisions for the mentally ill opens up a number of legal and moral dilemmas. Some of the troubling questions are these: Is it moral to place the mentally ill in institutions against their will simply because they might harm themselves or others? Is it moral to force treatment on them, most especially drugs or surgery or shock treatments, against their will? Is their informed consent for treatment truly voluntary if we have made it clear to them that they will be confined to an institution if they do not accept treatment?

Mental illness is not a clearly defined term. It covers a wide range of dysfunction from the severe to the relatively mild, and the categories used by the American Psychiatric Association are so general that physicians have considerable leeway in diagnosing patients' behaviors. This makes it all the more important to consider the ethical implications of how proxies make treatment decisions for those diagnosed as mentally ill.

We will consider but three issues in this complicated field: first, the relation of mental illness and decision-making capacity; second, decisions to commit or restrain the mentally ill against their wishes; and third, decisions to treat the mentally ill against their will.

Mental Illness and Decision-Making Capacity

A widespread misconception assumes that all mentally ill people are incompetent and have lost the capacity to make health care decisions. This is simply not true. As we pointed out in the last chapter, people are legally competent unless found incompetent by a judge. Most mentally ill people have not been found incompetent by a judge and hence remain legally competent.

Also, many mentally ill people retain decision-making capacity. Some mental illnesses do not override decision-making capacity, or, if they do, this state is only temporary, and periods of capacity remain wherein the patient is able to make decisions about treatment. Moreover, capacity, as we pointed out in the last chapter, is task specific, and a mental illness that destroys a patient's capacity to make some decisions does not necessarily destroy the capacity to make all health care decisions.

It is unwise then to assume that all mentally ill people have lost the ability to make their health care decisions. Rather, the decision-making capacity of people diagnosed as mentally ill should be determined the same way it is determined for the physically ill. That is, the physician will ascertain whether the patient is able to understand the important facts, to evaluate the illness and possible treatments in light of a framework of values; to reason about the impact that the various treatment options may have, and to give consent freely. Undoubtedly some mentally ill patients, as some physically ill patients, have lost the capacity to make health care decisions. But other mentally ill patients, as other physically ill patients, retain the capacity to give truly informed consent.

It is true, however, that mental illness often does affect the capacity to make health care decisions and to give voluntary consent for treatment. The illness can undermine any of the three aspects of decision-making capacity: understanding, evaluation, and reasoning. In some forms of schizophrenia, for example, a person may have a fixed belief that medications are really poisons or that health care providers are part of a plot to trap and imprison him. These beliefs interfere with his ability to understand the diagnosis and the true risks of various treatment options.

In other forms of mental illness—severe depression, for example—the person's ability to evaluate a course of action can be lost because the illness weakens the person's ability to care about any of the goals and projects in life that provide a framework for value judgments. And some manic stages of bipolar illness can distort the reasoning process by introducing a totally unrealistic picture of what can be done.

Although mental illness can attack the specific cognitive and volitional abilities needed to make health care decisions, it does not always do so and, if it does, does not always permanently destroy those abilities. Hence, the physician must assess each patient carefully to determine decision-making capacity and, if it has been lost, to determine whether it might return. The important thing is to avoid thinking that once a person has been diagnosed as mentally ill a proxy must make all the treatment decisions from that point onward. This kind of thinking all too easily disenfranchises a human being who retains the capacity to make decisions about his treatment.

Deciding to Commit or to Restrain the Mentally Ill

In recent decades the number of hospitalized mentally ill people has dropped significantly, from more than half a million in 1955 to a little more than one hundred thousand now. Many factors prompted this decline; among them are the development of drugs that control or reduce the dangerous or antisocial symptoms of patients and the growing awareness that patients have liberty interests and should not be hospitalized unless absolutely necessary. In addition, some institutions housing the mentally ill were such wretched places (partly because so many patients acted out in the era before psychotropic drugs were widely used and partly because so many people had become frustrated with the exasperating nature of mental illness) that society was content at times simply to "warehouse" patients so it could live in peace. And finally, there was a cost factor. Many of the mental health institutions were state hospitals, and few taxpayers wanted to spend a lot of money on caring for those whom they perceived as hopeless and unproductive members of society.

The deinstitutionalization of mentally ill people has resulted in fewer long-term mentally ill inpatients. Still, decisions by proxies to commit mentally ill persons must be made, and the decisions are both morally and legally difficult. Involuntary confinement is a direct attack on personal liberty. The involuntary confinement is not really a treatment but a detention. Depriving a human being of the freedom to live in society is a major restriction on his life, and we need a strong reason for doing it.

Two reasons are usually given when a proxy decides to commit a mentally ill patient against his will: He is a danger to others, or he is a danger to himself. We will examine the strength of these reasons.

Danger to Others

Certainly, some mentally ill people are dangerous to others, and their erratic behavior can be a source of great fear. But the "danger to others" reason for involuntary commitment has to be put in perspective. We have to remember that many people not mentally ill are dangerous to others—violent crimes are a fact of life—yet we do not detain people simply because there is some reason to believe that they might be a danger to others. If anyone proposed locking up every person who might commit a violent crime, we would be shocked at this proposed violation of personal freedom without cause and due process. People who might commit violent crimes have to be left alone unless they actually commit those crimes. Yet the attitude toward the mentally ill is often quite different. Many think that they should be confined when there is some reason to believe they might be a danger to others. It is this attitude that must be questioned, lest the important constitutional right of liberty and the moral value of freedom be prematurely compromised.

Moreover, the commitment of all mentally ill persons who might harm others will obviously be an injustice to some of them. Suppose, for example, there is an 80 percent chance that patients with a certain diagnosis will harm other people if left free in society. For some this percentage would be sufficiently high to justify involuntary commitment in order to prevent the violence. But think of this: If we force involuntary commitment on one hundred people with this diagnosis, then we are confining twenty people who, if left free, will never harm anyone. In order to justify morally confining one hundred people with an 80 percent chance of harming others, we will also have to justify forcing twenty people into confinement who did not harm anyone and will not harm anyone if they are left free in society. This is obviously a question of justice and an ethical dimension of involuntary commitment seldom considered when a decision is made to commit a mentally ill person because it is thought that she might be a danger to others.

The same factors have to be considered when there is a question of restraining hospitalized persons either by physical restraints that restrict their movements or by confining them to a secluded place other than their normal inpatient space. This is also a serious deprivation of freedom and can be justified only in emergencies or where providers are convinced that harm to others will actually occur.

So although it is certainly possible to justify involuntary confinement of mentally ill people on the grounds that they are a danger to others, it is not, in the absence of a history of violence, an easy case to make. It is very difficult to predict who will be violent if left in society and very hard to justify restraining or confining people simply because they might be violent. In order to protect personal rights and avoid injustice to the innocent, society has to leave free many people who might commit violent crime. For the same reasons, society has to leave free many mentally ill people who might be dangerous. The fact that some mentally ill people actually will commit violent actions does not justify confining every mentally ill person who might commit violent actions any more than the fact some people will commit violent crime justifies confining everyone who might commit violent crime.

Danger to Self

The second reason proxies use for the decision to commit mentally ill patients against their will is to protect them from harming, or even killing, themselves. Now some mentally ill people certainly are a danger to themselves, but, again, the moral reasoning justifying the commitment on the basis of the patient's best interest is complicated.

First, consider the mentally ill person with the capacity to make health care decisions, including the specific decision about commitment to a mental health institution. Suppose his family and physicians have reason to believe that the person is a danger to himself—does that belief justify their committing or restraining him against his will? We might be tempted to reason this way: The person is mentally ill and a danger to himself; therefore, confinement in a hospital is the best place for him.

Such reasoning is rooted in the laudable desire to protect the mentally ill person, but it is seriously flawed. If an adult has the capacity to make decisions about hospitalization, there is no sound reason for violating his liberty and confining him to an institution against his will simply because others think that he is a danger to himself. It would be a great tragedy if such an adult were not confined and restrained and then harmed or even destroyed himself, but it would be a greater tragedy if, as a matter of course, we committed to institutions competent people with decision-making capacity against their will. Forced confinement of sick people who retain decision-making capacity is a major violation of their personal liberty and dignity. Just as hospitals cannot force physically sick people to become patients or to remain in the institution against their will, neither can hospitals force mentally sick people to become patients or to remain in the institution against their will as long as the mentally sick people retain the capacity to decide for themselves about hospitalization.

The mentally ill person may well be a danger to himself, but this is not enough of a reason to confine him involuntarily if he still has the capacity to make his own decision about hospitalization. And if perchance the mentally ill person is in the hospital but retains the capacity to make decisions about the hospitalization and wants to leave, it is not morally justified to prevent the discharge. Confining a competent human being with decision-making capacity against his will is a most serious choice, and the possibility that he presents a danger to himself is seldom a strong enough reason to justify it.

Second, consider the mentally ill person who is a danger to herself and who lacks the capacity to make health care decisions. In this case a proxy will make the decision whether or not to commit the patient. For a mentally ill person who never had decision-making capacity, or once had it but left no advance indications of what she wanted, the proxy will use the best interests standard when deciding about commitment.

But for a mentally ill person without decision-making capacity who had, during a previous period of capacity, formulated advance directives or given clear indication of her wishes, the proxy will use the substituted judgment standard for the decision. And if the mentally ill person had indicated, during a previous period of lucidity when she had decision-making capacity, that she would not want confinement, the substituted judgment standard now constrains the proxy to decide against confinement despite the possibility that the patient may harm herself.

Hence, it is entirely possible that sound moral judgment directs a proxy to decline confinement for a mentally ill patient without decision-making capacity who is a danger to herself. This judgment is not a comfortable one, but the alternative is even more uncomfortable: confining someone who had, by advance directives, made it clear that she did not want the confinement. This is little more than imprisoning an innocent person against her will.

In some cases, however, prudential reasoning can by way of exception justify confining a mentally ill person to prevent her harming herself despite the patient's advance directives against it. One such case is when the mentally ill person is actually behaving in a self-destructive way. Perhaps she is engaged in violence against herself; or perhaps she is refusing to eat.

The confinement of the mentally ill against their previous wishes expressed during earlier periods of decision-making capacity is easiest to justify when the confinement is brief and temporary. If they have become so agitated or upset that they have lost the capacity to understand, evaluate, or reason and now pose a danger to themselves, it would seem morally justified to confine or restrain them involuntarily if they are expected soon to regain the capacity to make decisions for themselves. In some ways this resembles the protective custody used by some police departments to care for an inebriated citizen for a few hours. The police consider such a person a danger to himself and vulnerable to harm from others, so they confine the inebriated person in protective custody until his ability to take care of himself returns.

To sum up, there is seldom justification for the involuntary confinement of a patient suffering from any illness—mental or physical—if the person has decision-making capacity or, if he does not now have this capacity, once had it and had made it clear that he did not want confinement. Exceptions to this will be rare. One exception occurs when it is known with certainty that the person is a serious danger to others; another occurs when the person is actually engaged in harming himself or is in imminent danger of being harmed by others. The fact that a person might be a danger to himself, however, is not itself a sufficient reason to confine him against his present or previous wishes. Drug addicts are a danger to themselves, but this does not justify forcing them into institutions against their will. Many smokers are endangering their health, yet no one advocates confining them so they cannot obtain cigarettes.

And if a proxy does decide to institutionalize a mentally ill person on the basis of his being a danger to others, it is well to remember that the decision is not really a medical one, despite the fact that the person is confined to a medical facility rather than a prison. The confinement of the socially dangerous mentally ill person is not primarily for the benefit of the ill person but for the protection of innocent third parties. It is a decision primarily motivated by what is good for others, not by what is good for the sick person. The police power enjoyed by every society, and not medical benefit, is the source of the authority whereby those proven dangerous to others are confined against their will.

Deciding to Treat the Mentally Ill

Treatment is not the same as confinement. The reason for confinement is usually to provide treatment, but this is not always the case—sometimes people are confined because they are truly dangerous. And putting somebody in restraints or in seclusion is not really a treatment but a step taken to protect the patient from harming himself or others. This is why we consider the treatment of the mentally ill as something different from confinement or the use of restraints.

In general questions about treating the mentally ill can be resolved the same way questions about treating the physically ill are resolved. If mentally ill patients retain the capacity to make decisions about treatment, normally these decisions will be followed just as they would be followed for physically ill patients with decision-making capacity. And if mentally ill patients have lost the capacity to make decisions, then a proxy will make the treatment decisions based on substituted judgment, best interests, or the reasonable treatment standard.

Yet making decisions regarding treatment for the mentally ill can become rather complicated, as it does in the following situations.

Treatment for the Involuntarily Confined

For a long time, no one questioned treating involuntarily confined mentally ill patients without their consent. People simply assumed that the treatment was appropriate. If there were a good reason to hospitalize the mentally ill person over his objections in the first place, then there must be, it was thought, good reasons for providing treatments over his objections as well. Thus, shock treatments, psychosurgery, or drugs were often used without any effort to determine the involuntarily confined patient's capacity to give informed consent.

Some years ago, however, several legal challenges to this assumption were mounted. In a Massachusetts case that began in federal district court as *Rogers v. Okin* (1979) and was decided by the U.S. Supreme Court as *Mills v. Rogers* (1982), the Supreme Court acknowledged that mentally ill patients can refuse treatment, specifically psychotropic drugs, even if they are involuntarily hospitalized, provided they have not lost decision-making capacity and do not pose a serious threat of physical harm to themselves or to others.

From an ethical point of view, the U.S. Supreme Court's awareness that some people involuntarily confined to mental health institutions retain the capacity to make treatment decisions is sound. The person was involuntarily committed because there was reason to believe he was a danger to society or to himself, not because he had lost decision-making capacity. An involuntarily confined patient may not have lost decision-making capacity or, if he had lost it at the time of involuntary confinement, may have regained it subsequently. Unless it has been specifically determined that the involuntarily confined patient does not have the capacity to make health care decisions, his prerogative to give or withhold informed consent must be respected. If the involuntarily confined patient with capacity refuses consent for an intervention, it cannot be forced upon him unless extenuating circumstances are present.

Forced Treatment on the Incapacitated Patient

Sometimes an incapacitated patient, without advance directives, refuses treatments that the proxy and physicians believe are in his best interests. The proxy's first reaction in these situations may be to ignore the patient's objections and to give consent for psychotropic drugs, psychosurgery, or shock treatments. After all, the objections are from a mentally ill patient without decision-making capacity and therefore cannot be taken as authentic.

But there is an additional feature in these cases that is not present in most other proxy decisions, and it complicates the moral reflection. Unlike a proxy decision made for infants or for the unconscious or for the compliant adult, the incapacitated mentally ill patient will often challenge the treatment, sometimes strenuously. And frequently the objections are based on the patient's personal experience—the patient may have received the treatment or drugs before and thus knows first hand how unpleasant the side effects can be.

Forcing treatment on incapacitated patients when they resist it can cause them so much additional distress that the treatment that would have been in their best interests may no longer be a net benefit for them. Even if patients left advance directives for the treatment but now, in their incapacitated state, are strenuously objecting to it, their present objections may sometimes carry more weight than their previous directives and wishes.

One exception to this may occur when the unwanted treatment is the only alternative to unwanted confinement. In recent decades, more and more incapacitated mentally ill people are not confined to institutions. They are living in society, and some of them are being treated despite their objections. The central legal and moral argument used to justify treating these patients against their wishes is that the alternative—involuntary commitment—would be worse for them.

From a moral point of view if the incapacitated mentally ill person is truly a danger to others, this argument has some merit. Involuntary medication would not seem as bad as involuntary confinement and might be justified if it controls the social danger with fewer bad effects in the patient's life than involuntary confinement. If we can forcibly confine the dangerous mentally ill in order to protect others, it is reasonable to say we can forcibly treat them outside of the institution unless, of course, the side effects of treatment are so severe they outweigh the disadvantages of confinement.

If the incapacitated mentally ill person is not dangerous, however, and the treatment decision is not based on public safety but on the best interests of the patient, then, as we noted above, we have to consider carefully how the patient's objections may undermine any good the forced treatment might bring.

The important ethical point in these cases is the recognition that making treatment decisions for the incompetent mentally ill, whose prior wishes may be unreliable because of the mental illness, is not a simple case of relying on the best interests standard. Psychotropic drugs may well be in the best interests of a mentally ill patient, but if the patient objects to them, these objections must be taken seriously. Forcing treatments on a person, even an incompetent mentally ill person, is something that undermines his human dignity and can easily undermine the human dignity of the providers. It is not enough to say that we can override the patient's objections because he is "crazy." He may well be mentally ill and have lost decision-making capacity, but he is still a human being with awareness and values, no matter how distorted his perceptions and judgments may be.

On the other hand, paternalism in the care of the incapacitated mentally ill is more easily justified than it is for those not mentally ill. This makes it difficult for proxies and providers to withhold beneficial treatment when the patient refusing treatment is mentally ill. It is distressing to withhold helpful treatment when the patient refusing it is known to be mentally ill. The inclination is almost always to disregard the objections of these patients and to provide the treatments.

What, then, can we say about the ethics of providing treatment for mentally ill people without decision-making capacity when they object? Only that the situation is ambiguous and that the moral deliberation in each case requires most careful prudential reasoning. Proxies must be ever aware that the objections of the patient may well undermine the otherwise beneficial treatment and that forcing treatment on unwilling human beings creates a situation that can easily undermine respect for them and the self-respect of the provider as well.

Yet there may be times when a limited paternalism can be defended, and the proxy can approve the treatments over the patient's objections. Some mentally ill patients, for example, may object to the medication as part of a game when, in fact, they really are not objecting to it. Other mentally ill patients may object to treatment when they are agitated and need it but then acknowledge that they welcome the drugs that quiet them down.

Manipulating the Patient with Capacity

When we discussed informed consent in the last chapter, we pointed out that the consent must be voluntary; that is, the patient cannot be manipulated, coerced, or forced to accept the treatment. The shadow of manipulation sometimes haunts treatment decisions that affect the mentally ill. Suppose, for example, the mentally ill outpatient with decision-making capacity is given a choice: Either accept the psychotropic drugs or be committed to a hospital for the mentally ill. If she really does not want the drugs but consents to the treatment to avoid confinement, is her consent truly voluntary?

Again, suppose a hospitalized mentally ill patient is given a choice: Either accept the psychotropic drugs or be confined in a secluded room. If he really does not want the drugs but consents to them to avoid being confined, is his consent truly voluntary?

In effect the providers have already made a major decision affecting the mentally ill patients in these cases. They have decided that the patients will either accept treatment or be confined. This does not give the patient much room to maneuver, nor does it put the patient in a good position to give truly voluntary consent. It is very close to manipulation. But for reasons of social good, and perhaps for the good of the patient, it may sometimes be justified for providers or the courts to make these kinds of decisions. Manipulating patients to get consent for treatment is normally unethical, but it may be reasonable in some cases where mental illness is involved. If patients are restricted to a choice between treatment and confinement, however, it would seem that every effort should be made to avoid presenting the confinement as punitive. Rather, it should be presented as a necessary last resort if the patient will not accept treatment compatible with his freedom.

DECIDING FOR PATIENTS OF ANOTHER CULTURE

An interesting moral dilemma arises with patients, usually elderly, from another culture where attitudes of patient self-determination and informed consent do not play the important roles they do in our culture. When these people become ill in our country, their children will often step forward and begin to make decisions for them even when the parents are not incapacitated. The children may point out that medicine is paternalistic in their parent's country, that older people do not expect to be told about their diagnosis and prognosis, and that the responsibility of the physician and family is simply to do what they think is best. They may further insist that the older people will be totally confused if they are fully informed and then asked to make their own decisions. Moreover, a language problem often exists preventing the physician from communicating directly with the patient.

The ethical question here centers on whether the physician can go along with the children and (1) not tell the patient what is wrong and (2) decide with the children what will be done, even though the parent is not incapacitated and did not waive the right to give informed consent. If we invoke our standard doctrine of informed consent and insist that the diagnosis and prognosis should not be kept from patients, then the physician could not accept proxy decisions from the children as long as the patient still had decision-making capacity.

However, in an ethics attuned to circumstances and dedicated to doing what best achieves the human good, it is possible to justify a limited form of family and physician paternalism in this kind of situation. For it is true that some people have been raised in cultures where the major decisions in life are family decisions, where medicine is paternalistic, and where children do decide what is best for their parents when they reach a certain age. The children in these situations are, therefore, asking nothing more than to have their parents treated as they would be treated in their own country. In some cases at least, it would seem morally reasonable for the physician caring for these patients in what is for them a foreign country to respect their cultural heritage. A practical strategy in these situations is to ask the patient to waive informed consent and to let the children make the decisions.

FINAL REFLECTIONS ON DECIDING FOR OTHERS

In general, the three standards of proxy decision making—*substituted judgment*, *best interests*, and what we have called *reasonable treatment*—reflect an ethics of right reason. They are reasonable ways to achieve the human good as best we can in situations in which the patient is incapacitated. Before we conclude this chapter, however, two remarks are in order. First, the substituted judgment and best interest standards of proxy decision making do not absolve the proxy of his or her responsibility to act reasonably and morally. Second, we will live a better moral life if we appoint a proxy while we are still able to do so and if we communicate what we want done in the event we one day lose the capacity to make our health care decisions. We now say a word about each of these remarks.

Limitations of Substituted Judgment and Best Interests

The substituted judgment and best interests criteria of proxy decision making are most often all we need to justify morally the treatment decisions one person makes on behalf of another. They are not, however, the ultimate criteria of what is morally right or wrong. They are important standards, but they are limited because they are patient-centered standards. The proxy is communicating the patient's decision, if there is one, or deciding what is in the patient's best interests. We can never forget, however, that the proxy is a moral agent and therefore responsible for what she does.

In most cases the proxy acts ethically when she uses the substituted judgment standard or, if that is not possible, the best interests standard. Sometimes, however, this is not so. There are cases, rare to be sure, in which a proxy will decline to follow the substituted judgment and best interests standards for ethical reasons of her own.

A proxy behaves in a morally reasonable way in overriding the substituted judgment standard whenever the patient left treatment instructions that the proxy considers clearly immoral or unreasonable. For example, a patient may have left instructions that an order not to attempt resuscitation never be written for him, and now he is permanently unconscious, ventilator dependent, and dying of widespread cancer. There are good moral reasons for saying a proxy could give consent for the DNR order in such circumstances.

A proxy is also morally justified in overriding the best interests standard whenever what is in the best interests of the patient is clearly immoral or unreasonable. For example, it may be in the best interests of the patient to have a kidney transplant, but the only way to obtain a kidney for transplant is from a black market that pays desperate poor people to sell one of their kidneys. Obtaining a black market kidney would be in a patient's best interests if no other kidney is available, but the proxy may well refuse to give consent if someone offers to provide a black market kidney for the patient on the grounds that this practice is unethical.

Both substituted judgment and best interests are standards centered exclusively on the patient, but sound moral decisions about the patient may embrace other factors as well. The interests of others (especially of the family, of the providers, and of society itself) are sometimes not negligible and have to be factored into the decision about how incapacitated patients are treated. The doctrine of triage in emergency situations, a doctrine that allows withholding treatment from some so it can be provided for others with a better chance of survival, is a reminder of how treatment decisions are not always focused on a single patient.

Therefore, although substituted judgment and best interests are important criteria and very helpful to a proxy who is making decisions for another person, the proxy still has a moral responsibility to act in a morally reasonable way in his or her role as proxy. The ultimate moral criterion of the proxy's action remains right reason, and sometimes this means that she will not follow the patient's instructions or will not decide according to what is in the patient's best interests. A proxy is not a puppet but a moral agent in her own right, and the morality of virtue encourages her always to seek her good, even when acting as proxy for someone else.

The Moral Responsibility to Designate a Proxy

The difficulties our families and physicians may encounter if we become incapacitated without leaving instructions about who will be our proxy and how we want to be treated suggest that it is morally good for us, in a spirit of kindness and love, to help them by designating a proxy and discussing with that person how we would like to be treated if we ever lose capacity. Appointing a proxy who knows us well, and who has the authority to make decisions on our behalf, will make things much easier for our families and for the people caring for us. It will relieve them of the burden of trying to figure out who should decide and what treatments should be provided.

Aristotle reminded us that we study ethics not simply to know what is virtuous but to act virtuously. The study of proxy decision making, then, encourages each of us to designate a proxy and to make advance directives. These actions are virtuous because they help us to achieve what is good for ourselves by extending our wishes into a time when we may no longer have capacity and by making it easier for others who someday may have to make decisions for us.

In the ethics of virtue that we are developing in this book, we would not say that we have a moral obligation to appoint a proxy and to make advance directives. In a morality of the human good, it is enough to remind a reasonable person that these actions are noble and virtuous and that noble and virtuous actions are what make a life a good life.

SUGGESTED READINGS

A very helpful book on the topic of this chapter is Allen Buchanan and Dan Brock, 1989, *Deciding for Others: The Ethics of Surrogate Decision Making*, Cambridge, UK: Cambridge University Press. Also helpful are chapters 2 and 3 of the President's Council on Bioethics 2005 report *Taking Care: Ethical Caregiving in Our Aging Society*, available at *bioethics.gov*; the 1992 report of the New York State Task Force on Life and Law titled *When Others Must Choose: Deciding for Patients without Capacity*; Part IV of the President's Commission 1982 report *Making Health Care Decisions*, titled "Decisionmaking Incapacity"; Ezekiel Emanuel and Linda Emanuel, "Proxy Decision Making for Incompetent Patients: An Ethical and Empirical Analysis," *JAMA* 1992, *267*, 2067–71; John Hardwig, "What about the Family?" *Hastings Center Report* 1990, *20* (March–April), 5–10; and "The Problem of Proxies with Interests of Their Own: Toward a Better Theory of Proxy Decisions," *Journal of Clinical Ethics* 1993, *4*, 20–27; Carson Strong, "Patients Should Not Always Come First in Treatment Decisions," *Journal of Clinical Ethics* 1993, *4*, 63–65; Rebecca Dresser and John Robertson, "Quality of Life and Non-Treatment Decisions for Incompetent Patients: A Critique of the Orthodox Approach," *Law, Medicine & Health Care* 1989, *17*, 234–44. See also the nine articles in the special supplement titled "Practicing the PSDA," *Hastings Center Report* 1991, *21* (September–October), S1–S15; and the special section on substituted judgment in the *Journal of Clinical Ethics* 1995, *6*, 14–43. Often, proxies relying on substituted judgment need to be guided so they will faithfully report the patient's wishes. See Daniel Salmasy et al., "The Accuracy of Substituted judgment in Patients with Terminal Diagnosis," *Annals of Internal Medicine* 1998, *128*, 621–29; Marie Nolan et al., "When Patients Lack Capacity: The Roles That Patients with Terminal Diagnosis Would Choose for Their Physicians and Loved Ones in Making Moral Decisions," *Journal of Pain and Symptom Management* 2005, *30*, 342–53; Daniel Sulmasy, "How Would Terminally Ill Patients Have Others Make Decisions for Them in the Event of Decisional Incapacity? A Longitudinal Study," *Journal of the American Geriatric Society* 2007, *55*, 1981–88.

The story of Beth is taken from *Care and Protection of Beth* 587 N.E.2d, 1377 (1992).

For the important legal background of making decisions for minors, see James Morrissey et al., 1986, *Consent and Confidentiality in the Health Care of Children and Adolescents*, New York: Free Press, especially chapters 1–3; and Angela Holder, 1985, *Legal Issues in Pediatrics and Adolescent Medicine*, 2nd ed., New Haven: Yale University Press, chapters 5–10. Both books consider the ethical as well as the legal dimensions of making decisions for minors. J. Rozovsky, 2007, *Consent to Treatment*, 4th ed., New York: Aspen, chapter 5, is also very helpful.

For the seminal work in the moral development of the child, see Jean Piaget, 1965, *The Moral Judgment of the Child*, M. Gabain, trans., New York: Free Press. The English translation was first published in 1932. For an introduction to Kohlberg's research see Lawrence Kohlberg, 1981, *The Philosophy of Moral Development*, volume 1, San Francisco: Harper & Row, and "Moral Stages and Moralization: The Cognitive-Developmental Approach," in Thomas Lickona, ed., 1976, *Moral Development and Behavior*, New York: Holt, Rinehart and Winston, pp. 31–53. The best-known work identifying the sexual bias in Kohlberg's early research is Carol Gilligan, 1982, *In a Different Voice: Psychological Theory and Women's Development*, Cambridge, MA: Harvard University Press.

Helpful texts on deciding for minors include Sanford Leiken, "Minors' Assent or Dissent to Medical Treatment," in the President's Commission Report titled *Making Health Care Decisions*, volume 3, pp.

175–91; Buchanan and Brock, *Deciding for Others*, chapter 5; and Tomas Silber, "Ethical Considerations in the Medical Care of Adolescents and Their Parents," *Pediatric Annals* 1981, *10*, 408–10.

The American Academy of Pediatrics has urged a greater role for minors in their health care decisions. See "Informed Consent, Parental Permission, and Assent in Pediatric Practice," *Pediatrics* 1995, *95*, 314–17. For a commentary urging caution, see Lainie Ross, "Health Care Decisionmaking in Children: Is It in Their Best Interest?" *Hastings Center Report* 1997, *27* (November–December), 41–45. Also helpful in the same issue is Robert Weir and Charles Peters, "Affirming the Decisions Adolescents Make about Life and Death," pp. 29–40. See also Howard Kunin, "Ethical Issues in Pediatric Life-Threatening Illness: Dilemmas of Consent, Assent, and Communication," *Ethics and Behavior* 1997, *7*, 43–57; and Loretta Kopelman, "Children and Bioethics: Uses and Abuses of the Best Interests Standard," *Journal of Medicine and Philosophy* 1997, *22*, 213–17.

The legal citations for the paragraphs on contraception and abortion are *Griswold v. Connecticut*, 381 U.S. 479 (1965); *Eisenstadt v. Baird*, 405 U.S. 438 (1972); *Carey v. Population Services International*, 431 U.S. 678 (1977); *Roe v. Wade*, 410 U.S. 113 (1973); *Doe v. Bolton*, 410 U.S. 179 (1973); and *Bellotti v. Baird*, 424 U.S. 952 (1976) and 443 U.S. 622 (1979). The case cited in reference to parents' not making martyrs of their children is *Prince v. Massachusetts*, 321 U.S. 158 (1944).

Three important cases allowing involuntarily confined mentally ill people to refuse treatment if they have decision-making capacity and are not dangerous are *Rennie v. Kline*, 720 F.2d 266 (3d Cir. 1983); *Rogers v. Okin*, 738 F.2d 1 (1st Cir. 1984); and *Rivers v. Katz*, 495 N.E.2d 337 (1986). In Rivers, the supreme court of New York (the Court of Appeals) required physicians to establish legal incompetence before they can treat involuntarily confined patients against their will. In Rogers (a Massachusetts case) the first circuit also ruled judicial intervention was necessary if the patient was objecting; in Rennie (a New Jersey case) the third circuit required safeguards but did not insist on judicial review. Case law continues to develop in this difficult area. The story of Richard Roe is taken from *In the Matter of Guardianship of Roe*, III, 421 N.E.2d 40 (1981).

For discussion about making decisions for mentally ill people, see the excellent book by Norman Cantor, 2005, *Making Medical Decisions for the Profoundly Mentally Disabled*, Cambridge, MA: MIT Press. Cantor argues persuasively that there are times when the patient's best interests standard is too narrow and that other interests, those of the family or of research, should be factors in decision making. See also Clarence Sundram, "Informed Consent for Major Medical Treatment of Mentally Disabled People: A New Approach," *New England Journal of Medicine* 1988, *318*, 1368–73. Sundram's article reports that volunteer committees in New York are making treatment choices and giving informed consent for some categories of mentally ill people who do not have family proxies. See also Thomas Finucaner et al., "Establishing Medical Directives with Demented Patients: A Pilot Study," *Journal of Clinical Ethics* 1993, *4*, 51–54; Erich Loewy, "Treatment Decisions in the Mentally Impaired: Limiting but Not Abandoning Treatment," *New England Journal of Medicine* 1987, *317*, 1465–69; Nancy Rhoden, "The Presumption for Treatment: Has It Been Justified?" *Law, Medicine & Health Care* 1985, *13*, 65–67; Thomas Gurtheil and Paul Appelbaum, "The Substituted Judgment Approach: Its Difficulties and Paradoxes in Mental Health Settings," *Law, Medicine & Health Care* 1985, *13*, 61–64; Michael Irwin et al., "Psychotic Patients' Understanding of Informed Consent," *American Journal of Psychiatry* 1985, *142*, 1351–54. Also helpful is the special section containing six articles on making decisions for persons with mental retardation in the *Cambridge Quarterly of Healthcare Ethics* 1994, *3*, 174–235; and another special section with nine articles on ethics and Alzheimer disease in the *Journal of Clinical Ethics* 1998, *9*, 1–91; and J. Rozovsky, *Consent to Treatment*, chapter 6.

SIX

Determining Life and Death

Knowing exactly when one of us begins and ends would be very helpful in health care ethics. Our ethical judgments about fertilization in laboratories, freezing and splitting embryos, cloning, embryonic stem cell research, research on fetuses, the transplanting of fetal tissue, and abortion are all shaped by our views on when an embryo or a fetus becomes one of us. And our ethical judgments about withdrawing life-sustaining treatment from human bodies lacking brain function and about retrieving organs from dead donors are shaped by our views on when one of us dies.

Unfortunately neither biology, biochemistry, genetics, neurology, nor any other science can tell us exactly when we begin or end our earthly existence. All we can do is select a reasonable stage in the development of human life as the beginning of one of us and another stage in the subsequent deterioration of human life as the end of one of us. Determinations of the beginning and of the end of human existence are not facts but interpretations of facts.

These interpretations are difficult for two reasons. First, despite great progress in the past few decades, we are still learning the physiological facts of life and death. Second, interpretations always reflect our previously embraced, and often never analyzed, frameworks of meaning and value—that is, our prejudices.

Nonetheless, interpret the facts we must, since determining when a new one of us begins and when one of us dies is of utmost importance for ethics, law, and public policy. It matters a great deal whether a fetus is or is not one of us if we are thinking of destroying it. It matters whether an embryo is one of us if we are thinking of freezing it or using it for research. It matters whether a body with no brain function is one of us if we are thinking of keeping it alive or of removing the heart for transplantation.

Determining the beginning and the end of one of us is an interdisciplinary effort. We need science to provide the facts, and we need philosophy to interpret those facts. It is not enough to know that an embryo is human life with forty-six chromosomes and a specific genetic code to say it is one of us—a brain-dead patient on life-support equipment is similarly composed. And it is not enough to know someone's heart and lungs have permanently ceased to function to say she is dead; she may still be living thanks to a heart-lung machine or transplant. We have to know the facts, but we also have to interpret the facts to determine when one of us begins and when one of us ends.

The stages in the development of human life currently proposed as markers for the beginning of a new one of us are (1) fertilization, (2) implantation (completed by the fourteenth day), (3) appearance of the "primitive streak" (the band on the embryonic disk that begins to appear about the fifteenth day and marks the longitudinal axis of the embryo), (4) fetal brain life (thought to begin about the eighth week), (5) viability (once considered to occur about the beginning of the third trimester, but now recognized as beginning somewhat earlier), (6) birth, and (7) the end of infancy.

The confusing and frequently disputed current public policy in the United States tends to an interpretation whereby one of us begins somewhere between viability and the expulsion or extraction of the living fetus from the uterus. U.S. Supreme Court decisions allow states to make third trimester abortions illegal unless they are necessary to preserve the woman's life or her health.

However, an illegal third trimester abortion is not considered murder unless the fetus is removed alive and then destroyed. This approach leads to a confusing notion: deliberately destroying a third trimester fetus in the uterus is not killing one of us, but deliberately destroying a third trimester fetus outside the uterus is killing one of us.

The stages of biological deterioration proposed as markers for the end of one of us, which is death, are (1) the permanent loss of cardiopulmonary functions, (2) the permanent loss of all brain functions, including the functions of the brain stem, and (3) the permanent loss of the higher brain functions necessary for awareness and feeling. The present public policy in the United States reflects interpretations whereby we are dead once we have suffered the permanent loss of cardiopulmonary functions, or of all brain functions, or of both. The permanent loss of the higher brain functions associated with awareness is not considered a sign of death.

Many proposals for determining the beginning and the end of one of us run into serious difficulty for one of two reasons. Either they are reductionist (reducing the problem to scientific facts) or they introduce nonscientific ideas such as soul, mind, self, selfhood, person, personhood, bearer of rights, and the like.

The problem with the reductionist interpretations is that many of us think, with some reason, that we are something more than what science observes. And the problem with the nonscientific ideas is the impossibility of verifying them, and hence people can deny them or use them in different ways, often with hidden agendas. If you are familiar with the history of philosophy, you know that "soul" did not mean the same for Plato as it did for Aristotle, that "mind" did not mean the same for Hume as it did for Hegel, that "self" did not mean the same for Locke as it does for Ricoeur, that "person" did not mean the same for Reid as it did for Strawson.

Later in the chapter we will develop positions on the beginning and the end of one of us that will reflect an attempt to avoid both a reductionist position and a position employing ideas that cannot be verified. Before we outline our positions on the beginning and on the end of one of us, however, we first examine the major concepts of human life and death in our culture and the criteria used to determine when one of us begins and when one of us dies.

As we do this, it will be helpful to keep in mind the important distinction between concepts and criteria. Concepts are how we think and talk about things. You and I can think and talk about disease, health, life, and death in a meaningful way because our minds and language are sufficiently developed to handle the concepts of disease, health, life, and death.

Criteria, on the other hand, are the observable facts verifying the reality of what we are thinking and talking about—they tell us something is indeed the case. Suppose we are talking about infection for example. We have a concept of infection—we know what infections are and can describe them. But the concept of infection does not tell us that this leg or this arm is actually infected. The criteria do this and the criteria by which we determine an infection is present are the symptoms: fever, tenderness, inflammation, white cell count, and so forth.

When we turn to determining when one of us begins and ends, the concepts are not the problem. We already share them—we know what life and death are. If someone says there was an accident in which four people lived and two died, we know what that means. What we want to know are the criteria—how we can tell when a new one of us has begun or when one of us has died? When we ask "How do I know something is one of us?" or "How do I know one of us is dead?" we are asking for criteria. The criteria are the signs indicating that something is indeed one of us or that someone who was once one of us is no longer one of us.

The concepts and criteria of life and death, however, are not the whole story. Concepts and criteria are embedded in conceptual frameworks, and we need to know something about the presupposed conceptual frameworks if we are to understand the concepts and criteria of life and death.

The Classical Conceptual Framework

Until recently, discussions about the beginning and end of human existence would have presupposed some knowledge of how the classical theologians and philosophers conceived of "man." We would have considered their "philosophy of man," their views on the nature of "man," and what they thought marked his beginning and his end.

Today, we would like to find a better term than "man" when we discuss these ideas of classical philosophy. Some suggest "person," but person is a troublesome term. People do not agree on what it means to be a person. Moreover, the modern notion of person did not exist in Greek philosophy, and it played only an inchoate role in medieval thought. For want of a better term we will employ phrases such as "one of us" or "each of us," phrases we have already been using, to describe what the classical philosophers were talking about when they wrote about "man."

We will look briefly at the classical theologies and philosophies describing what we are, and their views on when each of us begins and ends. It is important to do this because so many features of their thought are still operative in our culture today.

The Mystery Religions: Socrates and Plato

The very earliest philosophers (sixth century B.C.E.) considered us as nothing more than our material bodies. But some of the "mystery" religions (not the civil religion dedicated to Zeus, Athena, and the other gods and goddesses, but the religious beliefs and rituals some ancient people held in private) suggested that we were something more than our bodies. The mystery religions usually called this "something more" a "soul," and some of them included doctrines about the soul's leaving the body at death and then coming back into another body. The doctrine of the soul gained influence in the second half of the sixth century with the emergence of a scholarly and religious group in southern Italy—the Greek-speaking Pythagoreans.

Although the mystery religions and the Pythagoreans did not survive, some of their ideas did. Two major philosophers, Socrates (470–399 B.C.E.) and Plato (427–347 B.C.E.), were influenced by them. According to their theory, each of us is a composite of body and soul. The body is material and biological, but the soul is neither material nor biological. Because the soul is immaterial, it cannot be seen, or touched, or observed in any way. Nor does it have a beginning or an end—it is eternal. The soul animates the body—keeps it alive and provides for its growth and movement—and enables the human being to know things and make choices. The immaterial soul enables us to know the things that are not of this material world, things such as numbers and other mathematical notions, as well as universal and unchanging ideas such as justice, courage, and the like. And it allows us to escape some of the determinism of the material world in which we are enmeshed to make choices and, thereby, to have some control over our lives.

In this Socratic-Platonic conceptual model, the soul had no beginning; it always was. Its existence is eternal. Each of us begins when the preexisting immaterial soul enters the human body, and we die when the soul departs from this body. Since the soul animates the body, the self-movement of the body indicates that the soul is present, and the lack of movement indicates it has escaped. In general terms, then, the criterion of human life was the spontaneous movement of a human body, and the criterion of human death was the permanent cessation of that spontaneous movement.

So powerful was this Socratic-Platonic model of the material body–immaterial soul that many early Christian thinkers adopted it. The Christians did make one important change—they rejected the eternal preexistence of the soul and said, instead, that God created a human soul for each of us at some point in our fetal development. However, the Christians retained, as we will see, the same material body–immaterial soul duality. They explained the beginning of life as the infusion of an immaterial rational soul into the human body, and the end of that life as the departure of the soul from the body.

Aristotle

Plato did not try to determine when the soul came into a developing fetus, but his pupil Aristotle (384–322 B.C.E.) did. Although Aristotle rejected many of Plato's ideas about the soul, including its preexistence and its survival after death in any personal way, he retained the basic concept of an immaterial soul in a material body. More important for our purposes, he proposed criteria for determining just when a developing fetal body gains a human soul. His work was based on observation as well as theory. He was familiar with various writings by the Hippocratic physicians, which contained descriptions of spontaneously aborted fetuses, and he may well have studied some fetuses himself. His explanation of human reproduction and fetal development, as well as the criteria he developed for determining when one of us begins, were to dominate both secular and religious thought for two thousand years. The main features of his account are as follows.

When semen mixes successfully with blood in the uterus, the mixture congeals, preventing further menstruation. The semen or seed retained in the uterine blood begins to develop, much like a seed develops once it is planted in the ground. The seed first develops in a vegetative way, growing and becoming differentiated into distinct parts, much as a plant develops its stem, branches, and leaves. At this first stage, the fetus has a vegetative soul.

Later, this vegetative fetus acquires the ability to feel. The feeling of touch develops first, and then seeing, hearing, smelling, and tasting follow as the bodily parts supporting these sensations appear. With the beginning of feeling the fetus passes from the vegetative stage to the second stage of its development—the animal stage. It now has an animal soul.

A third stage—the specifically human stage—appears when the fetus acquires what Aristotle called the "rational soul," the source of rationality. Unlike sensation, which resides in a part of the body such as the eye or the skin, rationality is not identified with any part of the body but with the immaterial soul. The immaterial rational soul not only thinks but animates the human body. It makes the fetus one of us, and each of us continues to exist as one of us until the rational soul ceases to animate the body. At this point there is still a human body, but it is dead. The rational soul is so closely entwined with the body that it ceases to exist when the body dies or, conversely, we could say that the body is so closely associated with the soul that it dies when the soul ceases to animate it.

Aristotle's answer to the question "When did I begin?" is therefore this: A fetus becomes one of us when the rational soul permeates the developing fetal seed sometime after the appearance of sensation or feeling, which marks the animal stage. Just how long after the animal stage the rational soul appeared, Aristotle did not, and could not, say. But he was sure that the rational soul could not appear before the animal soul. And just how long after the seed began to grow did the animal soul or sensation develop? Aristotle's answer strikes us as bizarre today: sensation developed after forty days of growth if the fetus is male, after ninety days if it is female.

What led him to this conclusion? We do not know for sure, but it seems to have been prompted by his observations of sexual development in fetuses. Apparently he assumed that the fetus had to be sexually differentiated before sensation could appear. Since he thought—erroneously—that the penis appeared on about the fortieth day (he was probably observing the little tag that was still intact on some early aborted fetuses, and thought it was the penis) and the vaginal opening about the ninetieth day, he concluded a male fetus could acquire a rational soul any time after the fortieth day, but the female fetus could not acquire the rational soul until at least the ninetieth day. The delayed appearance of the rational soul in the female fetus was accepted practically without question in our culture for almost two thousand years.

Aristotle's concept of a new one of us, and the criteria he used to verify the presence of one of us, are now clear. Each of us began as a seed planted in the uterus. The seed first grew as a vegetable, and then, some time after the biological development of sexual differentiation, sensation appeared. At some point after sensation, the rational soul appeared. The emergence of the rational soul in the male fetus at about the sixth week, and in the female fetus at about the thirteenth week, is what makes the fetus one of us.

It should be no surprise that Aristotle's explanation of the beginning of human life was an important factor in his moral evaluation of abortion. Simply put, he thought abortions became a serious moral problem once sensation occurred, since the invisible rational soul, and therefore one of us, could be present any time after that. In practice, since he could not determine whether a fetus was male or female, this meant he considered most abortions after the fortieth day unethical because the fetus might possess a rational soul and be one of us.

Hebrew Bible

The first book of the Hebrew Bible, the book of Genesis, records two versions of the myth of creation, including the creation of Adam and Eve. In both versions, however, the first humans appear as adults, so the biblical accounts of the beginning of the human race do not address our concern, which is the fetal beginning of each of us.

The most relevant biblical text for our purposes occurs in Exodus 21:22, which reports a legal question about a man who attacked a pregnant woman. She lived but miscarried. The biblical question centered on what should be the penalty for the criminal who caused the destruction of her fetus. If he killed one of us, he is a murderer, and the penalty is death; if the fetus is not one of us, a lesser penalty is sufficient. Exodus advocates the lesser penalty, suggesting that the Hebrews considered the unborn fetus important but not yet one of us.

Beginning around 250 B.C.E., at Alexandria in Egypt, the ancient books of the Hebrew Bible were translated into Greek. The translators, however, changed the text of Exodus 21:22 in a significant way. Whereas the original Hebrew text simply stated that the penalty for a criminal action resulting in the destruction of a fetus is a fine and not the death penalty, the Greek translation of this passage says that destroying a developed fetus, one with a human form, is punishable by the death penalty. Making the penalty for destroying a formed fetus the same as the penalty for murder is important because it implies the formed fetus is one of us.

Since the Hebrew text makes no distinction between early and formed fetuses, the statement in the Greek translation advocating the death penalty for the destruction of a formed fetus does not belong in the Bible. It reflects, rather, the position of the Greek translators of the Hebrew Bible working at the Greek library and research center in Alexandria, a position that could have been shaped by Aristotle's well-known doctrine that the rational soul, which defines what is one of us, does not appear until weeks into the pregnancy.

In any event, the Greek version of the Hebrew Bible agrees in large measure with Aristotle's idea that an early fetus is not one of us, but that a more developed fetus, one that is formed, *is* one of us. And it was the Greek translation of the Hebrew Bible, along with Aristotle's similar account, that influenced so many later Jews and Christians living in the classical Greek-speaking world. When the Latin language began to replace Greek in the vast Roman Empire, the early Latin versions of the Hebrew Bible were actually translations of the Greek translation and not of the original Hebrew. Only in the late fourth century, more than six hundred years after the Greek translation, did St. Jerome make the first major Latin translation of the Hebrew Bible directly from the original Hebrew text.

By this time, however, it was too late for the biblical position (destruction of a fetus is not killing one of us) to dislodge the Greek idea that a fetus becomes one of us when the rational soul enters the fetus during pregnancy and its implication that destroying a fetus months after the pregnancy is under way is actually killing one of us. Thus, the prevailing idea of our culture became the more conservative philosophical position of the Greeks: an animated or formed fetus is one of us, and aborting such a fetus is equivalent to homicide.

Early and Medieval Christianity

Early Christian theologians such as Jerome (340?–420) and Augustine (354–430) accepted, along with almost everyone else, the Greek conception wherein a fetus becomes one of us at some point in its development. They thought the destruction of a fetus at any stage of development was immoral but that it was not the destruction of one of us unless it occurred after the point in its development when God created a human soul and infused it in the developing fetal body. No one knew when this happened, but the tendency was to think it did not happen before there was sufficient development of the fetus to support feeling or sensation. The most widely held idea in Christianity seems to have come not from the Bible but from Aristotle: The rational soul was formed in the male fetus during the sixth week and in the female fetus during the thirteenth week, and only the destruction of these formed fetuses counts as killing one of us.

The classical Greek doctrine of the delay before a fetus became one of us received the official support of the Roman Catholic Church in the great collection of church law completed by Gratian around 1140. This collection, and the decrees subsequently added to it, had a long-lasting influence—it remained the foundation of church law until a new Code of Canon Law was published in 1917. Gratian's *Decretum*, as the collection was called, accepted the standard explanation: A fetus did not become one of us until the human soul entered the fetal body some weeks after conception.

Gratian's position was subsequently confirmed in one of the official papal decrees, or "decretals" as they were called, approved by Pope Gregory IX during his reign from 1227 to 1241. A previous pope, Innocent III, had ruled that a monk causing a miscarriage of his mistress's early fetus was not subject to the ecclesiastical penalties for murder unless the fetus had been "vivified." In Gregory's collection of laws, a fetus was considered "vivified" from the point in its development at which the soul was infused into it.

The idea of the rational soul's delayed arrival in a fetus received further confirmation in the twelfth and thirteenth centuries when Aristotle's works, long largely unknown in the Europe of the Dark Ages, were rediscovered and quickly became central texts in the curricula of the new universities. Thomas Aquinas (1224–1274), the scholar many recognize as the most influential thinker of this time, did not hesitate to embrace a position consistent with Aristotle as well as with Jerome and Augustine: The early fetus is not one of us. "In the generation of man first there is a living thing, then an animal, finally a man" (*Summa Theologiae* II II, q. 64, a. 1). The fetus becomes one of us when the rational soul is infused, an event he thought happened after at least six weeks of fetal development in the male, and thirteen weeks in the female.

Thus, consistent with the Christian tradition up to this point, Aquinas thought the deliberate destruction of a fetus before it is animated with the rational soul was morally wrong but not murder. Commenting on the famous passage in Exodus, Aquinas wrote: "A person who strikes a pregnant woman does something wrong, and therefore if the death of the woman or of the *animated* fetus follows, he does not escape the crime of murder" (*Summa Theologiae* II II, q. 64, a. 8 ad 2, emphasis added).

To sum up, in the classical conceptual framework, each of us is considered a combination of body and soul. The body is material and organic, and the soul is immaterial and inorganic. The body arises from a seed mixing with bloody fluid in the uterus. This mixture congeals, and the seed grows and begins to take on a life of its own. Its life is first vegetative, then it becomes sentient as it achieves the ability to feel, and finally it becomes one of us when the rational soul arrives. In this conceptual framework each of us is a composite of a human body and an immaterial rational soul, a composite that first appeared no sooner than forty days into the pregnancy.

Of course the fundamental metaphor is all wrong. The metaphor for the beginning of one of us is not a planted seed, but a fertilized egg. Vegetables and flowers begin from planted seeds, but animals do not, and each of us definitely does not so begin. The father of a child is not analogous to a farmer sowing seed in the ground, but to a cock fertilizing eggs. The mother of a child is not analogous to the ground where the seed grows, but to a hen producing eggs.

Breakdown of the Classical "Seed" Explanation

In the seventeenth century two major factors began to undermine the two-thousand-year-old explanation of when one of us begins. The first was the effort of some to move the time of the soul's infusion into the body earlier and earlier, almost to the very beginning of fetal development. The second was the series of discoveries in the biology of human reproduction that forced us to revise radically the classical conceptions of human reproduction.

Since no one working with the classical explanation could say just when the human or rational soul arrived in the zoological fetus, the exact time when a fetus became one of us was always open to debate. In the early part of the seventeenth century some physicians began to argue for a very early infusion of the rational soul. A Flemish physician, Thomas Feyens, thought the soul was infused the third day after the semen mixes with the blood in the woman's body, and a Roman physician, Paolo Zacchias, thought the soul was infused almost immediately after the semen came in contact with the blood. The opinion of Zacchias gained credibility for many European Catholics when he was honored by the pope as the outstanding physician of the Roman Catholic Church in 1644.

Moving the arrival of the human soul to the first few days or hours after the semen mixes with the blood makes the beginning of each of us practically coincide with what we now call fertilization. At that time of course nobody yet knew that a spermatozoon fertilizes a human egg. In fact, no one knew the human female had eggs! But this discovery and others were about to come.

By the end of the seventeenth century scientists were becoming aware of the flaws in the classical biological understanding of human (and animal) reproduction. A major technological breakthrough, the microscope, helped them tremendously. As we know, grinding lenses a certain way can magnify objects and let us see things we never saw before. Galileo, using these lenses in a telescope, explored the night sky and produced the evidence showing that the fundamental classical assumption of cosmology—that the sun and other stars circle the earth—was simply false, even though it looks true and has biblical support.

Others used ground lenses in microscopes to explore bodily fluids. They soon discovered that the classical assumption of reproduction—that we begin as a seed—was also simply false. From the study of reproduction in birds, where rather large eggs obviously play a pivotal role, they began to suspect that a human female might have eggs and that a new fetus began when sperm fertilized one of these eggs, not when semen mixed with blood in the uterus. At this point, however, no one had ever seen the tiny human egg, so the process was still poorly understood. If the human female had eggs as large as those of a small bird, undoubtedly the riddle of human reproduction would have been solved much earlier.

It was not until 1827 that scientists achieved good observations of the microscopic human egg, or ovum, and produced the first rough scientific model of our modern understanding of human reproduction. They now realized that the sperm was not a seed that would grow in the moist environment of the uterus but one of two biological pieces, the other being the ovum.

Later it was discovered that the spermatozoon and ovum each have only half the chromosomes of the other human cells and that the merger of the male and female sex cells is what produces a normal human being with forty-six chromosomes. Then, about half a century ago, the structure of the DNA molecule was discovered. We later learned that the fertilized ovum contains a unique genetic structure of about thirty thousand genes and that every cell of the human body that develops from that fertilized ovum will manifest that same genetic identity.

The discovery that new human life originated from the fertilization of an egg, and not from a seed planted in the woman's body, was provocative. The transition from two germ cells (ovum and spermatozoon) to one zygote in fertilization is undeniably a momentous development, and it suggested to some that it must be the moment when the rational soul arrives. If this explanation is accepted, then it is logical to say that the destruction of a fertilized ovum is the destruction of one of us. And if each of us has a right to life, then it is logical to say this right to life is being violated if the embryo or fetus is arbitrarily destroyed.

None of those embracing the body-soul model of describing who we are can ever know for sure, of course, when a soul would be infused in a fetus because both the philosophical and Christian traditions have always insisted that the soul was immaterial and hence beyond empirical observation. Because no one can ever produce any empirical or scientific evidence that a soul has arrived, the moment of the soul's infusion will always remain a somewhat arbitrary interpretation. The radical change that happens at fertilization, and the resulting zygote with its complete set of human genes, could well be the moment, but it could just as well not be. In any event, since they can never know for sure, some argue that to be on the safe side in our respect for human life we should treat every fertilized ovum as a new one of us.

Others, of course, disagree. They agree with the biological facts, but they argue that we cannot call the early embryo—something invisible to the naked eye and lacking a brain—one of us. They suggest we should not consider the embryo or fetus truly a member of our species until a later stage of development appears, perhaps brain life, or viability, or birth, or even the end of infancy. This disagreement is bound to continue for some time because what is at issue is no longer the biological facts—we understand them pretty well—but people's interpretations of them.

Modern Concepts of Who We Are

Unhappy with the classical philosophical and Christian concepts of the immaterial soul–material body composite, some modern philosophers and psychologists have suggested the concept of person or personhood as the best way to think of each of us. But we run into all sorts of problems about defining what a person is. Some conceive person so broadly that it includes everything from a fertilized ovum to a human body that has been irreversibly vegetative for decades. Others define person so narrowly that it includes only those with self-consciousness, or with rationality, or with moral agency, or with rights that must be respected, or with some combination of these features.

If we cannot agree on a conception of what constitutes a person, then we cannot agree on the criteria to verify when a fertilized egg becomes a person, and when a permanently unconscious patient ceases to be a person. The debates about personhood are so interminable it seems best to avoid the concept altogether.

Another modern concept is that of the "self," a concept closely associated with person and exposed to its difficulties as well. For the influential philosopher John Locke, our personal identity is not secured by a "thinking thing" or mental substance that endures while we experience the many and various thoughts in our lives but by the consciousness that accompanies our thinking. I not only think of a house, but I am conscious of my thinking of the house. My thoughts and actions come and go and are of all different kinds, but my consciousness of the different thoughts and actions, past and present, remains ever the same, and this is what secures my personal identity. This consciousness is my "self." All this points to a position claiming a human being is not simply a body, nor simply a body with a substance called mind, but a body with something more, a self.

The concept of self, however, no less than the concept of person is also the subject of great controversy, so it seems best to avoid using it. What we want to retain, however, is the notion of the "something more" that is captured in the ideas of soul, mind, person, and consciousness. Our concept of what we are will have to account for this, for otherwise it will collapse into the counter-intuitive extreme we have identified as reductionist—the tendency to say that we are nothing more than biological organisms.

Critique of the Classical and Modern Conceptions

The most widely employed classical concept of ourselves is the material body–immaterial soul model originating with Socrates and Plato and modified by subsequent philosophies and Christian theologies. The classical concept remains firmly entrenched in the thoughts and language of many. It is supported by various Christian teachings insisting that, although the body dies, the soul lives on for eternity. It also underlies the modern philosophical concerns about what is called the mind-body problem.

The classical body-soul conceptual framework has merit, but, unfortunately, there are no criteria to verify when something human gains or loses the immaterial soul or mind. Although those accepting the conceptual framework will agree that you or I are undoubtedly composites of a material body and an immaterial soul and that the soul has departed from the body taken to the morgue, there is no such agreement about the early stages of human development, nor about later stages of deterioration where some signs of life are still present.

We can all perceive an embryo under a microscope, and we can verify that it has forty-six human chromosomes, but does it have an immaterial soul? Some proponents of the body-soul concept believe it does; others believe it does not. Again, we can all see the permanently unconscious patient in the hospital, but does that body have an immaterial rational soul? Some will say yes, but others, knowing all feeling has been irreversibly lost, will see no reason for saying her body retains its immaterial rational soul.

The concept of the material body–immaterial soul composite fails us when we need it most; that is, at the edges of life when we ask when one of us begins and when one of us dies. And it fails us because there are no criteria to show that a rational soul is present in any human body, especially a human body not manifesting any signs of sensation or thought.

At the root of the difficulty is the nature of the soul. It is thought to be immaterial, and the immaterial by definition cannot be perceived. There is simply no way we can empirically confirm the presence of an immaterial soul in a human body, which, of course, is why some people simply deny the existence of souls and advocate a materialism whereby we are nothing but our bodies. For those accepting the concept that each of us is a composite of body and soul, there is no way to settle the arguments about whether the soul arrives at fertilization or at implantation or at the development of the primitive streak or at the beginning of brain life or at some other point. And there is no way to settle the arguments about whether or not a permanently unconscious human body still retains its immaterial soul.

And the modern concepts of mind, person, and self do not fare any better than the classical concept of soul. There is no way of knowing whether a fetus or neonate has become a person or a self, or whether a PVS patient is still a person with rights or a self that is one of us.

The problems generated by the classical and modern concepts suggest that we need a new concept describing and defining what we are. We need to begin again the effort to develop a concept of ourselves and to define, at least to some extent, what each of us is. Once the concept is developed, we can ask about the criteria to verify when something is one of us and when it ceases to be one of us.

A New Conceptual Framework

If the classical and modern conceptions of human nature and personal identity are not working well, we can try to forge a new one. In so doing we will not begin with popular but troublesome notions such as "soul," "mind," "person," or "self" but the more simple expression already mentioned—one of us. We want to know what makes an entity one of us and not something else so we can determine when one of us begins and when one of us ends, that is, dies. These determinations are important for numerous issues in health care ethics; among them, embryo and fetal research, cloning, abortion, withdrawal of life support, the harvesting of organs, and so on.

We want to avoid two current extremes in developing a working concept of one of us. At one extreme are the dualistic philosophies conceiving of each one of us as partly material and partly immaterial and claiming that the immaterial element is what makes us specifically human. The second extreme goes in the opposite direction and reduces each one of us to nothing more than a body that can be explained in terms of biology, the chemistry underlying that biology, and the physics underlying that chemistry. Contemporary approaches such as behaviorism, cognitive science, evolutionary psychology, and sociobiology assume this general position.

Neither of these positions does justice to what most people experience in life. Most of us do not experience human bodies—our own and everyone else's—as biological containers housing minds. And most of us experience ourselves—and others—as more than bodies that can be explained in terms of science.

A new conceptual sketch might help, especially if it is open to some confirmation (unlike the notions of "soul" and "mind") and more in tune with our experience (unlike the various forms of scientific reductionism). We could begin by considering one of us as an *individual human organism existing in the world with us*. Analyzing the components of the phrase "individual human organism existing in the world with us" can provide us with a working concept describing one of us.

Human Organism

Each one of us is primarily a human organism. A human organism is first of all a multicellular organism with a full complement of human DNA in the nucleus of its cells. Contrary to the dualistic philosophies making something called a human soul or mind the primary marker of humanity, this concept makes the human organism primary.

We add the phrase "full complement of human DNA in the nucleus" because experiments in the late 1990s showed that human embryonic stem cells began developing after being inserted into bovine cells with the nuclei removed. If these bovine cells with human DNA in the nuclei ever developed into fetuses, all of their nuclear DNA (which is where most DNA is located) would be human, although some mitochondrial DNA outside the nucleus of the bovine cell might persist and thus give the cells of the embryo or fetus a small amount of nonhuman (bovine) DNA. The resulting organism would still be human and thus could become one of us. However, we do not yet understand how this procedure might affect the development of the embryo, so these experiments do raise a new set of serious ethical issues.

What would be a problem for our notion of human organism is any development of a true hybrid—an embryo with germ cells from two different species, for example, an embryo produced by in vitro fertilization with baboon sperm and a human ovum or human sperm and a baboon ovum. Our notion of human organism does not embrace hybrids of this kind, and we would need to develop new concepts for this very worrisome possibility if it ever occurred.

The notion of human organism covers fetuses and embryos as well as bodies after birth. A human embryo is a human organism—an organized collection of cells with a full complement of human DNA. Hence, a human embryo is human life. Given its human DNA, it could be no other kind of life. It is also a human being, understanding "being" in a strict sense as, roughly, any distinguishable separate entity. As we will see, however, being a living human organism does not necessarily mean that the organism is "one of us." A human organism that has lost all brain function, including that of the brain stem, is no longer "one of us." Such an organism, thanks to life support, is still living, but we consider it legally dead, a sure sign that we no longer think of it as "one of us."

Individual

Each one of us is an individual human organism. Normally we have no trouble identifying individuality because we see a human organism that we can identify as an individual. But is a human embryo truly an individual? The embryo is obviously a living human organism with human DNA, but is it an *individual* human organism? Not for its first few weeks of life, as we will see. This is so because early embryos sometimes spontaneously split and become two babies. Researchers can also divide them and produce two or more embryos, and some suggest that you could produce another human being from any one of the as-yet undifferentiated cells of early embryos. And sometimes two embryos can fuse, producing one baby. Hence, the early embryo, although certainly a human organism and hence human life, is not yet definitively an individual human organism and hence not yet "one of us." On the other hand, a single human body could support two individuals, as when twins are conjoined.

Existing in the World with Us

Thus far we have identified two essential characteristics for something to be one of us: That something must be a human organism, and it must be an individual. Now we want to add a third characteristic: That something must exist in the world with us. The verb "exist" does not carry the same meaning as the verb "is." Human (and animal) existence means more than an organism simply "is" somewhere in the world; it means the organism "exists" or, as the etymology suggests, "stands out from" itself in an engagement with the world that matters for it.

And things matter for a human organism only if the organism can sense the world. The transition from human life that simply "is" to human life that "exists in the world with us" occurs when the organism becomes aware of its worldly environment. A human organism that does not yet include or has irreversibly lost the organic functions needed for the sentience or awareness necessary to connect, however weakly, with our world is not "one of us."

Sentience or awareness means that the organism feels itself in touch with its world. It is not simply acting and reacting to stimuli but acting and reacting with some awareness however rudimentary; the organism now *feels*. The dawn of awareness in a developing human organism provides a clear point when the human organism becomes *one of us in our world* and the final sunset of this awareness, something that has occurred in human bodies that were once sentient but are now back in an irreversible presentient or vegetative state, provide a clear point when the human organism, despite its cardiopulmonary organic life, is no longer one of us.

The suggestion that human organisms are one of us only if they have the neurological capability for awareness is, of course, controversial. But any attempt to develop a conceptual framework to define one of us will be controversial, so all we can do is offer some reasons why this concept might be more appropriate for what we know about ourselves today than other alternatives.

One advantage of a concept such as *individual human organism existing in the world with us* is that it avoids the two counterintuitive extremes in today's debates about the beginning of personal life. It represents a middle ground between those opining that a new human person occurs at the moment of fertilization (sometimes called conception), or at implantation, or when the primitive streak appears and those opining that a new person does not occur until viability, or birth, or even the end of infancy.

A second advantage is that, unlike theories invoking soul or mind, the concept of *individual human organism existing in the world with us* (a perceiving body) provides us with three clear tests for identifying one of us: We can test for human DNA, we know when an embryo becomes definitively one individual, and we know how much neurological development is needed for awareness. An organism without a full complement of human DNA in the nucleus of its cells is not one of us, nor is an organism with human DNA but without definitive individuality, nor is an organism with both human DNA and individuality but without any capability for awareness. One of us is any *individual human organism existing with awareness*. Unlike claims that a human body becomes one of us when it acquires a soul, the claim that a human body becomes one of us when it achieves awareness and thus begins to exist in the world is something that can be determined with a high degree of accuracy by neuroscience.

A third advantage of the concept is that, unlike concepts reducing our personal identity to no more than material reality, it allows—although admittedly it does not require—more than a strictly materialist understanding of one of us. The development of our existing with awareness into the realms of art, literature, religion, and morality suggests that there may well be something more to human existence than organic materiality. Awareness begins in organic pleasure and pain but does not stop there. It embraces, in many lives at least, a complex of goals, values, choices, responsibilities, and feelings that no strictly materialistic explanation explains well.

For practical reasons we can shorten the phrase "individual human organism existing with awareness" to *perceiving body, psychic body,* or *sentient body*. A perceiving or sentient body is a body that is more than vegetative; it is a body with the capability of awareness; it can feel. Hence, the two questions of this chapter—When does a new one of us begin? and When does one of us die?—become questions of when a human organism develops and when it loses the capability for sentience, that is, for existing in the world with us. We turn now to the first of these two important questions.

WHEN DOES ONE OF US BEGIN?

When I conceive of myself as a psychic or sentient body, the question "When did I begin?" really asks "When did the individual psychic body that is me begin?" To answer the question, we need science to tell us about the development of a fertilized ovum into an individual psychic body. The individual that is me did not begin until the fertilized egg became an individual psychic body. Thus, we want to know when the fertilized egg becomes an individual body and when that individual body becomes psychic or sentient.

The Fertilized Egg Becomes an Individual Body

A few recent discoveries help us to understand when it is appropriate to say an individual human body has developed from a fertilized ovum. First, fertilization is a complicated interaction lasting about twenty-four hours. The sperm and ovum normally fuse into a genetic entity of forty-six chromosomes called a zygote in a process spanning about a day. This means any position claiming that a new one of us begins at "the moment of conception" or "the moment of fertilization" is misleading; there is no *moment* of conception or fertilization.

Second, the fertilized ovum or zygote is not yet something that will inevitably develop into an individual human body and become one of us. We now know that a high number of zygotes, more than a third, are lost in the first few days of life. Fertilization normally occurs in a fallopian tube, and implantation of the fertilized ovum in the uterus begins several days later. Evidence now indicates that many zygotes do not implant successfully. Many fertilized eggs pass through the uterus and are sloughed off with the endometrial lining two weeks after ovulation during what appears to be simple menstruation.

If the fertilized egg or zygote is understood as one of us, then these women carried a baby but never knew it. If the zygote is understood as one of us, then tragic deaths occur with astonishing frequency—about as many zygotes die this way as there are pregnancies. If a baby is present in the uterus once fertilization is completed, then millions of babies die each year in the United States as they are spontaneously discarded in the first few days of life. Although this terrible waste of early human life is not a definitive argument that a zygote is not one of us, there is something suspect about claiming a zygote is one of us when so many are naturally lost because they do not implant in the uterus.

Third, we know the zygote is not necessarily the beginning of a new *individual* body, despite its unique genetic structure. The zygote will sometimes, albeit rarely, split in two, and each side of the split can become one of us—an identical twin. Usually the splitting of the human embryo is spontaneous, but sometimes, as we learned in 1993, the splitting can be the result of deliberate intervention. And two zygotes will sometimes, albeit rarely, fuse to become one entity that develops into one of us.

If we say a zygote is one of us, then we are also saying that one of us can become two of us, and that two of us can become "one of us." This makes no sense. The possibility of zygotes splitting or fusing suggests the zygote is not yet what we mean by one of us. The zygote is obviously human life, but it is not so obviously a human *individual* because it has not yet reached the stage where it cannot become two instead of one, or become one after it was two. In the first week or so after fertilization, the embryo has not yet reached a stage of development where it has established itself as an individual body. Some ethicists, supporting the view that an embryo is a person or equivalent to a person from the "moment of conception," argue that two of us do not become one of us when the embryo splits. Rather, they say, an original one of us gestates a second one of us in somewhat the way a woman gestates a child. But this approach is not without serious problems. For example, if the first embryo generates the second embryo, then one identical twin has generated the other, and this makes the original embryo a kind of parent of the younger twin, who is his or her off-spring. It is difficult to know how this makes sense.

The biological facts about wastage, splitting, and fusion suggest that one of us has not yet begun before implantation and also suggest a stage of development where the embryo will be but one of us. This analysis shows how implausible it is to say one of us begins the first week or so after fertilization when so many embryos are lost and when the individual identity of the embryo is not yet definitively established.

The Individual Body Becomes Psychic or Sentient

More important, we want to know when the individual body becomes sentient because that is when a fetus no longer simply *is* but now *exists* as one of us. It may not be possible, at least for a while, to pin down just when perception or awareness begins in a fetus, but growing evidence from neuroscience indicates many weeks of development are needed.

The neural pathways for perception or awareness run from sensory receptors in the skin to sensory areas in the cerebral cortex. The first sensory receptors in the skin appear about the seventh week of fetal development around what will be the mouth and then spread to the rest of the body. The fetal neocortex appears in the eighth week and achieves its full complement of neurons by the twentieth week. Most important the pathways connecting the sensory receptors to the sensory areas in the cerebral cortex are also completed at about the twentieth week. Only when these pathways are operative does a fetus begin to perceive.

Perception or awareness occurs at the cortical level, and it requires both a considerable degree of cortical maturity and the establishment of neural pathways from the sensory receptors in the body to the sensory areas in the cerebral cortex. This suggests that perception certainly does not begin before the eighth week of fetal development and probably not until some time later. If we describe each of us as a psychic body, then a new one of us does not begin until the psychic body appears, that is, until the fetus perceives, something that cannot happen until some months into the pregnancy.

This may seem like a revival of the older body-soul or body-mind developmental theories embraced by many philosophical and theological traditions. Indeed, there are similarities, but there are also important differences. First, in the traditional theories a fetus with awareness but lacking a rational soul—the view of Aquinas, for example—is not yet one of us. Nor is a fetus with awareness but lacking a *res cogitans*, a thinking thing or a mind—the view of Descartes—yet one of us. In a psychic body theory a fetus becomes one of us when it becomes more than a vegetative body and acquires a psychic dimension that allows it to *feel* even though it does not yet *think*.

Second, in the traditional theories the fetal body becomes one of us when the immaterial soul or mind arrives by divine creation or some other mysterious process. In our theory the fetal body becomes one of us when its sensory receptors are linked with its cortical sensory areas and it begins to perceive. The arrival of one of us is not a mysterious, unexplained event, as it was for Aristotle, or a direct creative intervention by God, as it was in Christian theology, but a natural development of the fetal body itself. The fetus simply becomes a perceiving body at the appropriate stage of its development, and a perceiving human body is what we mean by one of us.

The body of one of us *is* psychic. We are not saying that our body contains a psychic entity called a soul or a mind, nor that our body is a composite of body and soul, nor that our body is matter informed by a divinely created rational soul during pregnancy, as suggested in the philosophical doctrine of hylomorphism, the matter-form model Aquinas ingeniously suggested to account for the individuality of the body-soul composite each of us is. Rather, we are saying that our body is at once biological and psychological. The psychological is not infused into the biological, and the biological does not somehow contain the psychological; both aspects are entwined in a mutual and complementary way. Each one of us is a "perceiving body."

The biological and the psychological are two sides of the human body. Human existence is not exclusively or even primarily biological, nor is it exclusively or even primarily psychological. Philosophies of materialism and of idealism both slight the full concept of a human being. Each one of us began when the fetus became a psychic body, a body that is at once biological and psychological; that is, each one of us began when the genetically human fetus became an individual perceiving body.

The claim that each one of us begins many weeks into fetal development is derived from how I conceive myself. Once we conceive of ourselves as psychic or sentient bodies, we can provide a plausible and verifiable response to the question of when one of us begins. Each of us began when the individual body with our genetic code became sentient; that is, when it began to feel, to be aware, to perceive.

This view of what each one of us is and when each one of us begins to be will be, as are all other interpretations, highly controversial. Some will insist the fertilized ovum is a new one of us; they run the risk of devaluing the psychic dimensions of human existence. Others will insist human existence cannot begin until much later, perhaps at viability (which is achieved around the beginning of the third trimester), or perhaps as late as infancy; they run the risk of devaluing prenatal and neonatal human existence. The end of these controversies is nowhere in sight.

The suggestion that we should conceive of ourselves as psychic bodies and that a new one of us begins when the fetal body becomes psychic is simply one of many answers to the question "When did I begin?" It is an answer based on the idea that each of us is an individual human body sufficiently developed so that it is not capable of dividing or fusing and is capable of perception. This approach will not please everyone, but neither will any other approach. No one expects that everyone will agree on when one of us begins. All we can hope is that the question will be approached in an orderly and thoughtful way, first by developing a concept of ourselves and then by looking for criteria that will show when a fetus becomes one of us and when one of us dies. The classical conceptions of body and soul, and the modern conceptions of body and mind, no longer serve us well. Perhaps some such concept as psychic body or perceiving body will help.

WHEN DOES ONE OF US DIE?

The end of life is also an important determination in health care ethics. We do not want to treat dead human bodies as if they were patients, nor do we want to make the horrible mistake of considering a living patient dead.

Determining death has become even more pressing in recent decades because of two advances in medicine: life-support systems and organ transplantation. Life-supporting technology can sometimes sustain cadavers for weeks, and the need for organs encourages us to determine the exact moment of death so organs can be removed as quickly as possible.

In discussing the determination of death, the distinction between concept and criteria is once again important. The concept of death is what we mean by "death" and "dead." We all have a good idea of the concept of death. We know what it means when a friend or relative has died. We think of death as meaning someone has "left this world," "passed away," "departed," "passed on," or "is gone."

The criteria of death refer to the evidence that indicates someone is dead. Criteria enable us to verify that death has occurred. Sometimes the criteria are obvious. Anybody looking at a human body that has been dead for a few hours observes a whole series of changes that lead to one conclusion—the person died some time ago. A significant drop in body temperature, loss of normal color, rigor mortis, and biological disintegration are all clear criteria for indicating death.

These indications, however, are not sufficiently refined for medicine because they appear only several hours after death, and if life-support equipment is being used, they may not appear for weeks or even months after death. Medicine therefore uses two more refined criteria for determining when someone is dead. The first has a long history; the second was developed in the last few decades. The first criterion centers on circulation and respiration; the second on brain function.

The Cardiopulmonary Criterion of Death

According to the cardiopulmonary criterion of death, a person is dead if the functions of the cardiopulmonary system have irreversibly ceased. The pulmonary system provides oxygen, and the cardiac system distributes the oxygenated blood. The contributions of these systems are crucial for life. If air is not taken in by the lungs, and if blood is not pumped by the heart, organs begin to die. It matters little which function—cardiac or pulmonary—ceases first because the cessation of either will soon cause the cessation of the other.

Note that we did not say that the destruction of the heart or lungs is a criterion of death because it is not. We know today that we can remove a person's heart and lungs, and she can remain alive as long as something else, perhaps a heart-lung machine or a transplant, provides the functions of the heart and lungs. Note also that we said *irreversible* cessation of cardiopulmonary functions is the criterion for death. Temporary cessation of the cardiopulmonary functions does not mean the person is dead. Some cessations of pulse and breathing are reversible, although seldom after twenty minutes or so. In rare cases such as drug overdoses or hypothermia (low body temperature, usually caused by submersion in cold water), people can be revived after several hours without air or detectable pulse. Often, unfortunately, their neurological recovery will not be complete because irreversible brain damage is likely after prolonged oxygen deprivation.

The lack of pulse and breathing can be observed by physicians and other trained medical personnel with great accuracy, and except for cases of drug overdose or low body temperature, it does not take long for the cessation of cardiopulmonary functions to become irreversible. In most situations, then, the cardiopulmonary criterion of death provides adequate evidence of death within a few minutes after it occurs. It serves us well in most cases.

Several decades ago, however, a problem emerged. The development of life-support systems enabling unconscious people to live for extended periods of time meant respiration could be prolonged long after it would have naturally stopped. Techniques for long-term feeding were also developed. Patients were fed through a tube entering the nose and running down into the stomach or through a tube surgically inserted into the gastrointestinal system. With good care and antibiotics to fight infection, irreversible cessation of the cardiopulmonary functions could now be prevented for long periods of time.

Some patients on advanced life-support systems had experienced the loss of all brain function. Were it not for life-support systems, they would have irreversibly lost cardiopulmonary functions and been declared dead. With the life-support equipment, they lived for weeks and even months. This led many to wonder whether the life-support systems were preserving life or preventing natural death. The cardiopulmonary criterion of death did not seem appropriate for cases where life-support systems kept hearts and lungs working for people without any brain function. This suggested that another criterion of death was needed. The obvious candidate was the irreversible loss of all brain functions.

The Brain-Death Criterion of Death

In 1959 French neurophysiologists observed that some unconscious patients sustained by respirators lacked all awareness and all electrophysiologic activity in their brains. Moreover, when these patients finally died of irreversible cardiopulmonary arrest despite the life support, autopsies revealed extensive areas of necrotic brain tissue. This showed that their brains had been dead for some time, just as any organ of the body can die if it is not properly nourished by oxygenated blood. In fact sometimes the tissue had been dead for so long that it had begun to digest itself in a process called autolysis, a phenomenon that normally occurs in a dead body some time after death.

The French physicians concluded that these patients had not really been in a coma while they had been on the life-support systems but in a state "beyond coma," a state they called *coma depassé*. Their brains were dead, but the technology was sustaining cardiopulmonary function so their bodies were alive. Thanks to a respirator the bodies absorbed oxygen and were able to maintain the body temperature, pulse, and color of the living. The big question was: Are patients with dead brains and living bodies alive or dead?

At about the same time as life-support systems were creating a class of patients in coma depassé, another development was beginning—organ transplantation. In the early kidney transplantations, organs were retrieved from living donors with close tissue matches to the recipient, but it was immediately recognized that most organs would come from cadavers once drugs could be developed to fight rejection by the recipient's body. Using organs from cadavers presents a problem because the organs have to be fresh, that is, as fully nourished by a healthy blood supply as possible. Without this nourishment the organs rapidly degenerate and become unusable.

In other words, transplant teams want living organs, but they can only take them from dead patients. They need a way to determine death as soon as possible after it occurs, and they also need a way to determine when a patient dies while life-support systems are still nourishing the body.

In 1968 an ad hoc committee of the Harvard Medical School published an important report outlining criteria for determining what it called "irreversible coma," the *coma depassé* first described by the French physicians. It outlined several clinical tests and also called for the use of an electroencephalogram (EEG) to show the absence of electrical activity in the brain. It recommended that these tests be repeated in twenty-four hours. These criteria became known as the Harvard criteria. Their accuracy was demonstrated repeatedly in the ensuing years, for no patient diagnosed to be in "irreversible coma" according to these criteria ever recovered. These criteria of course were not really verifying the presence of an irreversible coma but of something else, something that would soon come to be called brain death.

A consensus began to emerge that patients whose brains had permanently ceased to function should not be described as in an irreversible coma, but as dead. Their cardiopulmonary functions supported by respirators made it look as though they were alive, but they were not. They were not living in a state "beyond coma" or in an "irreversible coma"—they were simply dead. In other words, a new criterion of death was emerging. If vital signs such as pulse, respiration, and normal body temperature were being maintained by life-support systems, but the brain had irreversibly ceased to function, then it was thought that we should consider this as evidence the person was dead. Along with the original criterion of death—irreversible cessation of the cardiopulmonary function—there was now a second criterion—irreversible cessation of all brain functions.

When life-support equipment is not being used, brain and cardiopulmonary functions will cease almost simultaneously, so the brain-death criterion is of little practical value in most deaths. But when life-support equipment is being used, the mutual dependency of the cardiopulmonary and brain functions can be broken. The life-support equipment can sometimes maintain the cardiopulmonary functions for days and even months after all brain functions have ceased. The new criterion of death, irreversible cessation of all brain functions, is designed for just such a situation. It allows us to say that people with adequate circulation and respiration (thanks to life support), but with irreversible loss of all brain function, are truly dead.

For a time there was extensive debate about the brain-death criterion, but a consensus soon emerged. In 1970 Kansas became the first state to recognize brain death as a legal criterion of death. Today almost all states recognize the brain-death criterion, either by legislation or by case law derived from court decisions. Unfortunately the laws are not identical in every state, and revisions are still being made. Some state laws, for example, speak of the cardiopulmonary and brain-death criteria as two separate but equal criteria, whereas other states make the cardiopulmonary criterion primary and accept the brain-death criterion only when the cardiopulmonary criterion cannot be used because life-support systems are in use.

In the early 1980s a Uniform Determination of Death Act (UDDA) was approved by the Uniform Law Commissioners, the American Bar Association, the American Medical Association, the American Academy of Neurology, and others and adopted verbatim by a number of states. It reads as follows: "An individual who has sustained either (1) irreversible cessation of circulatory and respiratory functions, or (2) irreversible cessation of all functions of the entire brain, including the brain stem, is dead."

Although this statement is actually quite clear, confusion over the brain-death criterion of death persists. People use the words "brain dead" and "brain death" in misleading ways. It would be well if we could abandon these phrases and speak, instead, of the neurological criterion for death, but it is undoubtedly too late for that. Since people will likely continue to use the expression "brain death," we should attempt to be clear about what it means.

First, when we speak of brain death, we are speaking of the whole brain. We are saying that the entire brain, including the brain stem, has irreversibly ceased to function. The brain stem is about three inches long and joins the spinal column to the brain itself. It is considered a part of the brain and is the primary center for the control of respiration and blood pressure. If it has ceased to function, there will be no spontaneous breathing, and cardiopulmonary functions will cease almost immediately unless a ventilator is used. The bodies of brain-dead people always need this equipment—no truly brain-dead person is being kept alive simply by a feeding tube. Irreversibly unconscious patients breathing without a ventilator are not brain dead. (Conversely, not every irreversibly unconscious patient on a ventilator is brain dead.) The brain-death criterion of death, therefore, never refers to what some misleadingly call cerebral or neocortical death, the death of the cerebral hemispheres or the neocortex. It refers always to complete brain death, the irreversible cessation of all functions of the entire brain, including its stem.

Second, brain death is a definitive criterion of death; that is, it is an observable fact that allows us to say someone is dead. If someone has suffered brain death, then he is not alive. If he is on life-support systems, he will look very much alive because cardiac and pulmonary functions, as well as normal body temperature and skin color, continue. But if physicians have correctly diagnosed brain death, then the person is truly dead. This means he does not die when the life-support technology is disconnected and his breathing suddenly stops; he was already dead when the life-support system was removed. In effect, the life-support system was removed from a corpse.

Unfortunately, many people continue to think life-support systems keep brain-dead patients alive. Newspapers, for example, sometimes print stories about brain-dead pregnant women being kept alive in an effort to save the fetus and brain-dead babies being kept alive while suitable organ recipients are sought. If these women and babies are truly brain dead, then they are simply dead, and it is incoherent to say that they are being kept alive. It looks as if the life-support equipment is keeping them alive, but this is not so because dead people cannot be kept alive. What is really happening is this: The life-support equipment is supporting the biological life of a corpse in an effort to save the fetus or to salvage fresh organs. People become confused because they see the classic signs of life—pulse, temperature, color, and breathing—but once we know all brain functions have irreversibly ceased, we know the individual is really dead.

Third, the role of the EEG in determining brain death is often misunderstood. It is not true to say that a "flat" EEG, one that shows no electrical activity in the brain, indicates that people are brain dead. Nor is it correct to say that an EEG showing electrical activity indicates that people are alive. The EEG was a requirement in the tests set forth by the Harvard criteria of 1968, but since then most published criteria for determining brain death rely on a clinical diagnosis, usually by a neurologist, and use the EEG only in a secondary role for confirmation. One reason for this is that the EEG is not always a good indicator of brain death. Sometimes people with a flat EEG are actually not brain dead, and sometimes the EEG indicates activity when in fact brain death has occurred.

Fourth, brain death is difficult to diagnose in children, especially in the first year of life when neurological development is incomplete. In the mid-1980s a special task force on brain death in children produced helpful criteria tailored to three age groups: over one year; between two months and one year; and between seven days and two months. The task force recognized the difficulty in applying brain-death criteria to children and declined to recommend criteria for infants less than a week old.

Fifth, despite widespread public acceptance of the brain-death criterion, some problems still linger. Among them are the following.

1. Some states have not yet passed laws defining neurological indications of death, and this leaves some physicians living in those states uncomfortable about using the brain-death criterion.

2. Some religious groups, including Orthodox Jews, object to the brain-death criterion. This has led some to suggest that people should be able to refuse the use of the brain-death criterion for determining their death, or the death of family members, if they so desire. Such a proposal, however, while considerate for individuals, would cause social problems. Societies need to know clearly whether someone is dead or not, and third-party payers for treatment understandably do not want to pay for treatment on legally dead patients.

3. Some people associated with right-to-life or pro-life groups still feel uncomfortable with the brain-death criterion, although their opposition to it is not as widespread as it was a decade or so ago. The underlying fear was, and to some extent still is, that acceptance of the brain-death criterion encourages a tendency to accept euthanasia and abortion.

RECENT CONTROVERSIES OVER DETERMINING DEATH

Despite widespread agreement with the criteria for determining death after the debates of the 1960s and 1970s, major disagreements surfaced once again in the 1990s and continue into the twenty-first century. These disagreements center on two issues: first, problems with the whole-brain-death criterion, and second, efforts to modify the cardiopulmonary criterion.

Problems with the Whole-Brain-Death Criterion

One major difficulty with the whole-brain-death criterion is people's failure to understand it. A 1989 study showed that two-thirds of the nurses and physicians prepared to retrieve organs from the newly dead did not really understand the brain-death criterion of death. These results are upsetting because the brain-death criterion is needed to determine death in most organ retrievals.

However, they come as no surprise—more than twenty years later many physicians are still recording the time of death as the removal of life support from a patient diagnosed as brain dead rather than the time of the diagnosis itself. If health care professionals still cannot fully understand brain death clearly, there is a problem associated with the use of the criterion.

A second difficulty with the whole-brain-death criterion arose when the insistence on "irreversible cessation of all functions of the entire brain" for declaring brain death came under increasing attack. Early discussions of whole-brain death acknowledged that some scattered electrical and cellular activities could persist after the whole brain had ceased to function. However, as the 1981 President's Commission Report titled *Defining Death* pointed out, these activities were not considered relevant because they no longer contributed to the operation of the organism as a whole.

It was not long, however, before physicians realized that the "nonfunctioning" brains of brain-dead people could retain some activities contributing to the functioning of the whole organism. The brains of some brain-dead patients, for example, continue to secrete hormones regulating identifiable bodily functioning. And surgeons harvesting organs for transplantation from brain-dead patients sometimes noticed increases in pulse and blood pressure when they made their incisions. These circulatory changes can be traced back to regulatory centers in the brain, suggesting that some brain functions affecting the operation of the body as a whole have continued despite the diagnosis of whole-brain death. Observed events such as the continuation of hormone secretions and the increases in pulse rates and blood pressure in response to trauma do undermine the definition of brain death as the "irreversible cessation of all functions of the entire brain" and reopen the brain-death debate that most everyone thought had been settled.

A third difficulty with the whole-brain-death criterion is worrisome: A large study presented at the annual meeting of the American Neurological Association (ANA) in late 2007 found that physicians in many well-regarded hospitals were routinely ignoring the American Academy of Neurology (AAN) guidelines for determining death by the whole-brain-death criterion. Although the UDDA allows hospitals to develop their own protocols for determining death, the AAN guidelines published in its journal *Neurology* in 1995 have served as a kind of gold standard for determining death by the whole-brain-death criterion. The 2007 study found that physicians were ignoring key features of the AAN guidelines and not performing some of the accepted tests to determine whether unconscious patients on life support were truly dead. The lack of a standard protocol for determining death by the whole-brain-death criterion not only leads to confusion about who is dead but opens the medical profession to the criticism that it is compromising the determination of death in efforts to harvest organs or to reduce financial losses by withdrawing life support.

A fourth difficulty with the whole-brain-death criterion is the so-called "conscience clauses" that exist in some jurisdictions. In New Jersey, for example, the law directs physicians not to declare people dead according to the whole-brain criterion if the physician knows it violates their religious convictions. Although such a law is sensitive to the religious plurality that exists in the United States, such an approach has a social downside that is illustrated by a recent case at the Beth Israel Deaconess Medical Center in Boston.

The family of a man who was a Buddhist insisted that the hospital continue life support for the patient after he had been declared dead by the whole-brain-death criterion. They argued that he was still alive according to their Buddhist religious tradition. Massachusetts does not have a "conscience clause," but the hospital delayed withdrawing the ventilator while it tried to negotiate with the family. After a few days, however, the body's extremities, despite the advanced life support, began to show signs of necrosis and decay similar to what one would see in a cadaver. Obviously this was extremely upsetting for the caregivers. The hospital then informed the family that the life support would have to be stopped. The family refused to consent and threatened legal action. The predicament was resolved when the hospital did convince the family to agree that medications to sustain blood pressure could be withheld, and the patient's heart soon stopped despite the ventilation. Cases like this show how the "conscience clause" that accommodates a family's religious beliefs can compromise the consciences of nurses and doctors by directing them to provide medical care for what is a corpse according to the whole-brain-death criterion.

In view of the difficulties with the whole-brain criterion of determining death, some authors suggest abandoning the brain-death criterion altogether and using only the cardiopulmonary criterion. It is difficult to predict how the reopened debate about brain death will affect the legal definitions of death. Changing laws and legal definitions is not easy, so perhaps nothing will happen. On the other hand laws and legal definitions written in language that is poorly understood and inconsistent with reality often cause so many problems that change is inevitable.

Problems with the Cardiopulmonary Criterion of Death

Driven by the laudable interest in obtaining more organs for transplantation, some have pushed for what amounts to a new understanding of the cardiopulmonary criterion, although some deny that their approach is really a new interpretation. Organ transplantation will be more fully discussed in chapter 15, but we need to provide some background here to understand new developments affecting the cardiopulmonary criterion of death.

There have never been enough donated vital organs for the people who need them, and the situation is getting worse. Unfortunately, organs from donors whose death is determined by the cardiopulmonary criterion are seldom usable because the cardiopulmonary functions in a dying body often fail slowly, and thus the organs are compromised before the arrest finally occurs. Moreover, physicians have to wait some time after the last heartbeat to be sure the arrest is irreversible. They cannot really determine that an arrest is irreversible until it is past the point where emergency CPR and ventilation might restart the cardiopulmonary functions.

In response to the organ shortage, transplant centers began exploring better ways to harvest organs after death from potential donors who happen to be on life support that is going to be withdrawn because it is no longer a reasonable treatment. The life support is keeping these organs well nourished with oxygenated blood. After life support withdrawal, these people, who have some brain function, can only be declared dead by the cardiopulmonary criterion. However, if physicians wait to be sure the cessation of cardiopulmonary function is irreversible, the organs will probably no longer be suitable for transplantation.

In an effort to retrieve usable organs from these donors, the University of Pittsburgh Medical Center (UPMC) developed a controversial protocol in 1992 that vastly increased the chances of obtaining usable organs from these donors who were then known as "non-heart-beating donors," and the procedure was known as "non-heart-beating donation." Today, in order to stress that the donor is really dead, the procedures are usually called "donation after cardiac death," "donation after cardiocirculatory death," or "donation after circulatory death." Sometimes the initials "DCD" are used to describe the procedures.

The protocols developed by UPMC and used by other transplant centers generally work in the following way. A dying patient on life support, or his proxy, consents to life-support withdrawal and agrees to organ donation after death. The patient, of course, has an order in place indicating that CPR will not be attempted. When everything is set for organ retrieval, the patient is taken to an operating room where physicians give appropriate sedation and withdraw the life support. If the cardiac function ceases within thirty minutes after the life support is withdrawn, the person is a viable candidate for DCD. Physicians then wait a minimum of two minutes after the heart has stopped or, more usually, five minutes and then declare the person dead. The transplant team waiting outside the OR immediately enters and begins removing the still-fresh organs.

The big question that interests us here, of course, is whether or not the patient is really dead according to the existing criteria of death when surgeons start harvesting his organs. He is certainly not dead according to the brain-death criterion because the functions of the entire brain will not have ceased in such a short time. Moreover, standard brain-death protocols require two neurological examinations at least several hours apart.

Is this patient dead according to the cardiopulmonary criterion? That depends on how you interpret the phrase "irreversible cessation of circulatory and respiratory functions." If the phrase means the cessation is *absolutely* impossible to reverse then he is not dead, because CPR initiated after the second or fifth minute might restore some cardiopulmonary function. However, if the phrase means the cessation is *in fact* impossible to reverse because (1) a spontaneous reversal has in fact never been known to occur after one minute and (2) a medical reversal will not occur because no one is going to try resuscitation, then one could say he is truly dead. This second reading is what the advocates of donation after cardiac death want the phrase to mean, and they buttress their argument by pointing out that it would be unethical for anyone to try CPR because the patient or proxy had already decided there would be no resuscitation efforts after cardiac failure.

Thus, it comes down to whether "irreversible" means *absolutely* not reversible, the usual way of understanding the word, or *factually* not reversible because no one is going to try to reverse the cardiac arrest, and, after two minutes, spontaneous reversal has never been known to occur. Using this *factual* interpretation of "irreversible" is uncomfortable to some because it appears to be giving the cardiopulmonary criterion a "spin" for utilitarian purposes—gaining more usable organs.

The discomfort became very public in April 1997 when the television show *60 Minutes* and the national media carried stories suggesting that organs were being taken from dying but not yet dead patients at some clinics. In response, the Department of Health and Human Services asked the Institute of Medicine (IOM) to look into the medical and ethical issues of retrieving organs from NHBDs. The IOM released its report titled *Non-Heart-Beating Organ Transplantation: Medical and Ethical Issues in Procurement* in December 1997. It supported the process of retrieving organs by donation after cardiac death as medically effective and ethically acceptable. It also made several important recommendations, including increasing the time period after the cardiopulmonary arrest to five minutes, a time frame adopted by most transplant centers. The IOM report was welcomed by some and attacked by others who claimed it allowed violation of the "dead donor rule."

One of the problems with the IOM report is that its major focus was on procuring more organs and not on defining death. It insisted on the "dead donor rule," which states that the donor must be dead before organ harvesting begins, but then seemed to gerrymander interpretations of the cardiopulmonary criterion of death to accomplish its primary interest of making more organs available.

A second problem with the IOM position is that we can easily imagine scenarios in which its interpretation of the cardiopulmonary criterion creates inconsistent conclusions about who is really dead. Imagine two patients in essentially similar conditions. One has indicated he wants to be a donor after cardiac death and has consented to an order withholding resuscitation efforts when physicians withdraw his life support. The other does not want to donate organs and wants resuscitation efforts if he arrests.

The first patient is in the OR awaiting organ retrieval. He arrests as soon as doctors stop his life support. Physicians wait five minutes and then declare him dead. Can they say he is really dead according to current criteria? The IOM report says they can make that determination. Hence, transplant surgeons are not killing him when they start taking his organs right away.

The second patient is in his room. He arrests when his life support malfunctions. A monitor records the time. The nurses were already busy with another emergency but one responds as quickly as he can, checks for a pulse, verifies that the patient does not have an order not to be resuscitated, calls for the special code team, and starts CPR. The code team arrives a few minutes later with the drugs and equipment. As they start CPR efforts, the physician notices it is now five minutes and ten seconds since the life support failed and the patient arrested. Would the physician say the patient is surely dead? No physician in these circumstances could say for sure that a patient is truly dead only five minutes and ten seconds after his arrest. The patient is probably dead, but sometimes in cases like this enough cardiopulmonary function can be restored for life to continue. We would expect the code team to begin CPR efforts.

And so the IOM report reinforces a new interpretation of the cardiopulmonary criterion that sets up incoherence in the determination of death. If the DCD patient in the OR is certainly dead five minutes after his arrest, so is the other patient, and conversely, if the patient in his room is possibly still alive five minutes after his arrest, so is the DCD patient in the OR. If we agree with the IOM and DCD protocols that organ donors are dead five minutes after their arrest, then it seems that we have to declare that everybody is dead five minutes after an arrest, which is an untenable position given the fact that CPR has restored cardiac function in some people five minutes or more after their arrest.

Thus some say that what the DCD protocols and the IOM report really provide is a cardio-pulmonary criterion for determining when a person is dying and not when he is certainly dead. Based on the best knowledge we have, they say it can be said a person is certainly dying five minutes after an arrest if no effort is made to reverse the arrest but insist we cannot say that he is certainly dead because in a few cases some cardiac function could be restored after five minutes by CPR efforts.

If the physicians advocating DCD are convinced that a patient is truly dead after five minutes, one wonders why they do not try to keep the organs as fresh as possible by putting the dead donor on full coronary bypass equipment after waiting the five minutes. At least one physician-ethicist has noted that no one wants to do this because they fear it might revive cardiopulmonary function or even awareness. This suggests that those determining death so soon after an arrest for the laudable purpose of obtaining organs may have some lingering doubts about the conformity of their actions to the dead donor rule.

Prudential reasoning suggests that any interpretation of the criteria of death giving rise to incoherence and playing into the public's fear that surgeons will start taking organs from the dying and not just the dead will do more harm than good despite the increase in organs it will produce. If the fear that surgeons are taking organs from the dying becomes widespread, it will undermine efforts to increase the number of organ donors. Transplant teams, as we will see in chapter 15, have traditionally been very careful to avoid negative publicity. Most will not, for example, take organs from the body of a donor who gave consent if family members object, lest the program be undermined by bad publicity initiated by upset family members.

A challenging question emerges in determining death in cases of DCD when the organs to be transplanted are the heart or lungs. Clearly a serious question arises if we determine that the donor is dead because he has sustained irreversible cessation of circulatory and respiratory functions and then transplant his heart and lungs into another body where we restart them to provide circulatory and respiratory functions once again! This is why some say that a DCD heart donor was not really dead if his heart and lungs can provide circulation in another body.

Yet another challenging question occurs in connection with the use of extracorporeal membrane oxygenation (ECMO) in conjunction with CPR efforts after an arrest. ECMO is a process used mostly with infants and children experiencing inadequate cardiac or respiratory function. The patient's blood flows through a machine that oxygenates the blood and then pumps it back into the body where it nourishes the organs, keeping them and the person alive.

The use of ECMO raises a challenging question about the determination of death in two major ways. First, recent studies have shown that ECMO employed with emergency resuscitation efforts can sometimes extend significantly the time a cardiopulmonary arrest can be reversed. Normally after twenty or thirty minutes of unsuccessful CPR efforts, a doctor will determine that cardiopulmonary arrest is irreversible and hence that the person is dead. However, when ECMO is used in CPR efforts, it has resulted in the restoration of cardiopulmonary function after a much longer time, in some cases more than an hour after the arrest (in one case the arrest lasted ninety-five minutes, yet the patient lived). This calls into question the UDDA cardiac criterion of death: Can we truly say that a person has sustained "irreversible cessation of circulatory and respiratory functions" twenty or thirty minutes after unsuccessful CPR efforts when CPR efforts with ECMO can reverse the cessation of those functions in some people more than an hour after the arrest?

The second way ECMO introduces a challenging question about determining death arises in some DCD transplantation protocols where ECMO is used to provide oxygenated blood to the organs after death is declared. The incoherence emerges because the person is declared dead on the basis of irreversible cessation of circulatory and respiratory functions, and then the circulation of oxygenated blood is restored to the body, which is now a cadaver, by ECMO. This obviously suggests that the person has not really sustained irreversible cessation of circulatory and respiratory functions because oxygenated blood is now circulating in the body and nourishing the organs, including the heart and lungs, which will soon function in another body when they are transplanted. Some transplant centers, the University of Michigan for example, avoid this incoherence by blocking ECMO-induced circulation above the diaphragm in the cadaver. Physicians confine the circulatory function provided by ECMO to the pelvic organs with the result that both cardiac and respiratory functions do not recur in the cadaver. This protocol satisfies the cardiopulmonary criterion of death but limits organ retrieval because the lungs and heart can no longer be used. However, it does allow retrieval of pelvic organs (e.g., kidneys and liver) without compromising the dead donor rule.

The debate over DCD and the cardiac-death criterion received renewed and intense media attention in the summer of 2008 after publication of a clinical trial in the *New England Journal of Medicine* involving three infants who received hearts from other babies declared dead by the cardiac criterion. Surgeons performed the transplants between May 2004 and May 2007 at Denver Children's Hospital. When life support was withdrawn from the first child, physicians waited three minutes after the heart stopped to declare the baby dead according to the irreversible cessation of circulatory function criterion and then transplanted the heart into another baby where it is currently providing circulation. For the second and third babies they waited only seventy-five seconds after the heart stopped before declaring the baby dead. Were these babies truly dead under current law; that is, did they suffer irreversible cessation of circulatory function? After all, their hearts are now providing circulation for other babies years after the donor babies were declared dead by the cardiac criterion of death. Some commentators say that these babies were not legally dead under current criteria and that their vital organs should not have been harvested. Others agree that the babies should not have been declared dead but recommend that we allow taking organs from severely neurologically damaged dying people with appropriate informed consent.

If we approach the issues relevant to the cardiopulmonary criterion of death generated by DCD how might prudential reasoning proceed? Changing the law so we can take hearts and lungs from the dying but not yet dead would generate tremendous controversy and might make some people reluctant to sign organ donor cards. Changing the criteria for determining death would also probably generate tremendous controversy

A more reasonable approach might be to stay with the UDDA determination of cardiac death—irreversible cessation of cardiopulmonary function—and understand it in a *factual* rather than an absolute sense. Thus, the irreversible cessation of cardiopulmonary functions will then denote the impossibility of a *spontaneous* resumption of circulatory and respiratory functions in the body, not the possibility that CPR might enable these functions to reoccur. Once ventilator withdrawal becomes morally reasonable for neurologically damaged and dying people who will not receive CPR and the patient or proxy wants organs donated, then determining death as soon as we can be morally certain that spontaneous revival of cardiac function will not occur would seem reasonable for a determination of death. When the cardiac *function* has ceased for so long that spontaneous resumption is no longer a medical possibility in this body, and CPR efforts, including CPR with ECMO, are not going to be attempted, then the body has *factually* undergone irreversible cessation of cardiac function.

The fact that a patient's heart and lungs can sustain cardiac and pulmonary functions in another body or could be restored in this body with ECMO does not matter at this point. All that matters is that the heart-lung function will not resume in this body because the time has passed for spontaneous resuscitation, and it would be unethical to attempt medical resuscitation because there is a DNR order. People with cardiac arrest are dead when the circulatory and respiratory functions have *in fact* irreversibly ceased in their body because spontaneous restart is impossible and interventions that might restart those functions are not going to be employed.

You can see from this discussion that both criteria of death—determining death by the cardiac criterion or by the whole-brain-death criterion—once thought to be well settled are in fact subject to ongoing and intense controversies driven in large measure by the laudable desire to obtain more life-saving organs. What we need is continuing moral, legal, and political discussion and debate to learn how to balance the important values involved: the protection of living human beings and the great good accomplished by organ transplantation after death.

Neocortical or Cerebral Death

Brain death (that is, the irreversible cessation of all brain functions, including those of the stem) is the only acceptable neurological criterion of death at this time. There are proposals, however, that we should accept another neurological criterion for death—neocortical or cerebral death. As the Multi-Society Task Force on Persistent Vegetative States (PVS) noted in its 1994 consensus statement, the term neocortical death is limited in its usefulness because it does not denote a distinct clinical entity. For those advocating acceptance of a neocortical criterion of death, however, the notion of neocortical death centers on the permanent loss of functioning sensory areas in the cortex. The neocortical functions that support awareness irreversibly cease when certain parts of the brain, usually the neocortex or the thalamus (a small area inside the brain beneath and somewhat surrounded by the neocortex), are permanently damaged, perhaps by lack of blood for more than a few minutes because of a cardiac arrest or a cerebral accident, perhaps from a severe head trauma.

The major neocortical function that interests us here is awareness. The ability to be aware depends on cortical areas in our brains. If this part of the brain has permanently ceased to function, the person will never again become aware of anything. People suffering what is called neocortical death are permanently unconscious. They are in either an irreversible coma or an irreversible vegetative state. They are not brain dead because at least some of the brain stem continues to function. Sometimes enough of the stem functions so that they can live without life-support equipment.

Although coma and vegetative state are sometimes confused, most of the literature describes them as distinct phenomena. One exception to this is the anomalous position taken by the National Institute of Neurological Disorders and Stroke (NINDS), which is a part of the NIH. The Institute's website in 2008 stated that PVS is a "synonym" for coma and that "some patients may regain a degree of awareness after persistent vegetative state."

Coma patients look as if they are in a deep sleep. Their eyes remain closed and they cannot be aroused. Patients in vegetative state usually go through alternating periods of sleep and arousal. When aroused, their eyes are open and their facial expressions can vary from something akin to smiling to something akin to crying. Sometimes they can make sounds as if they were trying to talk. Although aroused, they are unaware. Patients in either a coma or a vegetative state are totally unconscious. It is very important not to confuse the arousal observed in PVS patients with awareness.

Some patients in a coma will recover some awareness; others will suffer cardiopulmonary arrest in a relatively short time without recovering any awareness. Sometimes, however, the coma will become a vegetative state, and vegetative states can last for years or even decades. Once a vegetative state is established, it is known as a *persistent* vegetative state or PVS. Most instances of PVS are actually permanent vegetative states. The loss of all neocortical functions is irreversible. The 1994 Multi-Society Task Force on Persistent Vegetative States took the position that a vegetative state that lasted twelve months after a traumatic brain injury or three months after a nontraumatic brain injury could be considered permanent.

Because most vegetative states follow a period of coma, the family often interprets the appearance of arousal associated with a vegetative state as an indication that the patient is recovering from the coma. Unfortunately, the arousal associated with vegetative state is not a sign of recovery; the patient remains totally unconscious, and the longer a patient is unconscious, the less likely is recovery.

Some people suggest that patients suffering the irreversible loss of all neocortical functions, which means the loss of all awareness, should also be considered dead by a criterion they call neocortical death. These patients are "gone," since all that remains is a human body living irreversibly on a vegetative level. At the present time, however, neocortical death, unlike brain death, is not recognized as a criterion of death.

On the theoretical level there is no reason why the permanent loss of all capability for awareness could not be an accurate indication that one of us is no longer here; that is, that one of us has died. If we accept the idea that each of us is a psychic body, then the end of the psychic body is the end of one of us. True, the human body may live on in a vegetative state, sometimes for years or even decades, thanks to the use of feeding tubes for medical nutrition and hydration. But a permanently vegetative body is not a psychic body; it is not one of us. Each of us is more than a vegetative body—each of us is a perceiving body. Once all capability for perception is irretrievably lost, the body, although still a living human body, is no longer one of us. A permanently vegetative human body is but the remains of what was one of us.

Even if one does not accept the concept of a psychic body, there are good reasons for believing that the neocortical criterion for death is actually consistent with what most people think of life and death. As we have seen, many people think each of us is more than a human body. They speak of a human being as some kind of compound involving body and soul, or body and mind, or body and something called "personhood." The neocortically dead are not such compounds—they are simply vegetative bodies. There is no evidence of a human soul, or mind, or personhood. In fact, there is not even any potential for feeling on the sensory level, let alone on the rational, mental, or personal level. All that remains is a vegetative body, a living organism that will survive, if nourished, but without the ability to feel anything.

Nonetheless, there are good reasons for arguing against supporting any effort to make what some call neocortical death a legal criterion of death, at least at this time. First, we have learned from the experience of using brain death as a criterion for death that any neurological criterion of death can be easily misunderstood. Although brain death has been widely accepted as a legal and moral criterion of human death for more than three decades, a great deal of confusion still lingers in the minds of health care providers and of the general public.

It is not easy for some to accept the fact that an individual on life-support systems with normal pulse, color, and temperature is dead. Many still think that brain-dead patients on respirators die when the life support is removed and the breathing stops. This is why some physicians still make the time of life-support removal the time of death, despite the fact it may have been determined days earlier that the patient had suffered brain death. The continuing confusion over brain death, years after public policy has accepted it as a criterion of death, is a powerful argument for not making any effort at this time to have neocortical death accepted as a criterion for death, at least not in the near future.

Second, any move to make neocortical death a criterion of death at this time will be needlessly divisive in our society. Many opposed to euthanasia can be expected to argue against a neocortical-death criterion either because they believe it is a form of euthanasia or because they see it as a slippery slope that will lead to euthanasia. Many opposed to abortion can also be expected to resist the neocortical criterion. Their fear is that the support of a position whereby bodies suffering neocortical death are considered dead would make fetuses without neocortical development vulnerable to abortion.

Given the problems that would arise if we tried to have something like a neocortical criterion of death accepted as social policy, it seems better to leave things as they are. And there is no compelling reason to change the social policy. People can leave advance directives stating they do not want their vegetative bodies sustained after they have suffered the permanent loss of all awareness, and in the absence of such directives, good ethical reasoning supports a proxy's making the same decision for a patient.

Instead of presuming these patients would want their bodies maintained indefinitely in a vegetative state, we should assume the opposite is true unless there is clear and convincing evidence to the contrary. And if people do want their permanently vegetative bodies maintained indefinitely, it would not be unreasonable to require them to arrange funding for what might last for years and cost from $350 to $500 a day ($126,000 to $180,000 a year). Keeping neocortically dead bodies alive in PVS for years or even decades is simply unreasonable. It provides no benefit for the patient and is a burden for many others.

ETHICAL REFLECTIONS

Determining just when an individual human life begins and ends is difficult. The beginning of a new genetic human entity is now relatively easy to fix at the end of the fertilization process, but, as we saw, this entity is not yet a definitive individual entity—one of us—because it might fuse with another embryo or split into two embryos. After about fourteen days it does become a definitive individual no longer able to fuse or split, but, except for those who view human beings solely in physical or biological terms, this is not enough to provide a definite answer for when one of us begins. Sometime after several months into the pregnancy the fetus becomes capable of sensation. Although we do not know exactly when the fetus begins to perceive, the development of perception may well be the transition in the process that began with fertilization best suited to indicate the presence of a new one of us. Before this time, the fetus is a human being but does not possess human existence. It has not yet developed beyond a vegetative body, and a vegetative human body is not yet one of us.

We have to admit, however, that designating transitions in embryonic and fetal development remains a somewhat arbitrary exercise. We do know that a spermatozoon just beginning to penetrate an ovum is not yet a new genetic human being, and most of us readily admit that a viable fetus is very much one of us. But the intervening weeks between the beginning of fertilization and the beginning of viability are a gray area. Since science cannot say when one of us begins, it remains a matter of interpretation. And, as we know, people have their own reasons (and agendas) for choosing various points in the process as the precise moment when the developing entity becomes one of us.

To some extent, then, there is a time in the process of fetal development when we cannot say for certain whether or not we are faced with an individual human life that is one of us. This gray area raises an ethical concern. Some would say human life is so important that, even if we are not sure a developing embryo or fetus is one of us, we must treat it as if it were. Others feel that morality does not require us to treat what might be one of us in the same way as what is certainly one of us. Here, again, our response rests with what is reasonable. The more probable it is that we are dealing with one of us, the more careful we have to be. We undermine our own good when we cause harm without adequate reason to what is, or could be, one of us.

Two further remarks about the beginning of life are in order. First, our moral well-being depends to some extent on treating all human life, even before it becomes individuated and sentient, with respect. A recently fertilized embryo in a laboratory is not just another cluster of cells. It is a new human life, and it will be good for us to treat it with respect. The morally virtuous person treats all life, especially all human life, with a high degree of dignity and care. Destruction of human life before it becomes one of us would still be a moral matter of considerable significance, something not to be dismissed lightly.

Second, our suggestion that we consider the appearance of the sentient fetus as the appearance of a new one of us suggests an analogy with brain death. The analogy says that just as we consider whole-brain death an indication that human existence is over, so we should consider the absence of brain life in a fetus as an indication that human existence has not yet developed. Thus, some say we should consider human life as beginning with brain life and ending with brain death. This implies we should consider a fetus without brain life as if it were a body without brain life, that is, as if it were dead.

The symmetry is neat and provocative, but the analogy has serious drawbacks. There is a significant difference between a fetus without brain life and a human being who has lost brain life and is brain dead. The fetus is alive and the brain-dead patient is dead. The brain-dead patient is dead because he has suffered the irreversible loss of all brain functions. The fetus has not suffered any such loss and therefore is not dead. A brain cannot be considered dead if it never lived—death always follows life. True, neither the six-week fetus nor the brain-dead individual has brain life, but the former is alive (although not one of us), and the latter is dead. The fundamental difference between life and death undermines the analogy between an early fetus and a brain-dead patient.

For these reasons, comparing an early fetus with a whole-brain-dead patient does not seem to be a good idea. The early fetus is not dead but alive; it simply has not yet developed awareness. The lack of any awareness may mean, as we suggested, that the fetus is not yet one of us, but it does not mean the fetus is dead. The fetus is very much alive, very much human life with a potential for awareness, and we achieve our good by treating it with the respect we have for human life, which is something more than the respect we have for the dead. Good moral reasoning presupposes that we can separate the dead from the living. A patient declared dead by the whole-brain-death criterion is dead; a developing fetus, or even an embryo for that matter, is living.

Suggested Readings

A very helpful book for material covered in the first part of this chapter is Norman Ford, 1988, *When Did I Begin: Conception of the Human Individual in History, Philosophy and Science*. Cambridge, UK: Cambridge University Press. Ford believes a new human individual begins with the appearance of the "primitive streak" in the embryo at about the fifteenth day of its development. The primitive streak is a thickening of cells at the caudal or tail end of the embryonic disk, and it marks the future longitudinal axis of the developing embryo. Ford argues, convincingly, that the development of the primitive streak marks the beginning of the human individual. We have argued that a human individual is not yet one of us until it becomes a psychic body, an event that occurs several months after the primitive streak appears.

Also helpful are Bonnie Steinbock, 1992, *Life before Birth: The Moral and Legal Status of Embryos and Fetuses*, New York: Oxford University Press, chapters 1 and 3; Clifford Grobstein, "The Early Development of Human Embryos," *Journal of Medicine and Philosophy* 1985, *10*, 179–82; Hans-Martin Sass, "Brain Life and Brain Death," *Journal of Medicine and Philosophy* 1989, *14*, 45–59; Richard McCormick, "Who or What Is the Preembryo?" *Kennedy Institute of Ethics Journal* 1991, *1*, 1–15; Thomas Shannon and Allan Wolter, "Reflections on the Moral Status of the Pre-Embryo," *Theological Studies* 1990, *51*, 603–26; Lisa Cahill, "The Embryo and the Fetus: New Moral Contexts," *Theological Studies* 1993, *54*, 124–42; Carlos Bedate and Robert Cefalo, "The Zygote: To Be or Not to Be a Person," *Journal of Medicine and Philosophy* 1989, *14*, 641–45; Thomas Bole, "Metaphysical Accounts of the Zygote as a Person and the Veto Power of Facts," *Journal of Medicine and Philosophy* 1989, *14*, 647–53, and "Zygotes, Souls, Substances, and Persons," *Journal of Medicine and Philosophy* 1990, *15*, 627–35; Joseph Donceel, "Immediate and Delayed Hominization," *Theological Studies* 1970, *31*, 76–105; Mario Moussa and Thomas Shannon, "The Search for the New Pineal Gland: Brain Life and Personhood," *Hastings Center Report* 1992, *22* (May–June), 30–37; Lorette Fierning, "The Moral Status of the Foetus: A Reappraisal," *Bioethics* 1987, *1*, 15–34; and M. C. Shea, "Embryonic Life and Human Life," *Journal of Medical Ethics* 1985, *11*, 205–9.

The concept of the "psychic body" is suggested by a number of contemporary philosophies, among them the process philosophy of Alfred North Whitehead and the existential phenomenology of Maurice Merleau-Ponty. Whitehead's process philosophy, sometimes called the philosophy of organism, is strongly opposed to any bifurcation of reality into physical and mental substances such as body and soul. Rather, all reality is described as comprising both physical and mental processes entwined in various degrees. The processes fall into six major categories: the microscopic events of atomic physics, macroscopic inorganic things (e.g., stones), living cells, vegetative life, animal life, and human existence. Both animal life and human existence have sufficient mental feelings so that they have what Whitehead called, in his technical language, "hybrid prehensions," that is, a physical-mental consciousness or awareness. Before it develops these hybrid prehensions, the embryo is not a process we recognize as human existence; after it loses them irreversibly, it is no longer a process we recognize as animal or human existence. See Whitehead, 1968, *Modes of Thought*, New York: Free Press, pp. 156–57, and 1967, *Process and Reality*, New York: Macmillan, pp. 163–67.

Merleau-Ponty's philosophy also eschews the classical dualities of body and soul or body and mind; it makes the perceiving body primary. Our body is both object and subject, thing and consciousness, perceived and perceiving. A body that is not an object (a body unable to be perceived) does not enjoy human existence. And a body that is not a subject (a body unable to perceive) does not enjoy human existence. Hence, the embryonic bodies unable to perceive and the bodies locked in PVS do not enjoy human existence. "There is a human body when, between the seeing and the seen, between touching and the touched . . . a blending of some sort takes place—when the spark is lit between sensing and sensible, lighting the fire that will not stop burning until some accident of the body will undo what no accident would have sufficed to do." (Maurice Merleau-Ponty, "Eye and Mind," Carleton Dallery, trans., 1964, *The Primacy of Perception*, James Edie, ed., Evanston: Northwestern University Press, pp. 163–64). See also Merleau-Ponty, 1968, *The Visible and the Invisible*, Alphonso Lingis, trans., Evanston: Northwestern University Press, pp. 130–55. For the primacy of the psychic body in Whitehead and Merleau-Ponty, see Raymond Devettere, "The Human Body as Philosophical Paradigm in Whitehead and Merleau-Ponty," *Philosophy Today* 1976, *10*, 317–26.

For a plausible account claiming that the rapidly developing field of cognitive science is confirming empirically the ideas that the human body philosophers such as Whitehead and Merleau-Ponty were developing earlier in the century, see George Lakoff and Mark Johnson, 1999, *Philosophy in the Flesh: The*

Embodied Mind and Its Challenge to Western Thought, New York: Basic Books. Some Christian theologians are also moving away from the body-soul dualism so prominent in the tradition. See, for example, the view of James Keenan: "I resist any tendency to think of the person as something other or more than a human body. I believe that the human soul and the human body are so fully one that to distinguish them (in this life) is to miss the true understanding of personhood. Thus I cannot imagine personhood without the human body, nor can I imagine a living human body without conveying personhood" (James Keenan, 1995, "Genetic Research and the Elusive Body," in *Embodiment, Morality, and Medicine,* Lisa Cahill and Margaret Farley, eds., Dordrecht: Kluwer Academic Publishers, p. 59).

The most important source for Aristotle's ideas on reproduction is his *Generation of Animals.* Although he was influenced by the recorded observations of the Hippocratic physicians, Aristotle rejected their views on reproduction. The Hippocratic texts hold that both the man and the woman contribute seed that forms the embryo. See G. Lloyd, ed., 1986, *Hippocratic Writings,* trans. J. Chadwick and W. Mann, New York: Penguin, pp. 315–46. As we saw, Aristotle believed that only the man contributes seed. The woman contributes the material for the seed to act on. The famous second-century physician Galen thought both the man and the woman contributed seed, but it was the model of Aristotle that dominated the Western tradition. Unfortunately, it is a model that views the woman as passive in the generation of new life and makes her analogous to the dirt in which the valuable human seed is planted. The Islamic tradition, however, followed Hippocrates and Galen and held that both the man and the woman contribute semen to the offspring. See B. F. Musallam, 1983, *Sex and Society in Islam: Birth Control before the Nineteenth Century,* Cambridge, UK: Cambridge University Press, pp. 39–59.

Sometimes Aquinas's position that the fetus is not one of us before the infusion of the rational soul weeks after the pregnancy began is slighted when his work is translated into English. The passage cited in the text about an attacker being guilty of homicide if he kills either a pregnant woman or her *animated* fetus reads in Latin "si sequatur mors vel mulieris vel puerperii *animati,* non effugiet homicidii crimen." A well-known English translation, however, leaves out the word "animati" and makes the passage say: "if either the woman or the foetus dies as a result, he will be guilty of the crime of homicide" (Aquinas, 1974, *Summa Theologiae,* Marcus Lefebvre, trans., New York: McGraw-Hill, volume 38, p. 47). This inaccurate translation leaves the reader with the impression that Aquinas is saying that the destruction of a fetus at any stage of development is homicide, and this simply is not true. According to the Latin text, only the destruction of a fetus after it is animated by the rational soul many weeks into the pregnancy is considered homicide. The correct translation is: "if the death of either the woman or of the *animated* fetus follows, he does not escape the crime of homicide" (emphasis added).

An excellent starting point for understanding the issues and current debates associated with determining when one of us actually dies is the PCB's White Paper *Controversies in the Determination of Death* released in December 2008 and available online at bioethics.gov. See especially chapter 3 on whole-brain death, chapter 4 on the philosophical debate, and chapter 6 on non-heart-beating organ donation. For a commentary on this important document see Franklin Miller and Robert Truog, "The Incoherence of Determining Death by the Neurological Criteria: A Commentary on *Controversies in the Determination of Death,* a White Paper by the President's Council on Bioethics," *Kennedy Institute of Ethics Journal* 2009, *19,* 185–93.

See also the President's Commission report titled *Defining Death,* Washington, DC: U.S. Government Printing Office, 1981; and the report of the New York State Task Force on Life and the Law titled *The Determination of Death,* Albany: Health Education Services, 1986. See also Robert Veatch, 1989, *Death, Dying, and the Biological Revolution,* rev. ed., New Haven: Yale University Press, chapters 1 and 2; David Lamb, 1985, *Death, Brain Death and Ethics,* Albany: State University of New York Press; Karen Gervais, 1986, *Redefining Death,* New Haven: Yale University Press; Richard Zaner, ed., 1988, *Death: Beyond Whole-Brain Criteria,* Norwell: Kluwer; Robert Taylor, "Reexamining the Definition and Criterion of Death," *Seminars in Neurology* 1997, *17,* 265–70; Linda Emanuel, "Reexamining Death: The Asymptotic Model and a Bounded Zone Definition," *Hastings Center Report* 1995, *27* (July–August), 27–35; and Stuart Youngner et al., eds., 1998, *Defining Death in a Technological Age: The Interface between Medical Science and Society,* Baltimore: Johns Hopkins University Press. For brain death in children, see "Report of a Special Task Force: Guidelines for the Determination of Brain Death in Children," *Pediatrics* 1987, *80,* 298–300.

The following articles are also helpful: Christopher Pallis, "Whole-Brain Death Reconsidered—Physiological Facts and Philosophy," *Journal of Medical Ethics* 1983, *9,* 32–37; Daniel Wikler, "Conceptual Issues in the Definition of Death," *Theoretical Medicine* 1984, *5,* 167–80; Raymond Devettere,

"Neocortical Death and Human Death," *Law, Medicine and Health Care* 1990, *18*, 96–104; Michael Green and Daniel Wikler, "Brain Death and Personal Identity," in Marshall Cohen et al., eds., 1981, *Medicine and Moral Philosophy*, Princeton: Princeton University Press, pp. 49–77; Eelco Wijdicks, "The Diagnosis of Brain Death," *New England Journal of Medicine* 2001, *344*, 1215–21; and Alexander Capron, "Brain Death—Well Settled Yet Still Unresolved," *New England Journal of Medicine* 2001, *344*, 1244–46.

The article showing that two-thirds of nurses and physicians likely to be involved in organ retrieval did not understand the brain-death criterion is Stuart Youngner et al., "'Brain Death' and Organ Retrieval: A Cross-Sectional Survey of Knowledge and Concepts among Health Professionals," *JAMA* 1989, *261*, 2205–10. For the revived debate on brain death, see Robert Truog and James Fackler, "Rethinking Brain Death," *Critical Care Medicine* 1992, *20*, 1705–13; James Bernat, "How Much of the Brain Must Die in Brain Death?" *Journal of Clinical Ethics* 1992, *3*, 21–26; Robert Veatch, "The Impending Collapse of the Whole-Brain Definition of Death," *Hastings Center Report* 1993, *23* (July–August), 18–24; Daniel Wikler, "Brain Death: A Durable Consensus?" *Bioethics* 1993, *7*, 239–46; Amir Halevy and Baruch Brody, "Brain Death: Reconciling Definitions, Criteria, and Tests," *Annals of Internal Medicine* 1993, *119*, 519–25; Josef Siefert, "Is 'Brain Death' Actually Death?" *Monist* 1993, *76*, 175–202; Jeff McMahan, "The Metaphysics of Brain Death," *Bioethics* 1995, *9*, 91–126, and "An Alternative to Brain Death," *Journal of Law, Medicine & Ethics* 2006, *34*, 44–48; Robert Truog, "Is It Time to Abandon Brain Death?" *Hastings Center Report* 1997, *27* (January–February), 29–37; James Bernat, "A Defense of the Whole-Brain Concept of Death," *Hastings Center Report* 1998, *28* (March–April), 14–23, and "The Whole-Brain Concept of Death Remains Optimum Public Policy," *Journal of Law, Medicine & Ethics* 2006, *34*, 35–43; and Robert Truog, "Brain Death—Too Flawed to Endure, Too Ingrained to Abandon," *Journal of Law, Medicine & Ethics* 2007, *35*, 273–81.

The lack of consistency in determining death by the whole-brain-death criterion is reported by David Greer et al., "Variability of Brain Death Determination Guidelines in Leading US Neurologic Institutions," *Neurology* 2008, *70*, 284–89. See also Kurt Samson, "Top Hospitals Routinely Ignore Brain Death Guidelines, Study Finds," *Neurology Today* 2007, *7*, 13–14, available at aan.com/elibrary. The AAN guidelines for determining whole-brain death appeared in *Neurology* 1995, *45*, 1012–14. For a consideration of religious objections to the whole-brain-death criterion see Robert Olick, Eli Braun, and Joel Potash, "Accommodating Religious and Moral Objections to Neurological Death," *Journal of Clinical Ethics* 2009, *20*, 183–91.

The University of Pittsburgh procedures for organ retrieval from non-heart-beating donors (NHBDs) appears in the *Kennedy Institute of Ethics Journal* 1993, *3*, A-1–A-15. The determination of death after two minutes of an arrest is on p. A-6. All fifteen articles in this special issue of the journal are devoted to the ethical and social issues of taking organs from NHBDs. Most of the essays are excellent, and they are reprinted in Robert Arnold et al., eds., 1995, *Procuring Organs for Transplant: The Debate over Non-Heart Beating Cadaver Protocols*, Baltimore: Johns Hopkins University Press. The Institute of Medicine (IOM) report is 1997, *Non-Heart-Beating Organ Transplantation: Medical and Ethical Issues in Procurement*, Washington, DC: National Academy Press. For a criticism of the IOM report, see Jerry Menikoff, "Doubts about Death: The Silence of the Institute of Medicine," *Journal of Law, Medicine & Ethics* 1998, *26*, 157–65. John Potts, the principal investigator of the IOM study, and others wrote a brief reply on pp. 166–68. For some background on the IOM project see Roger Herdman et al., "The Institute of Medicine's Report on Non-Heart-Beating Organ Transplantation," *Kennedy Institute of Ethics Journal* 1998, *8*, 83–90. Discussions of organ procurement from NHBDs often neglect to discuss the ethical issues surrounding the determination of death. See, for example, Yong Cho et al., "Transplantation of Kidneys from Donors Whose Hearts Have Stopped Beating," *New England Journal of Medicine* 1998, *338*, 221–25; and Paul Hauptman and Kevin O'Connor, "Procurement and Allocation of Solid Organs for Transplantation," *New England Journal of Medicine* 1997, *336*, 422–31.

For the controversial transplantation of infant hearts after determining death by the cardiac criterion, see Mark Boucek, "Pediatric Heart Transplantation after Declaration of Cardiocirculatory Death," *New England Journal of Medicine* 2008, *359*, 709–14. The same issue contains three commentaries and an editorial: James Bernat, "The Boundaries of Organ Donation after Circulatory Death," 669–71; Robert Veatch, "Donating Hearts after Cardiac Death—Reversing the Irreversible," 672–73; Robert Truog and Franklin Miller, "The Dead Donor Rule and Organ Transplantation," 674–75; and Gregory Curfman et al., "Cardiac Transplantation in Infants," 749–50. Bernat argues that seventy-five seconds is not long enough to satisfy the cardiac criterion, Veatch argues that restarting the heart shows that the cessation of circulation was not irreversible, and Truog and Miller argue that we can make exceptions to the dead donor rule and take organs from dying patients with devastating and irreversible neurological injury as long as we have informed consent. The key study showing that ECMO allows survival long after cardiac arrest in some children is Alsoufi Bahaaldin et al., "Survival Outcomes after Rescue Extracorporeal Cardiopulmonary Resuscitation in Pediatric Patients with Refractory Cardiac Arrest," *Journal of Thoracic and Cardiovascular Surgery* 2007, *134*, 952–59. See also Douglas Schuerer, "Extracorporeal Membrane Oxygenation: Current Clinical Practice, Coding, and Reimbursement," *Chest* 2008, *134*, 179–84.

For an interesting article on death and the permanently unconscious, see Alan Shermon, "The Metaphysics of Brain Death, Persistent Vegetative State, and Dementia," *Thomist* 1985, *49*, 24–80. This article is noteworthy because Shermon, employing the classical medieval Christian concept of body and soul, suggests that it is more appropriate to say a patient in irreversible coma or PVS is dead than to say he is still living. This is so because there is no reason to think a rational soul still permeates the irreversibly unconscious body, and the departure of the rational soul is what marked death in medieval Christian thought. However, Shermon later moved away from this view in "Recovery from 'Brain Death': A Neurologist's Apologia," *Linacre Quarterly* 1997, *64*, 30–36, and "Chronic 'brain death': Meta-analysis and Conceptual Consequences," *Neurology* 1998, *51*, 1538–45. Shermon now rejects the whole-brain-death criterion and insists that a person is not dead until circulation has irreversibly ceased. See his "The Brain and Somatic Integration: Insights into the Standard Biological Rationale for Equating 'Brain Death' with Death," *Journal of Medicine and Philosophy* 2001, *26*, 457–78.

The consensus statement of the Multi-Society Task Force on PVS (with membership drawn from the American Academy of Neurology, Child Neurology Society, American Neurological Association, American Association of Neurological Surgeons, and American Academy of Pediatrics) is a valuable review of thinking about the persistent vegetative state and related conditions such as coma, brain death, locked-in syndrome, and dementia. It appears as a two-part report titled "Medical Aspects of the Persistent Vegetative State," *New England Journal of Medicine* 1994, *330*, 1499–1508 and 1572–79. The NINDS (NIH) site conflating coma and persistent vegetative state (as of September 2008) is at ninds.nih.gov/disorders/coma. One of the problems is that some studies show that PVS is sometimes misdiagnosed, often because it is confused with what has been recently identified as a "minimally conscious state." For an excellent overview of coma and PVS by a neurosurgeon who coauthored with Fred Plum the first edition of the landmark *The Diagnosis of Stupor and Coma* in 1972, see Bryan Jennett, 2002, *The Vegetative State: Medical Facts, Ethical and Legal Dilemmas*, New York: Cambridge University Press. The fourth and latest edition of *The Diagnosis of Stupor and Coma* is Jerome Posner et al., 2007, New York: Oxford University Press. The book includes helpful up-to-date information on both the vegetative and minimally conscious states and distinguishes these from comas.

SEVEN

Life-Sustaining Treatments

A LIFE-SUSTAINING OR life-prolonging treatment is a medical intervention designed to prolong the patient's life rather than to cure the problem threatening his health. Of course the distinction between life-sustaining treatments and other medical and surgical treatments is not a sharp one. Treatments promoting the restoration of health often prolong life, and treatments prolonging life often promote the restoration of health.

Nonetheless, the distinction is a helpful one in situations in which the major impact of a treatment is more the prolongation of life than the restoration of health. A ventilator, for example, supports respiration but does not always contribute to the restoration of health—sometimes it merely enables the patient to live longer with his disease. The same may be said for dialysis when the patient is not a candidate for a transplant—the dialysis merely enables him to live longer with renal disease. On the other hand, some treatments—a kidney transplant or chemotherapy—are treatments designed to restore health.

The life-sustaining aspect of some interventions is most easily noticed when the restoration of health is no longer possible. Consider for example a patient suffering from multiple life-threatening problems associated with advanced AIDS and approaching the end of her life, which is expected at any time. If she begins to suffer respiratory distress, a ventilator will keep her alive a little longer but will not restore her health. Consider, again, an infant born with anencephaly and having difficulty breathing. Ventilation can sustain his life, perhaps for months, but will not contribute anything to the amelioration of the anencephaly. In situations such as these the ethical question centers on when it is reasonable to employ life-sustaining treatments and when it is not.

Our main concern in this chapter will be respirators and ventilators. Every life-threatening disease, even those not directly affecting the respiratory system, will eventually threaten respiration. Now that we have the technology designed to support respiration when spontaneous respiration is no longer possible, a major moral problem has emerged over when it is good to use it.

We will also consider briefly two other examples of life-sustaining therapy—dialysis and surgery. Dialysis is designed to support kidney function by purifying blood when the renal system can no longer perform this function adequately, and some surgeries are directed more to prolonging life (and delaying death) than to curing the disease threatening to shorten life.

VENTILATORS

Early in the twentieth century, an American engineer named Philip Drinker designed the first respirator. The patient was placed inside an enclosed tank, and cycles of positive and negative pressure were used to push air into the lungs and then evacuate it. The popular name for the cumbersome and now obsolete Drinker respirator was "iron lung."

Smaller machines providing air under positive pressure, through tubes in the patient's throat, were soon developed. They were called respirators, although today they are more often called ventilators. In this chapter we use the words *respirator* and *ventilator* interchangeably to designate the electrically powered devices providing air through a tube inserted either down the throat (intubation) or into an opening cut into the neck (tracheotomy). These respirators and ventilators are marvelous life-saving inventions, but they have created a host of moral dilemmas.

Sometimes ventilators are clearly necessary for survival—if they are withdrawn, the patient will soon die. At other times they play a subsidiary role, either assisting the patient's breathing or providing a backup should the breathing falter. If a patient cannot live without the ventilator, it is truly a life-sustaining treatment.

Those still using the distinction between ordinary and extraordinary treatments in medical ethics invariably consider the respirator an extraordinary means of preserving life. As we noted in chapter 3, however, this distinction is ambiguous and thus not always helpful in ethics. The ventilator is a good example of this ambiguity. When the respirator was introduced, ethicists, moral theologians, and judges (impressed by the advanced technology) tended to consider it an extraordinary treatment. This made it more comfortable for them to say withdrawing a ventilator could be morally justified in some situations.

In one important sense, however, a respirator or ventilator is not extraordinary treatment—in fact, it is quite ordinary. A respirator does not provide medicine but air, an ordinary basic need of human life. It is most often used not to correct a medical problem but to enable a person with a medical problem to breathe. Mechanical ventilation thus resembles medical nutrition and hydration supplied by feeding tubes. The ventilator tube supplying air to the lungs through an incision in the throat is analogous to a gastrostomy tube supplying nutrition and hydration through an incision in the stomach. And the ventilator tube inserted through the mouth is analogous to a nasogastric feeding tube inserted through the nose. If we remove a needed feeding tube, the person dies from lack of nutrition and hydration; if we remove a needed ventilator, the person dies from lack of air.

Ventilation is frequently initiated in emergency situations when there is little or no time for careful decision making. If the need is temporary, ventilation seldom presents a moral dilemma. Sometimes, however, the need is long term or even permanent, and the patient will remain on a ventilator indefinitely, perhaps for life. It is the long-term uses of ventilators that create most of the ethical issues. Many patients kept alive by ventilators are suffering from life-threatening medical problems. Some of them do not want their lives prolonged by the machine, yet declining mechanical ventilation means an earlier death for those who cannot breathe without it. It can be distressing for a physician to withdraw a respirator when she knows her patient will thereby suffer respiratory arrest, often soon after the withdrawal.

Many ventilator-dependent patients are so sick they can no longer make decisions for themselves, and this complicates the moral issue. If they have not given advance directives, their proxies must determine what is in their best interest. If the proxy believes mechanical ventilation is not in the patient's best interest, she has little choice but to request withdrawal. Many proxies are reluctant to do this, especially if the patient will be conscious when the ventilator is removed. It is difficult for a proxy to request something that will result in the death.

Withdrawing a ventilator from a ventilator-dependent patient is, and should be, an extremely serious affair. The people doing it, as we saw in chapter 3, are not simply "allowing the disease to cause death." They are playing a causal role, along with the disease, in the patient's death at this time, although their actions are not necessarily unethical or immoral.

So unnerving is the connection between withdrawing the needed ventilator from a patient and the patient's death that many still insist that their actions of withdrawing the life-support equipment do not play any causal role in the subsequent death. They insist that the withdrawal of a ventilator merely "lets the patient die," and that the disease is the sole significant cause of death. We have already suggested the questionable nature of this description in chapter 3. It is more accurate to acknowledge that both the respirator withdrawal and the disease play causal roles in the death. Thinking this way enables us to see more clearly our responsibility for the death resulting from the withdrawal.

We must be careful of the word "responsibility" here. The word means we are morally and legally accountable for what we are doing; it does not mean we are doing something wrong. The key ethical question is not whether the action of withdrawing a treatment that is actually keeping someone alive plays a causal role in the death—it does—but whether the withdrawal is reasonable (that is, morally virtuous) in the situation. Acknowledging that the action of withdrawing life support is one of the causes of the person's death is important because it better enables us to think carefully about the moral seriousness of what we are doing.

How a ventilator is withdrawn is also morally important. Several methods exist. The tube can be removed, the ventilator can be shut off, or the functions of the ventilator (its rate, oxygen levels, and so forth) can be continually reduced until arrest occurs. Some authors have suggested the last because it makes it easier for physicians, nurses, and family to cope—they see the patient dying while still on life support and thus can avoid thinking he died because they withdrew the ventilator. Although one can understand their feelings, reducing the functions of the equipment instead of removing it or shutting it off makes no significant moral difference. The major concern in ventilator withdrawal once physicians have determined that the withdrawal is morally reasonable should be to comfort the patient if the patient has any awareness. And no matter what method is used, sedation sufficient to relieve discomfort is morally important.

We now consider some moral issues associated with several important legal cases involving ventilators. As we mentioned in chapter 4 in connection with the Hazel Welch story, although the cases are presented in a standardized format, this is not to suggest a rigorous method. The format serves rather as an illustration of just one way prudential deliberation and moral judgment might unfold in situations suggested by the cases.

The Case of Karen Quinlan

The Story

This is one of the most famous cases in health care ethics. It marks the beginning of the widespread public debate about stopping life-sustaining therapies and of court interventions in health care decision making.

In April 1975 Karen Quinlan, then twenty-one, felt faint after drinking at a local bar. Her friends took her home and helped her into bed. When they checked on her a short time later they found she had suffered a cardiopulmonary arrest, probably caused by the combination of alcohol and the prescription drugs she was taking. An ambulance responded, and the emergency personnel administered cardiopulmonary resuscitation, restoring her pulse. She was transported to a local hospital and placed on a ventilator. After some complications developed, a tracheotomy was performed the next day.

Nine days later she was transferred to St. Clare's Hospital, a larger facility. Here she was kept alive in the intensive care unit by the respirator and by a feeding tube that ran through her nose and into her stomach. She remained unconscious, although she displayed alternating periods of sleep and arousal. When her eyes were open, they moved randomly.

The months dragged on with no improvement. Parts of her body became rigid, and she lost weight, dropping from one hundred fifteen to about seventy pounds by September. As nearly as could be determined, she would never regain any awareness of anything.

Karen's family asked that the respiratory support be withdrawn. A local priest helped them to see the technology as an extraordinary means of preserving life and therefore not morally required according to the opinions of Catholic moral theologians and of Pope Pius XII himself in a 1957 address to anesthesiologists. The hospital insisted it could not honor the family's request unless the person making it, Karen's father, was legally appointed Karen's guardian.

The Quinlans went to court, and Karen's father, Joseph Quinlan, asked to be appointed her guardian with the power to authorize "discontinuance of all extraordinary procedures" for sustaining life. Hearing this, the court appointed him guardian of her property but not of her person. This meant Joseph could make decisions about his daughter's property but could not authorize the withdrawal of the respirator. The court then appointed another guardian, a guardian *ad litem*, to represent Karen in the case. Karen's guardian *ad litem* saw his role as preserving her life and, therefore, argued against withdrawal of the respirator. The legal process had now become (as so often happens) a battle. The patient's family wanted the respirator removed; the guardian *ad litem* wanted it continued.

During the legal hearings, the lawyer for the attending physician joined with the guardian *ad litem* in opposing removal of the respirator. He argued that removing respirators from living patients was not standard medical practice. Now there was another battle: a battle between the family and the physician.

In his decision of November 1975 the judge sided with the guardian *ad litem* and the attorney for the physician; he declined to give Karen's father the authority to have the respirator stopped. The Quinlans then appealed, and the case went to the New Jersey Supreme Court. Before looking at this court's landmark decision and how Karen was subsequently treated, we will pause to examine the ethical issues. We will try to determine what behavior is "according to right reason," where right reason is the prudence of the moral agents involved in the dilemma. We want to know how the moral agents involved in this tragic situation can find a way to live well, or at least to avoid the worse.

Ethical Analysis

Situational awareness. We are aware of the following facts in the Quinlan story.

1. After several months Karen was irreversibly unconscious in a persistent vegetative state (PVS). She could not, and would never again, feel anything. She was beyond experiencing the burden of pain or the benefit of any treatment or nourishment. She was, according to testimony, not lying peacefully in bed as if asleep but was "emaciated, curled up in what is known as flexion contracture. Every bone was bent in a flexion position and making one tight sort of fetal position. It's too grotesque, really, to describe in human terms like fetal." She was expected to die if the respirator were removed.

2. Karen had not prepared any written directives or communicated any specific instructions to her family about withdrawing respirator support for her if she ever became irreversibly unconscious. This is not surprising; few people were making advance directives at the time, and even today, it is not something most young people think of doing.

3. Since Karen had lost decision-making capacity, proxies (in this case her parents) had to make decisions for her. Since Karen's wishes had not been clearly communicated, her parents could not really use the substituted judgment standard for proxy decision making. They could say, based on their experience of living with their daughter, what they thought she would have wanted. They may have been convinced of this, but they could not report her explicit instructions about respirators because she had never left any. Nor could they use the other usual standard for proxy decision making, the best interests standard, because permanently unconscious persons have no interests—they cannot experience anything. A proxy making a decision for the permanently unconscious Karen can only ask what is the reasonable treatment for the vegetative body. He has to rely on what we have called the reasonable treatment standard.

4. The physician was reluctant to withdraw the respirator, and this is understandable. Respirator withdrawal from living patients was not a widely accepted medical practice in 1975. Moreover, the New Jersey attorney general was opposed to the withdrawal, and the threat of possible criminal charges would make anyone nervous about withdrawal. And the physician's lawyer later argued in court that he believed withdrawing a respirator from someone who needs it imposes a death sentence on the person.

We are also aware of the following good and bad features in the story.

1. We would expect Karen's death if the respirator were removed. Dying and death are bad, although in this case the person dying would not experience the process in any way, and the bad associated with the death was reduced by the massive damage already suffered by the brain. Nonetheless, every human death is bad; that is why we regret and mourn death.

2. Karen's life, as all life, was good, although it was not a good for her since she was not aware of it. Nonetheless, human life, even very damaged and very old human life, is an important good.

3. The suffering of the family was bad. Their suffering was caused by Karen's tragic condition, but also by the opposition of the physicians to their wishes for their daughter and by the stressful ordeal of the legal proceedings.

4. The distress the physicians would experience if they withdrew the respirator is another unfortunate aspect of the case. They had to deal with fear of prosecution, with ominous advice from attorneys, with a situation for which there was not yet a recognized medical tradition, and with their own recognition that stopping life support does play a causal role in bringing about a patient's death.

These are just some of the good and bad features in the story thus far. Most are directly linked to the central question—is it ethical to withdraw life support from a permanently unconscious patient? To answer this question we will ask what behaviors of the major moral agents in the case (here the parents and the physicians) would be reasonable behaviors; that is, what response in the situation would enhance their living well. And if any of their deliberate behaviors would bring about what is bad, we will ask what overriding reasons would justify this.

Prudential Reasoning in the Quinlan Story

We begin reasoning in an ethics of prudential judgment by asking two fundamental questions: What is truly good for the moral agents, and how can they achieve it? We have distinguished two ways a moral agent achieves the good and lives well. First, he enhances the good whenever he can reasonably do so. Second, he eliminates the bad features in the situation whenever possible. And if his deliberate behavior gives rise to anything bad (that is, anything causing suffering, damage, or death), it is always for overriding reasons that are strong enough to compensate for the bad features resulting from his behavior. This is the mindset we adopt in each case we consider.

We will now look at this dilemma about whether or not to withdraw a respirator from the perspectives of the patient (Karen), the proxy (her father), and the physicians.

Patient's perspective.   Karen was unable to function as a moral agent. She was forever beyond being a moral agent because she was beyond making decisions for her own good. In fact she was beyond experiencing any good or bad. There is no patient perspective in this kind of situation when the patient has left no advance directives.

Proxy's perspective.   Joseph Quinlan was a primary moral agent in this story. If his decision were carried out, the expected result would be the death of his daughter. He knew this and still wanted the respirator withdrawn. The death of a person is bad. His decision to stop life support for his daughter would be immoral unless he had an adequate reason to justify the bad outcome, death. Did he have a reason capable of justifying the death his decision would cause?

A proxy in this situation could begin by realizing how the bad features accompanying Karen's death are much less than they would be in the death of a normal person her age. The usual harms we associate with death will not occur when Karen dies. First, much of her brain is already destroyed, and there is no reasonable hope that she will ever regain consciousness. People dying in a state of permanent unconsciousness have already lost much, and they do not suffer. Death will not take that much more from Karen—she has already lost everything except vegetative life. And if Karen ever did regain consciousness, it would be terrible for her—her rigid, contorted body would cause her significant discomfort and pain.

Second, Karen's actual death will cause only minimal harm to her loved ones, since so much of Karen has already been destroyed by the brain damage that reduced her life to a vegetative state.

Third, Karen's death will cause no social harm; society has already lost any possible contributions she could have made. Moreover, society's interest in preserving life, an important interest we must not forget, is not undermined when the life has become irreversibly unconscious and is sustained by a mechanical respirator and feeding tubes.

The proxy might also ask how much good the life-support treatment is achieving. It does no good for Karen—she is beyond experiencing any good or bad. Nor is it doing good in the eyes of the family because the use of ventilation to sustain a vegetative body without any capacity for awareness makes no sense. Nor is it accomplishing any good for society or the common good; in fact it can be argued that this kind of a situation actually undermines the common good by its unreasonable use of financial resources contributed by others in the society.

In the ethics of Aristotle and Aquinas each moral agent follows the guideline: "act (and feel) according to right reason" where the right reason is prudence, and the reasonable is what achieves the agent's good in the circumstances. Joseph Quinlan's basic options were two: continue the ventilation sustaining a permanently unconscious body or discontinue ventilation, an action that would result in the death of a permanently unconscious body. He was convinced that withdrawal of the respirator was the more reasonable response—the less worse option. It is hard to fault his moral reasoning.

Providers' perspective.   The attending physician Dr. Robert Morse and other members of the health care team at St. Clare's Hospital were not convinced that withdrawing the respirator could be morally justified. Their position is not unreasonable, especially if we situate the story in its proper moment in history. At the time this story unfolded in the mid-1970s, many physicians and nurses were understandably upset about removing life-sustaining treatments from living people, and for good reasons. It was not a widely accepted action in medical practice, a thorough ethical analysis justifying respirator withdrawal in appropriate situations had not yet been developed, and the threat of legal action was real. Many physicians would have found withdrawal of life-sustaining treatment morally disturbing at the time. It would be considered less so today, however, because so much ethical dialogue and progress on the matter have taken place, along with some supportive court decisions.

Based on these considerations, there are sound reasons for the physicians' reluctance to withdraw the respirator. The reasonableness of their position is, on the other hand, weakened by the fact that they were forcing treatment on a helpless patient over the proxy's strong objections.

The clash between proxies and providers creates another twist in the story. It is one that occurs frequently. What is the most reasonable way for physicians to respond when a proxy asks them to do something they think is seriously immoral? The answer is relatively straightforward: Since they cannot compromise their moral integrity and do what they think is morally wrong because somebody asks them to, they will arrange for alternative provisions for care and then withdraw from the case. This response was already well worked out by the time the Quinlan drama unfolded. A few years before in 1973 the U.S. Supreme Court had declared most restrictions on abortion by state legislatures unconstitutional. What then should physicians and nurses opposed to abortion do when their patients sought an abortion? It was generally agreed that they could, and morally should, step aside.

If the physicians had a moral problem with the withdrawal of Karen's respirator, one reasonable response would have been to turn her care over to others and then step aside. The physicians chose not to do this, however, and thus another chapter in the Quinlan story began. Before we consider the moral issues embedded in this chapter of the story, however, we return to the state supreme court's decision in the case.

The New Jersey Supreme Court Decision

The Supreme Court of New Jersey reversed the decision of the lower court in March 1976. It allowed the appointment of Joseph Quinlan as Karen's guardian with the authority to have the respirator discontinued. The court found that the state certainly had an interest in preserving human life but that the constitutional right to privacy extends to decisions about medical treatment. It found that the state's interest in preserving life weakens, and the person's right to privacy grows, as medical interventions become more invasive and the prognosis for recovery diminishes. It further found that a person's right to privacy can be asserted by a guardian when the patient is incompetent.

Joseph Quinlan then requested removal of the respirator. Apparently the physicians were still unhappy with this decision. Instead of simply removing the machine, they began a process of weaning Karen from it. They withdrew the respirator support, for brief periods at first, and then gradually extended the time until, a month later, she was breathing without it. In June she was transferred to a nursing home where, twisted into an unnatural position and totally unconscious, she lived for another ten years in a PVS. Eventually she developed pneumonia, and her parents requested that antibiotics be withheld. She died in June 1986 from overwhelming infection.

We will never know for sure whether Karen would have died in 1976 if the respirator had been simply removed. But it was not. The physicians at St. Clare's apparently decided that every effort should be made to preserve her vegetative life despite her father's request, which was supported by the New Jersey Supreme Court and by a long Catholic moral tradition allowing people to forgo means of preserving life that are considered extraordinary.

Ethical Reflection

Here we take the perspective of an ethicist. We try to make moral judgments about some of the ethical dilemmas faced by moral agents in the story. The proxy's decision to withdraw the respirator in these circumstances seems reasonable. So does the decision of the New Jersey Supreme Court to allow the proxy to make such a decision. The initial decision of the physicians to continue the respirator can also be justified as reasonable if we remember that the situation happened in the 1970s, when the issue of respirator withdrawal had not yet been extensively deliberated and debated. However, once the court decision was given, the decision of the physicians to stay on the case and try so hard to wean Karen from the respirator does not seem reasonable. Their efforts were successful—Karen survived without a respirator for another ten years—but it was of no benefit to her.

The physicians' decision to wean rather than simply withdraw the respirator was morally problematic in that it brought no good to the patient, was not consistent with the desires of the proxy, and imposed a decade of expensive and useless care on a vegetative body. It is difficult to defend the physicians' actions after the state supreme court decision. If the physicians could not in good conscience withdraw the respirator in accord with the proxy's directions, the reasonable ethical response at that point would have been withdrawal from the case.

As we might well imagine, this case generated enormous publicity, and all sorts of opinions were voiced. Some people thought it would be tantamount to murder if the life-sustaining treatment were stopped. Others thought it was cruel for patients and their families to be trapped by a medical establishment so fixated on treatment that it would impose life-prolonging interventions regardless of their benefit for the patient or the wishes of the family. The public uproar was to be expected because new ground was being broken in legal and medical morality, and it takes time for new situations to be absorbed by the medical, legal, and ethical professionals as well as by the rest of society. Today the removal of a respirator from a permanently unconscious patient at the request of an appropriate proxy would not create a legal or moral problem for most people. But it was not so easy for those involved in the Quinlan case; they were breaking new ground.

The Case of Brother Fox

The Story

Brother Fox, a member of a Catholic religious order, arrested during surgery for a hernia repair in October 1979. It left him unconscious, and shortly thereafter he was diagnosed as being in a vegetative state with no chance of recovery. He was eighty-three years old at the time. His religious superior, Father Philip Eichner, asked that the respirator be withdrawn. When the hospital and the physicians caring for Brother Fox refused, he turned to the courts. He argued that Brother Fox had explicitly said more than once in discussions about the Quinlan case that he did not want to be kept alive on a respirator if he were in a similar condition.

The trial court judge approved the respirator withdrawal, but the district attorney appealed the ruling. On appeal, the case went to the Appellate Division of the New York Supreme Court. This court affirmed the lower court ruling, but its decision was also appealed. During this appeal process, Brother Fox died while still on the respirator. In order to establish a legal precedent, New York's highest court, the Court of Appeals, agreed to hear the case even though Brother Fox was now dead. Before looking at the decision of the highest New York court, we will consider the story from an ethical point of view.

Ethical Analysis

Situational awareness. We are aware of the following facts in the Fox story.

1. Brother Fox was permanently unconscious with no hope of recovery.

2. He had made it clear that he did not want a respirator used to keep him alive if this situation ever befell him.

3. His proxy was thus able to use the substituted judgment criterion of proxy decision making and report that Brother Fox had previously indicated he did not want a respirator in these circumstances.

4. The hospital and physicians refused to abide by the patient's request as reported by the proxy, and this refusal brought the case to court.

We are also aware of the following good and bad features in the Fox story.

1. Brother Fox was expected to die when the respirator was removed, and death is always bad. Death was not, however, a bad thing for Brother Fox because his permanent loss of consciousness had removed him from experiencing any bad or, for that matter, any good. Nor was it bad for others at this point because he was already permanently unconscious.

2. The expense of treatment that provided no good the patient could experience and that the proxy wanted stopped is a bad feature of the case. Somebody was spending money for health care services that would never provide any benefit the patient could experience.

3. The hospital and the physicians were distressed about withdrawing the respirator, and their distress was not surprising at this point in history. The Quinlan case had happened in New Jersey, not New York, and there was no guarantee that New York would not try to prosecute the medical team if they removed life support from a living patient and the patient died. The Fox story happened soon enough after the Quinlan story that we really cannot say at this point that removing respirators from permanently unconscious patients was a recognized medical practice.

Prudential Reasoning in the Brother Fox Story

What is good for the people involved in this situation, and how can they achieve it?

Patient's perspective. Brother Fox was unable to communicate anything, but he did leave instructions about what he thought was reasonable. He had decided that withdrawing his life-support equipment after the permanent loss of consciousness was a reasonable thing to do. He was correct—there are no reasons for using medical technology to sustain permanently unconscious patients.

Proxy's perspective. Father Eichner was also acting reasonably by reporting Brother Fox's instructions to the providers. This is exactly what a proxy is supposed to do. Anything else would have been unethical.

Providers' perspective. The hospital and physicians were against the withdrawal. Their position is not totally unreasonable, especially given the moment in history when the case happened. But it is not a very strong position either given the legal precedent (the *Quinlan* case) in the neighboring state and a growing body of commentary at the time indicating that there are strong moral reasons supporting respirator withdrawal when the treatment provides no benefit that the patient will experience and it is clear as well that the patient would not want the treatment.

The New York Court of Appeals' Decision

The highest court in New York, the Court of Appeals, approved the proxy's decision to withdraw the respirator. It confined its ruling to cases where the incapacitated patient is fatally ill with no reasonable chance of recovery and where we have "clear and convincing evidence" that the patient had given instructions to withdraw the respirator in this kind of situation.

This story differs somewhat from the Quinlan story because, thanks to the extensive publicity surrounding the *Quinlan* case, Brother Fox had left clear instructions about what he wanted. Once this was evident, the courts had no trouble granting Father Eichner's request. Other courts had long recognized a person's right to refuse medical treatment, and the New York courts sensibly argued that such a right should not be lost just because the person becomes incapable of exercising it.

We should note, however, the court's insistence that there be "clear and convincing evidence" of the incapacitated person's previous wishes. "Clear and convincing evidence" is a legal phrase denoting the highest level of evidence in civil cases. It is very difficult to obtain unless the patient has left explicit instructions about treatment. Most states do not require such a high standard of evidence for proxy decision making. Years after the *Fox* case, the U.S. Supreme Court was asked whether Missouri's insistence on "clear and convincing evidence" was so strict that it was unconstitutional—that is, so strict that it deprived citizens of their constitutional right to refuse medical treatment. The U.S. Supreme Court found, in the *Cruzan* case that we will consider in the chapter on medical nutrition and hydration, that it was not unconstitutional for states to insist on the strict "clear and convincing" standard in these cases. Fortunately, most states do not insist on such a high standard of evidence for establishing what we think the now-incompetent patient would want.

Ethical Reflection

The court's argument based on the patient's right to reject medical treatment does not, of course, settle the moral question. The moral question is whether or not Brother Fox's prior decision to reject life-sustaining treatment in the event of permanent unconsciousness was morally reasonable. As was stated earlier, it seems clear that it was, as was the behavior of his proxy, Father Eichner, morally reasonable. The reluctance of the hospital and physicians to abide by the information given them by the proxy was also a reasonable position in 1979 when many health care professionals were not morally comfortable with respirator withdrawal. Today, however, it would not be easy to defend morally a refusal to withdraw a respirator in a case such as this.

The actions of the district attorney, however, were more problematic. He chose to appeal the trial court judge's decision, thus dragging out the ordeal. Still, the patient was not suffering, and the appeal did move the case to the appellate level and eventually to the highest state court. This provided an opportunity to set a legal precedent for this kind of case. The decision thus added burdens to the proxy and caregivers, but it also contributed to a legal clarification for people living in New York.

The Case of William Bartling

The Story

William Bartling was a sick man in 1984. The California resident was seventy years old and had been hospitalized six times in the previous twelve months. His problems included severe emphysema, hardening of the arteries, an abdominal aneurysm, and inoperable cancer of one lung. His lung had collapsed during the initial biopsy that had found the lung cancer, and a ventilator was necessary to support his breathing. In view of his serious condition, doctors had no reasonable hope that he would ever again live without the ventilator. Since patients on ventilators in 1984 were usually kept in intensive care units (ICU), this prognosis meant that he would probably be confined to the ICU of the hospital for the rest of his life. Although he was suffering from depression, there was general agreement that he had not lost his capacity to make his health care decisions.

William's ability to communicate was hindered by the ventilator tube surgically inserted into his throat, but he was able to indicate repeatedly that he wanted the ventilator removed. After he had pulled the tube out several times, his hands were tied to the sides of the bed. He also wrote a statement saying he did not want the life support continued, appointed his wife proxy with durable power of attorney so she could order the respirator removed, and signed documents releasing the physicians and hospital from liability if they withdrew the treatment.

His physician seemed ready to respect his decision to refuse treatment until legal counsel advised the hospital administration to continue the ventilator. Bartling's lawyer then went to court in an effort to have his client's decision to refuse treatment respected by the hospital. He also filed a complaint against the physicians and the hospital for treating Bartling without his consent and for violation of his constitutional rights.

The day before the court hearing in June 1984, attorneys visited William Bartling in the ICU to take his testimony in a legal deposition. His attorney asked him three questions:

1. "Do you want to live?" Bartling indicated that he did.
2. "Do you want to continue to live on the ventilator?" Bartling indicated that he did not.
3. "Do you understand that if the ventilator is discontinued or taken away you might die?" Bartling indicated that he did.

The court found that Mr. Bartling was seriously ill but competent. Before considering its decision, however, we reflect on the ethics of the case.

Ethical Analysis

Situational awareness. We are aware of the following facts in the Bartling story.

1. Despite some depression, William was capable of making important decisions.

2. He was seventy years old and had several serious medical problems, including inoperable lung cancer. It was unlikely that he could ever live without the ventilator or leave the ICU.

3. His decision to withdraw the respirator had remained constant over many months. It was also supported by his effort to use every means possible to have his wishes carried out by himself or by others.

4. The physicians and the hospital refused to honor Bartling's decision to withdraw the respirator.

We are also aware of the following good and bad features in the Bartling story.

1. If the ventilator were removed, everybody expected Bartling's death. Unlike Karen Quinlan and Brother Fox, he would experience his dying because he was conscious. His suffering and death are clearly bad.

2. If the ventilator were not removed, Bartling's distress would continue. To prevent him from withdrawing the ventilator himself, his hands had been tied. Continuing the respirator and tying his hands were frustrating to William Bartling; they conflicted with his wishes, and he was aware of what was happening.

3. If the ventilator were not removed, his family would be distressed; they wanted his wishes carried out. The whole frustrating process was an additional bad situation for Bartling's family, who were already distressed over his life-threatening illness.

4. The physicians and the hospital were worried about adverse legal consequences if the ventilator were removed because of the legal advice they had received. Such worries are understandably upsetting but, as we will see, were not well grounded in this case.

Prudential Reasoning in the Story of William Bartling

What is good in this situation, and how can the persons involved achieve it?

Patient's perspective. William was in the best position to judge whether, all things considered, this treatment was really reasonable for him. He did not want to die, but neither did he want to continue the uncomfortable life-sustaining respirator. The respirator would not cure any of his diseases, and one of them (the inoperable lung cancer) was ominous, especially given his problem with emphysema. He had sought hospital treatment six times in the past twelve months, but he had now decided it was better to stop the life support than to live with the two new factors: the ventilator and the cancer. It is difficult to think his position was unreasonable, that is, unethical. The life support was providing some good—it was preserving his life for the moment—but it was also causing him a great deal of physical and emotional suffering. He did not want to kill himself; he simply wanted the treatment that was bringing him more burden than benefit to be stopped.

Proxy's perspective. Since William was still capable of making his decisions, there was no role for a proxy at that time. Ironically, if he had lapsed into irreversible unconsciousness, a judge might well have accepted his wife's testimony that there was clear evidence that he did not want the ventilator and then have allowed its withdrawal under the precedent set in the Fox case. Thus, Bartling's decision might very well have been accepted if he were unconscious, but it was not being accepted while he was still conscious and able to indicate exactly what he wanted. It is difficult to see the reasonableness of this because it makes the patient's wishes more significant when he does not have decision-making capacity than when he does have it.

Provider's perspective. From a legal point of view, one could claim that the physicians had some reason to fear litigation if they removed the ventilator and this conscious man died. However, it is hard to think they were worried about criminal prosecution—only a year earlier a California court had found that charges of murder could not be brought against two physicians who had ordered first a respirator and then tubes providing nutrition and hydration to be removed from an unconscious patient at the request of the family.

Moreover, the highest courts in New Jersey and New York (the *Quinlan* and *Fox* cases) had already established the right of people to refuse ventilators, and a decision in Florida for a case very similar to Bartling's (the *Perlmutter* case, which we will mention shortly) had also favored this right. In addition, the California living will law (the California Natural Death Act) was in place at the time of Bartling's request. It would have allowed William to refuse the respirator if he were considered terminally ill, something his physicians declined to say since they thought he might live for more than a year. All things considered, the worries of the physicians and of the hospital about legal liability were more imaginary than real. Nonetheless, the questionable legal advice they received did make the fear of litigation real to them, and exposure to prosecution is certainly something people want to avoid.

From a moral point of view, however, the decision of the attorneys to recommend against withdrawing the ventilator was problematic. The patient did not want it, and his physicians did not want to force it on him, but that is precisely what the legal advice encouraged them to do. Moreover, the decision of the hospital to fight Bartling's request in court is highly unreasonable behavior. It set up an unfortunate relationship of conflict between the institution and a patient, and the conflict could easily have been avoided. The attorneys for the hospital and the physicians did not have to fight for continuation of the ventilator in court; in fact they could have supported the right of patients to refuse burdensome life-sustaining treatment and simply sought a declaration of immunity to protect themselves if the respirator were withdrawn.

The Court Decisions

The trial court refused to support William's decision to remove the ventilator. It said the right to remove life-sustaining treatment extends only to the comatose or to the terminally ill. The court also refused to grant a subsequent request of Bartling's lawyer—he had sought to have the hospital untie Bartling's hands so he could withdraw the ventilator himself.

The case received widespread publicity in September 1984, when Mike Wallace showed dramatic documentary footage of Bartling in his ICU bed, giving his deposition on the television program *60 Minutes* and also reported how the judge had refused to let his wishes be followed.

Bartling's lawyer appealed the decision of the trial court judge. During the appeal William Bartling died, still tied up and on the respirator. Later the California Court of Appeals reversed the lower court. It ruled that the right to refuse treatment is not confined to the comatose or to the terminally ill but is based on the constitutional right of privacy enjoyed by all citizens. This decision would have allowed withdrawal of the respirator if William had still been alive.

Ethical Reflection

There seems to be no reason for saying William Bartling was behaving immorally by deciding to stop the uncomfortable treatment that was providing so little benefit for him at this point in his life. Another person in his position might decide differently, however, and that could also be a morally justified position. Prudential judgments often vary among individuals. In this kind of case, an ethicist could very well acknowledge two reasonable decisions: One patient may want the respirator continued; another may want it withdrawn. The primary moral agent, the patient, is thus not making a decision between two options, one ethical and the other unethical, but between two ethically reasonable options.

This does not mean that there is no right answer in this kind of case because there is. The right answer in this kind of case is the answer given by the patient, the person in the best position to determine how to achieve his good or, in this tragic situation, how to avoid the worse. For Bartling as for so many others, the respirator could not cure his life-threatening problems; it could only sustain his breathing in the face of severe emphysema and lung cancer. He decided that the burdens of the life-sustaining treatment in the ICU as his life ebbed away simply were not worth the benefit that treatment provided.

Let us look at those opposing Bartling on legal grounds, which were later shown to be invalid. There are serious questions about whether the great harm the legal delay and court actions caused the patient and his family can be morally justified. It is difficult to think of any adequate reasons for putting the patient and his family through this ordeal when other options were legally available. Instead of using the courts to fight the patient's wishes, the physicians and hospital could have presented themselves to the court as parties seeking legal protection for respecting a patient's decision to refuse treatment. This legal approach would have been more kind to the patient and his family. And it may have affected the trial judge's decision because, once the hospital stopped opposing withdrawal of the respirator, the central legal issue would emerge more clearly—the patient's legal right to refuse unwanted treatment.

There was no need for the hospital to use the legal system to force unwanted treatment on the patient. This is especially so since an earlier case in Florida had already resolved the issue in favor of the patient with decision-making capacity. In the 1980 landmark case known as *Satz v. Perlmutter*, the Florida Supreme Court affirmed the decisions of lower courts to honor the request of a conscious patient (suffering from amyotrophic lateral sclerosis—Lou Gehrig disease) to have his respirator removed. The earlier Florida case had another similarity to the Bartling case—Mr. Perlmutter had also tried to remove the respirator himself but hospital personnel had tied his hands so he could not.

Although the first ethical dilemmas about the use of ventilators centered on patients or proxies trying to remove them, lately ethical issues have emerged when proxies have insisted on prolonging ventilation long after it benefits the patient. Two such cases have received nationwide publicity. We consider the first, involving an elderly woman named Helga Wanglie, next; and we will consider the second, involving a baby known as Baby K, in the chapter on neonatal life.

The Case of Helga Wanglie

The Story

In December 1989, eighty-six-year-old Helga Wanglie broke her hip. She was successfully treated at the Hennepin County Medical Center in Minnesota and then discharged to a nursing home. In January 1990 she was back in the hospital with respiratory distress, and a respirator was necessary. In early May, still on the respirator, she was transferred to a chronic care facility where, two weeks later, she suffered a cardiopulmonary arrest. She was resuscitated and readmitted on May 31 to the medical center, where she was diagnosed as being permanently unconscious with chronic lung disease that would require a respirator for the rest of her life. It soon became clear that she was in a PVS.

By the end of 1990, almost a year after Helga had become respirator-dependent and months after the diagnosis of PVS, her attending physicians felt strongly that the ventilator and other life-support systems were medically inappropriate treatments since they could not serve any of the patient's interests. Helga's husband Oliver, however, wanted the life-sustaining treatment to continue. He felt that only God should take life and said that Helga would not have wanted anything done to shorten her life.

In December 1990 the medical center advised Mr. Wanglie in writing that it did not believe treatment considered inappropriate by physicians should continue but that it would continue the life-sustaining treatment if he obtained a court order mandating it. During this time both the hospital and the family tried to find another facility willing to accept Helga as a patient. None would accept her.

When the Wanglie family made no move to seek a court order for treatment, the medical center filed a legal petition on February 8, 1991, seeking appointment of a conservator for the patient. Ordinarily, a guardian *ad litem* would be appointed to perform this function, but Minnesota did not have a guardian *ad litem* process, so the hospital sought appointment of the conservator to protect the interests of the patient.

The medical center had serious doubts that Helga's proxy, her husband, was making the right decision, so it was seeking to have the court appoint a conservator to represent her. The center hoped the court-appointed conservator would say that the ventilator was not beneficial to Helga, paving the way for its removal. The hospital's legal move was undermined when Helga's husband filed a petition asking that he be appointed the conservator.

On July 1, 1991 the court did appoint a conservator for Helga—her husband. He continued to insist on the ventilator, and the medical center continued to provide it. Three days later, Helga died. During the last fourteen months of her life, Helga, a permanently unconscious woman in her late eighties with no hope of recovery, had her vegetative body sustained by a respirator at the medical center. It was reported that Medicare paid about $200,000 for her first hospitalization at the center, and that a private HMO paid over $500,000 for the second admission that ran from May 1990 to July 1991.

Ethical Analysis

Situational awareness. We are aware of the following facts in the Wanglie story.

1. Helga was in a PVS. She could experience neither benefit nor burden from life-sustaining treatment.

2. She had not made it clear that she would want a ventilator keeping her alive if she ever lapsed into a PVS, but there are several reasons to think that she may well have wanted it. Although her husband first said he did not know what she would have wanted, he later indicated in a letter to the medical center dated December 3, 1990 that she had always said she did not want anything

done "to shorten or prematurely take her life." Moreover, it was known that her religious views included the idea that only God gives and takes life and that her moral views were strongly pro-life. Unfortunately, a precious opportunity to learn Helga's wishes was lost. She was a conscious patient in the hospital on a respirator from January until May 1990, yet published reports do not indicate that anyone attempted to determine her wishes while she was still capable of stating them.

3. Her husband was her proxy and, thanks to the court, also her conservator. He wanted the ventilator continued. His decision was apparently based on his familiarity with her wishes, although this did not become clear until physicians asked him to consider withdrawing the ventilator.

4. Her physicians came to the conclusion that ventilation was not appropriate medical treatment for Helga. Although Dr. Stephen Miles, an ethicist serving as consultant to the physicians caring for Helga, declined to characterize the ventilator as futile treatment because it was sustaining vegetative life, a newspaper story in the *Chicago Tribune* of January 10, 1991, reported that other physicians involved in the case sought relief in the court because they did think the ventilator was futile treatment after the diagnosis of PVS. And an attending physician who joined the case later spoke of the respirator as "nonbeneficial" in that it could neither heal Helga's lungs nor restore her awareness.

We are also aware of the following good and bad features in the Wanglie case.

1. Without the respirator Helga would die, and death is always bad.

2. Withdrawal of the respirator would cause distress to Oliver and to his two adult children, who also opposed the withdrawal.

3. Continuation of the respirator would cause distress to the providers, who felt it was inappropriate. The respirator, however, caused no distress or burden to Helga, nor any benefit, because she was totally and irreversibly oblivious to it.

4. Continuation of the respirator required considerable financial support, and this was eventually a burden on insurance plans and the people paying into them.

Prudential Reasoning in the Story of Helga Wanglie

What is good in this situation and how can the persons involved best achieve it, or at least avoid the worse?

Patient's perspective. It is hard to comment on this because we do not know for sure whether Helga would have insisted on the ventilator to sustain her life once it had deteriorated into a PVS. The fact that her husband of fifty-three years at first took the position he did not know what she would want and then after some months said that she had stated she would not want anything done to shorten her life is cause for concern.

If a patient did want a ventilator continued after months of irreversible vegetative existence, it is difficult to see how moral reasons could justify that desire. Patients in a PVS experience no benefit from treatment, and both the costs and the responsibilities of care it imposes on others are significant burdens. Burdening others with what offers no benefit to oneself is difficult to justify as a morally admirable position. This leaves only a religious argument to justify a patient's insistence that life support be continued for her vegetative body; namely, the belief that God, and not anyone else, is the one to decide when death should come.

Religious beliefs are notoriously hard to critique. Whereas some very important religious thinkers—the thirteenth-century theologian Thomas Aquinas is perhaps the most notable example—insisted that no moral position derived from religious faith could ever contradict reason, not every religious person embraces such a position. Many claim that what is unreasonable to the human mind is not unreasonable in the eyes of God and further claim that they can know how God sees certain apparently unreasonable situations. For these people, the religious argument becomes a trump card. It trumps reason. Once it is proffered, no other reason can undermine it. The religious belief, no matter how unreasonable, becomes, in the mind of the believer, the reason for the decision. No reasoning from moral philosophy or prudence will ever appear cogent to a person basing her apparently unreasonable position on a religious belief.

Proxies' perspective. If Oliver and his two adult children really thought Helga wanted the ventilator continued after months in a PVS, then this is a reason in favor of their requesting continuation of the treatment. However, it is not of itself a sufficient reason. Simply because someone wants something does not mean what is wanted is morally good. If she had wanted a treatment that was clearly absurd, they could not in good conscience be a party to providing it for her. When a proxy acts on the basis of substituted judgment (that is, when a proxy makes the decision based on what he or she knows the patient wanted), there is a presumption that the proxy is presenting a decision that is morally acceptable or at least morally plausible.

Although some would argue that respirators for PVS patients in their eighties is an immoral use of personnel and resources because the treatment provides no benefit the patient can experience, some people do see the preservation of human beings in persistent vegetative life as morally good, or at least not morally evil. Helga's family apparently did believe the treatment was morally correct, so it was proper for them to request it. Their moral beliefs, judging from published reports, were based more on a religious conviction than moral reasoning, but religion is an important source of moral judgment for many people.

To carry out their religious conviction, however, they had to ask a hospital, physicians, and nurses to provide treatments these people did not think were appropriate. In effect they were forcing their morality on others, yet they had little choice but to do so because Helga needed professional care and hospitalization. Helga's vegetative life was a value to them, a good they saw through the eyes of their religious conviction, and a good they wanted to pursue.

Providers' perspective. The providers did not see any good in the treatment at this point, except for the possible comfort it gave to the family. Did they think continuing the treatment was therefore immoral? That is a separate issue. It is one thing to say the treatment is not doing the patient any good; it is another to say the treatment is immoral.

What did the providers think? Perhaps they thought using the ventilator on a PVS patient was immoral and that they had to stop it, but if this is so, one of their moves was curious. In December 1990, after Helga had been in PVS for about six months, the hospital's medical director wrote Mr. Wanglie and said that medical consultants, the attending physician, and he (the medical director) did not believe the hospital was obliged to provide inappropriate medical treatment but would do so if a court ordered it. If the medical director and consultants thought the inappropriate treatment was also unethical, they could not in good conscience make such a statement—legal immunity does not make something that is immoral moral. Thus, their position, assuming they are people of moral integrity, was that the treatment was medically inappropriate but not morally inappropriate.

Their position is coherent if we distinguish, as we should, between good clinical practice and clinical ethics. In this case a strong argument can be made that good clinical practice indicates that the ventilator supporting the irreversibly vegetative life of an elderly PVS patient for many months is not an appropriate clinical treatment and should be discontinued. This is not the same as saying, however, that continuation of the ventilator is unethical. Claiming that continued mechanical ventilation on this unconscious patient is not clinically good does not automatically mean it is not ethically good. What is clinically good is not always ethically good, and what is clinically bad is not always unethical.

Is the continuation of the ventilator not only medically inappropriate but unethical as well? Perhaps, but there are reasons for saying it is not. First, a ventilator does not cause PVS patients any burden or discomfort because they are not aware of anything being done to them. This removes a major source of ethical concern—the harm we may be causing a patient. Second, her family claims, or came to claim after several months, that she did not want life-sustaining treatments withdrawn before she died. Since we cannot ask her to verify this, the better course is to give them the benefit of the doubt and assume that she, unlike most people, would want to be kept alive indefinitely in a PVS. Apparently she considered vegetative life a value, and so does her family.

The view of some that vegetative life is valuable is not completely absurd. The value of vegetative human life is recognized in law. If, for example, a stranger walked into a hospital with a gun and shot a PVS patient dead, we know exactly what the charge would be—murder. Current law supports the idea that a PVS patient is still a living human being, and thus the idea that the ventilator is supporting something of value—human life—is not patently absurd.

In a pluralistic society respect has to be given (within reason) to the religious and moral considerations patients may have, but which their physicians may not share, as long as such considerations do not force the providers to compromise their moral integrity. In this case the physicians consider the ventilator medically inappropriate but, judging from their willingness to continue it if a court ordered them to do so, not morally evil. Thus, the providers would not be violating their moral convictions by continuing what they thought was unreasonable medical treatment.

This may have been an extraordinary situation where the hospital and the physicians should have continued the medically inappropriate treatment. There are several reasons bolstering this conclusion. First, the providers did not think the treatment was morally evil, only medically inappropriate; second, the proxy's refusal to accept withdrawal was for sincerely held religious reasons; third, the treatment was not causing the patient any suffering; and fourth, the treatment was not damaging the financial condition of the institution.

Ethical Reflection

The clash in the Wanglie case was ultimately a clash between the religious convictions of the family and the clinical convictions of the physicians. It could also have developed into a clash involving the insurance company, but that did not happen in this case because the HMO did not object to paying for life-sustaining treatment long after consciousness had been irreversibly lost.

The Helga Wanglie story is almost the exact opposite of the Karen Quinlan story. Both women were in a PVS, and neither had left clear advance directives. In Karen's case, however, the family wanted the respirator stopped and her physicians did not, whereas in Helga's case the family wanted the respirator continued and her physicians did not. Karen's case helped us clarify a proxy's ability to refuse treatment for a permanently unconscious patient; Helga's case raises questions about a proxy's ability to insist on treatment that is considered, with good reason, medically inappropriate by physicians. This is a new kind of situation, and unlike the right to refuse treatment, we have not yet developed a consensus about the right of a patient or proxy to demand treatment that physicians do not consider appropriate.

From the ethical perspective we have been developing, it can be argued that treating Helga is reasonable, given her religious beliefs and the instructions of her family, and the fact that treatment caused no harm to her. However, the actions of the hospital—asking the family to get a court order to sustain treatment and then, when the family refused, trying to have the court appoint a conservator who would authorize the treatment withdrawal—are strategies difficult to understand as morally reasonable. The efforts of the hospital to find another institution to care for her, however, were reasonable. And it was morally appropriate for the hospital to continue her care—which was reported as excellent—when no other institution would accept her as a patient.

Certainly it is troubling for physicians to give expensive life-sustaining treatment when they feel it is inappropriate, but when the treatment causes the patient no harm, the bad features of providing the treatment are significantly reduced. Of course, other bad features remain. Among them are the high costs of treatment providing no benefit to the patient and the distress health care professionals experience when they are asked to provide treatments that they consider unreasonable. But as long as the physicians and nurses cannot establish that these disturbing factors provide reasons sufficiently strong to override the family's reasons for treatment, they are not compromising their ethics by providing a treatment that causes the patient no harm. Here, what is at least arguably bad clinical practice—using respirators on PVS patients for many months—is not necessarily immoral because of the respect one tries to have for sincerely held religious beliefs.

Of course, if the hospital were being forced to provide for the care without compensation, then the drain on hospital funds would be a significant factor for consideration. But that is not the case here—the third-party payers made no move to question the treatment. In some ways, the payers of the treatment have stronger reasons for being morally disturbed over the treatment than the physicians. It is certainly harmful for insurance programs to pay out significant sums of money for inappropriate medical treatments of no benefit to the patient.

The day may come when third-party payers and HMOs will limit payments for the life-sustaining treatments they will agree to provide. Perhaps, for example, they will explain to their membership that payments for life-sustaining treatment will cease a certain number of months after a confirmed diagnosis of PVS. The family of a PVS patient would then have the option of withdrawing the treatment or seeking other sources of funding.

Finally, it must be said that an ethics of right reason finds nothing to justify the position taken by Helga's husband and family and perhaps by Helga herself. It simply does not seem reasonable for a patient or family to want ventilation continued indefinitely once PVS has been definitively diagnosed. Nonetheless, given the religious issue, continuing the harmless treatment—despite its expense and the upset it caused physicians and nurses—may have been the less unreasonable response in this case.

Helga Wanglie's case is morally challenging but at least the continuation of life support on her vegetative body could not cause her any harm. The situation becomes more challenging when a proxy insists on life support for a family member who is neither in a vegetative state nor comatose, as the following case shows.

The Case of Barbara Howe

The Story

In 1991 Barbara was diagnosed with ALS. She was admitted to Massachusetts General Hospital (MGH) six times in 1998 and seven times in 1999. In November 1999 she began her final stay at MGH. She became ventilator dependent and would remain on life support for the rest of her life. While she still had decision-making capacity, she had signed a form designating her daughter, Carol Carvitt, as her legal health care agent. The Massachusetts health care proxy law, unlike that of some other states, empowers the agent to make any decision that a patient could make, including the withdrawal of life-sustaining treatments. It also instructs the agent to follow the wishes of the patient if they are known. Barbara told her daughters repeatedly that she wanted "everything possible so long as she could appreciate her family." Her daughter believed that her responsibility was to be sure her mother received all possible care as long as she could recognize her family.

In August 2000 Barbara told her doctor that she wanted the aggressive treatment to continue and that being alert was more important than being free of pain. A year later she could no longer mouth words or move her fingers. Her communication was reduced to blinking her eyes in response to questions.

In April 2001 Dr. Andrew Billings, chief of the Palliative Care Service, informed the family that the ventilator should be removed because Barbara was suffering needlessly and had such a serious cognitive impairment that she could no longer communicate meaningfully with her family. When Carol filed for a restraining order to prevent the ventilator withdrawal, MGH decided to continue it.

Meanwhile Carol's father was a patient at MGH dying of colon cancer. Carol was also his health care proxy, and he had given some indication that he wanted aggressive care. However, when he lost his decision-making capacity and became extremely uncomfortable with pain, Carol declined further life-sustaining treatments for him. He died in June 2001. This is important because it suggests that Carol did accept the possibility of withdrawing life support from a parent in some circumstances.

In October 2001 the MGH Optimal Care Committee (OCC), an ethics committee that focuses on end-of-life issues, considered Barbara's case at the request of her primary physician. The OCC reviewed a neurologist's assessment that suggested Barbara might not be so cognitively impaired that she could not recognize her family. Rather, she might have cognitive ability but suffer from "locked in" syndrome, that is, be unable to communicate. Hence, the neurologist reported, we cannot tell whether or not she is still conscious of her family. The OCC then made two recommendations: the ventilation should be continued, but Barbara should receive a DNR order so resuscitation would not be attempted. Carol objected to the DNR order, and when she sought a court order to prevent it, doctors thought it best not to write the order.

By the spring of 2003 Barbara's condition had so deteriorated that she could no longer even blink or close her eyes. This meant her eyes did not receive proper lubrication, and, as a result, one eye ruptured and had to be surgically removed at the bedside in June 2003. To prevent this happening to the other eye, it was taped shut, and the tape was removed only when Carol or her sister came to visit. Barbara also developed severe osteoporosis and at one point, during routine turning, suffered broken bones—fractures of her ribs and a leg.

After her eye rupture, the OCC again reviewed the case and this time concluded that continuing the aggressive life-sustaining treatment in these circumstances was in conflict with "standards of ethics, morality, human decency, and common sense." The OCC chair wrote: "There is now 100% unanimous agreement that this inhumane travesty has gone far enough. This is the Massachusetts General Hospital, not Auschwitz." Moreover, the OCC noted that Barbara apparently did feel pain because she grimaced when she was moved, touched, or suctioned. Carol, however, did not want her to increase her pain medication lest it dull her responses to her family's presence. Carol vigorously disagreed with the OCC recommendation to withdraw ventilation, arguing that her mother still recognized family when they entered the room and would not want to die at this point. Carol did say that she would authorize ventilator withdrawal when her mother no longer could appreciate or react to her presence.

In March 2003 Barbara's insurance company, Blue Cross and Blue Shield of Massachusetts, notified MGH that it would stop paying for her hospital care as of June 21, 2003. Barbara's Blue Cross policy covered medical care but not custodial care, and the insurer took the position that Barbara was receiving only custodial care at this point. Published reports indicated that the cost of custodial care at MGH was probably between $1000 and $2000 a day.

In June 2003 the chair of the OCC wrote that "the patient's status has surpassed an acceptable limit endangering integrity, humanity, and basic human rights." After Carol still refused to allow withdrawal of the ventilator, the hospital petitioned the Probate and Family Court on June 18, 2003, requesting removal of Carol as Barbara's proxy or a determination as to what would be the appropriate level of care for Barbara in these circumstances. In effect, the hospital wanted the court to approve withdrawal of the ventilator. The court assigned two attorneys to investigate the case, one to represent Barbara Howe in a general way and one to act as her guardian *ad litem* in this specific case.

Courts sometimes move slowly, as we have seen. The formal hearing in the Barbara Howe case did not occur until February 9, 2004. The guardian *ad litem* recommended that the Court direct both parties to take steps that would allow the ventilator to be withdrawn. This recommendation was a bit unusual; often guardians *ad litem*, somewhat erroneously, view their job as keeping the patient alive no matter what the circumstances.

The Probate Court issued its ruling on March 22, 2004, nine months after MGH had sought relief. It found that it was no longer possible to know whether or not Barbara could appreciate her family and that not giving her heavy pain medication was reasonable since the medication could numb her consciousness and thus eliminate her reason for living—appreciating her family. The Court did conclude that Carol should "refocus her assessments from Barbara's wishes to Barbara's best interests," and this suggests the judge thought the ventilation should not continue. However, the judge did not give MGH what it asked for—authorization to remove Carol as Barbara's health care proxy or to withdraw the ventilator, which its ethics committee unanimously agreed was contrary to good ethics and good medical practice. And so Carol continued as her mother's decision maker, and the ventilator continued to keep Barbara alive.

On January 13, 2005, MGH again asked the court to authorize withdrawal of the ventilator because Barbara was in danger of losing her other eye, but Carol objected. She did tell the judge, however, that she would allow the ventilator to be withdrawn if her mother lost her remaining eye because eye contact was the one remaining way she interacted with her family.

Barbara's condition, as expected, continued to deteriorate. In February 2005 the hospital invoked a recent policy that it had adopted to resolve disputes about "futile" medical treatment. At a meeting with the probate judge, it informed Carol that she could transfer her mother to another facility, but if Barbara remained a patient at MGH, the hospital would unilaterally withdraw the life support. Carol objected strenuously. Her attorney again petitioned the Probate Court to issue a restraining order to prevent ventilator withdrawal. The judge declined, but he also declined to authorize the removal of life support. After Carol called a press conference to denounce the hospital for trying to end her mother's life, MGH decided to continue the ventilator "until a judge considers objections from the woman's daughter."

Probate Court judge John Smoot then summoned the disputing parties to a closed door meeting on March 12 in an effort to find some common ground. On that day the parties finally reached a compromise agreement: MGH would provide ventilation until June 30, 2005, at which time Carol would voluntarily relinquish her legal authority as Barbara's health care agent. At this point the hospital could make the decision to withdraw the ventilator, which it fully intended to do. In the written agreement MGH acknowledged that Barbara's family members had acted out of love and concern for their mother, and the family acknowledged that MGH had acted with similar concern and that Barbara would not have received better care anywhere else.

However, the saga of nearly six years as a ventilator-dependent patient at MGH did not end as planned on July 1, 2005. On June 4 Barbara Howe died while still on life support. She was 80 years old.

Ethical Analysis

Situational awareness.   We are aware of the following facts in the story of Barbara Howe.

1. Barbara had a terrible incurable terminal illness—ALS. There is no cure; she would deteriorate inexorably until death. She became ventilator dependent and steadily declined as her life drew to a close. The disease had ravaged her body for more than ten years. She had been hospitalized on a ventilator for more than five years, becoming progressively less responsive.

2. While she still had decision-making capacity, Barbara repeatedly said that she wanted aggressive treatments to stay alive as long as she could appreciate her family.

3. She designated her daughter Carol as her health care agent under the Massachusetts Health Care Proxy Act and instructed her daughter to provide aggressive treatments as long as she could "appreciate her family." The standard Massachusetts health care proxy forms instruct agents to carry out the wishes of the patient if they are known. For Carol this meant that she had a moral responsibility to carry out her mother's wishes.

4. Her daughter Carol cared deeply about her mother and wanted to carry out her wishes. She visited her in the hospital regularly and participated in caring for her. She was convinced that her mother still recognized her when the tape was removed from her mother's remaining eye.

5. MGH physicians and the OCC came to believe that Barbara, who was obviously dying from ALS, was experiencing practically no benefit from the treatments that were causing her significant discomfort. Caregivers at MGH believed that advanced life support year after year in a case like this is neither good medicine nor good ethics. For them, there was a moral responsibility not to provide inappropriate care for one of their patients.

Prudential Reasoning in the Barbara Howe Story

What is good in this situation, and how can the persons involved best achieve it or at least avoid the worse?

Patient's perspective. From all reports Barbara was a very strong person with definite ideas about how she wanted to live. After learning that she had ALS, she made it clear that she wanted aggressive treatment and reduced pain medication, even though it might cause her discomfort, as long as she could pursue what mattered most to her: appreciate her family and relate to them. She designated her daughter as her proxy and told her what she wanted.

Proxy's perspective. Carol believed that, as her mother's proxy, her first responsibility was to advocate for her mother's wishes. This is what the ethical literature calls "substituted judgment" and is also the instruction given to proxies in the Massachusetts Health Care Proxy law. Carol believed her mother appreciated her presence when she visited; she said that she saw it in her eyes. Carol was also willing to forgo ventilation for her mother when her mother no longer appreciated her family; when, for example, she no longer responded to the family's presence or was able to see them. Carol also believed, based on her mother's statements at the beginning of her illness, that she wanted to forgo medication for her pain in order to retain awareness of her family.

Providers' perspective. After years of ventilation for a patient dying of ALS whose discomfort seemed to outweigh the limited benefits she could experience as her life dwindled away, many providers became disturbed and began thinking that palliative care was the more appropriate medical response. As Dr. Billings, the chief of the palliative care service, put it in his letter of April 27, 2001 to Carol: "I know you and the family want to do what is right by the patient, but keeping her alive by extraordinary means seems only to offer her opportunity to suffer greatly, and to be more like torture than respectful medical care." The language is strong—torture is a very provocative term—but it captures the way caregivers were beginning to think of what was happening with this patient in 2001.

In June 2003 MGH had to confront yet another issue when Barbara's health insurance company ceased to reimburse the hospital because her care was no longer considered medical but custodial, and her insurance plan did not cover that type of care. Published estimates of the costs for her custodial care at MGH began at $1000 a day, which means they could run over $365,000 a year. Hence MGH, the provider of her care, found itself not only providing care Barbara's doctors thought was medically and morally wrong but providing wrongful care without any reasonable expectation of receiving compensation.

Judge's perspective. The judge was faced with a difficult situation. As a judge he would probably have been very much aware of previous ventilator withdrawal cases that had gone to court, especially the Helga Wanglie case where Helga's husband wanted the ventilation continued and the facility did not. As we saw, the court was reluctant to replace Helga's husband as her proxy, and Helga, who was diagnosed with PVS, died while still on the ventilator. Barbara's case was even more difficult for several reasons. Unlike Helga she was conscious and had also left clear instructions for aggressive care. A judge would understandably be hesitant about authorizing removal of life-prolonging treatment, even treatment that he might not have thought wise, from a conscious patient against her stated wishes and the wishes of her family. And he would be hesitant to remove Carol as her mother's surrogate decision maker simply because she was trying to carry out her mother's wishes. The judge made a great effort to bring the parties together in a solution both could live with, and he finally succeeded. This avoided a situation wherein a court would be making treatment decisions which really belong with physicians, patients, and families.

Ethical Reflection

This type of case is very difficult to resolve because both parties to the dispute are sincere, doing what they think is the right thing, and have plausible reasons for their decisions. Judging from published reports, Carol was dedicated to her mother—she spent hours tending to her needs in the hospital—and was convinced that her moral and legal responsibility, as her mother's health care agent, was to make sure her wishes were carried out. MGH, its physicians, and the members of its Critical Care Committee were also dedicated to their patient and were convinced that their responsibility was to make sure their patient was treated in a medically and morally appropriate way. If Barbara had not been conscious and not able to experience the harm of discomfort, the issue for MGH would not have been so acute, but Barbara did experience pain, pain that her daughter argued should not be totally masked because that would render her unable to experience her family, the major reason why she said she had wanted to continue existing.

What might be an insight from the perspective of virtue ethics in a case like this? A moral agent in Carol's shoes might reason this way: Mother made it clear that she wanted to be kept alive as long as she could appreciate her family, but mother was also a reasonable enough person not to want to be kept alive when a situation developed where it really made no sense or when it forced other people to act against their sincerely held moral convictions. An extreme example may help us see this point. Suppose there were a great disaster in the vicinity of MGH in early 2005, and hundreds of casualties were rushed to the hospital. Overwhelmed, providers would inaugurate a triage program to help those who could be saved. Now suppose a ventilator were needed immediately for a victim expected to survive, but none was available. Suppose also that this victim happened to be one of Barbara's children. In that case it would seem reasonable for Carol to conclude that Barbara, despite her original request for life support as long as she appreciated her family, would no longer want to keep the ventilator that could save the life of her child.

There is, of course, a vast difference between this imaginary scene and what was actually happening at the hospital, so the analogy limps badly. It does, however, illustrate an important point. Barbara's directive to provide ventilation as long as she could appreciate and interact with her family should not be taken as an inviolable absolute; there are situations where Carol could reasonably assume her mother would want the ventilator withdrawn, and the actual situation just described might be one of them. Carol might reasonably assume that her mother would not want her directive carried out literally if doing so would cause serious moral problems for numerous doctors and nurses or would cause many people dedicated to providing her with good care to behave against their moral and medical values.

In a word, a prudent decision maker in this case could reasonably assume that the mother would not want her directive followed to that point at the end of her life where the advance directive was becoming seriously harmful to others and could be classified as selfish and uncaring. In virtue ethics an agent for a patient who wanted "everything done" can reasonably assume that a patient would not want that directive pursued if it moved way outside the parameters of rationality and caused many people serious moral distress. In fact, if the proxy thought that the patient did want her to insist on something that was highly irrational and caused significant moral distress for many caregivers, then it is hard to see how a person of good character could accept the role of proxy decision maker for that person.

The autonomy of the patient is not the last word in virtue ethics. It is not virtuous (morally excellent) when patients, either directly or through their proxies, autonomously demand treatments that providers and experienced ethics committees, unable to transfer the patient, sincerely believe are morally and medically wrong. Nor is it virtuous for families to demand that a hospital provide expensive medically inappropriate care and make no serious effort to provide funds to pay for that care.

Ultimately the solution to cases such as this will depend not on judicial resolution as individual cases arise because, as we saw, the courts do not want to remove properly designated proxies or to order removal of ventilators keeping conscious people alive. What is needed is some sort of legislative relief that will protect caregivers when patients or families demand treatments beyond the standards of medical care. Some states have such laws. Texas, for example, has such a law called the Advanced Directives Act. After going through a clearly defined process the hospitals may unilaterally cease treatments without fear of civil or criminal liability. However, as we point out in chapter 17, the Texas law has caused some unfortunate and morally upsetting situations. Better laws are possible, but they will not prevent every conflict that arises when families demand unreasonable life-prolonging treatments. We simply do not yet have a good solution to these dilemmas beyond encouraging more public education about end-of-life issues.

Plato insisted in his late works (*Statesman* and *Laws*) that the primary goal of political leaders and laws is educating people toward virtue, especially the virtue of prudence, so they become wise enough to make reasonable decisions that enhance the human good. Perhaps more widespread education is our best hope to reduce these unfortunate dilemmas.

DIALYSIS

Although research on rabbits suggested as early as 1913 that a machine could perform some kidney functions and thus reduce the chemical imbalances associated with kidney failure, it was not until the 1940s that efforts were made to use such a device for patients with chronic renal disease. Less than twenty years later, hemodialysis became a reality. The dialysis machine does the work of a kidney, purifying the blood by removing waste products from it. Normally, the procedure takes about five hours and is repeated three times a week.

When dialysis was perfected in the late 1960s, there were more patients than machines, and difficult decisions had to be made about who would be given the treatment. Selection committees were soon formed. In some areas these committees were called "God squads," since their decisions were, indeed, decisions of life or death for those with serious kidney disease who were unable to obtain a kidney transplant.

In 1972 Congress responded to the shortage of dialysis machines by amending the Social Security Act to guarantee dialysis treatment for all those needing it, regardless of age or other disability. Within a short time, a sufficient number of dialysis centers opened (there are now over 3,600 centers with fewer than 10 percent of these in nonprofit hospitals), and the number of patients grew to over 341,000 by 2005. The current annual cost of treating kidney failure in the United States is over $23 billion. Over 60 percent of the patients suffer from diabetes or high blood pressure.

Dialysis is not a perfect answer to the problem of serious kidney disease. It does not cure the disease, and the patient experiences frequent discomfort during the treatment. Moreover, dialysis cannot quite match the work of healthy kidneys, and as time goes on, the disease gains ever so slowly. For example, one statistic shows that the life expectancy of a forty-nine-year-old dialysis patient is less than ten years, compared with more than thirty years for the general population.

After years of dialysis, some patients experience mounting health problems. In a few cases they decide to decline the treatment, judging that the mounting burdens outweigh the benefits. Sometimes, as the following story shows, family members must decide when the burdens of dialysis outweigh the benefits.

The Case of Earle Spring

The Story

Earle Spring was a vigorous man in his seventies when he developed serious kidney disease. He consented to dialysis and underwent the treatments despite the dizziness, leg cramps, and headaches they caused. As time went on, he became senile and lost his decision-making capacity. He began to resist transportation to the dialysis center and to pull the tubes out of his arm. Heavy sedation was necessary to control his disruptive behavior. His physicians thought he could live for months with dialysis. Survival for five years was conceivable but not probable. He was not a candidate for a kidney transplant. There was no hope his senility could be reversed, so he would remain in a state of mental confusion the rest of his life.

Since his wife was also advanced in years, the court appointed his son as temporary guardian in January 1979. Earle's son, with the consent of his mother (Earle's wife), immediately asked the probate court to issue an order stopping the dialysis. The judge appointed a guardian *ad litem* to investigate the facts in the case. Within a few weeks, the guardian *ad litem* finished his investigation and filed a report recommending continuation of the dialysis.

The judge deliberated until May 1979 and then issued an order for the cessation of dialysis. The guardian *ad litem* objected and filed an appeal.

While the appeal process was under way, the probate court judge had second thoughts about his order directing cessation of dialysis. In July 1979, realizing that he should not be making the treatment decision for Earle, he vacated his original order for ending the dialysis. He then issued a new order directing Earle's wife and son, with the attending physician, to decide whether or not to continue the dialysis. The guardian *ad litem* also appealed this ruling.

In December 1979 the appeals court affirmed the probate judge's July ruling directing the family and physician to make the decision about withholding dialysis. The guardian *ad litem* again objected and filed another appeal, this time to the Massachusetts Supreme Judicial Court. Meanwhile, of course, three times a week, the incompetent and protesting Earle was heavily sedated and given his dialysis treatment. It was now eleven months since his son, his legally appointed guardian, had first requested stopping his father's dialysis.

Unlike the two lower courts, the Massachusetts Supreme Judicial Court acted swiftly. In January 1980 it ruled that the probate judge's original order issued in May, the order for the cessation of dialysis, was correct and that his subsequent ruling in July (directing the family and physician to make the decision), later affirmed by the appeals court, was not correct.

The Supreme Judicial Court said dialysis should be stopped but not because the family and physician believed it to be more of a burden than a benefit. Rather, the Court ruled, it should be stopped because Earle "would, if competent, choose not to receive the life-prolonging treatment." The basis for withdrawing the dialysis from a patient who willingly accepted it when he had decision-making capacity cannot be, in the eyes of the court, the family and physicians determining what is now in his best interests. Instead, a judge must determine, thanks to substituted judgment, that the patient changed his mind about dialysis after he lost his decision-making capacity and now would, if competent, choose to stop his dialysis.

At this point, after more than a year, the legal system was at last allowing the family's wishes about Earle's treatment to be followed, and the dialysis should have been stopped. But nurses at the nursing home where Earle was now a patient raised questions about his incompetence. They claimed he was competent and that he was indicating he wanted to live. They took their concerns to the press, and it became a headline story. A right-to-life group asked the court to let them enter the case to fight for Earle's life.

The guardian *ad litem* brought this to the attention of the court. It immediately ordered the dialysis continued while it arranged for a panel of five physicians to determine whether or not Earle was truly incompetent. These physicians examined Earle and reported that he was indeed entirely and irreversibly incompetent. Before the court acted on this report, Earle died on April 6, 1980, still receiving dialysis. The cause of death was listed as cardiopulmonary failure. The Spring family sued the nursing home and was awarded a financial settlement to compensate for the actions of the staff who made their loved one's case a public spectacle and thereby delayed the cessation of treatment they believed was not in Earle's best interests.

Ethical Analysis

Situational awareness.   We are aware of the following facts in the Spring story.

1. Earle was seventy-eight and suffering from irreversible renal failure. Dialysis could extend his life for months, perhaps years. While he had decision-making capacity, he had agreed to undergo dialysis, but a court later determined he was incompetent. There is no evidence about whether or not he would want dialysis continued in the circumstances he faced—increasing age, bothersome side effects, and organic brain syndrome, the source of his confusion. We simply cannot say on the evidence presented whether he would have wanted the dialysis continued until the day he died, or whether he would have wanted it stopped at some point in his mental and physical deterioration. His vigorous protests against the dialysis cannot be taken at face value because they are the protests of a man without decision-making capacity or legal competence. He was so confused he no longer recognized his wife or son. Nonetheless, his struggles did indicate that the treatments were causing him significant emotional stress.

2. His primary proxy was his son. Although Earle's wife believed, based on her knowledge of him gained in their marriage of fifty-five years, that he would not want to continue to live in his

condition of senility and dependence on dialysis, the son did not have any explicit evidence of what Earle would have wanted for himself in these circumstances. The basis of the son's decision to forgo further dialysis, then, was largely what he thought was in his father's best interests at that point in his father's life. He believed that dialysis was no longer appropriate for him and that he probably would not have wanted it. His mother agreed, as did the nephrologist.

3. None of the three courts thought the dialysis had to be continued. Only the guardian *ad litem* continued to argue for it. It was his legal actions—the appeals he made from the decisions of the lower courts, and then his reopening the question of Earle's competency after the Supreme Judicial Court decision—that kept Earle on dialysis for fifteen months after his family, with the approval of the courts, decided it should be stopped.

We are also aware of the following good and bad features in the story.

1. We would expect Earle's death relatively soon if dialysis were stopped. The loss of a human life is always bad.

2. Earle was suffering side effects from the dialysis and protested vigorously when efforts were made to place him on the dialysis machine. The treatment was thus a significant burden to him and offered no cure for his disease. In his state of confusion, it was impossible to explain to him how the treatments could help him, so the discomfort had no meaning to him.

3. The family was suffering distress because they could not have their senile husband and father treated the way they thought he should be treated and the way the courts agreed he could be treated.

4. Newspaper reports indicated that some providers in the nursing home were upset that the dialysis would be stopped, and their discomfort was a bad feature, albeit not a significant one if the withdrawal was morally reasonable. The guardian *ad litem* may also have been personally upset by the possibility of stopping the dialysis and thought he had to exhaust every legal option to keep Earle on the life-sustaining treatment.

Prudential Reasoning in the Story of Earle Spring

What is good in this situation and how can the persons involved best achieve it, or at least avoid the worse?

Patient's perspective. Earle had lost decision-making capacity. He had earlier decided dialysis was worth the burden, but we have no evidence indicating what he would have decided about the dialysis in the situation he eventually confronted, and we will never know. There is no patient perspective in moral reasoning when a patient has lost decision-making capacity and has left no indications about how he would want to be treated in the future.

Proxy's perspective. Earle's son was the legal guardian of his father; he was the primary moral agent. He had the difficult task of figuring out what was in the best interests of his father, a man suffering from incurable but controllable renal failure and organic brain syndrome, or senility. Dialysis was causing Earle distress, but it could keep him alive a little while longer. The son believed it was reasonable to stop dialysis at this point. His father had already experienced renal failure and could not receive a new kidney. His rational faculties had collapsed as well, so the burdens and benefits of the treatment could not be understood by him. His body and mind were irreversibly disintegrating. Given his strong reactions against the dialysis treatment and the uncomfortable burdens it imposed on him without any meaningful benefit to him, the son concluded it was reasonable to stop the treatments. It is hard to argue that his position is unreasonable.

Providers' perspectives. There is no indication in the Supreme Judicial Court findings that any physician involved in Earle's care had any problem with discontinuing the dialysis. Some of the staff in the nursing home where he spent the last months of his life, however, did disagree with the decision. They claimed that he might be competent and that he told them that he did not want to die. Every indication, however, indicated that he was truly incapable of making health care decisions and legally incompetent, so it is difficult to understand the reasonableness of their claim.

The courts' perspective.   All three courts allowed the dialysis to be discontinued. This seems a reasonable position. Heavily sedating a senile seventy-eight-year-old patient with no hope of either mental or renal recovery in order to provide the life-prolonging treatment is not a reasonable course of action when the treatments are so upsetting to the patient.

The guardian *ad litem's* perspective.   Perhaps his first appeal was reasonable, but his subsequent efforts, even after the Supreme Judicial Court decision, are not easy to judge reasonable. A guardian *ad litem* in a treatment case has no legal obligation to use every legal ploy possible to keep a patient alive. His primary responsibility is to investigate the facts in the case, to report them to the judge, and to recommend to the judge what treatments he thinks are best for the patient. In its decision, the court noted that a guardian *ad litem* is expected to present only reasonable arguments for treatment and has no duty to present arguments for treatment that are not meritorious or to seek endless appeals in cases.

Ethical Reflections

The decision to discontinue dialysis on an elderly patient with irreversible kidney disease when the treatment obviously causes him great distress is a reasonable one. The treatment is burdening him significantly but doing little more than prolonging life in a nursing home for a patient who has lost, because of senility, meaningful contact with reality and his loved ones. If he had quietly acquiesced to the treatment and was living in peace, the decision to stop dialysis at this time would not be so readily defensible, but it might still be reasonable at some point. It is not reasonable to attempt reversal of every renal failure any more than it is reasonable to attempt reversal of every respiratory or cardiac failure. In some cases it is in a patient's best interests to forgo life-sustaining treatments, especially if they are causing her significant burdens with little gain beyond the continuation of a severely compromised life.

A word needs to be said about the reasoning of the courts. The first probate decision and the final Supreme Judicial Court decision insist that judges should be the ones to order treatment stopped or continued once the case comes to court. On the other hand, the second probate decision, confirmed by the appeals court, said the family and the physicians should decide on the appropriate medical treatment. The second approach is more reasonable. Although the courts must protect the lives of vulnerable people who have not left advance directives, they are not in a good position to determine proper medical treatment for a person whom they do not know. When appropriate proxies are available, and when there is evidence that they are acting in good faith and with good reasons, the courts should allow the normal process of treatment decisions to unfold.

Since the Spring case, efforts have been made to acknowledge this approach in legislation by granting civil and criminal immunity to proxies making health care decisions in good faith on the basis of best interests for patients without advance directives. Such a law did not exist in the Spring case, but the Supreme Judicial Court could have followed the appeals court and allowed the family to make the decision, a decision the court agreed was acceptable. This would avoid the situation whereby courts are saying to families: "Your decision is correct, but we are the ones to make it."

We should also remember that the basis of the Supreme Judicial Court's reasoning is suspect. It acknowledged that "there was no evidence that while competent he had expressed any wish or desire as to the continuation or withdrawal of treatment in such circumstances." Yet it claimed to know what Earle would have wanted in such circumstances if he were competent. If the court found no evidence as to what Earle would have decided in such a situation, it is difficult to see how the court can say he would have decided on withdrawing dialysis. As we noted, the Massachusetts court takes this approach because, although it recognizes the right of a patient to decline treatment, it will not allow anyone but the patient to make the decision. If the patient is incompetent, then it falls to a judge to decide what he would have decided if he were competent, a rather difficult challenge whenever the court acknowledges there is no evidence about the patient's desires before he became incompetent.

Underlying this position is a fear about introducing judgments about the quality of life in such cases. In a previous Massachusetts case, known as *Superintendent of Belchertown State School v. Saikewicz* (1977), the first major treatment-decision case in the state, the Supreme Judicial Court had rejected the idea that the value of life can be equated with the quality of life. It said that a poor quality of life can never be a deciding factor in a proxy's decision to withdraw treatment from the patient. This means that the court will not allow a proxy to use the best interests standard for the withdrawal of life-sustaining treatment. All cases pertaining to the withdrawal of life-sustaining treatment, then, must be construed as instances of substituted judgment, and it makes no difference whether the wishes of the incompetent patient are known or whether the patient is a child who was never able to express any wishes about treatment.

In an ethics of right reason, however, judgments about the quality of life are inevitable. They are the only way we can say what is reasonable or unreasonable in the circumstances. As the quality of life irreversibly deteriorates, the reasons for burdensome life-sustaining treatments become less cogent. It is hardly reasonable, for example, to subject very elderly and frail patients without advance directives or decision-making capacity to respirators or dialysis to keep them alive as long as we can.

In the final analysis then, the decision to stop dialysis in this situation belonged with the family, and their decision was prudent. Given the best interests of the patient, the decision to withhold the life-sustaining treatment was more reasonable than the decision to continue it in the very difficult circumstances.

SURGERY

Sometimes surgical interventions are associated more with life-sustaining efforts than with correcting medical problems. The surgeries to insert gastrostomy or tracheostomy tubes are cases in point. And the amputations necessary to prolong the life of diabetic patients are another example of life-sustaining surgery. We cannot really say that the amputation of a limb cures the gangrene affecting it, nor can we say that the amputation contributes to a cure of the disease causing the death of the tissue.

Sometimes patients do not think the life-sustaining surgery is a reasonable intervention in the circumstances, and they decline it. The following case illustrates how this can happen and shows how difficult it can be for families.

The Case of Rosaria Candura

The Story

Seventy-seven-year-old Rosaria came to this country from Italy in 1918. She married, raised a family, and was living in her own home when the case began in late 1977. She had been depressed and unhappy since her husband's death in 1976 and suffered from diabetes. Her relationship with her children (a daughter and three sons) was marked by a degree of conflict, and she really did not want to live with any of them.

Struggling against gangrene in her extremities, she had consented to the amputation of a toe in 1974 and to a part of her foot in November 1977. In April 1978 gangrene was found in the remainder of her foot, and she consented to the amputation of her leg.

On the morning of the surgery she changed her mind, and the operation was canceled. She was discharged to her daughter's home. Around May 9 after encouragement from a physician she had known for years, she again consented to the amputation but then reversed her decision a second time.

It was clear from her testimony and from the testimony of others that she was confused on some matters. Her train of thought sometimes wandered, and her conception of time was distorted. She was sometimes hostile with certain physicians and combative when questioned about the possibility of surgery. She expressed a desire to get well but, discouraged by the failure of the earlier amputations to stem the gangrene, was afraid the amputation of her leg would not be successful in controlling the problem. Her opposition to the surgery soon became definitive. She became quite clear on this point and gave every indication that she understood the consequences of declining the amputation.

Her daughter, Grace Lane, was understandably upset over her mother's refusal of the life-sustaining surgery. Grace asked the probate court to appoint her the guardian for her mother with the authority to give consent for the surgery. The court approved her request, but the guardian *ad litem* appealed the ruling. He felt it had not been proven that Rosaria was incompetent and therefore argued that she, and not a guardian, should make the decision about her own surgery.

Before looking at the outcome of his appeal to a higher court, we consider the case from an ethical perspective.

Ethical Analysis

Situational awareness.   We are aware of the following facts in the Candura story.

1. Rosaria suffered from diabetes and life-threatening gangrene. Only the amputation of her leg could save her life. Two previous amputations had failed to stem the spread of gangrene in her leg.

2. She was confused about some things and was somewhat unhappy and depressed. She had vacillated about the amputation, twice agreeing to it and twice changing her mind. In the final analysis, however, she seemed clearly opposed to it.

3. Grace believed that her mother should have the life-prolonging surgery and sought guardianship so that she could give consent to what she, the physicians, and most everyone else believed was appropriate medical treatment.

4. The judge in probate court agreed with Grace, and appointed her guardian of her mother so she could give consent for the surgery.

We are also aware of the following good and bad features in the case.

1. Rosaria's death, which could probably be delayed by the surgery, would be unfortunate.

2. The amputation of her leg would cause pain, suffering, and a difficult sense of loss. It would also undermine the ability of this strong-willed seventy-seven-year-old woman to live in her own home.

3. Her daughter was naturally distressed and upset that her mother was declining life-prolonging treatment. At least one physician was also upset and had tried to have Rosaria change her mind.

Prudential Reasoning in the Candura Case

Patient's perspective.   Rosaria was in the best position to determine whether, all things considered, the amputation of her leg was reasonable. She would be experiencing the pain resulting from the surgery, and she would have to live with the loss of her leg. There was no indication that she wanted to die; in fact, she told the judge she would like to get better. But she did not want the life-prolonging surgery. In her mind the burdens of another amputation and its consequences in her life outweighed the benefits of life without her leg. For the past few years she had felt great loss over the death of her husband and the amputation of her foot. Well aware that the two earlier amputations were not enough to prevent the life-threatening problems associated with gangrene, she simply did not see the sense of undergoing another great loss, her leg.

It would be hard to argue that her decision was unreasonable. Of course, another person in her position might think the surgery would be reasonable, and it would also be hard to argue with his decision. Often in ethics, especially when we are coping with difficult choices when both courses of action are burdensome, one can defend the reasonableness of both. In other words Rosaria's decision to decline the surgery is morally justified because the burdens she would experience outweighed the benefits, but another person's decision to have the surgery could also be morally justified if he would experience more benefit than burden from the amputation.

The only remaining moral question, then, is whether or not she has the capacity to make such a decision. Evidence indicated she was sometimes confused about some things, but there was no indication that she had lost the capacity to make the decision about amputation. In fact, the evidence indicated the contrary. When her physician sought informed consent for the surgery, he did not hesitate to obtain it from her, something he never would have done if he thought she had lost decision-making capacity or was incompetent.

Daughter's perspective. Rosaria's daughter was naturally upset that her mother was declining the surgery. She thought Rosaria should have the amputation that was expected to prolong her life. So she decided to ask the probate court to appoint her the guardian for her mother so she could authorize the surgery. If she was convinced that her mother had lost the capacity to make decisions, her efforts to be appointed guardian and make the decision for her were appropriate since children are usually the proper proxies for their parents.

The physician apparently refused to accept the daughter's consent for the surgery, so she took the matter to probate court. Here the judge agreed with her by concluding that Rosaria was "incapable of making a rational and competent choice to undergo or reject the proposed surgery to her right leg." The judge's finding reminds us that the daughter's belief that her mother had lost her capacity to decide about the surgery had some merit. Thus, her move to be appointed guardian was a reasonable one from a moral point of view.

The Court Decision

The appeals court did not agree that Rosaria was incompetent. It noted that a person is presumed competent unless and until it is established by evidence that he or she is not competent. And the burden is on the person petitioning for guardianship to prove the person is incompetent. The court acknowledged that Rosaria was confused on some matters but not on the issue of the surgery, where she "exhibited a high degree of awareness and acuity." The court also acknowledged that her decision may well have been irrational from a medical perspective, but the irrationality of a decision does not prove a person is legally incompetent. As we all know, competent people make irrational decisions every day.

The court also pointedly remarked that nobody had questioned Rosaria's competence the two times she had consented to the surgery. And it noted that surgeons were still prepared to amputate if she gave consent, an indication that they still considered her capable of giving informed consent for the surgery, despite the ruling of the probate judge.

Because the court did not find Rosaria incompetent, it dismissed her daughter's petition that she be appointed guardian. It acknowledged that Rosaria's decision may be regarded as unfortunate but insisted that she could not be forced to have the surgery. The law protected Rosaria's right to accept or reject treatment, whether or not the decision was a wise one.

Ethical Reflection

If Grace really thought her mother had lost decision-making capacity, and we have no reason to believe she did not, then her efforts to be named proxy were reasonable. If a parent cannot make decisions for herself, then it is laudable for the children to try to make the right decisions for her.

We must remember, however, that a proxy first tries to make a decision based on what she thinks the patient wants—the substituted judgment standard. If Grace thought her mother had lost decision-making capacity and that she had to function as her proxy, her first efforts should have been to report what her mother's wishes were. Only if she had no way of knowing what this might have been could she have proceeded to make decisions for her mother based on what she thought was in Rosaria's best interests.

As we might expect, the appeals court based its decision on the constitutional right to privacy that allows a person to decline life-sustaining treatment in most cases. The law allows people to accept or reject treatment regardless of whether the decision is wise or unwise. This is not enough for good ethics, however, because the ethicist will not consider a decision acceptable unless it is reasonable. But in this case, as we noted above, there are good grounds for thinking Rosaria's decision was a reasonable one for a person in her circumstances.

OTHER LIFE-SUSTAINING TREATMENTS

The ethical reasoning about accepting or rejecting other life-sustaining treatments is the same as we employ for ventilators, dialysis, and surgery. The moral agents involved, primarily the patient or proxy, and the physicians, will try to figure out what will achieve the balance of good over bad or at least what option is less worse.

This is true even if the life-sustaining treatment is simple and routine. Consider respiratory therapy, for example. In a situation where a person receiving respiratory therapy is found to have rapidly developing terminal cancer, a decision to withhold further respiratory therapy may be reasonable. Many patients would see no sense in prolonging life with this therapy when all it does is set up a situation in which they will suffer for a few more days or weeks as they die from the incurable cancer. In the last analysis, the ethics of all life-sustaining treatments revolves around what is reasonable or unreasonable, given the circumstances and the consequences of the treatment. The good and bad features—the benefits and burdens of what we deliberately do—have to be considered so we can determine as best we can what is reasonable under the circumstances.

Things get a little more complicated for some other forms of life-sustaining treatment. For example more and more people have implanted pacemakers or defibrillators, and some people have an implanted left ventricular assist device that helps their heart continue beating. In some situations their lives, despite the implanted devices, may have deteriorated terribly, perhaps because of other illnesses such as cancer, renal disease, or respiratory disease. And so the question arises: Is it reasonable at some point for a patient or proxy to have the implanted device shut off when, without it, fatal cardiac irregularities will develop? There is an ethical debate whether disabling these implanted devices is analogous to withdrawing a ventilator or whether it is a new kind of treatment-withdrawal case. Some have argued that disabling these implanted devices is not analogous to withdrawing external forms of life-sustaining treatment (ventilators, dialysis, even feeding tubes), whereas others have argued that they should be thought of the same way. The prudential reasoning of virtue ethics would suggest that moral agents act well by simply trying to figure out what is reasonable given the situation. If a person with a defibrillator is dying of cancer, it makes sense to honor a request to shut it off; otherwise, it will just keep reversing the fibrillation and cardiac arrest that occurs in natural death.

Unfortunately, most situations where life-prolonging treatments are an issue are tragic situations—no behavior really leads to a significant degree of well-being or happiness. People suffering from serious medical problems and permanently dependent on life-sustaining treatments have no attractive options. Prolonging a declining or sick life with these treatments or surgeries does not really result in a good life, and forgoing the life-prolonging treatment soon leads to no life at all. The only moral challenge of people trapped in these tragic situations is to determine whether accepting life-prolonging treatments is less worse than declining them. This is a highly subjective prudential determination and should be respected by others involved in their care.

SUGGESTED READINGS

For a succinct introduction to what ventilation entails, see Martin Tobin, "Mechanical Ventilation," *New England Journal of Medicine* 1994, *330*, 1056–61. The New Jersey Supreme Court decision in the Quinlan case is *In re Quinlan*, 355 A2d 647 (1976). Lengthy excerpts from the decision appear in many places, among them Tom Beauchamp and LeRoy Walters, 1982, *Contemporary Issues in Bioethics*, 2nd ed., Belmont, CA: Wadsworth Publishing, pp. 365–72 (later editions omit the excerpts); and Ronald Munson, 2008, *Intervention and Reflection*, 8th ed., Belmont, CA: Wadsworth Publishing, pp. 733–35. Eight years after Karen died, her family authorized publication of the neurological findings contained in the postmortem report. Perhaps the most interesting fact was that the most severe damage was not, as expected, in the cerebral cortex but in the thalamus, suggesting the critical role this area of the brain plays in awareness. See Hannah Kinney et al., "Neuropathological Findings in the Brain of Karen Quinlan," *New England Journal of Medicine* 1994, *330*, 1469–75.

There are many commentaries on the Quinlan case. See Joseph Quinlan and Julia Quinlan, with Phyllis Battelle, 1977, *Karen Ann: The Quinlans Tell Their Story*, New York: Doubleday Anchor; and Julia Quinlan, 2005, *My Joy, My Sorrow: Karen Ann's Mother Remembers*, Cincinnati: St. Anthony Messenger Press. See also Gregory Pence, 2004, *Classic Cases in Medical Ethics*, 4th ed., New York: McGraw-Hill, chapter 2, pp. 29–39; Richard McCormick, 1981, *How Brave a New World: Dilemmas in Bioethics*, Washington, DC: Georgetown University Press, chapter 19; and Robert M. Veatch, *Death, Dying and the Biological Revolution*, New Haven: Yale University Press, pp. 118–23.

See *In re Eichner* (*In re Storar*), 52 N.Y. 2d. 363 (1981) for the New York Court of Appeals decision in the *Brother Fox* case. Because Brother Fox was unconscious, the case was brought to court by his religious superior, Father Eichner. The name Storar refers to a second case involving treatment which the court resolved in the same decision. See also George J. Annas, "Help from the Dead: The Cases of Brother Fox and John Storar," *Hastings Center Report* 1981, *11* (June), 19–20; Richard McCormick and Robert Veatch, "The Preservation of Life and Self-Determination," *Theological Studies* 1980, *41*, 390–96; Paul Ramsey, "The Two Step Fantastic: The Continuing Case of Brother Fox," *Theological Studies* 1981, *42*, 122–34; and John Paris, "Court Interventions and the Diminution of Patients' Rights: The Case of Brother Joseph Fox," *New England Journal of Medicine* 1980, *303*, 876–78.

For the Bartling case, see *Bartling v. Superior Court*, 163 Cal. App. 3d 186 (1984), and *Bartling v. Glendale Adventist Medical Center*, 184 Cal. App. 3d 97 (1986) and 184 Cal App. 3rd 961 (1987) for the decisions. For background to the early court battle, see George Annas, "Prisoner in the ICU: The Tragedy of William Bartling," *Hastings Center Report* 1984, *14* (December), 28–29. The citation for the Perlmutter case is *Satz v. Perlmutter*, 379 So. 2d 359 (1980).

The court proceeding relevant to Helga Wanglie is *In re: The Conservatorship of Helga M. Wanglie*, No. PX-91-283 (Probate Court Division, 4th Judicial District, Hennepin County, Minnesota). A physician-ethicist who was involved in the case has written several articles on the family's demand for continued respirator support; see Steven Miles, "The Informed Demand for 'Non-Beneficial' Medical Treatment," *New England Journal of Medicine* 1991, *325*, 512–15; and "Legal Procedures in Wanglie: A Two-Step, Not a Sidestep," *Journal of Clinical Ethics* 1991, *2*, 285–86. See also two articles by Marcia Angell, "The Case of Helga Wanglie," *New England Journal of Medicine* 1991, *325*, 511–12; and "After Quinlan: The Dilemma of the Persistent Vegetative State," *New England Journal of Medicine* 1994, *330*, 1524–25.

The case of Barbara Howe is *In the Matter of Howe*, No.03 P 1255, 2004 (Mass. Prob. & Fam. Ct. Mar. 22, 2004). For an excellent overview of the legal history of major cases where family wanted life-sustaining treatment that providers wanted to stop, including the Howe and Wanglie cases, see Patrick Moore, "An End-of-Life Quandary in Need of a Statutory Response: When Patients Demand Life-Sustaining Treatment That Physicians Are Unwilling to Provide," *Boston College Law Review* 2007, *48*, 433–69. For a media account of the Barbara Hall conflict, see stories by Liz Kowalczyk in the *Boston Globe* for September 28, 2003, February 23, 2005, March 11, 2005, and March 12, 2005.

For the Massachusetts Supreme Judicial Court decision involving dialysis for Earle Spring, see *In the Matter of Earle Spring*, 405 N.E.2d 115 (1980). The citation for the Saikewicz case is *Superintendent of Belchertown v. Saikewicz*, 370 N.E.2d 417 (1977). A helpful commentary is George Annas, "Quality of Life in the Courts: Earle Spring in Fantasyland," *Hastings Center Report* 1980, *10* (August), 9–10. For a study of withdrawing dialysis, see Steven Neu and Carl Kjellstrand, "Stopping Long-Term Dialysis: An Empirical Study of Withdrawal of Life-Supporting Treatment," *New England Journal of Medicine*

1986, *314*, 14–20. The Massachusetts Appeals Court decision involving Rosaria Candura's refusal of surgery is *Lane v. Candura*, 376 N.E.2d 1232 (1978).

The literature about providing, withholding, and withdrawing life-sustaining treatment is, as can be imagined, very extensive. Among the helpful basic resources are: *Deciding to Forego* [sic] *Life-Sustaining Treatment*, President's Commission for the Study of Ethical Problems in Medicine and Biomedical and Behavioral Research, originally published by the U.S. Government Printing Office (1981) but now available from Indiana University Press. *Guidelines on the Termination of Life-Sustaining Treatment and the Care of the Dying*, a 1987 report of the Hastings Center, is also helpful. A more recent basic resource is the 2005 PCB report *Taking Care: Ethical Caregiving in Our Aging Society*, especially chapter 4, "Principles and Prudence in Hard Cases," available online at bioethics.gov. The NIH has an excellent site with many links on end-of-life and palliative care at bioethics.od.nih.gov/endoflife.

For an interesting overview of forgoing life-prolonging treatments by members of the Medical Ethics Department of the British Medical Association, see Veronica English, ed., 2007, *Withholding and Withdrawing Life-Prolonging Medical Treatment*, 3rd ed., Boston: Blackwell Publishing. An early article of historical interest is Charles Fried, "Terminating Life Support: Out of the Closet," *New England Journal of Medicine* 1976, *295*, 390–91. See also the historical development in two important articles by a group of physicians: Sidney Wanzer et al., "The Physician's Responsibility toward Hopelessly Ill Patients," *New England Journal of Medicine* 1984, *310*, 955–59; and Sidney Wanzer et al., "The Physician's Responsibility toward Hopelessly Ill Patients: A Second Look," *New England Journal of Medicine* 1989, *320*, 844–49. For an excellent study of shared decision making in the withdrawal of life-sustaining treatment (ventilation, dialysis, and vasopressors) from twenty-eight patients in an intensive care unit, see David Lee et al., "Withdrawing Care: Experience in a Medical Intensive Care Unit," *JAMA* 1994, *271*, 1358–61. See also Howard Brody et al., "Withdrawing Intensive Life-Sustaining Treatment— Recommendations for Compassionate Clinical Management," *New England Journal of Medicine* 1997, *336*, 652–57.

The perplexity and distress engendered by trying to determine when it is morally good for patients, physicians, nurses, and families to employ or forgo life-sustaining treatments, as well as the growing debate over euthanasia and physician-assisted suicide, have prompted a renewed interest in palliative care at the end of life. Recent efforts include the Robert Wood Johnson Foundation's *Last Acts* project, the AMA's *Education for Physicians on End-of-Life Care*, and the Institute of Medicine's 1997 report, *Approaching Death: Improving Care at the End of Life*. Washington, DC: National Academy Press.

The role of the courts in cases involving life-sustaining treatments has been both extensive and important. Although it is now somewhat dated, an article by a judge of the Massachusetts Appeals Court provides a good analysis of the trend in court decisions through 1986: Christopher Armstrong, 1987, "Judicial Involvement in Treatment Decisions: The Emerging Consensus," in *Critical Care*, Joseph Civetta, Robert Taylor, and Robert Kirby, eds., Philadelphia: J. B. Lippincott, pp. 1649–55. More current are Alan Meisel, "Legal Myths about Terminating Life Support," *Archives of Internal Medicine* 1991, *151*, 1497–1502, and "The Legal Consensus about Forgoing Life-Sustaining Treatment: Its Status and Prospects," *Kennedy Institute of Ethics Journal* 1992, *2*, 309–45; and Robert Veatch, "Forgoing Life-Sustaining Treatment: Limits to the Consensus," *Kennedy Institute of Ethics Journal* 1993, *3*, 1–19.

In 1992 the National Center for State Courts in Williamsburg, VA, produced its "Guidelines of State Court Decision Making in Authorizing or Withholding Life Sustaining Medical Treatment." These guidelines will undoubtedly be widely consulted by judges and attorneys involved in future cases. The New York State Task Force on Life and the Law has published 1987, *Life-Sustaining Treatment: Making Decisions and Appointing a Health Care Agent*, Albany: Health Education Services.

EIGHT

Cardiopulmonary Resuscitation

IN THIS CHAPTER we consider the ethical aspects of attempting cardiopulmonary resuscitation (CPR) in hospitals and nursing homes. We know that over three-quarters of the roughly two million people who die in the United States every year die in hospitals or chronic care facilities. Every person who dies suffers cardiopulmonary arrest, so we know that about 1.5 million potential CPRs can be attempted every year in our health care facilities.

Attempted resuscitation in a health care facility is an emergency procedure involving a high level of activity by a team of physicians, nurses, and technicians. One or two nurses insert IV lines and administer strong drugs, sometimes directly into the heart. Another nurse does chest compressions that may result in injuries, especially in the elderly. A respiratory therapist or anesthesiologist intubates the patient, and a physician applies electric shocks to stop the fibrillation, the useless fluttering of the heart, that often occurs. Despite the latest equipment and a high level of expertise, the effort often fails to revive the patient or, if it does revive the patient, leaves him with extensive brain damage caused by lack of adequate blood circulation in the brain.

Clearly there are reasons why some cardiopulmonary arrests in hospitals and other facilities should not trigger these resuscitation efforts. The dying person may be a hospice patient, for example, and not want resuscitation. Or the patient may be so sick and frail that the shock treatments and chest compressions of CPR would be unreasonable—the harm they would inflict would outweigh the slim chance of limited benefit they might offer.

After a brief consideration of terminology relevant to CPR, this chapter considers the history of resuscitation efforts, the effectiveness of these efforts, the move to withhold these efforts in some cases, the development of institutional policies for not attempting resuscitation, a typical hospital policy for withholding resuscitation efforts, and a look at some lingering ethical questions about attempting resuscitation. The chapter concludes with an analysis of several key cases involving CPR.

TERMINOLOGY

Strictly speaking, there is a difference between cardiac arrest and respiratory arrest. For our purposes, however, we can ignore the difference. The cardiac and pulmonary functions are closely linked. Loss of blood flow soon causes damage to the respiratory centers of the spinal cord and brain, so the person stops breathing. Conversely, lack of oxygen causes damage to the cardiovascular centers of the spinal cord and brain, so the heart stops beating. In other words a cardiac arrest leads very quickly to respiratory arrest, and respiratory arrest leads very quickly to cardiac arrest. Since cardiac and pulmonary arrests are so closely related, we will consider them as one and the same event and speak of *cardiopulmonary arrest*. We will also refer to the attempts aimed at reversing these arrests as a single action—*cardiopulmonary resuscitation*, often known simply as CPR.

Unfortunately, the terms cardiopulmonary resuscitation and CPR are misleading. Resuscitation means revival, yet the cardiopulmonary resuscitation often fails to revive the patient. Despite the efforts at CPR, the heart and lungs do not restart, and the person dies. We should really understand the treatments designed to reverse a cardiopulmonary arrest not as "cardiopulmonary resuscitation" but as "attempting cardiopulmonary resuscitation." And the physicians and nurses working at the scene of an arrest are not "doing CPR"; they are "attempting CPR."

This distinction may seem insignificant, but it is important in ethical considerations. Suppose for example you are making decisions for an elderly and sick parent, and a physician asks whether you want your mother to be resuscitated if her heart stops. The natural response to this question will almost always be affirmative; of course you want your mother to be revived. But if the physician asks whether you want nurses and physicians to attempt resuscitation if her heart stops, and if he explains what these attempts involve, and how often they fail to prevent death or, if they do prevent death, leave the patient with a damaged brain and body, you might not be so quick to give an affirmative answer.

It is well then to remember that CPR does not really mean cardiopulmonary resuscitation, but the *attempt* at cardiopulmonary resuscitation. And we should think of physicians' orders not to intervene in the event of a cardiopulmonary arrest not as "do not resuscitate" orders but as "do not *attempt* resuscitation" orders, and the abbreviation DNR (do not resuscitate) should really be DNAR (do not attempt resuscitation). This is important because study after study shows that CPR efforts in hospitals usually fail to restore heart and lung function or, if they do restore it, leave the patient in worse condition than before the arrest.

A BRIEF HISTORY OF RESUSCITATION ATTEMPTS

Attempts to resuscitate people have a long history in medicine. That history reached a turning point in the middle of the last century with advances in anesthesia and surgery. Chloroform, administered to mask the pain of surgery, sometimes caused cardiopulmonary arrests. Physicians naturally sought ways to reverse these arrests, but it was not until the middle of the twentieth century that effective treatments were developed. By the 1940s it was learned that a combination of drugs, electric stimuli, and heart massage could sometimes restart stopped hearts. At first the heart massage was internal—as a last-ditch effort surgeons opened up the chest so they could actually get their hands on the heart—but it soon became clear that the heart could be massaged effectively by external chest compressions.

Attempts at resuscitation became more frequent, first in hospital operating and recovery rooms, then in emergency rooms and intensive care units, especially cardiac care units, and finally throughout the institution. Hospitals trained special teams and positioned the equipment they would need in the event of an arrest. Since there is no chance to reverse a cardiopulmonary arrest after the first few minutes—recent figures indicate the chance of success drops significantly after six minutes—the resuscitation team must respond immediately.

Before the widespread use of electronic beepers, the fastest way to assemble the members of the resuscitation team was by announcement throughout the hospital over the loudspeaker system. Since it would be inappropriate to announce something like "Heart attack in room 329," the notification was usually given in a coded form. Some hospitals, for example, used the expression "Code Blue—room 329" to alert the code team without upsetting other patients and visitors. In time, attempting resuscitation became known as "coding" someone or "calling a code," and physicians' instructions not to attempt resuscitation were often called "no code" orders.

Gradually attempts at resuscitation spread to other areas of health care. Emergency medical technicians and paramedics were trained and provided with equipment that could be brought to the scene of an arrest. Nursing homes also trained their staffs in the procedure and provided the equipment needed to attempt resuscitation. Police officers and firefighters were also trained, and a vast public education campaign was mounted so anybody could begin emergency CPR by blowing in a person's mouth and by rhythmically pushing down on the chest to massage the heart. What began as an intervention by physicians in an operating room soon became a widespread emergency treatment.

THE EFFECTIVENESS OF ATTEMPTING CPR

Just how successful are the attempts at CPR in hospitals? The answer varies of course and depends on many factors. But a brief glance at several studies will give a general idea.

A 1983 report from the Beth Israel Hospital in Boston, a teaching hospital, traced 294 attempts at resuscitation and found that 166 patients died during the attempted CPR, 31 died within twenty-four hours, and another 56 died later in the hospital. Only 41 of the coded patients (14 percent) of those coded lived to discharge.

A 1988 study at the Houston Veterans Administration Medical Center traced 399 attempts at resuscitation and found that 238 patients died during the attempted CPR, 15 died within twenty-four hours, and another 124 died later in the hospital. Only 22 of the coded patients (6 percent) lived to discharge.

A 1991 study conducted at Rhode Island Hospital, a teaching hospital in Providence, found that of 185 patients brought to the Emergency Department in cardiac arrest with emergency personnel performing CPR, only 16 survived long enough for admission to the hospital. None of these patients improved sufficiently for discharge; they all died in the hospital. Fifteen of them never regained consciousness. The average time before death in the hospital for these sixteen patients was about 12 days, although one patient remained alive for 132 days. Authors of the study questioned whether it was good medicine for emergency department personnel to attempt CPR when the arrest happened outside the hospital.

A 1988 study of forty-nine very-low-birth-weight babies suffering cardiopulmonary arrest revealed that only four survived, and three of these suffered from neurologic deficits.

On average, attempts at CPR are successful about one-third of the time in hospitals, and fewer than one-third of the resuscitated patients live to be discharged. It must be remembered, of course, that many of these patients were in the hospital because they were very ill, and some of them would never have recovered sufficiently for discharge even if they had not suffered the arrest that led to the successful CPR.

The figures help us place resuscitation efforts in perspective. Since the emergency treatment often brings a burden to the patient and frequently fails, we have to ask when it is reasonable to initiate CPR in a clinical setting. And patients have to consider whether it makes sense for them to be subjected to it. For a patient to figure this out, of course, he needs some idea about how often attempted CPR brings little or no benefit.

An interesting study conducted at the Presbyterian–St. Luke's Medical Center in Denver in the early 1990s revealed the following. When patients over sixty were asked whether they wanted CPR attempted if they arrested, 41 percent said they did. But when they were informed of the probability of survival until discharge (somewhere between 10 and 17 percent), the number dropped to 22 percent. When the same patients were asked whether they wanted CPR attempted if they had a life expectancy of less than one year, 11 percent said they did. But when they were informed of the probability of survival until discharge (somewhere between 0 and 5 percent), the number dropped to 5 percent, fewer than one out of twenty.

This reminds us how unreasonable it is to attempt reversal of every cardiopulmonary arrest. In other words in many cases the reasonable ethical response action to a cardiopulmonary arrest is to make no effort to save the patient's life. Emotionally this is not easy. When physicians and nurses see an arrest and have the training and equipment designed to reverse it, it is not easy to do nothing when they know the probable outcome is death. On the other hand, attempting CPR in some cases strikes almost everyone as ridiculous. It makes no sense, for example, to work at reviving a dying cancer patient every time she arrests. Several decades ago it became clear that we would have to learn how to withhold efforts to revive some people experiencing a cardiopulmonary arrest.

LEARNING TO WITHHOLD CPR

As could be expected, once people learned how to attempt CPR, they tended to do it whenever a patient suffered an arrest. They soon realized, however, that this presumption of intervention was frequently a mistake because the treatment failed, left the patient alive but with neurological damage, or succeeded only in prolonging the life of a dying patient for a limited time. This left physicians and nurses in a difficult dilemma. If they attempted to revive every patient, they would often be providing inappropriate medical treatment; if they did not attempt to revive a patient, they might be letting someone die who could have benefited from being saved, and they could be subject to accusations from the family about medical negligence.

In 1974 a National Conference on Standards for Cardiopulmonary Resuscitation and Emergency Cardiac Care acknowledged both the value of attempting CPR in some cases and of withholding it in others, especially when it was a case "of terminal, irreversible illness where death is not unexpected." In such cases the conference recommended writing the DNR order in the patient's progress notes so all providers would be aware that CPR should not be attempted if an arrest occurred.

Despite these recommendations some providers felt morally obliged to continue making every effort to save life whenever a patient arrested. Others did acknowledge that attempting CPR was inappropriate in some situations but found it difficult to acknowledge that treatment was being withheld from patients suffering respiratory or cardiac failure. It became clear that some guidelines were needed.

In 1976 two Boston hospitals instituted written policies—known as DNR policies—guiding the withholding of efforts to revive patients suffering an arrest. The policy of Massachusetts General Hospital centered on the physician—it allowed physicians to decide when attempting CPR was not medically appropriate and then to write the DNR order in the medical record. The policy of Beth Israel Hospital, on the other hand, centered on the patient—it allowed patients to refuse CPR efforts, in advance, regardless of their medical condition, and it required physicians to have the consent of the patient or proxy before writing a DNR order.

The need for sound moral thinking and dialogue about attempting CPR as well as the need for good hospital policies became more apparent after a well-publicized New York grand jury investigation in 1984. The grand jury investigating the death of an elderly patient in the intensive care unit at La Guardia Hospital found that hospital administrators and representatives of the medical staff had decided, in an effort to minimize legal exposure, that patients and families would not be consulted about DNR orders and that the orders would not be written in the patients' medical records. Instead, the DNR orders would be signified by small purple dots affixed to file cards kept by the nurses. As a result no DNR order could be traced to any physician. The only record of it, the file card with the purple dot, was discarded when the patient was discharged or died.

The case investigated by the grand jury is summarized later in the chapter as "The Story of Maria M." It illustrates how the failure to face ethical dilemmas openly can create serious clinical and ethical abuses in patient care and in the relationships between physicians and nurses.

On February 8, 1984, the New York grand jury made a number of important recommendations regarding the withholding of attempted CPR. They included the following: (1) The decision not to resuscitate should be made jointly by the physician and the patient or by the physician and the patient's proxy; (2) the order should be a permanent part of the medical record; and (3) the physician, or the patient, or the proxy can revoke the order at any time.

The need for policies embodying these recommendations was underscored within weeks of the grand jury report. On March 25, 1984, eighty-seven-year-old Rose Dreyer died at New York Hospital after suffering an arrest. She had been admitted ten days earlier for pneumonia and, without consulting her or her family, the staff had determined that CPR would not be appropriate. The staff followed its custom of deciding unilaterally which patients would not be resuscitated. Their names were then circled in red on cards that were discarded after discharge or death. When Mrs. Dreyer arrested, no one attempted CPR.

The New York State Health Department brought administrative charges against the hospital, which admitted it had violated the woman's rights by withholding CPR without her or her proxy's consent. The charges were dropped when the hospital accepted a fine and agreed to develop written guidelines for withholding CPR, guidelines that included informed consent by patients or their proxies, and the entry of all DNR orders by the physicians in the permanent medical records of patients.

Today most hospitals and long-term care facilities have written DNR or "no code" policies in place. These policies are for the most part morally sound and very helpful. By considering the elements in a good DNR policy and an example of what a DNR policy looks like, we can learn much about the ethics of attempting and withholding efforts to revive people in cardiopulmonary arrest.

IMPORTANT ETHICAL ELEMENTS FOR A DNR POLICY

A morally sound DNR policy will include the following provisions.

1. Physicians have the responsibility of initiating discussion about CPR with the patient or proxy if there is some reason to think a cardiopulmonary arrest may occur. Examples of reasons for thinking an arrest might occur are: a previous arrest, known respiratory or heart problems, terminal illness, irreversible loss of consciousness, and so forth.

Attempting CPR is a medical treatment, and patients or proxies should be involved in choices about medical treatment. Many patients and proxies will not know that they can decline resuscitation efforts unless their physicians tell them. And they have to be told in advance because there is no time for discussion when an arrest occurs. If an arrest occurs when there is no DNR order, the providers will usually consider it an emergency and treat to save life. Physicians should therefore initiate discussions about treatment in the event of an arrest in order to avoid having CPR attempted when it is not wanted or when it is not medically appropriate. Unfortunately many physicians still delay or decline to initiate these difficult discussions, and this sets the stage for a situation where a patient who would not have wanted CPR is nonetheless coded. The importance of stressing that physicians should take the initiative in discussing DNR orders with their patients is underlined by several studies showing that only 20 percent of hospitalized patients with DNR orders discussed their wishes about resuscitation efforts with their physicians.

2. Patients (or their proxies) normally have the final word on accepting or rejecting CPR efforts. Attending physicians, however, will assist the patient or proxy in thinking through the risks and benefits of attempted CPR and in reaching an informed decision.

There is a strong legal and moral tradition against forcing unwanted treatment on people, and this gives the patient or proxy the last word on accepting or rejecting CPR attempts. The ideal, however, is to have the decision-making process shared by both patient or proxy and the physician. The participation of nurses in the decision-making process is often helpful as well.

3. If resuscitation efforts will be withheld, the physician will write the DNR order in the medical record.

Recording the DNR order in the medical record provides a permanent record of the order, the process leading to the decision, the reasons for it, and the person responsible for it. This eliminates the chances for the kinds of confusion and abuse that have surrounded some DNR decisions in the past.

4. The patient or proxy may cancel the DNR order at any time. The cancellation becomes effective as soon as the patient or proxy tells the physician or nurse of his decision to cancel the DNR order.

This provision allows the patient the opportunity to reconsider his or her refusal of treatment and to have any change of mind respected. It is important to note that the patient (or proxy) can cancel the order by simply telling a nurse of his desire to cancel it. The DNR order does not remain in effect while the nurse notifies the physician; it is cancelled as soon as the patient or proxy cancels it. The immediate cancellation of a DNR order at the request of the patient or proxy is morally necessary lest a code team be placed in the unethical position of refusing to provide wanted treatment for a patient. Of course the patient's physician should be notified of the cancellation as soon as practicable.

5. The physician will automatically review the DNR order at frequent intervals, perhaps as often as every twenty-four hours.

Regular review of the DNR order is necessary to prevent the continuation of the order after the circumstances prompting it have ceased to exist. A patient on DNR status may improve to the point that attempting CPR would be a reasonable intervention in the event of an arrest. If the order has not been reviewed and, where appropriate, canceled, the improving patient will not be given CPR and could be deprived of beneficial treatment.

6. If CPR is initiated, the attempted resuscitation will be genuine; that is, providers will do everything they can to revive the patient. In exceptional cases fully informed patients may have indicated a desire for limitations on the efforts to revive them. Perhaps they want some efforts at CPR but also want to exclude certain aspects normally associated with the procedure—intubation or defibrillation, for example. Their desires should be respected. In most cases, however, these prior limitations will not exist, and the resuscitation team will do everything it can to resuscitate the patient.

When patients without a DNR order suffer a cardiopulmonary arrest, providers almost inevitably attempt to save their lives. Sometimes, however, the resuscitation efforts are obviously inappropriate, and the providers feel terrible about performing CPR. In the past this dilemma was sometimes solved by what were called "show codes" (much activity but little that was effective) or "slow codes" (making the right moves so slowly that death would occur before any great harm from resuscitation efforts was done to the patient). These are not good solutions. Both slow codes and show codes are deceptive, and they compromise the ethical integrity of health care providers. Good ethics requires us to establish the DNR status of a patient likely to suffer an arrest as soon as possible. If this has not been done, and a patient whose condition is such that resuscitation efforts are not an appropriate response suffers an arrest, the morally sound response is to withhold the treatment if it is inappropriate, not to fake it.

7. A DNR order applies only to withholding CPR in the event of an arrest; it does not indicate in any way that other life-sustaining treatment should be withheld, diminished, or withdrawn.

Sometimes providers presume an order not to resuscitate implies that other interventions to sustain life need not be provided. This is not so. For example, a DNR order does not mean a ventilator should be withheld from a patient suffering respiratory distress, or that efforts should not be made to stabilize an erratic heartbeat. There may be good reasons for abating other treatments, but those decisions are separate issues, and a DNR order has no direct bearing on them.

8. A DNR order for a patient under anesthesia requires special consideration. If a patient has a DNR order, the surgeon and the anesthesiologist should discuss, during preoperative conversations, the question of attempting CPR in the OR and during the immediate postoperative period. Often, but not always, it is reasonable to suspend the DNR order during these times.

During anesthesia and surgery an arrest can be much more effectively countered by CPR efforts. Some of the equipment is already in place, and the physicians can take immediate action. Moreover, the arrest may well be the result of anesthesia, and the anesthesiologist is trained to reverse this. Yet there are cases where CPR would not be appropriate in the operating room. A hospice patient, for example, undergoing surgery for pain relief may wish to maintain her DNR order during the surgery. Such a request is morally reasonable and should be respected by surgeons and anesthesiologists. If they cannot agree to it, they should seek others to provide the surgery or anesthesia and then withdraw from the case.

9. Ordinarily a DNR order does not require court approval. In some cases, however, recourse to legal counsel and perhaps to a court is appropriate.

Seeking court decisions about medical treatment is very much the exception not the rule. Judges are not really in the best position to make decisions about medical treatment. Nonetheless, there are exceptions. Sometimes family members may be hopelessly divided over whether a DNR order should be written for a patient incapable of indicating what is desired; sometimes a proxy may want CPR, but the physician is convinced that attempting it is a medical error. These kinds of cases sometimes end up in court.

A good policy will include most, if not all, of these provisions. Institutional DNR policies are usually developed by hospital ethics committees and then approved by the medical staff and the administration.

Lingering Questions about DNR Orders

The Question of Unreasonable CPR Efforts

Sometimes proxies or patients refuse to give consent for a DNR order when resuscitation is clearly an inappropriate medical response to an arrest. By refusing a DNR order, the patients or proxies in these cases are really ordering, by default, other people to provide inappropriate medical treatment. This sets up a difficult situation.

In an effort to resolve the difficulty, some suggest that providers could say that the inappropriate CPR would be futile for a patient, and therefore it should not be attempted even if there is no DNR order. But as we saw in chapter 3, we have to be careful about the word "futile." Certainly CPR without the possibility of reversing the arrest is futile, but it is not so certain that successful CPR despite the expectation of future arrests would be perceived as futile by everyone. Some people think human life is so valuable that even a short gain is worthwhile.

The 1991 *Guidelines for the Appropriate Use of Do-Not-Resuscitate Orders* issued by the Council on Ethical and Judicial Affairs of the American Medical Association noted that futility is likely to be interpreted in different ways by different physicians and thus is not a judgment the physician or proxy can make. Rather, "judgments of futility are appropriate only if the patient is the one to determine what is or is not of benefit, in keeping with his or her personal values and priorities." This is an excellent point, and reminds us that the notion of futility is not really something a physician should rely on when refusing possible life-saving interventions.

What does a provider do when a patient or proxy refuses consent for a DNR order, and the provider is convinced the resuscitation efforts would be medically and morally wrong? Physicians and nurses cannot in good conscience behave wrongly even when a patient requests it. The solution, however, is not to refuse the treatment because it is futile—the distinction between futile and not futile treatment is too ambiguous—but because it is bad medicine and contrary to ethical clinical practice.

Refusal of inappropriate resuscitation efforts is not always easy in practice. The unique nature of CPR—patients automatically receive it unless a physician has written an order against it—enables patients and proxies to demand it, in effect, by simply refusing to give consent for a DNR order. Nonetheless, providers cannot abdicate their responsibility to provide only appropriate treatment and may have to refuse CPR efforts or try to withdraw from the case. This can be very difficult in practice, and thus, moral problems linger when patients and proxies expect CPR efforts in inappropriate situations.

No completely satisfactory answer can be given to this problem of unreasonable CPR, but physicians and nurses must try to find a way to avoid giving their patients unreasonable medical treatment. As we shall see in the Gilgunn case, some judges are beginning to recognize this. Physicians and nurses clearly cannot always go along with patients and proxies who want "everything done" for the patient. The circumstances in which providers can decline treatment against the wishes of the patient or proxy, however, are not yet worked out in the ethical conversation of our culture.

The Question of Conditions for DNR Orders

Early DNR policies and court decisions tended to restrict the DNR order to terminally ill patients or to those whose death was thought imminent. Newer policies acknowledge the prerogative of patients with decision-making capacity to decline CPR just as they would decline surgery or chemotherapy. In other words, they need not be faced with terminal illness or imminent death before declining CPR.

If the patient does not have decision-making capacity, however, the situation is still not clear. The 1988 New York law governing DNR orders, for example, does not allow a DNR order at a proxy's request unless the patient is terminally ill or permanently unconscious or unless the resuscitation will be medically futile or impose an extraordinary burden on the patient (N.Y. Public Health Law. Article 29-B, section 2965). Unfortunately, the law does not define "extraordinary burden" (perhaps because, as pointed out in chapter 3, it is impossible to define "extraordinary"), and so the extent of the restriction on the proxy's decision to request a DNR order is not clear.

Clearly, though, the New York legislation intended to make the proxy's authority to request a DNR order more narrow than that of the patient.

On the other hand the 1990 Massachusetts Health Care Proxy Act empowers the patient's health care agent (the proxy) to make any decision the patient could have made. Since a patient has the unconditional authority to refuse any treatment, there are no conditions that must be met before a properly designated Massachusetts proxy can refuse CPR on behalf of the patient, provided, of course, the proxy's decision adheres to the criteria of proxy decision making. In Massachusetts, then, a designated health care agent can decide on a DNR order even though the patient is not terminally ill or permanently unconscious.

Attempting CPR on Newborns

Attempting CPR on newborns poses special problems. CPR does not seem a reasonable intervention for very-low-birth-weight babies because it so often fails and hence probably should not be attempted. There is something morally worrisome about attempting to resuscitate, sometimes repeatedly, an infant who weighs about 750 grams (one pound, ten ounces) or less. The whole issue of CPR for premature or seriously defective infants is a delicate one that needs much more extensive analysis than it has received in the ethical literature. Parents and neonatologists have to balance providing helpful treatment with protecting the infants from traumatic treatment interventions of little real benefit.

Attempting CPR with Extracorporeal Membrane Oxygenation

As noted in the discussion of determination of death in chapter 6, in recent years there has been some success using extracorporeal membrane oxygenation (ECMO) when CPR efforts fail to reverse a cardiac arrest. ECMO is a system somewhat similar to dialysis: The patient's blood flows through a machine that oxygenates it and then sends the oxygenated blood back to the body so the organs can be kept alive even though the heart or lungs may have stopped working. It is used mostly for children; adult usage is controversial, and it is rarely used with CPR efforts on adults. In a study reported in 2007 involving eighty children of ages ranging from one day to over seventeen years, thirty-seven (46 percent) died despite the ECMO whereas forty-two (54 percent) survived thanks to the ECMO. However, eighteen of the survivors had an unfavorable outcome; only twenty-four of them survived with intact neurological status, and seven of these needed a heart transplant to survive. Some of the cardiac arrests lasted more than an hour.

Attempting CPR with ECMO raises numerous ethical questions. One has to do with determining death, as we noted in chapter 6. Another is the ratio of severely compromised survivors to healthy survivors (eighteen vs. twenty-four): At what point does it become unreasonable to reverse the dying of children after standard CPR efforts fail to reverse a cardiac arrest? True, twenty-four of the eighty (30 percent) survived with a favorable outcome, but eighteen (22.5 percent) survived with an unfavorable outcome that introduced serious difficulties for these children and their families. Yet another issue arises because the use of ECMO with CPR efforts is more of an experiment than a treatment, and, given the high number of unfavorable outcomes, it is a high-risk experiment on children. The research was conducted outside the United States (in Canada and in Saudi Arabia), but risky research on children would be tightly controlled by federal regulations and institutional review boards in the United States. At the very least prudential reasoning suggests that parents should give consent for experiments with ECMO-enhanced CPR efforts, and these parents should be well informed of the high percentage of children who will survive with unfavorable outcomes, children they will have to care for and who may outlive them. At the present time ECMO is rarely used to complement CPR efforts in children.

Attempting CPR during Transfers

Patients are often sent in ambulances to other facilities for treatment. If a patient with a DNR order arrests during a transfer, the ambulance crew will almost always start CPR despite the hospital DNR order. They will claim that it is an emergency, so treatment must be given. Moreover, many ambulance companies order their people to do everything they can to save a life.

It is very difficult to justify this practice from a moral point of view. If the DNR order was appropriate in the hospital, there is no reason to believe it should be ignored while the patient is temporarily outside the hospital. Some legislatures are beginning to address this issue and to formulate a public policy that will allow ambulance and other emergency personnel to abide by legitimate DNR orders without fear of liability.

DNR Orders after Discharge

Some patients are discharged from hospitals to other facilities such as rehabilitation hospitals or nursing homes. Such a move puts the status of the DNR order in question. Strictly speaking the hospital's medical order ceases on discharge; yet it may still be appropriate for many of these patients to remain on DNR status. If the new facility accepts the hospital DNR order, there is no problem; if it does not, then the process that led to the original DNR order has to begin again at the new facility. In other words the physician and the patient or proxy must go through the informed consent process all over again, even though the patient's condition may not have changed. This is a rather cumbersome exercise, and there is always the danger the patient may have an arrest before it is completed. This could mean resuscitation will be attempted despite the wishes of the patient or proxy not to have it.

More work needs to be done in this area so patients will not receive treatment they do not want or that is not appropriate. One solution is to have the new facility accept the hospital's DNR order on a temporary basis and then reformulate the order in accord with its own institutional policy.

Another solution, and some states have already done this, is to allow physicians to write a DNR order on a legal form and on a bracelet indicating out-of-hospital CPR is not to be attempted. Once emergency medical personnel see the DNR verification form or the bracelet, they are expected to forgo or to cease CPR efforts.

Overriding DNR Orders

Overriding a DNR order and attempting CPR on a "no code" patient is hard to justify because, in effect, the providers are forcing treatment on a patient against his, or his proxy's, wishes. One situation where some do acknowledge the possibility of ignoring the DNR order and of attempting CPR arises when the arrest was caused by the providers. For example, a physician may have mistakenly ordered, or a nurse may have mistakenly given, the wrong medication, thereby causing respiratory arrest.

There are good reasons for trying to reverse this arrest regardless of the DNR order. First, we can assume that the patient or proxy did not have this kind of arrest in mind when she consented to the DNR order. Second, it would be very difficult for the physician or nurse, now aware of the potentially fatal mistake, to live with the fact if he did nothing to correct it. If a mistake caused the cardiopulmonary arrest, there are good reasons for making attempts to save that life by overriding, if necessary, a DNR order.

The lingering questions surrounding CPR are not easy to resolve, but one of the first steps we can take to sort out these remaining moral issues is to distinguish between two kinds of cardiopulmonary arrest. The first kind of arrest is expected. If we know a person is seriously ill or dying or very elderly, we also know that a cardiopulmonary arrest will occur at some point soon. These arrests are not really emergencies. They are not surprises, and resuscitation efforts are seldom a reasonable response.

The second kind of arrest is unexpected. It occurs suddenly and without warning. Sometimes we do not know the cause—a person might just collapse. At other times we do know the cause—it might be an accident, a fire, a near drowning, or a shooting. When an arrest is unexpected, attempting CPR is often a reasonable response.

A second step that we can take is to correct the erroneous optimistic beliefs that many patients and families have about the benefit of attempting CPR, especially on older people. One study of one hundred hospitalized patients seventy or older (none of them in an ICU) showed that 81 percent of them thought that their chance of surviving CPR and being discharged from the hospital was better than 50 percent; in reality studies suggest that it is considerably less than 10 percent and probably approaches almost zero. Both families and patients often overestimate the success of CPR efforts, perhaps because of the high success rate on TV shows that do not depict the majority of CPR efforts ending in failure.

The fundamental approach to CPR is, therefore, one of prudence. Patients deliberate to decide what is good for them, given the circumstances. Proxies try first to acknowledge what the patient wanted. If this substituted judgment is impossible, they try to figure out what is in the best interests of the patient. And if the patient has no interests because of irreversible unconsciousness, then a DNR order is the only reasonable treatment decision. Physicians will share in this decision-making process by providing adequate information about what attempted CPR involves, its physical and neurological risks, and the rather slim chances of a truly beneficial outcome. They will also help the patient or proxy decide whether or not attempting CPR would be a reasonable response in the circumstances if a cardiopulmonary arrest occurs.

We will now consider several cases that illustrate the history and complexity of decisions not to attempt resuscitation. These cases will help make us familiar with the early problems associated with CPR efforts, problems that led to the policies we have today, and they will also provide us with opportunities for engaging in the process of making moral judgments about withholding or providing treatments to reverse cardiopulmonary arrest.

The Case of Maria M

The Story

On January 11, 1981, Maria M was brought to the emergency room at La Guardia Hospital and eventually admitted. She developed respiratory problems, and on February 11, with her daughter's consent for the tracheotomy, was placed on a respirator. Her condition worsened. In March, a feeding tube was surgically inserted because a fistula in her throat was allowing food to enter her lungs. The cause of her problems was not known, and hence no one was saying that she was terminally ill; and no one mentioned that CPR might be withheld if she arrested. Through all this Maria was coherent and able to communicate somewhat with her daughter and providers. Sometimes she indicated that she wanted to return home, with a respirator if necessary. At other times she disconnected the tubing of the ventilator, leading some to think she did not want the equipment used.

At one o'clock in the morning of March 27, the monitor at the nurses' station showed that the heart of this seventy-eight-year-old woman was failing. A nurse and a medical student went to the room (no physician or resident was in the ICU at the time) and found the respirator disconnected. The student started chest compressions as the nurse reconnected the tubing. Then, according to the testimony of two nurses, the student said: "What am I doing? She's a no-code." The student then stopped the CPR. In this hospital the resuscitation team was summoned by announcing "Code 33" over the public address system, and no code was called. The student later disputed the nurses' testimony, but a resident arriving a few minutes after the arrest testified that the student had ceased CPR and had called him not to help resuscitate Maria but to pronounce her dead.

When the resident examined Maria, he found her heart still beating faintly. He resumed chest compressions but in vain, and Maria died. Later, one of the nurses asked the student why he stopped CPR and why he had indicated Maria was not to be coded. He claimed a cardiologist had given him a DNR order orally; the cardiologist denied he ever gave such an order.

When physicians informed Maria's daughter of her mother's unexpected death, they told her everything possible had been done to save her life. They also requested permission for an autopsy, but the daughter refused. A few nights later, the daughter received a phone call from someone claiming to be a nurse at the hospital. The caller told her that her mother had died unnecessarily because she was considered a DNR patient. The daughter notified authorities, and an investigation, including an autopsy, followed. It showed that Maria had died of cardiac arrest after disconnection from the ventilator. How the ventilator was disconnected is a mystery the grand jury could not solve. Somehow the alarm switch had been turned off and the tubing neatly tucked behind and under her pillow, yet the patient herself was thought incapable of performing either action.

In the course of its investigation the grand jury became aware of the deliberate effort by the physicians at the hospital to avoid any tangible evidence that some patients would not be given CPR if they arrested. The subterfuges included the practice of sticking adhesive purple dots on the nurses' cards that we discussed earlier.

Many of the nurses were deeply concerned over withholding of resuscitation efforts from patients without informed consent and without any notation about the treatment decision in the patient's permanent medical record. Some also felt that the adhesive dot system was unreliable, and indeed it was. One nurse, for example, had a card for a patient named Daisy S who had died at the hospital on January 5, 1982. There were two purple dots on it, yet all the physicians treating Daisy denied any knowledge of these dots, which were, in effect, orders not to attempt resuscitation if she arrested. And some nurses also felt it was unfair for physicians to expect them to document the DNR decisions with the purple dots on the cards in their file when the physicians themselves were unwilling to document the decision in the medical records.

Clearly, as the grand jury indicated, this was an intolerable situation. One of the reasons for telling the story of Maria is to show how careless things had become in some hospitals before people took seriously the ethics of DNR orders and the need for hospital policies to secure an ethically credible response to cardiopulmonary arrests.

A second reason for telling the story of Maria is to provide us with the opportunity to consider a case where we can ask whether a DNR order would, or would not, be the reasonable and moral thing to put in place. We want to bracket the conduct of the providers and hospital in 1981 and consider the ethical issues surrounding CPR for a patient such as Maria.

Ethical Analysis

Situational awareness. We are aware of the following facts in Maria's story.

1. Maria is seventy-eight, ventilator dependent, and nourished by a feeding tube. She has serious respiratory problems, but we really do not know why, and therefore we cannot say she is terminally ill or that her death is imminent. In recent weeks she has had three surgeries: two were needed for the tracheotomy and one to insert the gastrostomy tube. Her prognosis is uncertain: She could improve, stabilize, or continue to decline.

2. Although she was coherent and able to communicate by writing notes and speaking during the brief periods the respirator was removed, no one attempted to discuss CPR with her. And, although the grand jury report indicates that she did discuss her general situation with her daughter and nurses, it makes no mention of discussions with her physicians.

3. Despite some coherence and ability to communicate, it is entirely possible that this seventy-eight-year-old respirator-dependent woman would not be able to understand enough about CPR and the chances of a beneficial outcome to make an informed decision to accept or reject it. If this is so, and her physician has to make this judgment call, then her daughter would have a key role to play as proxy. If this is not so, then she needs a chance to consider her options.

We are also aware of these good and bad features.

1. Withholding CPR efforts means death is inevitable within moments if an arrest occurs. Maria's death, as any human death, would be unfortunate.

2. Attempting CPR causes trauma and often damages a patient. If it succeeds only partially, it leaves the person alive but in a condition worse than before. And in about five out of six cases, patients receiving CPR either die or never recover sufficiently to leave the hospital.

3. Not attempting CPR on Maria when neither she nor her family had agreed to decline it caused distress to her family, as the legal suit later brought by her family showed.

Prudential Reasoning in Maria's Story

Prudence asks two fundamental questions: What is my good and how do I achieve it? My good is what truly constitutes my fulfillment in life, what makes my life a good life, and this is living virtuously. The ethical task in any situation is for each person to figure out how he can live a good life in the circumstances.

Patient's perspective.   The grand jury report indicates that, although Maria has some ability to understand and to communicate, her views on withholding or withdrawing life-sustaining treatment (the ventilator) and on withholding or attempting CPR cannot be conclusively determined.

Proxy's perspective.   Based on her knowledge of Maria, her daughter may have been able to make a good decision about attempting CPR and about other life-sustaining treatment, but she never had the chance. If she had the chance to make a decision about attempted resuscitation, she would make it on the basis of what her mother wanted or, if she did not know her mother's wishes, of what she thought was in her mother's best interests. And what would have been in her mother's best interests? Without knowing Maria, this is difficult to say. Since we do not know the nature of her medical problems, it is always possible she could recover from them. If so, attempting CPR if she arrested may have been reasonable. On the other hand, there are also reasons for thinking that resuscitation efforts would be unreasonable in these circumstances and that a DNR order to withhold CPR would have also been reasonable.

Providers' perspectives.   As we look back on this case today, we can see many areas where providers, chiefly the hospital administrators and physicians, suffered ethical lapses about the whole question of attempting CPR in the hospital. Good ethical reflection could have led them to realize that the system of subterfuge was not morally sound, and that any legal concerns about not attempting unreasonable resuscitations could be removed by taking appropriate legal steps. Physicians in Massachusetts had successfully sought judicial relief in a case involving the decision to withhold resuscitation efforts a few years earlier in the Dinnerstein case, and the physicians at La Guardia could have done the same.

The nurses on the floor when the arrest occurred were in a different situation. The circumstances surrounding Maria's arrest are murky. Somehow the respirator alarm had been shut off, and the tube had been withdrawn and tucked behind her pillow, yet she was not deemed capable of making these moves herself. How should the providers have reacted when the heart monitor indicated trouble and they found the respirator tube withdrawn?

If a nurse does not know what a patient or proxy wants, and finds a respirator withdrawn without a proper decision-making process, then she has good reason to restore the respirator and attempt CPR if necessary. It is difficult to think inaction can be ethically justified in such circumstances. Although it can be argued that it is unreasonable to attempt CPR on seventy-eight-year-old Maria whose respiratory problems require ventilation, the circumstances of this arrest—the disconnected respirator, the absence of any decision-making process involving the patient or proxy, and the unknown cause of her problems—all provide strong arguments for the nurses' attempts to resuscitate in this case.

Ethical Reflection

It is obvious that serious problems existed in this hospital relevant to withholding CPR efforts. There were real problems in many hospitals about CPR in the early 1980s, and it is good to remind ourselves of them so we can better appreciate the need for open dialogue and policy, not secrecy and purple dots, in these matters of moral concern. It should be noted that, as a result of Maria's case, the hospital took immediate steps to correct its CPR protocols.

For a patient in Maria's condition today, what would be the ethical decision about attempting CPR? The answer is not clear; this may be a case where there are two right answers. It is not difficult to see how some patients in her position might prefer to decline CPR efforts. Others, of course, might prefer CPR in the event of an arrest. If the patient in an ambiguous situation has decision-making capacity, the decision is hers to make, and neither option is morally unreasonable.

However, when a proxy has to decide and does not know whether or not a patient wants resuscitation efforts in the event of an arrest, the decision in this kind of case is a difficult one. It is hard to know what is in Maria's best interests. If a patient is receiving respiratory support, as Maria was, a DNR order is often a reasonable response. If a patient has a cardiopulmonary arrest while on life-support systems, it often indicates that the arrest is associated with the end of life rather than with an unknown or readily reversible condition.

On the other hand it may be reasonable to delay writing a DNR order for a patient in Maria's condition. The cause of her respiratory problems was not yet known, and there was no evidence that she was suffering from a terminal illness. However, if a DNR order is not written in this kind of case, and the weeks on the respirator stretch into months, or if the patient suffers an arrest but is revived, the reasons supporting a DNR order grow stronger. At some point it does become unreasonable for a proxy not to consent to a DNR order for an older patient who has lost decision-making capacity and is supported indefinitely, perhaps permanently, by a respirator.

What was clearly unreasonable in this case, of course, was the whole DNR situation at that hospital. As we noted, these situations are now largely a thing of the past in American health care thanks to the widespread adoption of thoughtful institutional DNR policies.

Based on the grand jury account, then, we have reasons for saying both a decision for CPR (declining a DNR order) and a decision against it (consenting to a DNR order) would be morally justifiable decisions for a proxy to make. Actual situations, however, are much richer than the reports we read of them, so it is entirely possible that a proxy actually involved in this kind of situation would be able to discern better the more appropriate moral response.

The Case of Shirley Dinnerstein

The Story

The first major court case directly involving CPR happened in 1978, a few years before the case of Maria. Shirley Dinnerstein was a sixty-seven-year-old woman suffering from Alzheimer disease. In 1975 her complete disorientation, frequent psychotic outbursts, and deteriorating ability to control her bodily functions required intensive nursing care in a nursing home. In February 1978 she suffered a massive stroke that left her paralyzed on one side. She was admitted to Newton-Wellesley Hospital, a teaching hospital located in a suburb of Boston, in a semicomatose state, unable to speak. She was fed by a nasogastric tube, and, in addition to her Alzheimer disease and stroke, she suffered from uncontrollable high blood pressure and life-threatening coronary artery disease. Her life expectancy was no more than a year, and the most likely immediate cause of her death was expected to be, if not another stroke, a cardiopulmonary arrest.

In view of the circumstances, her attending physician recommended that CPR not be attempted in the event of an arrest. Her son, also a physician, and her daughter, with whom she had lived, agreed. But the physicians and family had a problem. They were in Massachusetts, and a recent (1977) decision of the Massachusetts Supreme Judicial Court concerning chemotherapy for an incompetent patient named Joseph Saikewicz required "judicial resolution of this most difficult and awesome question—whether potentially life-prolonging treatment should be withheld from a person incapable of making his own decision." Judicial resolution means, of course, going to court so a judge can decide whether the treatments can be withheld.

At the time of the Dinnerstein case, many lawyers were telling physicians that the Massachusetts Supreme Judicial Court decision in *Saikewicz* required physicians to obtain judicial approval before withholding any potential life-prolonging treatment. Based on this perception, the hospital, the physician, and Shirley's two children sought in probate court a determination that a DNR order for Shirley could be written without judicial approval or, if that were not possible, that judicial approval be given for such an order. The court appointed a guardian *ad litem* for Shirley. He apparently thought a patient in this situation should be resuscitated if possible and opposed the DNR order. This set the stage for a court battle.

The probate court sent the case to the appeals court without a decision. Before looking at its decision, we will consider the case from an ethical perspective.

Ethical Analysis

Situational awareness. We are aware of the following facts in the story of Shirley Dinnerstein.

1. Shirley is without decision-making capacity and is a terminally ill patient whose wishes about CPR are not known.

2. Her children and physician think the DNR order is in her best interests. That is to say, they do not think attempting resuscitation would be in her interests if she arrests. Shirley is dying, and they expect an arrest may well be the immediate cause of her death.

We are also aware of these bad features:

1. The DNR order will result in Shirley's certain death if an arrest occurs, and any human death is bad.

2. Attempting CPR in the event of an arrest will probably result in discomfort and further damage to Shirley.

3. Attempting CPR would also, presumably, cause distress for the physicians and her family because they do not think that it is appropriate.

4. The Massachusetts Supreme Judicial Court in the *Saikewicz* decision apparently required judicial intervention in cases involving the withholding of life-prolonging treatment from patients without decision-making capacity, and this is a factor the hospital and physicians must consider.

Prudential Reasoning in the Shirley Dinnerstein Story

Patient's perspective. We do not know from the case what Shirley would have wanted.

Proxies' perspective. Her children have made what appears to be the more reasonable decision, given the circumstances. In fact, it is somewhat difficult to see how we could say the decision to attempt CPR is a reasonable one in this kind of case.

Providers' perspective. Their position is also reasonable. In view of Shirley's terminal condition, and the decision of her children, they are comfortable ordering resuscitation attempts withheld in the event of an arrest that, if it occurs, will not surprise anyone. In the legal climate of the time, however, they understandably perceive a legal risk if they order CPR efforts withheld. The hospital deserves credit for not sweeping the matter under the rug or using "purple dots" but for seeking declaratory relief from the courts in this matter. This helped clear the air for the hospital and physicians and also set a legal precedent acknowledging that the proper place for decisions about CPR is in the clinic, not the courtroom.

The Court Decision

The appeals court realized that because everybody has a cardiopulmonary arrest when they die, it made no sense to require court approval for withholding CPR efforts every time a patient is dying. It therefore agreed with the physicians and family and declared the DNR order in this situation would not violate the law. It further said that the question of DNR is "not one for judicial decision, but one for the attending physician, in keeping with the highest traditions of his profession, and subject to court review only to the extent that it may be contended that he has failed to exercise 'the degree of care and skill of the average qualified practitioner, taking into account the advances in the profession.'"

The court distinguished the Dinnerstein case from the Saikewicz case. In *Saikewicz* the issue was chemotherapy for an incompetent patient, and the court saw this as a treatment designed to bring remission from a disease—leukemia. In *Dinnerstein* the issue was CPR for an incompetent patient, and the court did not see this as a treatment that could bring any cure or relief from Shirley's medical problems, and thus it concluded that the requirement of judicial resolution in *Saikewicz* did not apply in *Dinnerstein*.

Other courts have seen it within their purview to decide whether or not the guardian for a patient can request a DNR order. This happened, for example, in a Delaware case known as *Severns v. Wilmington Medical Center* in 1980. At the present time however the placing of a patient on DNR status in accord with current hospital DNR policies seldom requires judicial overview if patient or proxy consent is given and the physician agrees that the DNR order is appropriate.

Ethical Reflection

An ethicist looking at a situation such as the one faced by Shirley Dinnerstein's family will conclude rather easily that, in the absence of knowing the patient's wishes, the most reasonable course of action is a DNR order. Attempting CPR is seldom reasonable for terminally ill patients at the end of life when an arrest is expected. If the resuscitation efforts fail, they needlessly burden a dying patient; if they succeed, the seriously ill patient remains alive, but little has been gained. The terminal illness has not been reversed, and the likelihood of another cardiopulmonary arrest has increased.

The Case of Catherine Gilgunn

The Story

By the time Catherine was seventy-two years old, she had had a long history of health problems including a thirty-year struggle with diabetes, breast cancer followed by a mastectomy, three broken hips rebuilt with surgery, and a stroke. In May 1989 she was alert but suffering from pernicious anemia, chronic renal insufficiency, Parkinson's disease, ulcers on her feet, and coronary artery disease. Then she fell and broke her hip yet again. This time she refused to go to the hospital. By June 7, however, her ulcers were infected, and she was having difficulty breathing, so her daughter Joan, who lived with her, called an ambulance that took her to Massachusetts General Hospital, where she was admitted.

After eight days of care she was stable enough for surgery and gave her informed consent for another hip operation. Then she began suffering numerous seizures, and by the time these were controlled five days later, she was almost totally unresponsive. The scheduled surgery was cancelled. Catherine had a husband and several children, but the family agreed that daughter Joan would be her principal proxy decision maker.

By the beginning of July there was no real improvement. The attending ICU physician recommended a DNR order, but Joan and the family refused to give consent. The physician con-sulted the chair of the ethics committee, known as the Optimal Care Committee (OCC), Dr. Edwin Cassem, who agreed that attempting CPR would be a violation of standard practice, a mistreatment of Catherine, and not a genuine therapeutic option. On July 5 the attending physician wrote the DNR order without the family's consent.

Joan protested, insisting that her mother always wanted everything done to save her life. Two days later the physician cancelled the order. Joan and the family then requested aggressive life-sustaining treatments, and physicians complied by starting both a ventilator and a gastrostomy feeding tube. The treatments had some impact—by July 13 Catherine became more alert, although she never regained decision-making capacity. Then more seizures occurred, and by the end of the month she was totally unresponsive, even to painful stimuli.

On August 1 a new ICU attending physician, Dr. William Dec, began managing her care. He and his ICU team met with Joan and told her that her mother's condition was "hopeless from a medical point of view and that further interventions were futile." Joan insisted on CPR if Catherine arrested. The discussion became heated, and Joan walked out of the meeting, obviously very upset and angry. Meeting notes indicate that she became verbally abusive, voicing death threats against Dr. Dec as well as obscenities.

Dr. Dec then consulted with Dr. Cassem of the OCC, who again agreed that a DNR was appropriate and wrote in the medical record that "CPR was medically contraindicated, inhumane, and unethical." Dr. Dec then wrote the DNR order. Over the next few days he tried in vain to speak with Joan. He did talk with two of her sisters and her brother, and also with Catherine's husband, who refused to discuss the situation. And he spoke as well with a family attorney about his treatment plans for Catherine and his willingness to have her transferred to another facility if one would accept her. Following the conversation with the family's attorney, Dr. Dec consulted a hospital attorney who assured him not only that the DNR was legally sound but, in addition, as long as he was acting in the patient's best interests, it would also be acceptable to withdraw the life support.

On August 7 Dr. Dec called the family home and told an unidentified person that he was going to withdraw the ventilation from Catherine. During the weaning from the ventilator her blood gases were not monitored to determine how she was tolerating the withdrawal of ventilation. After two days of weaning Catherine was breathing on her own but began experiencing cardiopulmonary distress on August 10. The ICU staff made no effort to perform CPR (the DNR order was still in place), and she died that morning.

Joan then sued Dr. Dec, Dr. Cassem, and the Massachusetts General Hospital. In May 1995 a two-week jury trial ensued in Superior Court. Before looking at the verdict, we shall examine this case from an ethical point of view. It is a classic drama highlighting how patients or proxies can demand CPR simply by not agreeing to a DNR order and why the debate about "futile" treatments has become so difficult to resolve.

Ethical Analysis

Situational awareness. We are aware of the following facts in the story of Catherine.

1. By the end of July Catherine was totally unresponsive, and neurologists had declared that her chances of cognitive recovery were nil. She also suffered from numerous other problems including a broken hip. She was a comatose person sustained by life support and a feeding tube with no realistic hope of recovery.

2. Catherine had left no clear advance directives but her daughter Joan claimed: "Mother wanted everything possible to save her life regardless of cost." At the trial the judge instructed the jury to determine whether Catherine would want CPR and ventilation until death. The jury found that she would want these treatments as long as she was alive. Hence Joan's position has some credibility: She was not making the decision to refuse a DNR but simply reporting her mother's decision to have CPR. If Joan was telling the truth, and if the jury's finding was correct, then the conflict is really between the views of the doctors and Catherine, not the views of Joan. Joan may have agreed with her mother but that is not the crucial issue if her mother had given advance directives. Her role is as the reporter of her mother's wishes.

3. Written records indicate Joan was, at least some of the time, abusive and uncooperative. Unfortunately, this factor complicates these situations.

4. Despite Joan's objections, Dr. Dec decided to write the DNR order and then withdraw ventilation. Less than a day after ventilation was removed, Catherine suffered a cardiac arrest; no one tried to reverse it.

We are also aware of these good and bad features in the case.

1. The preservation of Catherine's minimal human life was of some good. If she dies people will grieve because her death, as any death, is a loss of something good.

2. Employing advanced life-support technology indefinitely and performing CPR on coma-tose people who have no realistic hope of any significant recovery at the end of their lives is bad. It is bad clinical medicine, and it is bad when physicians and nurses are pressured to provide unreasonable treatments by patients or proxies.

3. Physicians unilaterally deciding to stop life support and prevent CPR against the proxy's wishes that are based on the patient's preferences sets up a bad scene that can lead to bitter disputes and litigation. Litigation about treatment issues, although sometimes inevitable and occasionally helpful, is always unfortunate for physicians and families.

4. Somebody was paying for Catherine's care and treatments, but these were not doing her any good if she was truly unresponsive with no hope of regaining awareness. Providing treatments and attempting resuscitation on a patient no longer able to benefit from them are bad because they make no sense.

Prudential Reasoning in the Story of Catherine Gilgunn

Patient's perspective. If Catherine truly wanted what Joan said she wanted in this situation, then Catherine's request was unreasonable and immoral. It is not morally good for a person to demand that everything, including CPR efforts, be done no matter how dismal her situation might become. Every person on this planet will one day suffer a cardiopulmonary arrest, and it is simply preposterous to say that we should attempt to reverse every arrest.

Proxy's perspective. If Catherine truly wanted everything, including CPR, then Joan's initial position is understandable. A proxy's first responsibility is to relay the patient's wishes to physicians whenever they are known. This is what bioethicists call substituted judgment. But what happens when the patient's wishes are unreasonable, as they are in this case? If a proxy thinks that the patient's wishes are unreasonable, she can certainly so inform the physicians when she reports the patient's wishes and then decline to pressure them into delivering the inappropriate treatments. Of course, if the proxy thinks the patient's wishes for "everything" make sense, then she will push for CPR, and the stage is set for a conflict. What was Joan's personal position about her mother's wishes? Published reports suggest that she may have been convinced that doing CPR on her mother was an intelligent move and a good choice. If so, it is difficult if not impossible to defend her position as reasonable.

Providers' perspectives. Here we see a difference of opinion. In July the first attending physician did think a DNR was appropriate, but after further discussions with the family, he then agreed to cancel his DNR order, writing in the chart: "I find it difficult to provide a medical reason to avoid CPR that is as powerful as their desire to have it done." He also agreed to start ventilation and a feeding tube. Assuming he was a person of moral integrity, he must have felt that it was morally reasonable to perform CPR and put life support in place at that time. However, the physician-chair of the OCC did not think CPR was appropriate. He wrote: "For this patient, CPR is not [a genuine therapeutic option] and she should be protected from it by specific written order."

In August the new ICU attending physician did not think CPR or the ventilation ordered by the previous attending physician was appropriate. His notes of August 1 state that "aggressive means to prolong life (including pressors, CPR, defibrillation) are not in the patient's best interests." He apparently agreed with Dr. Cassem, the chair of the OCC, who wrote on August 2 that CPR is "a procedure which is medically contraindicated, inhumane, and unethical." The opinion of Drs. Dec and Cassem at this point seems unassailable—CPR and ventilation bring no benefit to a patient in Catherine's position. She had become totally unresponsive and was developing other problems as well. At some point it makes no sense to attempt resuscitation on ventilator-dependent people who have multiple medical problems and are thought to be dying in a coma unlikely to be reversed, and Catherine was clearly past that point. It is not so clear, however, that attempting CPR and maintaining ventilation would be unethical. Good clinical judgments are usually good moral judgments, but not always. A virtue-based ethics of prudence is very situation sensitive, and it does not reason deductively from an objective definition of futility to a concrete judgment in a particular case.

Judge's perspective.   Six years later this case was in Superior Court for a jury trial. In his instructions to the jury the judge gave two special questions related to their role as finders of fact. One of these required the jury to determine with a "yes or no" answer whether or not CPR and ventilation were in fact futile. Thus, the judge took the position that an objective and factual definition of futility exists and that a jury could decide whether medical treatments were futile for Catherine in August 1989. Given that the debate about an objective definition of futility is still raging a decade later, the judge's position is questionable. Unfortunately it forced jurors to render a judgment about futility when no widely accepted definition of futility exists.

Ethical Reflection

Getting an acceptable objective definition of futility, of course, is at the heart of the problem. Who and what defines futility? If CPR may reverse an arrest, and if ventilation and a feeding tube can support life a little while longer, then these interventions are not, strictly speaking, futile. Unreasonable and unethical they may be, but they are not physiologically futile. The judge's position as reflected in his instructions to the jury presupposes that an acceptable definition of futility exists, whereas the current debate on futility shows clearly that it did not and does not. Maybe the day will come when society will agree on a definition of futility, but until it does, judicial instructions to juries that force them to declare that any specific treatment in an individual case is or is not futile are morally questionable.

This type of case presents a truly difficult situation for physicians and nurses. They, as well as the patients and proxies, are moral agents and therefore are responsible for their actions. If we look only at the clinical aspects of the doctor-patient encounter on August 1, it is fairly easy to agree that CPR and life support were not reasonable. True, the physician in charge of the case at the end of July apparently thought that CPR would be reasonable because he decided not to write a DNR order, but he may have been simply letting things go until his month in the ICU was finished.

But the doctor-patient clinical encounter is not the whole story. As sometimes happens, the proxy wants "everything done." Is this a good reason to perform medically inappropriate CPR on a patient? Usually the answer is no, but prudence suggests that exceptions are possible. One important question is whether the inappropriate treatment will be burdensome or harmful for the patient. In this case, on the basis of the neurological diagnosis made at the end of July, the CPR would be no burden to the patient because she is totally nonresponsive and not expected to recover any awareness. If patients are totally and irreversibly unresponsive, they really have no interests, and nothing is a benefit or a burden to them. CPR may cause bodily injury, but it will not matter to the patient because he or she will not be aware of any pain or dysfunction. These patients are beyond all harm. They are beyond all help as well, and that is why it makes no sense to treat them unless there are some extenuating circumstances.

The moral issue in this kind of case is wider than the clinical issue of unreasonable treatment. Acknowledging that CPR efforts are not medically reasonable does not necessarily mean that they should be withheld. Another key issue is whether it is prudent to write DNR orders despite strong family objections when performing CPR would not cause any distress to the permanently unresponsive patient. The situation would be totally different if the unreasonable treatments would cause the patient distress, but that was not thought to be the case here.

On the other hand it is virtuous to make reasonable efforts, and these were made in this case, to educate the family about the irrationality of their demands so they would take a more reasonable position. And aggressive efforts should also be made to transfer the care of the patient either to another physician or to another facility willing to abide by the family's wishes. We need to remember that the willingness of the attending ICU physician in July to maintain life support with no DNR order is telling the family something. It was the new attending physician who began managing the case on August 1 who saw things differently. It is conceivable that other physicians at Massachusetts General Hospital or at another institution would have been comfortable treating Catherine without a DNR order.

Unless and until society reaches a consensus on an objective definition of futile treatment, and this will be difficult to do if the futility debate is any indication, there is a moral danger in letting medical professionals unilaterally dictate what will not be done when there is conflict about the treatment of unresponsive patients who cannot be hurt. This is especially true as we enter the new era of managed care where there is often a financial incentive for physicians and hospitals not to treat. Physicians and hospitals need to think of the public trust as well as clinical medicine. The fear and even rage that some people will experience when they discover that physicians unilaterally refuse efforts at resuscitation and withdraw treatment keeping loved ones alive is a very real circumstance that prudential reasoning will consider. It is obviously not morally reasonable for physicians to harm their patients simply because a family demands unreasonable treatment, but patients such as Catherine Gilgunn and Helga Wanglie can no longer experience anything so they are not being hurt by whatever is done to them. It is at least arguable that they can be treated while troubled providers try to arrange a transfer. Although there are strong reasons for saying that CPR for someone in Catherine's situation is medically and morally unreasonable, there may be reasons for providing the medically unreasonable treatment in exceptional circumstances (such as when the proxy insists it is something the patient would want) when the patient will not suffer from the CPR.

The AMA Council on Ethical and Judicial Affairs took a positive step toward resolving at least some of these conflicts between patients or proxies and physicians in early 1999 when it proposed, as we saw in chapter 3, policies on futility that would put a fair and open hierarchy of steps in place that both sides should follow once a conflict emerges. The AMA proposal acknowledges that, although a policy based on an objective definition of futility is not possible, a policy presenting an orderly process of half a dozen steps can be helpful in resolving disagreements about life-sustaining treatment. Patients or proxies can be informed from the beginning that any conflict will trigger a multistep process aimed at resolution. Of course, if the patient or proxy will not participate in the process, as was the case here, then the physicians will be left in a terrible spot.

The Jury Decision

The jury, ordered by the judge to determine by "yes or no" whether attempting CPR and using ventilation were futile treatments for Catherine Gilgunn, determined that they were futile. Once they decided that these treatments were futile, it was all but inevitable that they would not find the physicians or the hospital guilty of negligence—it would be irrational to define treatments as futile and then say that physicians were negligent for not providing them. Joan lost her case. She filed an appeal but withdrew it in 1998 shortly before hearings were scheduled to begin in the Appeals Court. The jury decision is thus final. It is not, however, an appellate ruling so it does not create a legal precedent. Nonetheless, the Gilgunn case is important because it shows how one jury failed to find physicians negligent when they wrote a DNR order and removed life support from a dying patient over the proxy's objections.

SUGGESTED READINGS

Chapter 7 of the President's Commission report titled *Deciding to Forego Life-Sustaining Treatment*, 1981, pp. 231–55, is a good introduction to decisions involving resuscitation. The report includes a long appendix (pp. 493–545) presenting the DNR or "no code" policies of selected institutions. Although these policies are somewhat dated (they make no provision for retaining a DNR order in the operating room, for example), they do give the reader an idea of what a DNR policy is. The Joint Commission on Accreditation of Healthcare Organizations expects hospitals to have an appropriate DNR policy; see JCAHO, 1991, *Accreditation Manual for Hospitals*, pp. 77–78.

The report of the New York State Task Force on Life and the Law titled *Do Not Resuscitate Orders*, 1986, Albany: Health Education Services, is also a valuable document. The second edition (1988) includes the 1987 New York law on orders not to resuscitate, which became effective on April 1, 1988, making New York the first state to enact legislation governing the withholding of cardiopulmonary resuscitation. For comments on the New York law, see Tracy Miller, "Do-Not-Resuscitate Orders: Public Policy and Patient Autonomy," *Law, Medicine & Health Care* 1989, *17*, 245–54; and John McClung and Russell Kamer, "Legislating Ethics: implications of New York's Do-Not-Resuscitate Law," *New England Journal of Medicine* 1990, *323*, 270–72.

See also the section on "Guidelines on Emergency Interventions" in *Guidelines on the Termination of Life-Sustaining Treatment and the Care of the Dying*, Garrison, NY: Hastings Center, pp. 43–52; "Standards and Guidelines for Cardiopulmonary Resuscitation (CPR) and Emergency Cardiac Care (ECC)," *JAMA* 1986, *255*, 2945–46; and the "Guidelines for the Appropriate Use of Do-Not-Resuscitate Orders," *JAMA* 1991, *265*, 1869–71.

For the study of attempted CPR at Boston's Beth Israel Hospital, see Susanna Bedell et al., "Survival after Cardiopulmonary Resuscitation in the Hospital," *New England Journal of Medicine* 1983, *309*, 569–76. For the study of attempted CPR at Rhode Island Hospital, see William Gray et al., "Unsuccessful Emergency Medical Resuscitation—Are Continued Efforts in the Emergency Department Justified?" *New England Journal of Medicine* 1991, *325*, 1393–98; see also the editorial on pp. 1437–39. For the study of attempted CPR on babies of very low birth weight, see John Lantos et al., "Survival after Cardiopulmonary Resuscitation in Babies of Very Low Birth Weight: Is CPR Futile?" *New England Journal of Medicine* 1988, *318*, 91–95. Also valuable is G. Taffet et al., "In-Hospital Cardiopulmonary Resuscitation," *JAMA* 1988, *260*, 2069–72; and Robert Wachter et al., "Life-Sustaining Treatment: A Prospective Study of Patients with DNR Orders in a Teaching Hospital," *Archives of Internal Medicine* 1988, *148*, 2193–98. The study of patients changing their minds about receiving CPR if they arrest is Donald Murphy et al., "The Influence of the Probability of Survival on Patients' Preferences Regarding Cardiopulmonary Resuscitation," *New England Journal of Medicine* 1994, *330*, 545–49.

Many fine commentaries on the ethical issues involved in CPR have been published in recent years. We can mention several: Michael Cantor et al., "Do-Not-Resuscitate Orders and Medical Futility," *Archives of Internal Medicine* 2003, *163*, 2689–94; Jeffrey Burns et al., "Do-Not-Resuscitate Order after 25 Years," *Critical Care Medicine* 2003, *31*, 1543–50; Derrick Adams and David Snedden, "How Misconceptions among Elderly Patients Regarding Survival Outcomes of Inpatient Cardiopulmonary Resuscitation Affect Do-Not-Resuscitate Orders," *Journal of the American Osteopathic Association* 2006, 106, 402–4; Andrew Evans and Baruch Brody, "The Do-Not-Resuscitate Order in Teaching Hospitals," *JAMA* 1985, *253*, 2236–39; Leslie Blackhall, "Must We Always Use CPR?" *New England Journal of Medicine* 1987, *317*, 1281–85; Donald Murphy, "Do-Not-Resuscitate Orders: Time for Reappraisal in Long-Term-Care Institutions," *JAMA* 1988, *260*, 2098–2101; J. Chris Hackler and F. Charles Hiller, "Family Consent to Orders Not to Resuscitate: Reconsidering Hospital Policy," *JAMA* 1990, *264*, 1281–84; Tom Tomlinson and Howard Brody, "Futility and the Ethics of Resuscitation," *JAMA* 1990, *264*, 1276–80; Stuart Youngner, "DNR Orders: No Longer Secret, but Still a Problem," *Hastings Center Report* 1987, *17* (February), 24–33; Kathleen Nolan, "In Death's Shadow: The Meaning of Withholding Resuscitation," *Hastings Center Report* 1987, *17* (October–November), 9–14; Giles Scofield, "Is Consent Useful When Resuscitation Isn't?" *Hastings Center Report* 1991, *21* (November–December), 21–36; and K. Faber-Langendoen, "Resuscitation of Patients with Metastatic Cancer: Is Transient Benefit Still Futile?" *Archives of Internal Medicine* 1991, *151*, 235–39.

For a discussion of when it would be moral for physicians to override a patient's DNR order after an arrest caused by medical interventions (for example, an unexpected allergic reaction to a medication or a clinical error), see David Casarett and Laine Ross, "Overriding a Patient's Refusal of Treatment after an Iatrogenic Complication," *New England Journal of Medicine* 1997, *336*, 1908–9. Despite the wide ethical disapproval of "slow codes" on patients with no DNR order when physicians feel (usually with good reason) that CPR should not be attempted, the practice apparently still exists. See Gail Gazelle, "The Slow Code—Should Anyone Rush to Its Defense?" *New England Journal of Medicine* 1998, *338*, 467–69. The failure of the public to realize that most CPR efforts in hospitals fail may be the result of some popular television shows such as "ER" and "Chicago Hope," where most emergency CPR efforts are successful. See Susan Diem et al., "Cardiopulmonary Resuscitation on Television," *New England*

Journal of Medicine 1996, *334*, 1578–82, with a reply by Neal Baer, 1602–5. Several studies show most people overestimate the success rate of CPR, especially for those of advanced age.

For the debate over retaining DNR orders during anesthesia and surgery, see Robert Truog, "'Do-Not-Resuscitate' Orders during Anesthesia and Surgery," *Anesthesiology* 1991, *74*, 606–8; Cynthia Cohen and Peter Cohen, "Do-Not-Resuscitate Orders in the Operating Room," *New England Journal of Medicine* 1991, *325*, 1879–82; and Robert Walker, "DNR in the OR: Resuscitation as an Operative Risk," *JAMA* 1991, *266*, 2407–11. A sidebar in this article includes "Suggested Policy Guidelines for Intraoperative Do-Not-Resuscitate (DNR) Orders" (p. 2410).

The study reporting the use of ECMO with CPR efforts on children is Alsoufi Bahaaldin et al., "Survival Outcomes after Rescue Extracorporeal Cardiopulmonary Resuscitation in Pediatric Patients with Refractory Cardiac Arrest," *Journal of Thoracic and Cardiovascular Surgery*, 2007, *134*, 952–59. See also Douglas Schuerer, "Extracorporeal Membrane Oxygenation: Current Clinical Practice, Coding, and Reimbursement," *Chest* 2008, *134*, 179–84.

The story of Maria M was constructed from the "Report of the Special January Third Additional 1983 Grand Jury Concerning 'Do Not Resuscitate' Procedures at a Certain Hospital in Queens County," dated February 8, 1984. The Grand Jury was impaneled in January 1983 at the request of the Deputy Attorney General and Special Prosecutor for Nursing Homes, Health and Social Services. The story of Shirley Dinnerstein is based on *In the Matter of Shirley Dinnerstein*, 380 N.E.2d. 134 (1978).

The Gilgunn case is *Gilgunn v. Massachusetts General Hospital*, Massachusetts Superior Court (1995), No 92–4820. For an account of the case co-authored by Dr. Dec and Dr. Cassen of the OCC, see John Paris et al., "Use of a DNR Order over Family Objections: The Case of *Gilgunn v. MGH*," *Journal of Intensive Care Medicine* 1999, *14*, 41–45. For a critical analysis of the way the case was handled see Alexander Capron, "Abandoning a Waning Life," *Hastings Center Report* 1995, *25* (July–August), 24–26.

NINE

Medical Nutrition and Hydration

MEDICAL TECHNIQUES for providing nutrition and hydration have introduced another major area of ethical concern. Although providing nutrition and hydration for the sick is normally considered a part of good patient care, there are times when it can be questioned. For example, a dying patient experiencing considerable suffering may well question the reasonableness of prolonging life a little while longer by using feeding tubes. And the proxy for an irreversibly unconscious patient may well question the reasonableness of maintaining the unconscious body with feeding tubes for months, years, or even decades.

Providing nutrition by tubes or lines is not always morally reasonable. In fact it could be immoral if the burdens it places on the patient outweigh its benefits, or if it wastes resources while providing no benefit to the patient, or if the patient with decision-making capacity does not want it. Moral deliberation endeavors to discern those situations in which the provision of medical nutrition and hydration is reasonable and contributes to the human good and those situations in which it does not.

Before we consider some typical cases where supplying nutrition and hydration by medical interventions was morally problematic, two preliminary considerations are in order. First, we need some idea of the techniques and technologies used for supplying nutrition and hydration. Second, we need to examine the conceptual and linguistic presumptions underlying, and frequently distorting, much of the discussion about feeding tubes and IV lines.

The Techniques and Technologies

There are three major medical procedures for supplying nutrition and hydration.

Peripheral IV Lines

About a hundred years ago physicians began administering saline solutions directly into the veins of the arm. This was the beginning of the familiar IV lines running into arms that we see so often today. Because adequate long-term nutrition is not practicable with these IV lines because of infections and other problems, they are best viewed as temporary and not really adequate means for supporting human life indefinitely. Their use rarely presents major ethical concerns, although occasionally ethical questions do arise about starting or withdrawing them.

Feeding Tubes

Surgical insertion of a feeding tube into the stomach was first attempted in the nineteenth century, but the practice did not become widespread until several decades ago. Because a feeding tube introduces nutrients into the gastrointestinal system, it is sometimes called enteral nutrition. (Other ways of placing nutrients in the body, most notably those using veins, are called parenteral.)

There are two general types of feeding tubes, the gastrostomy tube and the nasogastric (NG) tube. The gastrostomy tube (often called a G tube or, more recently, a PEG or percutaneous endoscopic gastrostomy tube) is normally inserted under local anesthesia through the abdominal wall into the stomach or into the small intestine. The prevailing technique now inserts a thread into the stomach through a minimally invasive incision, captures the thread in the stomach with an endoscope, pulls the thread out through the mouth, attaches the tube to the thread, and then pulls the tube through the mouth into the stomach and out the incision by pulling on the end of the thread left sticking out of the stomach. The patient is left with a small tube protruding from the stomach area. Once in place, the tube is relatively comfortable.

The NG tube runs through a nostril and into the stomach by way of the esophagus. Once inserted, it stays in place and, unfortunately, can irritate the nasal passages and cause vomiting. Pneumonia sometimes follows as the aspirated contents of the stomach get into the lungs. Many semiconscious or sleeping patients manifest an instinctive reaction to pull the NG tube out; it is often necessary to tie their hands so they cannot dislodge it.

Gastrostomy and NG tubes are connected to a line from a bag of liquid nutrition, and the nourishment flows slowly under gravity at a controlled rate into the stomach. Both G tubes and NG tubes can provide total nutritional needs for indefinite periods of time, decades if necessary.

Total Parenteral Nutrition

In the 1960s, physicians were inserting a line into a large chest vein to measure pressure in the heart. It was soon discovered that specially prepared nutritional fluids could be inserted into this central vein, enough to supply complete nutrition for indefinite periods of time, and total parenteral nutrition (TPN) became a reality. Early problems with infections at the site were reduced by new types of catheters that separated the entry through the skin from the entry into the vein. The procedure provides a way to nourish patients whose gastrointestinal system cannot tolerate the nutrition introduced through feeding tubes.

The solutions used in TPN are less like food than the fluids used in tubal feeding. They are not really the kind of fluids we would ingest, and they must be prepared and delivered under sterile conditions. They contain the electrolytes, amino acids, sugars, fats, minerals, vitamins, and other nutrients that the body normally produces after digestion. Despite the additional complexity of TPN, however, patients receiving it are no longer confined to hospitals. Some now receive TPN in nursing homes and, with nursing care, even at home.

More recently another medical technique for parenteral nutrition has been introduced. A catheter is inserted into a vein in the arm and then threaded through this vein into the central vein in the chest. The fluid nourishment thus runs into what looks like a peripheral IV line, but the internal catheter is actually carrying it to the central vein in the chest. This new procedure can provide more nutritional support than a peripheral IV and for a longer time, but it has not yet been used for indefinite total nutrition. It is referred to as partial parenteral nutrition (PPN).

In this chapter when we speak of feeding tubes, we mean the G tubes and the NG tubes inserted into the gastrointestinal system; when we speak of lines, we mean the peripheral and central feeding lines inserted into the venous system. For reasons that will become clear, we will use the phrase medical nutrition for both the feeding tubes and the venous lines.

Before considering some of the moral issues surrounding these ways of nourishing people, we need to consider the language we use to talk about the medical techniques for providing nutrition.

CONCEPTUALIZING MEDICAL NUTRITION AND HYDRATION

Whenever we are confronted with new realities in medical practice, we tend to think of them in terms of the classifications and descriptive categories already familiar to us. When nutrition by tubes or lines became a reality, two familiar classifications were available; we could think of the process as feeding someone, or we could think of it as a medical treatment. The interventions are a kind of feeding because they provide nutrition and hydration rather than medicine or medication, and nutrition and hydration are things everyone needs to live whether ill or healthy. The interventions are also a kind of medical treatment because medical research and practice developed the procedures and because health care professionals first insert, and then monitor, the tubes and lines. Nourishing people this way is not something the untrained person can accomplish.

Yet the interventions are in important ways unlike both other forms of feeding and other forms of treatment. In assisted feedings with bottles, cups, spoons, or straws, the recipients are able to swallow what goes into their mouths. With feeding tubes and lines, the person is not swallowing—the nourishment flows directly into the stomach or veins.

On the other hand the tubes or lines are also unlike other forms of treatment. The procedures do not provide medicine or medication but what we all need to live—nourishment and hydration. If we withhold or withdraw the tubes or lines, the person will not die of the disease but will expire from malnutrition and dehydration, or from diseases such as pneumonia that would not be fatal were it not for the weakened state caused by the malnutrition and dehydration. Moreover, there is a symbolism attached to providing nourishment that is not found in providing treatment. Humans have always fed their children, and sharing nourishment with the needy or with guests has great personal and cultural significance. It makes us feel guilty to have nutritional substances and then not give them to those unable to nourish themselves.

Nourishment by tubes or lines, then, does not fit neatly into either traditional classification—it is neither a typical kind of feeding nor a merely medical treatment. If we try to use either classification, we have to force or "shoehorn" the procedures into it. Medical nourishment resists being classified with feeding the hungry, but it also resists being classified with other forms of treatment or medication.

It may seem that concern over how we classify nourishment by tubes or lines is a linguistic quibble without importance. But this is not so. The moral judgment of many people is significantly influenced and sometimes determined by how they classify the procedures they are evaluating. Thus, those classifying intravenous or tubal nourishment as medical treatment inevitably defend the morality of withdrawal whenever it seems unreasonable, and those classifying the procedures as feeding inevitably claim withdrawal is immoral as long as the body accepts the nourishment.

An example of how classifications play an important role in the moral evaluation of feeding tubes can be seen in the two different positions taken by Roman Catholic bishops on the nourishment of patients who are in a persistent vegetative state (PVS). Normally the bishops speak as one on moral matters, but they have taken different positions on medical nutrition, and each position owes much to the way they classify the procedures. In a brief filed with the state supreme court, the bishops of New Jersey described the nutritional support of PVS patient Nancy Jobes as clearly distinct from medical treatment and concluded withdrawal of the feeding tube would be immoral. In contrast, the bishop of Rhode Island described the nutritional support of PVS patient Marsha Gray as "artificially invasive medical treatment" and concluded withdrawal of her feeding tube would be moral. The bishops of Texas later aligned themselves with the bishop of Providence, whereas the bishops of Pennsylvania later sided with their colleagues in New Jersey. The 2004 papal allocution of Pope John Paul II sided with the bishops of New Jersey and Pennsylvania when it stated: "I should like particularly to underline how the administration of water and food, even when provided by artificial means, always represents a *natural means* of preserving life, not a *medical act*." The allocution went on to say, as noted at the end of the chapter, that feeding tubes must be used in principle even for PVS patients.

What is happening here is clear. If people describe the tubes and lines as feeding, then they will consider withdrawing them as starving people to death, and they will argue that the tubes and lines must always be used as long as the body will accept the fluids. If, on the other hand, people describe the tubes and lines as medical treatment, then they will consider withdrawing them as withdrawing a medical treatment, and they will argue that the tubes and lines may be withdrawn whenever life-prolonging medical treatments could be withdrawn. In many debates about nourishment by tubes and lines, the descriptive classification chosen before the debate even begins determines the moral judgment. Serious moral reasoning about the issue never has a chance to begin.

If nourishment by tubes and lines is not well described either as feeding or as medical treatment, how can we classify it? It is best understood as a new kind of human action, one that combines the notions both of feeding and of treating but is reducible to neither. We should not shoehorn these procedures into either of the more traditional descriptive categories (feeding or treatment), but develop a new classification, something like "medical nutrition and hydration." By not describing the procedures simply as feeding, withdrawal of the procedures will not be considered as "starving the patient to death." And by not describing the procedures as medical treatment, withdrawal will not be considered as if it were simply another case of stopping a medical treatment. In our analysis of cases involving feeding tubes and lines, we will not classify the interventions in either of the traditional categories of feeding or treatment but in terms of a new hybrid classification that we will call "medical nutrition and hydration" or, more simply, "medical nutrition."

In the past ten years numerous cases about medical nutrition have emerged from the courts, and we now review several of them.

The Case of Clarence Herbert

The Story

In May 1981, fifty-five-year-old Clarence Herbert presented at the emergency room of the Kaiser Foundation Hospital in Harbor City, California with intestinal problems. Two operations were required. He was recuperating at home in July when he developed kidney problems, and he spent another brief time in the hospital. By the end of August his progress looked good, and he was back in the hospital for surgery to close the ileostomy that had been necessary to allow his bowel to recover from its original problems. The surgery was, as expected, routine, but he suffered cardiopulmonary arrest in the recovery room. CPR saved his life, but his brain was so badly damaged that he lapsed into a coma. He was placed on a respirator and transferred to the ICU.

The next day, August 27, his physician, Dr. Barber, indicated in the medical record that Mrs. Herbert, who had been told her husband would not recover, wanted "no heroics." The following day he wrote that she wanted the respirator removed and that she had consented to an autopsy. He left an order for the nurses to remove respiratory support, but the ICU nurses refused to withdraw the respirator. When a consulting neurologist requested more tests on the comatose patient, Dr. Barber cancelled the order to remove the respirator.

The additional tests confirmed extensive brain damage, and the family renewed their request to withdraw the respirator. The next day Dr. Barber privately stopped the respirator for a few moments and observed that Clarence was unable to breathe on his own. He told the family that their husband and father would probably die very quickly when the respirator was removed. They understood and gathered around the bed for his final moments. Dr. Barber then disconnected the respirator tube from the endotracheal tube in Clarence's throat. Much to everyone's surprise, he started breathing on his own.

Other than breathing spontaneously, he remained in the same medical condition, and his family continued to feel that his comatose state should not be sustained by treatment. According to court testimony they even objected to certain routine procedures used by hospital personnel in caring for comatose patients. On August 31, after continual consultation with the family, Dr. Barber removed the peripheral IV lines. Six days later Clarence Herbert died. His autopsy report listed dehydration, brain damage, and pneumonia as the causes of death.

Immediately after Clarence's lapse into a coma, disagreements about his care had arisen between his doctors (Dr. Barber and his surgeon, Dr. Nedjl) and the nurse in charge of the ICU, Sandra Bardenilla. In particular she was upset about the failure of the physicians to order a misting device to prevent choking after the respirator had been removed and about the withdrawal of IV support so soon after the patient became comatose. Frustrated about her attempts to resolve the problems within the hospital structure, she filed a complaint with the Los Angeles Department of Health Services. After its investigation the Department gave the information to the Los Angeles District Attorney.

A year later, in August 1982, both doctors were charged with murder and conspiracy to commit murder. The murder charge made the case national news.

A magistrate reviewed the case and ordered the complaint dismissed, but the Superior Court of Los Angeles County ordered it reinstated. Attorneys for the physicians appealed. Before considering the decision of the court of appeals, we will examine the case from an ethical point of view.

We want to use the case as an example so that we can deliberate about the morality of withdrawing nourishment from an unconscious patient.

Ethical Analysis

Situational awareness. We are aware of the following facts in the Herbert story.

1. Clarence is unconscious but breathing without respirator support. Although the court described him as being in a vegetative state that was likely to be permanent, we know today that such a diagnosis was a little premature. Normally, the diagnosis of a vegetative state that is likely to be permanent takes more than a few days. Moreover, comas and vegetative states are not really the same. It does seem a fact, however, that Clarence was unconscious and unlikely to recover.

2. It is not entirely clear what Clarence would have wanted. The court did find that he had said to his family that he did not want to "become another Karen Quinlan." At this time (1981), Karen had been living in a vegetative state without respirator support for several years, so it is quite possible Clarence did mean to say he did not want to be hydrated by tubes or lines if he became permanently unconscious and lapsed into a state similar to Karen's.

3. The proxy decision maker, Clarence's wife, and the children signed a document, along with two nurses as witnesses, before the respirator was removed. It said: "We the immediate family of Clarence LeRoy Herbert would like all machines taken off that are sustaining life. We release all liability to Hosp. Dr. & Staff."

4. The physicians' actions do not indicate they had any problem with withdrawing the respirator and, when Clarence did not die, the IV lines.

5. The hospital's legal counsel had circulated a memo dated August 21, 1981, advising physicians to obtain legal consultation before withdrawing life-sustaining treatment. Clarence's physicians knew of this memo—the neurologist had attached a copy to the front of Herbert's chart—but they chose to ignore it, apparently because they believed treatment decisions were something between physicians and the family.

We are also aware of these good and bad features in the case.

1. If Clarence is truly irreversibly unaware, then no benefits or burdens, no good or bad, will affect him; he is beyond experiencing anything. His death, of course, as any human death, even the death of someone in a permanent coma or PVS, is bad, but not for him. And if he continues to live in a state of permanent unconsciousness, the preservation of his life is a good, but not for him, and it could well be a burden for others.

2. His family members, acting on his previous remarks and on their understanding of what is the best thing to do, think the treatment should be stopped. They will suffer distress if it is continued against their wishes.

3. At least some of the nurses were upset at the way the case was handled. Sandra Bardenilla later told an interviewer that she was disturbed that there were no guidelines for this kind of case, that the family had consented to an autopsy before Clarence was dead, that the respirator was to be disconnected before the neurologist had run a confirmatory EEG, that a misting device had not been ordered to keep his airway clear after the respirator had been removed and the patient continued to breathe, and finally, that hydration had been stopped after only a few days of coma. "God, you mean if you don't wake up in three days, this is what can happen to you?" she was reported to have said.

Prudential Reasoning in the Clarence Herbert Story

Patient's perspective. Clarence is no longer able to make decisions, but he may have concluded earlier that he would not want feeding tubes or lines to keep him alive indefinitely if he were like

Karen Quinlan, that is, in a permanently unconscious state. Most would agree that this is a reasonable position for a person to take. In fact, wanting to be kept alive indefinitely in a state of permanent unawareness strikes most people as unreasonable.

Proxy's perspective.   If Clarence had previously indicated he would not want his life sustained if he became permanently unconscious, then his wife's request to withdraw medical hydration is easily justified. In fact, it would be difficult to justify her failure to request withdrawal in these circumstances. If Clarence had not made his wishes known but was truly irreversibly unconscious, then the request to decline medical hydration is also easily justified. The problem, of course, is that it is difficult to diagnose permanent unconsciousness in the first few days after it begins.

Providers' perspective.   It is morally reasonable for physicians to honor a request from a patient or proxy to withdraw medical nutrition and hydration in appropriate circumstances, and permanent unconsciousness is certainly an appropriate circumstance for withdrawal. If a patient left advance directives for withdrawal, those directives should be followed. If he did not, then the appropriate proxy is morally responsible for making the decision. Some would say that the best interests standard would justify a proxy's decision to withdraw medical nutrition and hydration. Because a permanently unconscious patient has no interests in anything, however, it is better to base the decision on simple moral reasonableness—it is not reasonable to sustain a human body once all awareness has been permanently lost.

The Court of Appeals' Action

The California Court of Appeals ordered the county Superior Court to drop the murder charges. That ended the legal action. A murder trial never took place, but the close call made an indelible impression on many physicians.

Several aspects of the appeals court's findings are relevant to the ethics of health care:

1. The court conceived administering nourishment and fluid by IV lines as treatment akin to respirators and other forms of life support and not as feeding or providing food and water. As we pointed out, once nourishment and hydration by lines or tubes is described as treatment, the tendency is to acknowledge that this medical treatment is not always appropriate. And in matters of medical treatment, the courts tend to defer to the competence of physicians in determining whether to begin, withhold, or withdraw it.

2. The court interpreted the removals of the respirator and the IV lines not as withdrawing treatments, but as withholding them. Apparently the court thought withholding treatment was legally less sensitive than withdrawing it, and wanted to construe the physicians' behavior in a favorable light. After all, if the doctors merely withheld treatments that they thought were inappropriate, then it is difficult to think of them as murdering their patient.

But how could the judges consider disconnecting a respirator or ordering IV lines removed as "withholding" treatment? They explained it this way: Each pulsation of a respirator and each drop of IV fluid is a discrete or separate self-contained application of a treatment. Thus, the court conceived disconnecting the respirator not as withdrawing life-sustaining treatment but as withholding the next pulsation, and it conceived pulling out IV lines that supply fluid not as withdrawing hydration but as withholding the next drop that would have entered the line.

The court thereby held that the doctors did not perform any action that would have killed Clarence since their behavior consisted only of omissions. "[W]e conclude that the petitioners' *omission* to continue treatment under the circumstances, though intentional and with knowledge that the patient would die, was not an unlawful *failure* to perform a legal duty" (emphasis added).

Needless to say, conceiving the actions of respirator withdrawal and IV disconnection as omissions is very peculiar. It is also unnecessary. We have already pointed out in our discussion of the distinction between withholding and withdrawing treatments how the decision to withdraw is easier to justify than the decision to withhold from a moral point of view. Once we are using the life-sustaining treatment, we know what it can do and what it cannot do, and this places us in a better position to determine whether or not it is a reasonable treatment for the patient.

3. The court rejected the distinction between ordinary and extraordinary treatment, claiming it begs the question. Thus, it avoided the argument advanced by some that nourishment and hydration by tubes or lines must always be provided because it is ordinary treatment. It suggested that the crucial distinction is between proportionate and disproportionate treatment. This is determined by weighing the benefits gained by the patient with the burdens the intervention imposes. This position is very close to the ethical approach we have been advocating where the norm is what is reasonable in the circumstances.

4. The court acknowledged that a proxy decision maker should first base her decision on the patient's desires to the extent they are known and only then on what she thinks is best for the patient. Thus, the court embraced the widely accepted criteria for proxy decision making: the proxy first tries to use substituted judgment; if that fails, she resorts to best interests. Of course, if Clarence is truly irreversibly unconscious, he has no interests and the best interests standard will not apply. In this case, however, the court did find that Clarence had indicated he would not want to be kept alive by machines or "become another Karen Quinlan," and this allowed the court to say that his wife was relying on the substituted judgment standard.

5. The court remarked that seeking judicial intervention in treatment decisions is "unnecessary and may be unwise." In other words, the California court agreed with the *Quinlan* court in New Jersey (and disagreed with the *Saikewicz* court in Massachusetts) that the legal setting is not the proper place to make decisions about medical treatment.

This case is the first and only time to date that physicians have been charged with murder for withdrawing hydration from a patient at the request of the family. And the Court of Appeals protected the physicians by refusing to let the murder trial proceed. To this day some physicians and nurses and some attorneys believe that there is a real threat of criminal prosecution for withdrawing medical nutrition or hydration. This case in which the murder indictment was thrown out before the trial even began and the absence of any other cases where physicians have been charged with murder for removing feeding tubes or lines show that the threat of criminal prosecution is more imagined than real. Prosecutors simply have not been charging physicians with murder when feeding tubes or lines are withdrawn at the request of the patient or proxy.

Ethical Reflection

Withdrawal of medical nutrition and hydration from a patient known to be permanently unconscious is not difficult to justify morally, especially if we have indications that the person would not want to be kept alive this way.

Many of the circumstances in this case, however, were less than morally acceptable. Specifically the decision to withdraw hydration was made too soon after the coma began. It is not always easy to diagnose permanent unconsciousness, and prudence would indicate that at least a few weeks are needed to verify that a patient breathing without respirator support is truly irreversibly unconscious. Hence, the nurse's position—that things went a little too fast and without sufficient attention to supportive care—is more reasonable than the physicians' willingness to withdraw the IV lines so soon after the cardiopulmonary arrest.

Moreover, the communication between the physicians and nurses was inadequate, and the communication between the physicians and the family also seems to have been poor judging from the subsequent claims of the family that they did not understand Clarence's condition when they agreed to withdraw the treatments. The failures of communication between the physicians and family may have been the fault of the physicians, or of the family, or of both. The main point to note is that good ethics demands good communication. Physicians and nurses must make certain that patients and proxies really grasp what they are saying.

The Case of Claire Conroy

The Story

In 1979 Thomas Whittemore became the legal guardian for his aunt, Claire Conroy. She had lived a very simple life; in fact, she had lived all her life in the house of her childhood. She had never married, had worked for the same company all her life, and had few friends. She had been close to her three sisters, but they had all died. Thomas was her only surviving blood relative, and he had been visiting her weekly for a number of years. As far as he knew, she had feared and avoided doctors all her life. When his wife once took her to an emergency room, she had objected vigorously. By the time she was about eighty years old, she was suffering from an organic brain syndrome that caused periodic confusion. Thomas then placed her in a nursing home where she became increasingly confused, disoriented, and physically dependent.

In 1982 she was hospitalized for four months. One of her problems was a gangrenous left foot thought by her physicians to be life-threatening. Two surgeons recommended amputation, but Thomas refused to give informed consent because he was sure that she would not have wanted the surgery. Despite the dim prognosis, she lived. During the same hospitalization, an NG tube was inserted to supplement her nutritional intake. After three months it was removed, but attempts to feed her by hand were not sufficient, and so it was reinserted. She was discharged to the nursing home, where another attempt was made to nourish her without the tube in January 1983. This effort also failed.

Later that year, when it became apparent that the feeding tube would be permanently needed, Thomas sought to have it removed on the grounds that she would never have consented to its insertion in the first place. By this time Claire was suffering from arteriosclerotic heart disease, hypertension, and diabetes. Her left leg was gangrenous to the knee. She could not speak, and physicians were not sure just how much pain she felt. Perhaps she was uncomfortable because she did pull and tug at her bandages, feeding tube, and catheter.

Her attending physician, Dr. Kazemi, and the nursing home administrator, a nurse named Catherine Rittel, did not think the feeding tube should be removed. Thomas Whittemore then went to court. The case is important because no court had ever before authorized the removal of feeding tubes. He filed his petition on January 24, 1984, and the case was argued a week later. A consulting physician testifying on behalf of the nephew said he thought that it was appropriate to remove the feeding tube with the nephew's consent. He felt that Claire did not have long to live, could never experience significant recovery, and was possibly suffering. During the hearing a seminary professor of Christian ethics (Ms. Conroy was a Roman Catholic) testified that removal of the tube would not, in his view, be a violation of Catholic teaching because the medical nutrition should be considered extraordinary treatment and therefore optional in these circumstances.

The trial court judge decided the case on February 2, 1984. He allowed removal of the feeding tube, stating that prolonging Claire's life with its burdens by medical nutrition was pointless and might even be cruel. The guardian *ad litem* appealed to the superior court, appellate division. During the appeal process Ms. Conroy, still on the NG tube, died on February 15, 1984. Nonetheless, aware of the public need for judicial review on this kind of situation, the superior court agreed to hear the case.

The appellate court reversed the decision of the lower court, arguing that withdrawal of the NG tube would not simply be letting Claire Conroy die but would be tantamount to active euthanasia or killing her. This decision was appealed, and the case went to the New Jersey Supreme Court. Before examining its decision, we will look at the story from an ethical point of view.

Ethical Analysis

Situational awareness. We are aware of these facts in the Conroy story.

1. Claire, in her eighties, was suffering from several serious problems. She was failing and would not live long. She was conscious but mostly passive and incapable of making treatment decisions for herself. Her nephew was the appropriate guardian, and the court found he had no conflict of interest in requesting withdrawal of the NG tube.

2. Her proxy was requesting withdrawal of the feeding tube based on what he believed she would have wanted. She had never said explicitly that she would not want feeding tubes, but her lifelong aversion to medical care supported his position. Her physician was against the withdrawal.

We are also aware of these good and bad features in the case.

1. Without the NG tube, Claire would die, and a human death is always bad. Moreover, she may have suffered somewhat as she died from malnutrition and dehydration.

2. Using medical nutrition to keep her alive in her dying months prolonged her suffering and discomfort, yet it achieved little benefit beyond an added period of life that had already lost so much.

3. The NG tube could have been causing her distress. All her life she had declined medical treatment, and we have no reason to think that she had changed her mind and would want it now. Confused though she may have been, she may well have been upset with the NG tube but so weak and incapacitated that she could not refuse the interventions.

4. Keeping her alive was undoubtedly upsetting to her nephew because he believed it was against her desires. It is difficult for caring proxies to see their patient's wishes disregarded.

Prudential Reasoning in the Claire Conroy Story

Patient's perspective. Given the limited life expectancy and health problems (which include diabetes, a gangrenous leg, heart disease, high blood pressure, and no control over bodily functions), a patient not expecting to live long might well think that declining medical nutrition and hydration is the appropriate moral response. Of course, Claire was too sick to decide this at the time, but, judging from what we know of her, she did feel this way before she deteriorated, and it is not an unreasonable view.

Proxy's perspective. A proxy acts morally when he tries to present what the patient would have wanted, provided that what the patient would have wanted is not clearly immoral. In this case there are good reasons for believing that Claire would not have wanted her life prolonged with medical nutrition and hydration and, if this was her position, the proxy's request to stop the medical nutrition is easily justified; in fact, it would be rather difficult to justify any other proxy decision in this kind of case. If a proxy has good reason for thinking that the patient would not want the NG tube continued in the circumstances, his failure to request withdrawal would be morally questionable. Thomas was on solid moral ground when he requested that the feeding tube be withdrawn from his aunt.

Providers' perspective. There are also good moral reasons for doing what the providers did in this case. In the earlier stages of the patient's illness they provided needed nutrition with the NG tube, but they saw it as something temporary and twice tried to wean her from it. Temporary use of a tube for nourishment is morally justified in most cases. Of course, if Claire had clearly refused tubal feeding while she had decision-making capacity, either personally or through advance directives to her proxy, it would have been unethical for providers to force the tubal nourishment on her.

As it became apparent that Claire's medical nutrition and hydration would be permanent and that she would die within a short time even if it were continued, the reasonableness of the tubal nutrition declined to the point where its withdrawal can be morally justified. Moreover, if her proxy could show that she would not have wanted indefinite medical nutrition at the end of her life, it is arguably unethical for physicians to continue it.

It was also appropriate for the providers to seek a judicial opinion before withdrawing the feeding tube. In 1983 it was not well established that the withdrawal of a feeding tube would not be considered equivalent to illegal euthanasia, and, in fact, the superior court did so consider the proposed withdrawal. Even today withdrawing medical nutrition from conscious patients without evidence that this is what they would want is a very sensitive issue from a legal point of view. Prudent legal advice and judicial intervention were important protections for providers before any legislation or case law had established support for withdrawing medical nutrition from conscious patients without decision-making capacity.

The New Jersey Supreme Court Decision

In a long decision dated January 17, 1985, the New Jersey Supreme Court reversed the ruling of the Superior Court and concluded that a proxy may direct withdrawal of tubal nourishment in some cases provided certain procedures are followed. It argued that the right to self-determination can outweigh the state's interest in preserving life and that, as the *Quinlan* decision by the same court a few years earlier had shown, this right is not lost when a person becomes incapable of exercising it personally. The court ruled that a proxy can direct withdrawal of medical nutrition if any one of three tests or standards can be met. The court described these standards as follows.

1. *Subjective:* Here the proxy knows what the patient would have chosen to do. This knowledge can be the result of written or oral advance directives or come from knowing the reactions of the person to similar cases. The knowledge might also be deduced from a person's religious beliefs or from a consistent pattern discernible in prior decisions about medical treatment.

2. *Limited objective:* Here the patient's wishes are not as clear as they would be with the subjective standard, but there is some trustworthy evidence that she would have refused the treatment and, in addition, the patient is suffering unavoidable pain that outweighs the benefits of continued life.

3. *Pure objective:* Here we have no trustworthy evidence that the patient would have refused the treatment, but the burdens of pain and suffering are so great that the proxy can reasonably conclude they outweigh the benefits of continued life.

According to the New Jersey court, any one of these standards would in principle legally justify a proxy's decision to withdraw medical nutrition from a conscious patient. The question now is: Did the request of Claire's proxy meet any of these standards? According to the state supreme court, it did not.

The court felt that the evidence at trial was inadequate to satisfy any of the three standards. If Claire Conroy were still alive at the time of the decision, then, her nephew would have had to present additional evidence before it would have been legal to withdraw the NG tube. If he wanted to use the subjective test, he would have to show more clearly that she would not have wanted the tubal nourishment. If he wanted to use either objective test, he would have to show better that she was suffering so much that the suffering overrode the benefits of continued life. Perhaps he could have presented additional evidence that would satisfy the court's requirements, but since she had died almost a year earlier, there was no need for him to pursue the issue, and the court declined to remand the matter for further proceedings. Thus, the case of *Claire Conroy* ended at this point.

The court also commented on several distinctions that are now familiar to us. It rejected the distinction between actively hastening death by terminating treatment and passively allowing a person to die of a disease, claiming that the description of conduct as active or passive is a notion so elusive it is of little value in decision-making situations.

The court also rejected the use of the distinctions between withholding and withdrawing treatment and between ordinary and extraordinary treatments. The court recognized the emotional significance of feeding, but saw a distinction between feeding by bottle or spoon and feeding by tube and lines, which is a medical procedure. It also pointed out that receiving nourishment by means of a tube can be seen as equivalent to breathing by means of a respirator; both interventions enable a body to perform a vital function it can no longer manage on its own. Since withdrawing respirators is morally justified in many cases, so must be withdrawing feeding tubes.

We should note that the *Conroy* decision is rather limited in its application—it applies only to patients in nursing homes. It also required the physician to follow certain detailed procedures. These included notifying the New Jersey Ombudsman Office of the intended withdrawal and obtaining confirmation of the patient's diagnosis and prognosis by two physicians not affiliated with the nursing home. In addition, if either objective standard is being used, the patient's family members or, in their absence, the next of kin must concur with the decision to withdraw the medical nutrition.

The Conroy case was important because it was the first time a state supreme court ruled that in some circumstances medical nutrition and hydration could be withdrawn from a conscious patient who lacked decision-making capacity. The court also recognized that a competent person has the right, based on common law and on the Constitution, to reject medical treatment regardless of the person's medical condition or prognosis and that this right remains intact even when the person becomes incapacitated.

Ethical Reflection

An ethicist could rather easily conclude, along with the moral theologian who testified in the trial court, that it is morally reasonable for a proxy to request withdrawal of medical nutrition and hydration for a person in Claire's condition and with her history of refusing most medical interventions throughout her life. Keeping people in their eighties with limited life expectancy alive by using tubes and lines for nourishment at the end of their lives does not make a lot of sense when we have good reason to believe they would not want the interventions.

Some will consider the case of Claire Conroy as an argument for active euthanasia. If it is morally justified to withdraw medical nutrition and hydration from a conscious patient, they argue, then it seems reasonable and compassionate to give the person a lethal injection rather than to allow the slow death caused by malnutrition and dehydration. Unlike the cases where the patient is unconscious, a person in Claire's position might suffer when her feeding tube is withdrawn, and because the fatal outcome is inevitable without nourishment, waiting days for death seems senseless.

This argument has a certain appeal but is not a convincing argument for active euthanasia. The key is to prevent suffering when a feeding tube is removed, and if we can prevent suffering without taking the drastic step of having a physician kill the patient, then good ethics suggests we do so. Once we sedate a person, suffering is not a question, and no compelling reason for euthanasia remains. True, the sedation of a patient just waiting for death after nutrition is withdrawn creates a situation no one really likes, but euthanasia creates an even less desirable scenario—physicians killing patients.

The Case of Elizabeth Bouvia

The Story

In February 1986, twenty-eight-year-old Elizabeth was a patient at the High Desert Hospital in Lancaster, California. She had been afflicted since birth with cerebral palsy, and quadriplegia had left her immobile except for some movement in her fingers, head, and face. She also suffered from degenerate and crippling arthritis that caused so much pain that a permanent catheter had been placed in her chest for regular doses of morphine. It gave her some, but not total, relief. Her mind was clear, and she had earned a college degree. Her weight hovered around sixty-five to seventy pounds. She had stopped eating solid food when the food began causing her nausea and vomiting. The hospital's physicians, fearing her liquid diet would be inadequate, had inserted an NG tube.

She had dictated advance directives to her lawyers and signed them with a pen in her mouth that marked an "X" on the paper. These directives indicated she did not want nourishment by tubes, but her physicians ignored them.

Undoubtedly part of the reason why they inserted the NG tube was their knowledge of the circumstances surrounding her previous hospitalization in 1983. At that time—shortly after she had checked into the Riverside General Hospital—there was some indication that she had decided to starve herself to death and wanted medical support as she died. Physicians at Riverside prevented her suicide by inserting an NG tube, and a court had supported the hospital's position. Elizabeth did not appeal that ruling, and she eventually began eating again, so the NG tube was removed. Thus, the physicians at High Desert Hospital in 1986 may well have thought she was making another attempt to commit suicide, and they may have been trying to prevent it by using NG tubing, something the physicians at Riverside had done with court approval three years earlier.

Her lawyer asked the court to issue an injunction ordering physicians at High Desert Hospital to remove the NG tube. The court refused, arguing that disconnecting life-support equipment could only be done if the patient was unconscious and terminally ill. Elizabeth was neither unconscious nor terminally ill; testimony indicated that she might live another fifteen to twenty years if adequately nourished.

In April 1986, the California Court of Appeals reversed the trial court's decision and directed the lower court to order the NG tube removed. Medical nutrition was withdrawn, and the providers at High Desert Hospital began feeding Elizabeth as much as she could tolerate. This turned out to be sufficient. She left the hospital and remains alive as this is being written (2008).

The California Court of Appeals argued that competent adults have the right to refuse life-sustaining medical treatment even if they are not terminally ill and unconscious. It also reminded providers that "no civil or criminal liability attaches to honoring the refusal by a competent and informed patient of medical treatment."

Ethical Analysis

We now want to consider this case from an ethical point of view. It can serve as a paradigm case for people with decision-making capacity who are experiencing a high level of pain and suffering with little hope of any significant improvement. If spoon-feeding causes them additional distress, is it morally reasonable for them to decline it? And if they do decline the uncomfortable spoon-feeding, is it morally reasonable for them to decline medical nutrition as well?

Situational Awareness

We are aware of the following facts in the Bouvia story.

1. Elizabeth was severely ill, and her pain was only partially controlled by morphine. Her prognosis for improvement was slight, although her life could continue for decades. She was accepting some liquid nourishment but not enough to sustain her life indefinitely because the food caused her physical distress. She did not want medical nutrition by tubes or lines, but an NG tube was nonetheless inserted. Because of her illness, she was powerless to resist the insertion of the NG tube against her will. A gastric tube may have been more comfortable for her, but she had not given informed consent for the surgery to insert it. She wanted the NG tube removed.

2. Her providers and the first judge to review the case believed the tube should remain. They viewed the situation as an attempted suicide rather than as a refusal of medical interventions providing nutrition and hydration.

We are also aware of these good and bad features in the case.

1. Elizabeth was not able at this time to receive adequate nourishment orally. The feeding tube was preserving her life, and human life is good.

2. Removal of the NG tube would be a causal factor in her death, and human death is always bad.

3. Oral nourishment caused Elizabeth distress and discomfort, but so did the NG tube, which she did not want.

4. If providers believed she was once again trying to commit suicide, then withholding or withdrawing the tube could cause them distress. Many physicians and nurses would not want to help patients, especially those not terminally ill, to commit suicide.

Prudential Reasoning in the Bouvia Story

Patient's perspective. Elizabeth had been thrown into a terrible and tragic situation. As one judge wrote: "Fate has dealt this young woman a terrible hand. Can anyone blame her if she wants to fold her cards and say 'I am out?'" And in 1983 her intentions at Riverside apparently were to commit suicide.

In 1986, however, she was no longer trying to commit suicide; she was simply refusing the oral nourishment that was causing her distress and the medical nutrition supplied by an NG tube. Is the refusal to eat reasonable for someone in her position? It would be difficult to say it is not. Food caused her so much distress that her refusal to eat does not seem unreasonable, especially in view of her tragic situation. And if she declined to eat, must she accept a feeding tube? Again, it seems not. She knew, better than any of us, what a burden it is to live like this, and her desire not to use feeding tubes to prolong this painful life was not an unreasonable response. If a person can no longer eat naturally, then it may well be reasonable for her to decline feeding tubes in some situations, and this seems like one of them.

So incomprehensible to us is the position of a patient locked into such a terrible condition that it almost seems arrogant to second-guess her preferences. It would be difficult for anyone to say, given her unfortunate situation, that her decisions to refuse food her body does not tolerate well and to decline tubes for nourishment are morally unjustified.

Providers' perspective. What is the right thing for providers to do when patients cannot eat adequately and then refuse to accept feeding tubes? When the patients are as damaged as Elizabeth was and are experiencing significant pain and suffering, there seems little doubt that providers should acknowledge the patient's desires. This conclusion becomes clear when the alternative is considered. If a patient with decision-making capacity refuses a feeding tube and her wishes are ignored, it creates a situation in which physicians are forcing medical interventions on her. In this case they could physically do this because Elizabeth was too helpless to resist. But the thought of taking advantage of her paralysis to force an unwanted feeding tube through her nose is not a comfortable one, especially since her anguish at being treated this way was evident.

The motivation of people working in health care to save lives is a wonderful thing, but it cannot override the wishes of patients with decision-making capacity who are in a better position to know what is best for them. Forcing treatment or tubes for nutrition on competent adults against their wishes is difficult to justify. It violates respect for them and pushes medicine back into its paternalistic mode. Certainly it was difficult for providers to remove the NG tube, which they thought she needed to live, but it should be more difficult for them to force tubes into helpless people against their will and to refuse to withdraw them when the patient with decision-making capacity clearly wants them out.

Ethical Reflection

If we look on this case from the vantage point of our ethical approach, the patient's decision to forgo nourishment by tubes is reasonable, as would be the decision to accept medical nutrition. There is a point where a suffering person may reasonably decide that the burdens of treatment and medical nutrition fall so far short of the benefits that it is more reasonable to decline the interventions, even if it means death, than to accept them. Nothing Elizabeth could choose would help her live well or have a good life in any meaningful sense of these terms. She was trapped in a tragic situation and could only choose the less worse.

It is difficult to find cogent reasons for requiring a person suffering from an incurable painful situation to accept tubes and lines for nourishment. The idea that each person should live reasonably and take reasonable care of her life is not undermined when a person whose body is almost totally immobile and generating so much pain that continual morphine is required opts to decline treatment or nutrition. Nor is it unreasonable if a person in this situation opts for treatment and medical nourishment. In tragic situations such as these, providers can allow some leeway for the suffering patient to decide what interventions are acceptable. In some cases, and this may well be one of them, the patient has plausible reasons for both accepting and rejecting medical nutrition.

Not to be overlooked, however, is Elizabeth's earlier request for assistance in committing suicide. During her 1983 hospitalization she did want help in starving herself to death. In today's debate about physician-assisted suicide, some might argue that her providers should have helped her end her life. Although not terminally ill, she was suffering significantly and had little hope of meaningful improvement. Since she had decision-making capacity and was freely requesting assistance in suicide, compassion suggests to some that she should have been given that assistance.

But her physicians did not help her commit suicide when she was at Riverside General Hospital, and the fact that many years later she continues to eat suggests that we should be careful when suffering patients ask for help in killing themselves. Their requests cannot always be taken at face value. Sometimes the determination of these patients to kill themselves is only temporary.

Elizabeth had reasons other than her medical problems for being depressed in 1983. She had developed a pen-pal relationship with a man in prison, and they became a couple when he was released. A glimmer of good fortune came into her life, but he abandoned her when she became pregnant. Then she suffered a miscarriage. It is not surprising that significant depression would follow these experiences, especially for someone in her circumstances.

However, her survival to this day (an obituary in the *Los Angeles Times* in May 2008 mentioned that she was still alive) indicates a will to live that reasserted itself after that temporary desire to commit what some would call a "rational suicide." This reminds everyone in the debate about physician-assisted suicide just how difficult it is to know when the desire of a suffering patient with decision-making capacity for help in committing suicide is truly a definitive stance. Few people want to help a patient commit suicide when the patient would have changed her mind if she had had the chance.

In recent years there have been a number of legal cases involving the nourishment of patients in PVS, a neurological condition resulting in total loss of awareness that was explained in chapter 6. Many of these patients survive for years, even decades, thanks to feeding tubes and basic nursing care, yet they will never regain any consciousness. A trend has developed wherein courts allow proxies to stop the medical nutrition and hydration if there is evidence that these patients would not have wanted it continued in a PVS.

Among the most celebrated early cases where courts have allowed the withdrawal of medical nutrition and hydration from PVS patients are these:

1. *Paul Brophy*, Massachusetts Supreme Judicial Court, 1986
2. *Nancy Jobes*, New Jersey Supreme Court, 1987
3. *Marsha Gray*, Federal District Court (Rhode Island), 1988
4. *Carol McConnell*, Connecticut Supreme Court, 1989

However, there are other cases not involving PVS where the courts have refused to allow the withdrawal of feeding tubes. Two examples are the stories of Mary O'Connor and Michael Martin.

Mary O'Connor had worked in a hospital for years before her retirement in 1983. For years she had been telling her daughters that it was "monstrous" for patients to be kept alive by life-sustaining treatments when they were not going to get better and, after hospitalization for a heart attack in 1984, repeated how she would not want her life prolonged if treatments could not restore a reasonable degree of health. A year later she began suffering a series of strokes. At first her two daughters, both practical nurses, cared for her at home, but by February 1988 she needed nursing home care as she became bedridden, partially paralyzed, and severely demented. By June 1988 she had deteriorated so much that the nursing home transferred her to the Westchester County Medical Center, where physicians wanted to insert an NG tube, which would, they said, extend her life for several months or "perhaps a year or two."

Mary's daughters said that she would not want a feeding tube in these circumstances and asked that it be withheld. After the hospital ethics committee supported the physicians, Mary's daughters still refused permission for the feeding tube, and the hospital then sought authorization to insert the feeding tube from the court.

The Westchester County judge found Mary's wishes to decline life-prolonging medical interventions in her present condition were clear enough and declined to authorize the feeding tube. The hospital appealed the ruling, but the appellate division upheld it. The hospital then appealed to the Court of Appeals, which is the supreme court in New York. In a five-to-two decision dated October 14, 1988, this Court reversed the lower courts and allowed the hospital to insert the feeding tube, arguing that Mary's wishes were not sufficiently "clear and convincing." The dissenting justices stated that the majority had "trivialized" Mary's wishes, arguing that "Mary O'Connor expressed her wishes in the only terms familiar to her, and she expressed them as clearly as a lay person should be asked to express them. To require more is unrealistic, and for all practical purposes it precludes the right of patients to forgo life-sustaining treatment."

A second example where courts refused to allow feeding tube withdrawal is the 1995 Michael Martin case in Michigan. Michael had suffered serious brain damage in an automobile accident. He was severely paralyzed and needed a gastrostomy tube. He still had some awareness but no decision-making capacity. His wife Mary was his proxy decision maker. After it became clear his situation was irreversible, she requested that the feeding tube be removed. She said she knew that this would be what he wanted because he often said he did not want to be kept alive if he became dependent on people and machines.

The hospital ethics committee and a court were satisfied that Michael had made it sufficiently clear that he would not want a feeding tube keeping him alive in such a condition. Michael's mother and sister, however, objected to withdrawing the tube, so they appealed the court decision. The appeals court also agreed that Michael would not want to be kept alive in such a state, but Michael's mother and sister appealed this decision as well. The Michigan Supreme Court reversed the decisions of lower courts and ruled that there was not "clear and convincing evidence" that Michael would not want to be kept alive by a feeding tube in his present condition. Undoubtedly the court was uncomfortable with the idea of withdrawing medical nutrition from a person not unconscious and not terminally ill.

Although the withdrawal or withholding of feeding tubes and lines is often a difficult decision emotionally and ethically, there are times when it is reasonable, especially in cases where patients have expressed their desires not to have their severely compromised and deteriorating lives prolonged when there is no realistic hope of any meaningful recovery. As with any interventions, virtue ethics will ask whether what we are doing is a reasonable response given the circumstances. There often comes a time when the goal of medical interventions becomes palliative rather than the prolongation of severely damaged life with no realistic hope of recovery. This is seen most clearly in patients in PVS, but there are situations as well when feeding tubes and lines are not a morally or medically reasonable response to the situation.

The most noteworthy cases involving feeding tube withdrawal, however, are those of Nancy Cruzan in Missouri and Terri Schiavo in Florida. In both cases the patient was diagnosed as being in PVS. *Cruzan* is the only case involving the withdrawal of medical nutrition that was heard by the United States Supreme Court; its decision came in June 1990. Terri's parents tried to have the Supreme Court hear the *Schiavo* case, but the Court declined in 2001 and again in 2005. We will now look at these famous cases in detail.

The Case of Nancy Cruzan

The Story

In January 1983 Nancy's car veered off the road into a ditch. She was found lying face down and not breathing. Emergency personnel began CPR; it restored her breathing, but she never regained consciousness. A year later, it was clear that she was in a PVS. She could conceivably live for decades without any prospect of regaining the slightest level of awareness. After several years her parents, acting as her guardians, asked that the gastrostomy tube be removed; they claimed she had made remarks indicating she would not want any life support keeping her alive unless she could live at least halfway normally. Her physicians and the hospital refused to stop the medical nutrition. Her parents went to court in 1988.

The evidence indicating that Nancy would want the medical nutrition withdrawn consisted primarily of statements she had made to a roommate about a year before the accident. This person reported that Nancy had said she would not want to live if she ever faced life as a "vegetable." After hearing the evidence, Judge Charles E. Teel of the Jasper County Circuit Court authorized the withdrawal of the medical nutrition. His order was not carried out because a guardian *ad litem*, supported by several state officials, appealed to the Missouri Supreme Court.

The Missouri Supreme Court reversed Judge Teel's decision. It said that medical nutrition cannot be withdrawn from a PVS patient unless there is "clear and convincing" evidence that this was the patient's wish. The court also noted (correctly) that Nancy was not terminally ill and was not suffering. Thus, it saw no reason to act contrary to the state's interest in preserving life, no matter how minimal the life had become. "The state's interest is in life; that interest is unqualified." In other words, the quality of a life has no bearing on the state's interest in preserving that life.

The Missouri court acknowledged that the doctrine of informed consent gives people a right to refuse treatment and that this right persists even when they are incapacitated, but the court insisted that a proxy cannot exercise this right except (1) under the requirements of the state Living Will statute or (2) in situations where the evidence of the patient's wish to decline medical nourishment is "clear and convincing."

The phrase "clear and convincing evidence" is important, although there is no precise definition for it. "Clear and convincing evidence" falls somewhere between the evidential requirements in civil cases captured in the phrase "preponderance of the evidence" and the more strict requirement of evidence in criminal cases known as "evidence beyond a reasonable doubt." It is a very strict evidential requirement, as we saw in the O'Connor case.

After the Missouri Supreme Court ruled against them, the Cruzans appealed to the U.S. Supreme Court, and arguments were heard in December 1989. A major issue was whether Missouri's requirement of "clear and convincing evidence" was so demanding that it effectively violated a patient's constitutional right to refuse medical interventions. The due process clause of the Constitution gives one the liberty to refuse unwanted medical treatment, and most would argue that this liberty is not lost simply because a person has lapsed into unconsciousness. If unconscious people do not lose constitutional protection, then an environment must be maintained so their proxies can see to it that their wishes about treatment remain effective. The question is whether or not the demand that a proxy produce "clear and convincing evidence" is so strict that it, in effect, destroys the constitutional protection most people should enjoy when they become permanently unconscious.

Before looking at the decision of the U.S. Supreme Court in the *Cruzan* case and its aftermath, we examine the case from a moral point of view.

Ethical Analysis

Situational awareness.   We are aware of the following facts in the Cruzan story.

1. About a year before the accident, Nancy had made some reference to the fact that she would never want to live as a "vegetable." Now that had become her status, and it would continue for the rest of her life.

2. Her proxies (her parents) believed the medical nutrition should be stopped because she would not want it in her condition.

3. Her physicians and the state of Missouri believed it should be continued because they had medical and legal interests in preserving life. Since the evidence of her previous wishes was not clear and convincing as the state law governing living wills requires, and since she was not suffering, they saw no reason why their interest in preserving life should not prevail.

We are also aware of these good and bad features in the case.

1. Nancy's death, as any human death, would be unfortunate even though most of her brain had already ceased functioning.

2. Providing medical nutrition caused no burden or benefit to her because she could not experience anything. It did cause her parents distress, however, because they were convinced she would not want it, and this is a bad feature of the case.

3. Withdrawing the nutrition would cause her physicians and state officials (the court records name the administrator of the Missouri Rehabilitation Center and the director of the Missouri Department of Health, acting in their official capacities, as opposing the Cruzans) some distress, judging from their strong stand against withdrawal.

4. The treatment and care of Nancy burdened the taxpayers of Missouri; they were paying most of the medical bills. Unfortunately, the public funds could not provide any benefit Nancy would experience.

Prudential Reasoning in the Nancy Cruzan Story

Patient's perspective.   Nancy had no perspective at this point, but she did have some ideas before she lost consciousness about not wanting to live in a vegetative state. Were these ideas morally reasonable? Undoubtedly they were. The vast majority of people, most ethicists, and even the courts are in agreement that it is reasonable for people to want medical nutrition stopped if they fall into a PVS. One is hard pressed to find any plausible reason why a person would want his irreversibly vegetative body kept alive for years.

Proxies' perspective.   The proxies acted in an admirable way. They knew what their daughter did not want, and they knew, after several years, that the continuation of medical nutrition and hydration was senseless. Since they had reason to believe their daughter would not have wanted the medical intervention continued indefinitely, they were on solid ethical ground when they requested its removal.

Providers' perspective.   The physicians disagreed with the parents about withdrawing the nutrition. This position can be justified if they felt withdrawal would be illegal under Missouri law, because the evidence that Nancy would not want the tubal feeding was less than "clear and convincing." The physicians knew Nancy was not suffering, and if they thought the law required them to continue the feeding, this is a good reason for them to do so until a court resolved the legal issue.

Guardians *ad litem*'s perspective.   There were actually two guardians *ad litem* appointed in this case, and one of them took an interesting legal position. He thought that it was in Nancy's best interest to have the medical nutrition withdrawn, but he also thought it was important to have the case reviewed by the state supreme court. This was a new type of case in the state, what is called a case of the "first instance," and the state supreme court decision would therefore establish a legal precedent for Missouri. This guardian *ad litem* therefore took a rather contradictory position: He concluded Nancy's nutrition should be withdrawn, and then he appealed the judge's order allowing the withdrawal. And when the Missouri Supreme Court later ruled against withdrawal, the same guardian filed a brief urging the U.S. Supreme Court to reverse the decision of the Missouri court and to allow the withdrawal.

From a moral perspective, however, it seems that a guardian *ad litem*'s role is simply to determine what is right for the patient. Since the guardian in this case was satisfied with the lower court's decision to allow withdrawal of medical nutrition, his role in appealing its decision is difficult to justify from an ethical standpoint. Guardians *ad litem* are expected to determine what is best for the patient in the particular litigation; normally they would appeal a decision only if it goes against what they think is right for the patient.

Missouri's perspective. The state decided to fight the parents after the first court ruled that the medical nutrition could be withdrawn. Its position is difficult to justify morally. The state officials could have simply accepted the ruling of Judge Teel, but they did not. Why did the state of Missouri adopt an adversarial role against the family and appeal Judge Teel's decision to the state supreme court?

Perhaps the state officials felt obliged in conscience to do so. Perhaps they were also motivated by political considerations that extended beyond anything directly connected with the reasonable treatment of Nancy Cruzan. Published reports indicate that an intense political struggle between advocates of the right to life and advocates of the right to choose was unfolding in Missouri during the years when Nancy's family was trying to have the medical nutrition withdrawn, and Nancy's case happened to become a focal point of that political struggle.

In 1986 Missouri had amended its abortion act to read: "It is the intention of the . . . state of Missouri to grant the right to life to all humans, born and unborn." If unborn humans have a "right to life," then so does an adult on life-support systems. Permitting the withdrawal of life support from an unconscious adult could undermine the claim that not-yet-conscious fetuses have an inviolable right to life. The intense state interest in fighting the wishes of Nancy and the request of her parents may have had more to do with the strong position of many state officials against abortion than with the question of withdrawing nutrition from a PVS patient.

But good ethical reasoning can see the difference between abortion and withdrawing medical nutrition from patients in PVS, just as people can see the difference between abortion and killing criminals for capital crimes, a practice that exists in Missouri and in many other states where many people are strongly opposed to abortion on the basis of the right to life. To the extent the state officials' opposition to Nancy and her parents was motivated by their position on abortion, their actions were morally suspect, and the suffering they caused the family was a morally unjustified imposition. The Cruzan family may well have been a pawn in a burning political issue that has nothing to do with PVS—the politics of abortion.

The U.S. Supreme Court Decision and Its Aftermath

The U.S. Supreme Court decided in June 1990 that Missouri's insistence on clear and convincing evidence before a proxy could have a feeding tube removed was not so strict that it violated the Constitution, and it also noted that no such clear and convincing evidence is yet found in this case. In effect, then, the court ruled that the medical nutrition could not be withdrawn. The court stated that a competent person has "a constitutionally protected liberty interest" in refusing unwanted medical treatment. It also said that, for purposes of this case, it can be "assumed" that a competent person has "a constitutionally protected right" to refuse life-saving nutrition and hydration, but "this does not mean that an incompetent person should possess the same right." Thus, the court, by allowing states to adopt the "clear and convincing" standard, did little to protect the right of an incompetent patient to refuse medical nutrition and hydration, although much of the press seemed to read the decision as indicating otherwise.

On November 1, 1990, the Cruzans were back in Judge Teel's court in Carthage, Missouri. Three friends of Nancy's came forth to give "clear and convincing" evidence that she had told them she would never want to live like a vegetable, and her physician testified that it was no longer in her best interests to be medically nourished. The state of Missouri, which had originally opposed the withdrawal of medical nutrition, had by now withdrawn from the case.

On December 14, 1990, Judge Teel issued a new order, similar to his original order of 1988. He said again that the medical nutrition could be stopped. Only this time he was able to say, thanks to the new witnesses who had come forward, that the "court by clear and convincing evidence" finds Nancy's intent would be to terminate her nutrition and hydration, and thus her parents were authorized to have it stopped.

Despite strong protests at the hospital by groups supporting the right to life, the medical nutrition was stopped. On December 26 Nancy died while special state police details guarded her hospital room to keep the chanting and praying protestors at bay. It was almost eight years after she had lapsed into the irreversible unconsciousness of a PVS. A documentary of the case was subsequently shown on *Frontline* by PBS television. It is well worth seeing.

Ethical Reflection

The decisions of Nancy and her parents are morally reasonable. The nutrition and hydration offered no benefit that Nancy could experience. Medical nutrition given to a permanently unconscious person is meaningless to that person, and the presumption should be that it is reasonable to discontinue it when permanent loss of consciousness is definitively diagnosed. In rare situations, there may be a reason for continuing it briefly. The person may be an organ donor, for example, and it may be reasonable to continue life support in order to enhance organ transplantation.

Most people intuitively sense that withdrawal of medical nutrition is appropriate when a person is in PVS. When asked, few people want their bodies kept alive indefinitely after all awareness has been irreversibly lost. There is no point in maintaining a permanently unconscious and meaningless coma or vegetative state. Once a person has lost all capacity for any awareness, he is no longer really one of us. Truly human existence is gone, only vegetative life continues. Intervention becomes meaningless, and if it imposes a burden on others, as it does, then it is arguably unreasonable and unethical to continue it.

The state of Missouri apparently assumes, in effect, that most people would want to be kept alive in vegetative state. It requires a strong standard of evidence—the clear and convincing standard—before families or other proxies can have medical nutrition withdrawn from a patient in PVS. This makes the family's decision to withdraw medical nutrition look like the exception when, in fact, it is what most people consider a reasonable reaction to a PVS. The effort to keep an irreversibly vegetative body alive for years, and even decades, is what strikes most people as unreasonable, not the request to stop meaningless treatment of no benefit to the patient.

Treating a PVS patient creates many burdens on the family, on the providers who feel it is unreasonable, and on those paying for it. These burdens can be justified if they are balanced by proportionate reasons, and there are seldom any such reasons when a person has lapsed into PVS.

Some people, however, do not feel this way. A small but vocal and well-organized minority takes a strong position against withdrawing medical nutrition from PVS patients. The *amicus curiae* or "friend of the court" briefs filed when the Cruzan case went to the U.S. Supreme Court provide an indication of just how divided people are on this subject. Among those supporting the position against Nancy and her parents were these:

- National Right to Life Committee
- United States Catholic Conference
- National Association of Evangelicals
- Baptists for Life and Southern Baptists for Life
- Catholic Lawyers Guilds of Boston and New York
- National Federation of Catholic Physicians' Guilds
- Knights of Columbus
- Roman Catholic Archdiocese of New Orleans
- Missouri Doctors for Life

Among those supporting Nancy's parents were these organizations:

- American Medical Association
- American College of Surgeons
- American Nurses Association and the American Association of Nurse Attorneys
- National Hospice Organization
- Catholic Health Association
- Evangelical Lutheran Church in America
- American Academy of Neurology
- St. Joseph Health System
- Center for Health Care Ethics, Saint Louis University Medical Center

The Case of Terri Schiavo

The Story

Theresa Schiavo, known as Terri, suffered a cardiopulmonary arrest during the night in February 1990. She was twenty-seven years old. Her husband Michael found her unresponsive and called her father as well as 911. Emergency personnel performed CPR and restored her pulse. Her arrest had lasted about eleven minutes, long enough to cause significant brain damage according to most medical experts. After the resuscitation she was comatose and placed on a ventilator.

The cause of her arrest remains unknown; the autopsy showed no evidence of a heart attack or stroke. What is known is that she suffered from a significant potassium imbalance perhaps caused by her struggles to lose weight. In the six years preceding her arrest, she had lost 140 pounds, dropping from 250 to 110.

Two months after her collapse she began to show signs of arousal. Her coma was evolving into PVS with alternating states of apparent wakefulness and sleep. When she was able to breathe on her own, the ventilation was withdrawn. In May 1990, with no objection from her parents, Robert and Mary Schindler, a court appointed Michael as her legal guardian. For the next several years Michael and the Schindlers consented to aggressive treatments aimed at restoring awareness; at one point Michael even had Terri flown to California to receive an experimental treatment. Unfortunately, every attempt to restore awareness failed.

Friction eventually developed between Michael and the Schindlers after Michael received a financial settlement in February 1993. He had sued Terri's physicians, claiming their failure to diagnose and treat her potassium imbalance caused her collapse. The award provided him with $300,000 for loss of consortium (companionship) and placed some $700,000 into a court-managed trust to provide care for Terri.

The Schindlers and Michael began arguing about the money. The Schindlers thought that Michael should share some of the $300,000 award for loss of consortium with them. He refused, and soon they were not speaking to each other. Later, Judge George Greer, after listening to both sides, found that the breakup between Michael Schiavo and the Schindlers developed over money: "It is clear to this court that such severance was predicated upon money and the fact that Mr. Schiavo was unwilling to equally divide his loss of consortium award with Mr. and Mrs. Schindler." Eventually the disagreement over money developed into intense animosity. Published reports indicate that the Schindlers were also upset over Michael's desire for a DNR order for Terri, over his wishes to forgo treatment for infections, and over his relationships with other women.

The Schindlers repeatedly tried to remove Michael as Terri's guardian so they could become her guardians. They argued that they and not Michael had Terri's interests at heart. It may not have helped the Schindlers' efforts to gain guardianship when, at one point, Michael's attorney elicited testimony from them that, if it were necessary to keep her alive, they would authorize major surgeries including the amputations of her arms and legs. They also testified that, if Terri had left a formal living will indicating she would not want to be kept alive indefinitely with a feeding tube, they would try to have her directive overturned because such a living will was not, in their opinion, consistent with their beliefs or with hers. The court saw no reason to cancel Michael's guardianship, and he retained the right to make decisions on behalf of Terri.

In 1998, eight years after Terri was diagnosed in PVS and five years after the feud with her parents erupted, Michael petitioned the court to allow him to authorize withdrawal of the feeding tube. The Florida law stipulated, as does the Missouri law that we noted in the Nancy Cruzan case, that a proxy could direct withdrawal of tube feeding from a person in PVS only if there is that high standard of evidence called "clear and convincing evidence" showing that the person would not want to be kept alive by medical interventions. At the hearing Michael testified that after deaths of people in the family who had been on life support Terri had said she would not want to be kept alive this way. The Schindlers objected strenuously to the withdrawal of the feeding tube, and thus the case went to trial.

Judge Greer appointed a guardian *ad litem*, Richard Pearse, to protect the interests of Terri. Pearse recommended that the feeding tube not be withdrawn and noted in his report that Michael had a conflict of interest in that he stood to gain financially if Terri were to die because he was the sole heir to her estate and all the money from the fund set aside for her care had not yet been spent. At that point Michael asked the judge to remove Pearse as guardian *ad litem*. Judge Greer did dismiss Pearse but did not replace him until years later, in October 2003, when Jay Wolfson was named guardian *ad litem*.

At the trial there were five witnesses. Three witnesses (Michael, his brother, and his sister-in-law) testified that Terri had made statements indicating that she would not want to be kept alive if she ever became severely damaged. Mrs. Schindler also testified. She indicated that Terri had made remarks indicating she would want life support to keep her alive. At one point she testified that she heard Terri, when she was between seventeen and twenty years of age, say during the highly publicized Karen Quinlan ventilator withdrawal case that they should just leave her alone; that is, leave the ventilator in place. When it was pointed out that the Quinlan case was in the news in 1975–1976, long before Terri was seventeen, Mrs. Schindler admitted in later testimony that Terri must have been about eleven when she made these remarks, an admission that obviously weakened her claim that Terri would not want the feeding tube withdrawn. A fifth witness, a friend of Terri's, also testified that Terri had made remarks about the Karen Quinlan case indicating she thought her ventilator should not be withdrawn but Judge Greer stated that he did not find this witness credible because she said that Terri's remarks about the Karen Quinlan case were made in 1982 when, the judge pointed out, it seems more likely that they were made in 1975–1976 when the Quinlan case was in the news.

In February 2000 Judge George Greer responded to Michael's 1998 petition by ruling that there was indeed "clear and convincing evidence" showing that Terri was in PVS and that she would choose to stop the medical nutrition and hydration if she could make the decision. He authorized Michael, her legal guardian, to request withdrawal of the medical nutrition and hydration.

This could have ended the story but did not. Before looking at the dispute that dragged on for more than another five years and involved numerous state and federal judges, the U.S. Supreme Court, many politicians including President George W. Bush, Governor Jeb Bush, Florida legislators, members of the U.S. Senate and House of Representatives, as well members of several very vocal groups that supported Terri's parents, we will consider the case from an ethical point of view.

Ethical Analysis

Situational awareness. We are aware of the following facts in the Schiavo story.

1. By 1998, thanks to a feeding tube, Terri had been living more than eight years in what had been diagnosed as PVS. For the first few years her husband, who was her legally designated guardian, and her parents tried many therapies to help Terri regain awareness. They all failed.

2. After eight years Michael wanted the medical nutrition and hydration stopped because it was not providing any benefit that Terri could experience and because she had said that she would not want to be kept alive on life support if she became severely compromised.

3. Judge George Greer ruled that Michael's request was allowable under Florida law because there was "clear and convincing evidence" that Terri would not want to be kept alive this way.

We are also aware of these good and bad features (the values and disvalues) in the case.

1. Terri's life, severely damaged as it was, had definite human value, and her death would be unfortunate even though her brain was so gravely damaged that she had irreversibly lost all awareness.

2. Providing nutrition and hydration by feeding tube caused no burden or benefit for her because she could not experience anything.

3. Withdrawing the nutrition and hydration would cause Terri's parents tremendous distress because they had come to believe, among other things, that Michael no longer had their daughter's

best interests at heart, that Terri might not have been in PVS or, if she was, might have benefited from some additional therapy, that she never said she would not want to be kept alive this way, and even if she had said it this was inconsistent with her beliefs.

4. By 1998 Michael was the husband of a woman whose body has been vegetative for eight years. This is a terrible tragedy for her and her parents, but it is also a tragedy for him. He has lost her spousal companionship, and he has also lost the ability to live a normal life. Before feeding tubes became widely used he would have been widowed for years by now, certainly a tragedy for a young person, but it would have allowed him to do what many young widowed people would want to do: grieve and then seek another marriage partner and perhaps start a family. Ironically, despite a growing awareness that is pointed out in chapter 4 showing how the well-being of family is an important factor in health care decision making, there is practically no mention of the continuous damage to Michael's life that maintaining his wife's totally vegetative body is causing him. Michael is in his thirties and trapped in what has become only the formality of a marriage.

Prudential Reasoning in the Terri Schiavo Story

Patient's perspective. Terri had no perspective at this point but had, according to her husband, expressed some ideas about not wanting to be kept alive indefinitely in a vegetative state. These ideas are not, as was pointed out in the Cruzan story, unusual. Many people say that they would not want their vegetative body kept alive for years with no reasonable hope of any cognitive recovery because of extensive brain damage. In fact as more and more people make their wishes known to their families and physicians, it is almost unheard of for people to indicate they want their vegetative nonsentient bodies kept alive for years after suffering such extensive brain damage that they would never again be aware of anything, not even intense pain.

Proxy's perspective. Terri's husband Michael first thought that aggressive treatment might help Terri, but eight years later, when it did not, he thought it reasonable to withdraw the feeding tube, especially in view of the fact that she had indicated that she didn't want to be kept alive indefinitely if she was severely damaged and no recovery was expected. He believed, despite her receiving more therapy designed to restore feeling in her body than most PVS patients receive, that prolonging her vegetative body with a feeding tube made no sense anymore.

Parents' perspective. At first the Schindlers accepted the diagnosis of PVS and supported Michael's efforts to reverse it. By 1998, however, they had come to believe that PVS was a misdiagnosis and that Terri would want the feeding tube continued. They perceived Terri as minimally conscious with hope of some recovery, and they saw Michael as someone who was neglecting her and couldn't wait for her to die. If parents come to believe their child has not been correctly diagnosed and has a chance to recover, then their fight to continue nutrition and hydration is understandable. After all, no medical diagnosis is absolutely certain. The history of medicine is full of surprising outcomes, some good, some not so good. Good parents will want to do everything they can to give their children a chance for a good life. The moral hazard, of course, is conflating wishful thinking with a reasonable hope of improvement. Good moral decisions are not based on wishful thinking but on experience and critical thinking. That's the best we can do.

The arguments that Terri was not in PVS or that she would want feeding continued for years or decades even if she was in PVS or that she had some reasonable hope of significant recovery or that withdrawing medical life support providing no benefit a patient can experience is homicide are all unhelpful arguments unless supported by cogent reasons. The Schindlers suffered a great tragedy when Terri collapsed, and everyone can understand something of their suffering, their love for their daughter, and their desire to do everything to see that she could recover. But moral reasoning needs to be rooted in facts and advanced in a reasonable way that respects the positions of others who may disagree with us but have reasons for their position. It is hard to find the Schindlers' decision to continue the feeding tube after eight years of PVS despite extraordinary early treatments a wise decision from the perspective of virtue ethics. Given what we know about the chances of recovery for patients in PVS for many years, the decision of Nancy Cruzan's parents to withdraw nutrition and hydration from their daughter represents a more reasonable response than the decision of Terri Schiavo's parents to make every effort to force its continuation for their daughter.

Guardian *ad litem*'s perspective.   Richard Pearse reported that Terri was in PVS with no hope of recovery but recommended that the feeding tube be continued because there was no clear and convincing evidence of her wishes. He pointed out that there was no living will and that Michael had a conflict of interest: He would inherit Terri's estate, which Pearse reported was then over $700,000, if she died. He also pointed out that the Schindlers would have the same conflict of interest if they were made the guardians.

From a legal perspective attorney Pearse's position is understandable. If a state law requires "clear and convincing evidence" that a person in PVS had previously indicated she would not want a feeding tube, there is reason to conclude that this standard might not be met if the only evidence is testimony by her husband, who stands to inherit around $700,000 if she dies, and his brother and his brother's wife.

However, the appointment of a guardian *ad litem* is primarily to protect the interests of the person with respect to the matter in litigation. It would not have been inappropriate for Pearse to report that, in one important sense, Terri had no interests at stake. People correctly diagnosed in PVS really do not have interests. Nothing that happens to them makes a difference to them now or will make a difference to them at any future time.

Judge's perspective.   Judge Greer correctly defined his role as determining, based on evidence presented to the court, two fundamental issues: whether Terri was in PVS and whether there was clear and convincing evidence that she would not want to be kept alive in these circumstances and would, if she could, ask that the feeding tube be withdrawn. He decided that she was in PVS and that there was sufficient evidence that she would not want the medical nutrition and hydration continued. He authorized Michael to have it stopped. There were good reasons for his decision, and it was upheld on appeal.

The Aftermath

The story does not end here, however, because the Schindlers appealed Judge Greer's ruling. When the Florida appeals court affirmed the decision, they then appealed to the Florida Supreme Court, which declined to review the case. The Schindlers then appealed the decision to the U.S. Supreme Court, which also declined to hear the case. On April 24, 2001, more than fourteen months after Judge Greer's ruling, Terri's medical nutrition and hydration were finally withdrawn at the request of Michael, her husband and legal guardian.

The Schindlers immediately went back to the appeals court, claiming that they had new evidence undermining Michael's claim that he knew what Terri wanted and arguing that there were new treatments that might restore some cognitive function. Two days later, on April 26, the appeals court ordered the feeding resumed to allow consideration of these issues. The court then scheduled a hearing to determine whether Terri was truly in PVS and whether any treatment could improve her condition. The Schindlers also filed a complaint of abuse against Michael, the first of nine such complaints in the next three years. These complaints accused him of neglecting her hygiene and dental care, poisoning her, and causing her physical harm. Florida state agencies investigated all their complaints and found no evidence supporting any of them.

To evaluate the Schindlers' claims the court asked five physicians to examine Terri, two chosen by the Schindlers, two by Michael, and one by the judge. They all testified in October 2002, more than thirty months after Judge Greer's original ruling. Not surprisingly, the two experts chosen by the Schindlers, one of whom was a radiologist and the other a board-certified neurologist, testified that Terri was not in PVS. The neurologist, Dr. William Hammesfahr, also testified that he had treated thousands of patients with brain injury, including PVS patients, and had achieved some success with hyperbaric oxygenation therapy (HBOT). However, he could not produce any evidence documenting the success of this novel treatment, and there are no studies showing that it works for patients in PVS. The other three neurologists all testified that Terri was in PVS and could never regain any awareness.

The judge again concluded, on November 22, 2002, that there was "clear and convincing evidence" indicating that Terri was in PVS and would not want feeding tubes continued in this situation. He ordered that the feeding should be stopped as of January 3, 2003. The Schindlers appealed his decision once again so the withdrawal of nutrition and hydration was delayed. On June 6, 2003, the Florida appeals court again affirmed the lower court's decision and directed Judge Greer to schedule another hearing "solely for the purpose of entering a new order scheduling the removal of the nutrition and hydration tube." The Schindler's appealed this decision to the Florida Supreme Court, but once again it declined to review the case.

At the hearing on September 17, 2003, Judge Greer again ordered withdrawal of medical nutrition and hydration, and on October 15 the feeding tube was disconnected once again. Now the case leapt into the national spotlight as busloads of demonstrators gathered outside the facility where Terri was a patient and the national media intensified its coverage of the story.

Having failed to succeed in the courts, the Schindlers, with strong vocal support from conservative religious groups, turned to the legislative branch and to Governor Jeb Bush. On October 21, 2003, the Florida legislature rushed to pass what became known as "Terri's law." The law authorized the governor to override a court order allowing withdrawal of medical nutrition and hydration if (1) the patient left no written instructions, (2) a court has determined that the patient is in PVS, (3) nutrition and hydration have already been withheld, and (4) a member of the patient's family has challenged the withholding. Governor Jeb Bush immediately signed the bill and then ordered the feeding tube reconnected. After six days Terri Schiavo was back on the feeding tube.

On October 31, 2003, the court appointed Jay Wolfson, a professor at the University of Southern Florida recognized for his expertise in health care financing, guardian *ad litem* for thirty days and instructed him to prepare a report with recommendations for the court and the governor. He met with Michael, the Schindlers, Terri's siblings, the clinic staff, attorneys for both sides, and Governor Jeb Bush himself, and he reviewed the medical and legal records, which by now, according to his account, had grown to some 30,000 pages.

He reported that Terri had been repeatedly diagnosed as being in PVS after a coma that lasted two months and that the Schindlers had not challenged the appointment of Michael as her guardian or the diagnosis of PVS in the early years. He concurred with the courts that the medical evidence had produced "clear and convincing evidence" that Terri was in PVS and that her husband had acted in accord with her wishes and her best interests when he sought to have the medical nutrition and hydration withdrawn. However, he also stated that the governor's order to continue feeding under Terri's law should stand if there was any valid evidence indicating a reasonable hope that therapy could help Terri swallow or if there was any evidence indicating even minimal cognitive function. He also recommended that a permanent guardian *ad litem* be appointed to represent Terri's interests, but this was never done.

On May 5, 2004, the Florida appeals court struck down "Terri's Law" that had been signed into law in October 2003 by Governor Jeb Bush on the grounds that it violated the state constitution. Governor Bush appealed this ruling to the Florida Supreme Court. He lost again, on September 23, 2004, when the Florida Supreme Court upheld the appeals court ruling in a seven–zero decision, thus nullifying Governor Bush's order to provide nutrition and hydration of Terri by feeding tubes. The governor then appealed to the U.S. Supreme Court, but he lost again; in January 2005 it declined to hear his appeal. After the Supreme Court action, the trial court judge, George W. Greer, again ordered the medical nutrition and hydration stopped, this time as of March 18, 2005, more than five years after his original ruling. He was picketed and threatened with death and had to be protected by armed guards.

The Schindlers and their supporters tried to reopen the case in the Florida courts, claiming among other things that the 2004 statement of Pope John Paul II indicating that people in PVS should, in principle, be fed with feeding tubes, applied to Terri because she is a Catholic. (This papal statement is discussed in the next section of this chapter.) When the courts declined to reconsider the case, the Schindlers and their supporters turned again to the Florida legislature and asked for a new law that would prevent the feeding tube withdrawal but be so written that the state courts could not declare it unconstitutional. The Florida House actually passed such a bill, but it failed to win approval in the state Senate.

On March 18, 2005, Terri's feeding tube was disconnected once again. Unable to make headway in the Florida courts or in the state legislature, the Schindlers and their supporters next turned to Congress where they found support for passing a federal law that would allow them to pursue their case in the federal court system. On March 20 the U.S. Senate did pass such a bill and sent it to the House. That same evening the House began debating the bill at 9 p.m., with live coverage of the heated debate by C-SPAN. The bill allowing the Schindlers to present their case in federal court passed shortly after midnight and President Bush, waiting at his ranch in Texas, signed the bill into law about 1 a.m. on March 21, 2005.

Empowered by the new federal law, the Schindlers immediately asked the federal district court in Florida to issue a temporary restraining order that would require resumption of nutrition and hydration. However, a U.S. district court judge denied their request. The Schindlers appealed his decision to the federal appeals court in Atlanta (the 11th Circuit Court), but the Circuit Court upheld the district court's decision. It not only rejected the appeal but the chief justice, a conservative republican, wrote that the law passed by a republican congress and signed by the republican president was actually in violation of the U.S. Constitution. The Schindlers then appealed this decision to the U.S. Supreme Court, but on March 24 it declined once again to intervene. The court battles were over.

Meanwhile, back in Florida Governor Bush suggested on March 23 that he might order state law enforcement authorities to force the resumption of Terri's feeding. Judge Greer immediately issued an emergency temporary restraining order to prevent the state from doing this.

Terri Schiavo died of dehydration on March 31, 2005, as noisy protests, TV cameras, and police surrounded the site. The chaotic scene was much like the scene outside the hospital when Nancy Cruzan died in 1990. Terri was forty-one years old; she had been in a vegetative state for about fifteen years and might still be in that state if the feeding tube had not been disconnected. Her autopsy report was made public on June 15, 2005. It showed that her brain had shrunk to about half its normal size and was so seriously damaged that she had no capacity for any awareness. It also showed she must have been totally blind, yet the Schindlers had claimed repeatedly that she recognized them when they entered her room. The autopsy clearly confirmed the diagnosis of PVS and reported that her body showed no evidence of abuse or neglect, as the Schindlers had repeatedly claimed.

Ethical Reflection

Stopping the nutrition and hydration for a patient who has been repeatedly diagnosed for years as being in PVS is a morally reasonable decision. It is very difficult to argue that keeping vegetative bodies fed and hydrated for years at significant expense when there is no reasonable hope of recovery is wise, especially since we can assume most people would not want their vegetative body treated this way. Some will say that to maintain the nutrition and hydration is wise because it protects vulnerable human life but the real issue is whether years or even decades of providing nutrition and hydration to vegetative bodies is a *reasonable* protection of human life, especially since few people ever insist on it in their advance directives or in their conversations with loved ones. In fact the opposite seems to be true: Most people would not want to be sustained in this state for years until they die.

We should note that the courts, in their effort to protect vulnerable human life, invariably look for some evidence that the person would not have wanted to be kept alive indefinitely this way. In so doing they assume that the default position should be to provide nutrition and hydration for patients in PVS, and this default position can be defeated only if there is evidence the patient would not want his or her vegetative body sustained this way for years. There are some good reasons for this approach: The courts need to be cautious, and it may be better that they look for some indication that the person would not have wanted to be maintained in PVS for years before allowing withdrawal.

In moral deliberation, however, the more reasonable default position is the opposite: Keeping totally vegetative bodies alive for years and even decades is not a reasonable medical response, and we can assume that most people would not want their vegetative bodies sustained indefinitely when there is no reasonable hope of recovering any awareness. Thus, withdrawing nutrition and hydration from long-term PVS patients is reasonable even without any evidence of what the person would have wanted. In fact even if a person in PVS had left an advance directive insisting on medical nutrition and hydration after lapsing into PVS with no hope of regaining even minimal consciousness, a reasonable case could be made that the wise thing to do would be to stop the tubal feeding at some point, perhaps after a year or so, despite the advance directive because the person's wishes are so unreasonable.

AN EMERGING CONTROVERSY: THE VATICAN AND FEEDING TUBES

Toward the end of the Schiavo story a controversy erupted over remarks made by Pope John Paul II in a March 2004 address to participants at an international conference on "Life-Sustaining Treatments and the Vegetative State." The Pope stated that removing medical nutrition and hydration that is providing nourishment for PVS patients is morally wrong and tantamount to euthanasia. Supporters of Terri's feeding tube began citing the papal statement in their arguments for continuing the medical nutrition and hydration for Terri, who was a Catholic. The key language of the 2004 papal statement is as follows:

> I should like particularly to underline how the administration of water and food, even when provided by artificial means, always represents a *natural means* of preserving life, not a *medical act*. Its use, furthermore, should be considered, in principle, *ordinary* and *proportionate*, and as such morally obligatory, insofar as and until it is seen to have attained its proper finality, which in the present case consists in providing nourishment to the patient and the alleviation of his suffering (emphasis in the original). . . . Death by starvation or dehydration is, in fact, the only possible outcome as a result of their withdrawal. In this sense it ends up becoming, if done knowingly and willingly, true and proper euthanasia by omission.

Those familiar with the Catholic moral tradition will see important echoes in the emphasized words of the papal statement. In general, Catholic teaching has traditionally held that people are obliged to use *natural* means of preserving life but may forgo *medical* means in certain cases. Also, Catholic teaching has traditionally held that people are obliged to use *ordinary* means of preserving life but may forgo *extraordinary* means. Finally, Catholic teaching has more recently held that people are obliged to use *proportionate* means of preserving life but may forgo *disproportionate* means. By describing nutrition and hydration supplied by feeding tubes as "natural," "ordinary," and "proportionate" the papal statement comes down squarely on the side of holding that there is "in principle" a moral obligation to use feeding tubes for people in PVS "insofar as and until it is seen to have attained its proper finality"; that is, as long as the body tolerates the nutrition and hydration.

The papal statement prompted widespread reaction and considerable debate among Catholic moral theologians. Some welcomed it, some were puzzled by it, and some thought it should be ignored. In an effort to clarify the situation, the United States Conference of Catholic Bishops (USCCB) submitted two questions to the Congregation for the Doctrine of the Faith (CDF) on July 11, 2005. The CDF responded on August 1, 2007, and noted that its response was approved by Pope Benedict XVI.

The first question the USCCB asked was whether the administration of food or water by artificial means to a person in a vegetative state is morally obligatory except when it cannot be assimilated or when it causes "significant physical discomfort." The CDF answered "Yes." It explained that nutrition and hydration by artificial means is, "in principle, an ordinary and proportionate means of preserving life" and is therefore obligatory as long as it accomplishes its finality or purpose, which is the hydration and nutrition of the patient. It should be noted that the USCCB's inclusion of a "physical discomfort" exception for PVS patients in their question is puzzling; by definition patients in vegetative state do not, as vegetables do not, experience any discomfort or, for that matter, any comfort.

The second question the USCCB asked was whether nutrition and hydration supplied by artificial means can be discontinued when competent physicians judge with moral certainty that the patient will never recover consciousness. The CDF answered "No." It stated again that such patients must receive all ordinary and proportionate treatment, which includes, "in principle, the administration of water and food even by artificial means." The CDF commentary noted only three exceptions to the obligation to provide medical nutrition and hydration: (1) physical impossibility such as the unavailability of feeding tubes and rehabilitation facilities to care for people with them, (2) the inability of a patient's body to assimilate the nutrition, and (3) medical complications caused by the nutrition.

Some of the debate among moral theologians has centered on the papal qualifying phrase "in principle," which seemed to indicate there could be exceptions to providing medical nutrition and hydration for PVS patients. The challenge, then, would be to identify the exceptions. According to the USCCB Commentary on the 2004 papal allocution and the 2007 CDF response, however, those exceptions are limited to the following two for PVS patients: either the patient in PVS is in a part of the world where feeding tubes are not available because of poverty or limited medical care facilities, or the vegetative patient's body cannot assimilate the nutrition and hydration. The USCCB commentary mentions a third exception: The medical nutrition and hydration may be excessively burdensome or cause significant physical discomfort, but this puzzling exception is irrelevant for PVS patients who are beyond experiencing burdens or discomfort. The USCCB Commentary also makes it clear that the Vatican conceptualizes providing nutrition and hydration by feeding tubes or lines not as a medical treatment but as a natural way of preserving life. As we explained at the beginning of this chapter, once medical nutrition and hydration is classified as something natural and not as a medical treatment, the moral conclusion that it must be provided if it is available and can be assimilated follows immediately.

The CDF statements and the USCCB Commentary, however, have not resolved the issue for many Catholic theologians and for many people working in Catholic hospitals and health care facilities. Several prominent Catholic moral theologians have continued to object to a position requiring PVS patients such as Terri Schiavo to be kept alive indefinitely with feeding tubes, and two bishops, Cardinal Rigali of Philadelphia and Bishop Lori of Bridgeport, the chair of the USCCB Committee on Doctrine, have been publishing articles disagreeing with positions taken by these theologians.

The controversy will undoubtedly continue for some time, especially since the American bishops at their semiannual meeting in June 2008 have directed their Committee on Doctrine to revise the guidelines for medical nutrition and hydration in their official *Ethical and Religious Directives* that govern practices in Catholic hospitals. Underlying the controversy is a debate about moral reasoning that we identified in chapter 1: Whether the goal of living a good life is better achieved by employing situation-sensitive practical wisdom—the virtue of prudential reasoning—or by employing definitions such as "the artificial administration of nutrition and hydration is a natural, ordinary, and proportionate means of preserving life" followed by action-guiding rules such as "people are always obliged to employ ordinary, natural, and proportionate means to preserve life whenever possible."

ETHICAL REFLECTIONS

What ethical reasons do the opponents of withdrawing medical nourishment from irreversibly unconscious people give for their position? In general, several common threads run through their arguments. The first is a rights-based argument. They accept the political philosophy of Thomas Hobbes and John Locke and build an ethic on the right to life. It was this right, Hobbes argued, that secured everyone's self-preservation. If everyone has a right to life, then no one can kill anyone else. This right also gave the state its authority and power because the state must preserve this right to life, especially when the person cannot defend it himself. The government in all its branches must therefore oppose any movement that undermines or might undermine anyone's right to life.

A second thread often found in the arguments of those opposing the withdrawal of medical nutrition and hydration from people in PVS is the fear of a slippery slope—that is, the fear that allowing the withdrawal of nutrition will inexorably lead to other actions they consider immoral. Most of those opposed to withdrawing nutrition from patients in PVS know the nutrition is of no interest or benefit to the patient. Their concern lies elsewhere. They fear these withdrawals will open the door to euthanasia, which they vehemently oppose. And they fear, as the *Cruzan* case suggests, that withdrawal of nutrition from a human being in a vegetative state will open the door to abortion, especially the abortion of fetuses that have not yet achieved any awareness and therefore exist in a vegetative state.

A third thread running through the arguments of those opposing withdrawal of nutrition from PVS patients is the conviction that any consideration of the quality of a patient's life is irrelevant to moral questions about preserving that life. In other words, it is not relevant that the life of a PVS patient has deteriorated to a purely vegetative state because of extensive neurological damage. Human life is human life; its value is intrinsic. Most people embracing the right-to-life approach in ethics allow no room for judgments about the quality of that life.

These arguments will not appear convincing in the ethical approach inspired by Aristotle and Aquinas that we have been employing. Making the political doctrine of rights the foundation of ethics is not without serious problems. It is not at all clear, for example, where these rights, never really noticed until several centuries ago, originated. Some say they come from nature (they are "natural" or "human" rights); others speak as if they come from God or the "Creator." And a moral philosophy based on rights frequently ends up in irresolvable conflict. One reason the abortion debate remains so persistent is that both sides rely on a rights-based position. One side bases its position on the right to life; the other side bases its position on the right to choose. The result is gridlock. The rapidly emerging euthanasia debate is now trapped in a similar stalemate: Many opponents of euthanasia rely on the right to life; proponents rely on the right to choose and the right to die.

The slippery-slope argument is also weak. History simply cannot be predicted. The euthanasia practiced in Germany during the 1930s, for example, did not slide into an abortion movement. In fact, there was a strong antiabortion movement in the Germany of the 1940s, although it was not motivated by any respect for human life. There is simply no way to say that withdrawing medical nourishment from PVS patients will be followed by more abortions or by euthanasia. In fact, the contrary can be argued: The willingness to withdraw unreasonable life-prolonging treatments weakens the fear of losing control that motivates some supporters of euthanasia. Certainly, there are slippery slopes in life, and some have a limited validity in moral reasonings, but sometimes we cannot avoid facing a slippery slope. When this happens, we can only proceed with caution and take the necessary steps to avoid sliding out of control into moral disaster.

Finally, the refusal of any quality-of-life assessment in moral judgments about human life is simply impossible. Certainly, making quality-of-life assessments is open to abuse, but we cannot do good ethics without considering the quality of life in some cases. The quality of life is an important aspect of the ethical question in many situations; it cannot be ignored in any ethics of prudence and prudential moral judgment. It is one of the important circumstances, and ethical judgments ignoring the quality of life are hobbled by their ignorance of this significant feature in the situation.

SUGGESTED READINGS

An excellent, albeit somewhat dated, introduction to the ethical dilemmas of medical nutrition is Joanne Lynn, ed., 1986, *By No Extraordinary Means: The Choice to Forgo Life-Sustaining Food and Water*, Bloomington: Indiana University Press. It includes essays on the medical procedures, the moral and legal issues, and the religious perspectives. Also helpful is Richard McCormick, "Nutrition-Hydration: The New Euthanasia?" which appears as chapter 21 in his 1989, *The Critical Calling: Reflections on Moral Dilemmas since Vatican II*, Washington, DC: Georgetown University Press; Norman Cantor, "The

Permanently Unconscious Patient, Non-Feeding and Euthanasia," *American Journal of Law & Medicine* 1989, *15*, 381–437; William Curran, "Defining Appropriate Medical Care: Providing Nutrients and Hydration for the Dying," *New England Journal of Medicine* 1985, *313*, 940–42; Rebecca Dresser and Eugene Boisaubin, "Ethics, Law, and Nutritional Support," *Archives of Internal Medicine* 1985, *145*, 122–24; Robert Steinbrook and Bernard Lo, "Artificial Feeding—Solid Ground, Not a Slippery Slope," *New England Journal of Medicine* 1988, *318*, 286–90.

Some health care facilities are attempting to develop institutional policies on nutrition and hydration similar to the policies for cardiopulmonary resuscitation. For an interesting example, see Monica Koschuta et al., "Development of an Institutional Policy on Artificial Nutrition and Hydration," *Kennedy Institute of Ethics Journal* 1991, *1*, 133–38. The authors trace the development of the policy at Hospice of Washington. The actual policy is published, along with a brief commentary by John Robertson.

The court of appeals decision in the Clarence Herbert case is *Barber v. The Superior Court of Los Angeles County*, 147 Cal. App. 3d 1006 (1983). Dr. Neil Barber was one of the two physicians whose murder charge was reinstated by the Superior Court of Los Angeles after a magistrate ordered it dismissed. The Court of Appeals decision directed the Superior Court to vacate its order and prohibited it from taking any further action against the physicians. Good discussions of the case are found in David Meyers, "Legal Aspects of Withdrawing Nourishment from an Incurably Ill Patient," *Archives of Internal Medicine* 1985, *145*, 125–28; and Bernard Lo, "The Death of Clarence Herbert: Withdrawing Care Is Not Murder," *Annals of Internal Medicine* 1984, *101*, 248–51. The Meyers article also includes an analysis of the Conroy case.

The New Jersey Supreme Court decision in the Claire Conroy case is *In re Conroy* 486 A.2d. 1209 (1985). Among the many commentaries are these: Bernard Lo and Laurie Dornbrand, "The Case of Claire Conroy: Will Administrative Review Safeguard Incompetent Patients?" *Annals of Internal Medicine* 1986, *104*, 869–73; and the six articles that make up Part V of Lynn, *By No Extraordinary Means*.

The 1984 California Superior Court decision that refused to allow withdrawal of Elizabeth Bouvia's feeding tube lest hospital staff become accomplices in her suicide is *Bouvia v. County of Riverside*, No. 159780 (Sup. Ct. Cal.), 1984. The later decision allowing her to forgo tubal feeding based on the right of a competent person to refuse medical treatment, including treatment furnishing nutrition and hydration, is *Bouvia v. Superior Court* (Glenchur), 179 Cal. App. 3d. 1127 (1986). For commentaries see George Annas, "Elizabeth Bouvia: Whose Space Is This Anyway?" *Hastings Center Report* 1986, *16* (April), 24–25; and Robert Steinbrook and Bernard Lo, "The Case of Elizabeth Bouvia: Starvation, Suicide, or Problem Patient?" *Archives of Internal Medicine* 1986, *146*, 161–64.

The decision of New York's highest court, the Court of Appeals, in the Mary O'Connor case is *In re O'Connor*, 531 N.E.2d 607 (1988). Bernard Lo et al., "Family Decision Making on Trial: Who Decides for Incompetent Patients?" *New England Journal of Medicine* 1990, *322*, 1228–31, discuss this case and that of Nancy Cruzan. For other commentaries see Daniel Gindes, "Judicial Postponement of Death Recognition: The Tragic Case of Mary O'Connor," *American Journal of Law and Medicine* 1989, *15*, 301–31; and George Annas, "Precatory Prediction and Mindless Mimicry: The Case of Mary O'Connor," *Hastings Center Report* 1988, *18* (December), 31–33. The Martin case is *In re Martin*, 538 N.W.2d 399 (1995). For a commentary see Rebecca Dresser, "Still Troubled: *In re Martin*," *Hastings Center Report* 1996, *26* (July–August), 21–22.

The U.S. Supreme Court decision in the Cruzan case is *Cruzan v. Director, Missouri Dept. of Health*, 110 S. Ct. 2841 (1990). The commentaries on the case and the Supreme Court decision are innumerable. Some examples include these: George Annas, "The Insane Root Takes Reason Prisoner," *Hastings Center Report* 1989, *19* (January–February), 29–31, and "Nancy Cruzan and the Right to Die," *New England Journal of Medicine* 1990, *323*, 670–73; Marcia Angell, "Prisoners of Technology: The Case of Nancy Cruzan," *New England Journal of Medicine* 1990, *322*, 1226–28; Lois Snyder, "Life, Death, and the American College of Physicians: The Cruzan Case," *Annals of Internal Medicine* 1990, *112*, 802–4; David Brushwood, "Need for Clear and Convincing Evidence of a Patient's Wishes before Artificial Nutrition and Hydration May Be Withdrawn," *American Journal of Hospital Pharmacy* 1990, *47*, 2720–22; Alan Meisel, "Lessons from Cruzan," *Journal of Clinical Ethics* 1990, *1*, 245–50; and Robert Weir and Larry Gostin, "Decisions to Abate Life-Sustaining Treatment for Nonautonomous Patients: Ethical Standards and Legal Liability for Physicians after *Cruzan*," *JAMA* 1990, *264*, 1846–53. See also the four brief articles by William Colby, Pete Busalacchi, Charles Baron, and Joanne Lynn and Jacqueline Glover in *Hastings Center Report* 1990, 20 (September–October), 5–11.

The literature on the Schiavo story is very extensive, as any search online will show. A key site is the Schindlers' *terrisfight.org*. See also Robert and Mary Schindler, 2006, *A Life That Matters: A Lesson for Us All*, New York: Grand Central Publishing; and David Gibbs, 2006, *Fighting for Dear Life: The Untold Story of Terri Schiavo and What It Means for All of Us*, Minneapolis: Bethany House. For the perspective of Terri's husband see Michael Schiavo, 2006, *Terri: The Truth*, New York: Dutton Publishing. An interesting article by Jay Wolfson, the last court-appointed guardian *ad litem*, is entitled "Erring on the Side of Theresa Schiavo: Reflections of the Special Guardian" and appears in the *Hastings Center Report* 2005, *35* (May–June), 16–19. For the finding of Judge Greer that disagreements over money played a major role in causing the rift between Terri's husband and her parents see *In re: the Guardianship of Theresa Marie Schiavo*, File No. 902908GD-003; a summary of the legal proceedings is at *Schindler v. Schiavo, 851 So2d (Fla Dist. Ct. App. 2003)*.

The English translation of Pope John Paul II's statement on treating people in PVS can be found on www.vatican.va and in *The National Catholic Bioethics Quarterly* 2004, *4*, 367–79 and 573–76. The reply from the Vatican to the two questions submitted by the United States Catholic Conference (USCC) is also in the *National Catholic Bioethics Quarterly* 2008, *8*, 123–27. The USCCB commentary on the papal allocution and the CDF responses is at usccb.org/comm./hydrationcommentary. For examples of Catholic theologians supporting the morality of withdrawing nutrition and hydration from PVS patients, see Thomas Shannon and James Walter, "Assisted Nutrition and Hydration and the Catholic Tradition: The Case of Terri Schiavo," *Theological Studies* 2005, *66*, 651–62, and "Implications of the Papal Allocation on Feeding Tubes" by the same authors in the *Hastings Center Report* 2004, *34* (July–August), 18–20; Kevin O'Rourke, "Reflections on the Papal Allocution for PVS Patients" in Christopher Tollefsen, ed., 2008, *Artificial Nutrition and Hydration: The New Catholic Debate*, Dordrecht, The Netherlands: Springer Publishing, pp. 165–78. See also Ronald Hamel and James Walter, eds., 2007, *Artificial Nutrition and Hydration and the Permanently Unconscious Patient: The Catholic Debate*, Washington, DC: Georgetown University Press, for a collection of excellent articles; and Thomas Shannon, "'Unbind Him and Let Him Go' (JN 11:44): Ethical Issues in the Determination of Proportionate and Disproportionate Treatment," *Theological Studies* 2008, *69*, 894–917, for a good overview of the debate in the Catholic context.

TEN

Reproductive Issues

THERE IS SOME DISAGREEMENT about just when a pregnancy begins. Some think a woman is pregnant as soon as an ovum in her body is fertilized. This view, however, gives rise to several difficulties. First since more than one-third of fertilized ova fail to implant, it forces us to conclude that the number of spontaneous abortions is quite high—several million every year in the United States alone. Second, it conflicts with how we think about the embryo transfer that occurs during in vitro fertilization (IVF). A woman undergoing IVF procedures is not considered to be pregnant when the embryos are transferred to her uterus—she is considered to be pregnant only if one of the embryos implants. And when embryos fail to implant, which is more often the case, the failures are not considered miscarriages or spontaneous abortions but unsuccessful pregnancy attempts.

For purposes of discussion we will say pregnancy begins when a fertilized ovum implants in a woman's body. Pregnancy is something that happens to a woman, not an ovum. It seems reasonable to say that a woman becomes pregnant when her body "conceives" or "takes hold" of the fertilized ovum. The Latin etymology of conception is *concipio*, and the roots of *concipio* are *com* and *capio*. These roots indicate conception connotes a grasping, a laying hold of, a taking in. This suggests a pregnancy begins when the woman conceives, that is, when her body grasps the fertilized ovum.

The decision to consider implantation as the beginning of pregnancy does not mean the embryo is less than human before implantation. A human embryo is certainly a new human life before it implants, but the emergence of new human life does not mean a woman is pregnant. The human life of children resulting from IVF, for example, began in the laboratory, but their mothers did not become pregnant until the embryos were transferred and became attached to the uterus. The question of when a new human life begins and the question of when a pregnancy begins are two different questions. There is nothing inconsistent about saying that a new human life begins at fertilization and also saying that the pregnancy does not begin until implantation. And as we noted in chapter 6, there is nothing inconsistent about saying that a new one of us does not begin until some time after both fertilization and implantation.

The destruction of an embryo before implantation, whether that embryo is in the laboratory or in the woman's body, is a morally significant action. The deliberate destruction of human life is a serious matter and always immoral unless justified by an adequate reason. Destruction of an embryo before implantation, however, is not what we mean by abortion. Because abortion presupposes that a pregnancy has begun, destroying an embryo before implantation, however unethical it might be, is not really an abortion.

We will consider abortion in the next chapter. In this chapter we examine the techniques and technologies affecting reproduction. In the first part we will look at the medical interventions designed to prevent pregnancy (that is, contraception and sterilization), and in the second part we will consider the medical interventions designed to cause pregnancy.

CONTRACEPTION AND STERILIZATION

Contraception—a better word might have been "contra-conception"—describes any behavior where the intention is to prevent pregnancy. Thus, a condom or a tubal ligation is contraceptive, but so is abstinence or noncoital sex when the intention is to avoid pregnancy. In ordinary discourse, however, we usually associate contraception with heterosexual intercourse, and we use the term contraception to describe the effort to prevent conception resulting from heterosexual intercourse.

Some do not consider contraception and sterilization to be issues of morality. Indeed, most modern moral philosophers and health care ethicists scarcely mention contraception and sterilization. If they do mention sterilization, their concern is coerced sterilization—the sterilization of the retarded or of criminals or of irresponsible mothers.

Yet there are at least three reasons why we should consider contraception and sterilization the subject of moral reflection. First, from its very beginning until the mid-twentieth century, Christianity, the most influential religious tradition of our culture, always condemned contraception as immoral, and a few Christian churches still do. Since there is nothing in the Bible about contraception, thoughtful people will ask why Christians were so opposed to it.

Second, until recently many states in the United States had laws condemning the distribution and, in some cases, the use of contraceptives. Since laws are passed by elected representatives of the people, the laws against selling or using contraceptives suggested that many people thought something was wrong with contraception.

Third, many contraceptive interventions, and all sterilization procedures, are medical interventions posing some risk to the person, and whenever we do anything that risks damage to life, we are faced with an ethical issue. We now know that some contraceptive interventions have caused serious damage to women. Many women, for example, suffered great harm from using the Dalkon Shield, a type of intrauterine device (IUD). Behavior that risks causing damage to life is ethical only if we have adequate or proportionate moral reasons to balance the risks.

Contraception in History

Contraception has a long history. Ancient Egyptian, Greek, and Latin texts all reveal attempts to prevent conception, some of them quite crude. Contraception was also the subject of some early ethical concerns, especially when the survival of a people depended on reproduction. In a society needing a high birth rate to survive, preventing pregnancy was sometimes seen as immoral because it undermined the social good.

By the second century the Romans, despite their toleration of infanticide and the exposure of unwanted children, had laws against the ingestion of drugs thought to prevent conception or cause miscarriage. The reason for these laws is not entirely clear. Certainly the Romans were concerned about the declining birth rate as the empire deteriorated, but they may also have been concerned about the serious side effects women experienced from these rather crude, and often ineffective, drugs.

The Hebrew Bible emphasized having children, but it said nothing about the immorality of preventing them by contraception, probably because it was not widely practiced. The book of Genesis encourages people to increase and multiply, and most of the great biblical heroes reproduced with both wives and concubines. The twelve sons of Jacob destined to become the patriarchs of the twelve tribes of Israel, for example, were born of four women, two of them wives and two of them concubines. And the Bible shows no discomfort with Solomon's many wives and concubines both were numbered in the hundreds. With notable exceptions such as Jeremiah, the central biblical figures set an example of reproduction, not contraception, yet contraception was never explicitly condemned.

Some religious critics of contraception once pointed to the biblical story of Onan, a son of Judah, as an indication of God's displeasure with people who frustrate the reproductive aspect of sex. Onan had been told by his father Judah to have children with Tamar, the widow of his wicked older brother, whom God had slain. Onan did not want children by Tamar, so when he engaged in sexual intercourse with her, he withdrew before ejaculating. "Onan knew that the children would not be his own, so whenever he had relations with his brother's wife, he wasted his seed on the ground, in order not to raise up descendants for his brother" (Genesis 38:9). God then punished Onan the same way he punished his brother—he struck him dead.

Was Onan punished because his sexual behavior was contraceptive? Over the centuries many thought so, including Pope Pius XI, who used the biblical story in his 1930 encyclical letter on Christian marriage to support his condemnation of contraception. Today, however, most biblical scholars do not think Onan's death was a punishment for contraception. Nor do many of them think, as some have suggested, that it was a punishment for disobeying a law that required sons to beget offspring with a dead brother's widow—that particular law did not come until much later. God seems to have killed Onan not because he practiced contraception or broke a law but because he disobeyed his father, a major offense in a patriarchal society.

The early Christians did not continue the Hebrew emphasis on reproduction. In fact, many of them claimed that virginity was superior to fruitful marriage. Having a family was simply not a central Christian concern. Jesus, a Jew who neither married nor fathered a family, often encouraged his followers to leave their families and follow him. As for contraception itself, not a word about it is mentioned in the Christian scriptures; it is neither condemned nor condoned.

If neither the Hebrew Bible nor the Christian scriptures contain any texts proscribing contraception, why did so many Christians condemn it throughout the centuries, and why does a major religious denomination, the Roman Catholic Church, continue to condemn it to this very day? The roots of the contraception condemnation are not in the Bible but in Stoicism, the most powerful moral philosophy in the Greek and Roman traditions.

Stoicism dominated the ancient world from about 300 B.C.E. until Christianity began to emerge in 350 C.E. as the dominant religion of the vast Roman Empire. Two fundamental features of Stoic philosophy paved the way for a negative moral judgment about contraception. First, Stoics emphasized nature as the norm of morality. Living and behaving morally meant living and behaving according to nature. Second, they thought nature was imbued with reason, what the Greek Stoics called *logos*. Moral behavior is behavior according to reason, not behavior spawned by emotion or passion.

For the Stoic, then, sex will be moral when it is undertaken (1) according to its natural design and (2) in accord with reason, not passion. The morally good Stoic will not introduce into sexual intercourse any intervention contrary to nature and will not seek sex for passion or for pleasure but for a reason, and the most obvious reason for sexual intercourse is reproduction. On two counts then, the Stoic ethic was anticontraceptive: Contraception is artificial, not natural, and contraception indicates that the sexual activity springs from passion rather than its purpose—reproduction.

The influence of Stoicism on Christianity was greater than is often realized. Much of this influence was subtle, but there are some explicit references. For example, a prominent early Christian writer, St. Jerome (340–420), quoted with approval the Stoic philosopher Seneca as saying that a wise man ought not to love his wife with affection but with judgment, and that nothing is more foul than for a man to love his wife as one loves an adulteress (that is, with passion but without the desire to create children).

The person most responsible for shaping the traditional Christian theology that condemned contraception and permitted sexual activity only for reproductive purposes, however, was not Jerome but Augustine (354–431). Augustine converted to Christianity in his thirties. Before his conversion he had lived with a woman for over a decade and fathered a child. He dismissed this woman, the mother of his son, when his mother selected another woman, a girl of about thirteen, for him to marry. While waiting for her to mature, however, he converted to Christianity and embraced a celibate life. He became a priest and later a bishop. He wrote numerous theological works, although he is probably best known for his rather personal *Confessions*, a moving story of his conversion that is widely read to this day.

In his book on marriage, *The Good of Marriage*, Augustine drew a parallel between eating and sex. The reason for eating is survival, and as long as we are eating to survive, we may enjoy whatever pleasure eating provides. Similarly, the reason for sex is pregnancy, and as long as married couples are engaging in sex for pregnancy, they may also enjoy whatever pleasure sexual intercourse provides. All sex initiated when pregnancy is not the goal, even sex between husband and wife, is morally defective because it lacks the reproductive purpose. In *The Good of Marriage*, Augustine wrote that an unmarried woman having intercourse in order to have a child sins less than a married woman having marital intercourse with the hope of avoiding pregnancy.

Underlying Augustine's theology of sexuality, which was to dominate Christianity for a thousand years and which casts its shadow over some Christian theology to this day, is his rather idiosyncratic interpretation of Genesis 2:18. This biblical text depicts God's creating the first woman, Eve, after noting it was not good for man to be alone. Augustine asked why it was not good for man to be alone, and what help a woman could possibly provide for man. And he replied: "I do not see what other help woman would be to man if the purpose of generating were eliminated." In other words the existence of women is helpful only for their role in reproduction. Augustine understood both sex and the creation of women in terms of the same purpose: pregnancy. In such a theology there is clearly no room for contraception. The only thing that justifies sex is reproduction; in fact, the only thing that justifies the existence of women is reproduction.

In his later book *On Marriage and Concupiscence*, Augustine explained how sexual passion, what he called lust or concupiscence, is the effect of Adam's "original sin." He was convinced that God's original plan of human reproduction, even though it would have involved man and woman, did not require sexual arousal—that is, lust or concupiscence—on the part of either the woman or the man. Adam's original sin ruined all this, and so lust, Augustine thought, unfortunately now accompanies, at least in the male, sexual intercourse. Augustine also claimed in *On Marriage and Concupiscence* that the lust involved in intercourse is the specific disorder in the reproductive act that transmits Adam's sin to what will become a new human being. In Augustine's theology every new human life begins in sin, an original sin that only the waters of Christian baptism can wash away.

Thus, two bad features mark sexual intercourse—the concupiscence, a disorder caused by Adam's sin, and the transmission of Adam's sin to the embryo. Since every act of intercourse arouses concupiscence and multiplies sin in the world, it is something everyone should avoid unless there is an overwhelming reason for engaging in it. And there is one such reason, and only one: reproduction. Sexual intercourse is a terribly flawed action justified for only one reason, the intention to cause pregnancy, for without pregnancies the human species will die out.

There is no room for contraception or sterilization in such a theology. And not surprisingly, we find an explicit condemnation of both practices in *On Marriage and Concupiscence*. Those trying to prevent pregnancy, "although they be called husband and wife, are not; nor do they retain any reality of marriage, but use the respectable name [of marriage] to cover a shame. . . . Sometimes this lustful cruelty, or cruel lust, comes to this, that they even use sterilizing drugs." The phrase "sterilizing drugs" (*sterilitatis venena*) was to become the central phrase used in almost all the theological and ecclesiastical texts condemning contraception and birth control for the next thousand years. Augustine reinforced his argument against contraception by recalling the story of Onan, whose efforts to avoid pregnancy were, according to Augustine's mistaken reading of the story, punished by God.

The condemnation of contraception continued in Christian moral theology throughout the Middle Ages. We find it in the penitential books that guided priests' hearing of confessions, in the legal decrees of the Roman Catholic Church, and in the writings of the philosophers and theologians teaching in the universities. The fundamental idea underlying the condemnation of contraception was always the Stoic argument from nature or natural law—contraceptive behavior is against nature, and morality is always "according to nature" or "according to the natural law." Furthermore, for the Christian, nature was designed and created by God, and thus contraception, a violation of nature, is also an act against God. Contraception is not only a crime against nature but a rebellion against God's will; it is both unnatural and sinful.

By the sixteenth century, the original Stoic-Christian position against contraception came under increasing attack. A growing number of people, including some Christian theologians, began wondering whether contraception was always immoral. The Roman Catholic Church, however, stood firm. The great Council of Trent (1545–1563), called to reform abuses in this church and to clarify its position against the new Christian churches springing up in the Protestant reformation of Christianity, produced an official catechism. Unlike theological tomes read mostly by specialists, catechisms are used to educate the people at large about the central tenets of the Catholic faith. This catechism appeared in 1566 and, as might be expected, condemned contraception. But that is not all—the catechism considered contraception a form of homicide (that is, it equated it with murder). Lest this very strict position be overlooked, the editor-in-chief of the catechism, St. Charles Borromeo, issued a commentary on the catechism explaining how contraception is a sin against the biblical commandment "Thou shalt not kill." This placed contraception in the same moral category as murder.

The effort to consider contraception as an act of homicide was renewed by Pope Sixtus V in 1588. He condemned both abortion and contraception, calling them murder, and advocated both excommunication from the church and the death penalty for those convicted of these crimes. Many theologians dissented from this extremely rigid papal teaching, and shortly after Sixtus's death several years later, his successor repealed most of the penalties for contraception while continuing to insist the practice itself was sinful.

Contraception and Christianity in the Twentieth Century

Although some Christians continued to wonder whether contraception and sterilization were always immoral, most Christian churches maintained their absolute prohibition of contraception until the twentieth century, when a shift began to occur. The Anglican Communion had condemned artificial contraception in the Lambeth Conferences of 1908 and 1920. In the Lambeth Conference of 1930, however, the Anglicans reversed their position, holding that artificial birth control is ethical if practiced for morally sound reasons and if it is not motivated by selfishness.

Many other Christian denominations soon followed the Anglicans, and by 1959 the World Council of Churches took an official position advising Christian couples that responsible parents should consider many factors, including the population problems of their region, in the decision to reproduce. The World Council of Churches also took the position that once a responsible decision was made not to have a child, any appropriate method could be used. In other words the World Council of Churches saw no moral differences among natural family planning, artificial barrier methods (condoms and the like), sterilization, and anovulant drugs (birth control pills).

In 1930 the Roman Catholic Church also made a significant change in its centuries-old opposition to contraception. In the 1920s it was definitively established by medical science that a woman is fertile for only a few days each menstrual cycle and that these days occur about two weeks after menses. This had been suspected for some time but had never been established by scientific evidence. Now that the cycles of fertility were better understood a new question arose: Is it moral for married couples to abstain from sex voluntarily during fertile days in order to avoid pregnancy? If they avoid fertile periods, there will be no pregnancy, yet no "unnatural" sexual behavior is involved. Is such behavior moral?

In 1930, somewhat surprisingly, Pope Pius XI officially stated that intercourse deliberately undertaken during the infertile periods before and after ovulation in order to avoid pregnancy was not contrary to the order of nature and therefore could be practiced if there was a good reason for it. This represented a major change in traditional Roman Catholic teaching; the older theology had always insisted on the link between the purpose of sex (pregnancy) and the act itself. Now the Pope was saying that a couple, for a good reason, could deliberately choose to have sexual intercourse only during the infertile periods for the purpose of preventing pregnancy.

The deliberate effort to prevent pregnancy by having sexual intercourse during the infertile periods before and after ovulation was first called periodic continence or the rhythm method; today the practice is more commonly known as natural family planning.

Although the acceptance of deliberate but natural family planning represented a significant change in the traditional Catholic linkage of sex and reproduction, there was no change in the Catholic teachings against other ways of planning families (artificial contraception). All the traditional prohibitions against artificial birth control remained in force.

In the 1950s the controversy over birth control in the Christian churches rekindled with the development of "the pill." The birth control pill prevents pregnancy by preventing ovulation. Most Christian churches had no trouble accepting it, and a number of Roman Catholic theologians suggested the birth control pill could be accepted by the Roman Catholic Church as well. They argued that sexual intercourse was performed in a perfectly natural manner when a woman was on the pill. Using the birth control pill was, in their view, not that much different from the approved rhythm method or natural family planning.

In 1963 Pope John XXIII set up a commission to study questions of population in the world, something now recognized as a serious problem on the planet. The commission's investigations naturally led to questions of controlling births and thus opened up the whole issue of contraception. Some church leaders urged that the question should be debated at the Second Vatican Council that was meeting at the time (1962–1965), but Pope Paul VI ordered that the question of contraception be kept off the agenda. In 1966 the commission gave the Pope its findings: by a large majority it concluded that artificial contraception was contrary neither to Christian morality nor to the natural law. The commission acknowledged that contraception could be selfish and thus sinful but that it need not be if there were good reasons for limiting births.

In 1968 Pope Paul VI published the official Roman Catholic teaching on artificial contraception and sterilization in an encyclical letter titled *Humanae vitae*. The Pope rejected the findings of the papal commission and repeated the centuries-old position: All forms of artificial contraception, including the pill, are immoral.

The Pope also rejected the commission's view that nothing in natural law shows that contraception is immoral. He argued this way: Jesus made Peter and the Apostles the authentic interpreters of all moral laws, both the law of the Gospel and the law of nature. The Pope and the bishops are the successors of Peter and the Apostles, so they are the authentic interpreters of the natural law today. According to their authentic interpretation, the natural law does forbid all forms of artificial contraception.

By saying that natural law, and not just church discipline, forbids contraception, the Pope was saying that artificial contraception is immoral not only for Roman Catholics but for all human beings. This is so because the heart of the natural law doctrine is that all human beings are subject to it.

The idea that religious authority is needed to provide authentic interpretations of the natural law was a rather startling departure from the centuries-old tradition of natural law in philosophy and in Roman Catholic theology itself. Although natural law can be understood in a number of different ways, a key feature running through all the different versions is that it is knowable by *natural* reason; that is, it can be discerned by people using their own resources of understanding. Neither religious revelation nor religious authority is needed for us to know what natural law requires; it is natural precisely because it is discoverable by the natural reflection of intelligent people of good will. Biblical revelation and ecclesiastical authority were always understood as complementary to the natural law, but they were not needed to know what natural law allows and forbids. The whole point of "natural" law was that people could discern it by their natural powers of understanding and interpretation.

In the 1950s, however, some Catholic theologians had begun to back away from this traditional view of the natural law, largely because of the growing controversies over birth control. The more astute among them realized that no explicit natural law arguments against contraception exist. Thus, some began to argue that human beings cannot always discern the natural law by natural reason alone but need the Roman Catholic Church to explain it to them. In his influential *Medico–Moral Problems*, published in 1958, the prominent American theologian Gerald Kelley wrote: "Rather frequently, circumstances have made it necessary for the Holy See to explain the natural law as it applies to medical problems. . . . The Church not only claims divine authorization to interpret the moral law; it also claims that its teachings are a practical necessity for a clear and adequate knowledge of this law."

Ten years later this idea—that in practice we cannot know some aspects of the natural law by unaided human reason but need guidance from the Pope—reappeared as the crucial rationale for the papal condemnation of artificial contraception. In the final analysis then, the natural law is not so natural after all. In some cases, and contraception is one of them, it has to be interpreted by the Pope, and his interpretations are the authentic and authoritative interpretations binding for all human beings. Needless to say, many supporters of a natural law ethic, especially those not of the Catholic faith, have trouble accepting this view of the natural law. And of course many moralists, especially those of the last few centuries, do not take a natural law approach to ethics.

This detour into a consideration of artificial contraception and the traditional Christian stance against it may seem a little out of place in a text on health care ethics. After all, most people today do not consider birth control a moral issue. The failure to see contraception as a moral issue, however, is an unfortunate part of the all too familiar tendency in medicine to ignore the moral significance of reproductive questions. In recent years techniques were developed to prevent pregnancy—people wanted them, and so physicians provided them. And techniques were developed to enhance the chance of pregnancy—people wanted them, and so physicians provided them. But few people until recently saw the moral implications of these interventions.

Whether one agrees with the Roman Catholic Church or with the Anglican Communion and the World Council of Churches on artificial contraception, at least their statements serve as a reminder that artificial contraception and sterilization raise moral issues. Interfering with the normal reproductive process is not a morally neutral activity.

And it is important in a text on health care ethics to ask what underlies the traditional Christian position against artificial birth control. The ideas prompting the traditional religious prohibitions of contraception are of historical interest even today.

First, in a time when sex was considered mostly from the male viewpoint and chiefly as an outlet for passion, the effort of many people, among them the Stoics, was directed toward humanizing the sex drive. Philosophers and theologians were convinced men should not simply use women to satisfy their sexual hunger. Looking for a way to dignify human sexuality, they tried to link it with an environment of responsibility, the family.

Insisting on the link between sexual passion and family is a major factor in the humanization of sex. It elevates human sex above sexual activity in the forest and in the barnyard. The man having sexual intercourse with the intention of procreating a child is having intercourse with the woman he wants to be the mother of his child, and this generates a respect for her that would not be there if his actions were motivated by pure sexual need.

Second, the traditional Christian stance against contraception reminds us of the bad features associated with most contraceptive interventions. Many contraceptive interventions entail risks of unwanted side effects. Many of the early efforts to prevent conception caused health problems for women. Advances in medicine have reduced these problems significantly but not completely. Surgeries that sterilize by tubal ligation or vasectomy, IUDs, anovulant pills, and Norplant are all medically controlled contraceptive techniques with some degree of risk, and the bad features have to be recognized in an ethics of right reason. In fact, almost anything done to prevent a pregnancy, even the use of a condom, introduces a disorder into sexual intercourse.

Morality urges us to avoid disorders in human behavior unless we have an appropriate reason to justify them. The traditional Christian prohibition against contraception reminds us that we cannot simply charge ahead and engage in contraceptive practices without thinking about the impact they will have on our lives. Specifically, we have to ask whether the interventions will truly contribute to individual and social human good or undermine them; that is, whether contraceptive interventions are moral or immoral.

Contraception and the Law

The Christian churches were not the only major opposition to birth control in our culture; until recently laws in many states restricted contraception. The ease with which people can obtain contraceptive devices and medical interventions in our country today is a relatively new phenomenon. Not so long ago the distribution and even the use of contraceptives were illegal in many places. The fact that these laws existed until recently is one more reminder that many of our predecessors thought something was wrong with contraception.

The laws banning contraceptives came under attack in the middle of this century, shortly after most of the Christian denominations accepted the morality of contraception. In 1961 a pharmacist in Connecticut challenged the state laws in a case before the U.S. Supreme Court known as *Poe v. Ullman*. Although the court dismissed the case on technical grounds, two justices dissented. They believed that the Connecticut law against contraception violated the constitutional right of privacy and therefore should have been examined by the Court. One dissenting justice,

Justice Douglas, feared that the law banning contraceptives would lead to an intolerable situation: since it is the duty of police to enforce laws, we might "reach the point where . . . officers appeared in bedrooms to find out what went on." Justice Harlan, the other dissenting justice, echoed the same concern for privacy.

It is important to note that Justice Harlan did not favor overturning the Connecticut law against contraceptives because he thought that contraception was morally acceptable. On the contrary, he was convinced that contraception was immoral and that it encouraged such "dissolute actions" as fornication and adultery. His only concern was that he thought it unwise to bring "the whole machinery of the criminal law into the very heart of marital privacy, requiring husband and wife to render account before a criminal tribunal of their uses of that intimacy." The key word here is privacy; Harlan thought laws against contraceptives were bad because they make an intimate and private matter—what married couples do when they have sexual intercourse—a subject for criminal investigation and prosecution.

In 1965 Connecticut's law banning contraceptives was again challenged, this time in a famous case known as *Griswold v. Connecticut*. Under state law, Connecticut had imposed a criminal penalty on a physician for prescribing contraceptives for a married couple because he thought a pregnancy would be dangerous for the woman. The U.S. Supreme Court struck down the Connecticut law, explicitly recognizing a constitutional right of privacy, a right that was to play a major role eight years later in the even more famous *Roe v. Wade* abortion decision. Since *Griswold*, states can no longer prohibit married couples from using contraceptives because such a ban would "allow the police to search the sacred precincts of marital bedrooms for telltale signs of the use of contraceptives." In other words, using contraceptives is wrong, but invading the bedroom to enforce the law is a greater wrong because it would violate the couple's right to privacy during sexual intercourse.

This decision did not end the court battles about contraception. A few years later an outspoken advocate of birth control, Bill Baird, was arrested in Massachusetts for distributing contraceptives to anyone who wanted them. The Massachusetts law differed from the Connecticut law struck down in *Griswold* in two ways: It banned the distribution and sale of contraceptives, not their use, thus avoiding the repulsive idea of police checking whether people are using contraceptives when they have intercourse, and it banned the distribution of contraceptives only to unmarried people.

In the 1972 case known as *Eisenstadt v. Baird*, the U.S. Supreme Court struck down the Massachusetts law prohibiting the distribution of contraceptives to unmarried people. "If the right of privacy means anything, it is the right of the *individual*, married or single, to be free from unwarranted governmental intrusion into matters so fundamentally affecting a person as the decision whether to bear or beget a child." As the result of this decision, states cannot prevent the distribution of contraceptives to any adult, married or single.

In 1977 the U.S. Supreme Court struck down still another law restricting the distribution of contraceptives. New York had a law prohibiting the sale or distribution of contraceptives to minors under the age of sixteen. In its decision overturning this law, *Carey v. Population Services International*, the court emphasized that "the Constitution protects individual decisions in matters of childbearing from unjustified intrusion by the State." As the result of this decision, states cannot restrict the distribution of contraceptives to minors.

Several points emerge from this brief review of three U.S. Supreme Court decisions involving contraception. First, they remind us that many state legislatures had enacted laws against contraception, even for married people. The laws never could have existed unless a good number of elected representatives believed that their constituents thought there was something wrong with contraception.

Second, the court never disagreed with this view; it never said contraception was not immoral. It invalidated Connecticut's law because it was unenforceable without having police officers in the bedroom, and it invalidated the Massachusetts and New York laws because it thought that the decision of individuals to prevent children is a private matter they should be able to pursue without government intrusion, regardless of whether they are unmarried or under sixteen years of age. The court never invalidated the laws prohibiting contraception because those laws incorrectly implied contraception was wrong; it invalidated the laws restricting contraception because those laws violated people's privacy.

The many laws against contraception remind us, as does the traditional Christian stance against it (and undoubtedly the two prohibitions are related), that in many people's minds contraception was immoral and should be illegal. The very fact that so many people once considered contraception wrong helps to make us aware that moral issues might well be involved in contraceptive behavior.

Contraception and Ethics

Today a variety of contraceptive methods are available. They raise a special set of ethical issues in health care. Unlike standard medical treatments that are intended to correct what is dysfunctional, contraceptive medical interventions are intended to cause the dysfunction of what is functioning properly. Such interventions are morally acceptable only if they are justified by adequate reasons.

The most popular forms of contraception today are the following ones.

- Sterilization by tubal ligation or by vasectomy.
- Short-term barriers such as male and female condoms, diaphragms, cervical caps, contraceptive sponges, vaginal rings, and spermicides.
- Long-term barriers such as IUDs or a microinsert into the fallopian tubes that causes tissue to close the tubes (approved by FDA in 2002). Some barriers are effective up to six years; others for a year or more.
- Anovulants, which include (1) birth control pills, providing protection against pregnancy one month at a time; (2) injections of Depo-Provera, providing protection for three to four months at a time (another injected anovulant, Lunelle, has been withdrawn in the United States); (3) Ortho Evra patches placed on the body once a week for three weeks every cycle; and (4) the emergency "morning after pill" or Plan B (actually two pills taken twelve hours apart within seventy-two hours of intercourse). In 2006 the FDA, after a politically charged delay, allowed adults (those over eighteen) to obtain Plan B without a prescription. In March 2009 a federal district court judge in New York ruled that the age restriction was based on politics and not science and that the FDA should approve Plan B without prescription for women over seventeen. It is not really "over the counter" but "behind the counter," and young women must show a government-issued ID as proof of age to obtain the contraceptive. Women under seventeen still need a prescription for Plan B.
- Antiprogestin drugs such as RU-486 that can be used as a contraceptive to prevent uterine implantation of embryos. Since the major use of RU-486 is to dislodge implanted embryos, we will consider this drug in the section on abortion. Depo-Provera also has an antiprogestin effect on the uterus.

The moral implications of these interventions are not all equal. Using an IUD to prevent the implantation of an embryo is more morally serious than using a barrier to prevent fertilization or using anovulant drugs to prevent ovulation. And permanent surgical sterilization is more morally serious than various reversible methods of contraception.

But the key ethical issue in these interventions is when, if ever, they contribute to the human good of the couple and of society despite the disorder they introduce into the reproductive physiology and despite the risks and side effects that accompany most of them.

In deliberating about the morality of various contraceptive interventions, the following points may be helpful.

First, we now accord love in general, and sexual love in particular, a much more important role than did earlier peoples, who tended to see marriage in terms of procreation of children, social standing, political advantage, and so forth, and sex in terms of appetite and lust. Perhaps the greatest signs of this are the assumptions we all make that we can simply choose our mates and that we will mate with the one we love. In earlier times parents arranged marriages, and love was not a crucial factor.

The personal history that Augustine records in his *Confessions* sums up the earlier practice: His mother picked a girl for him to marry, so he dismissed the woman he said he loved and with whom he had lived with their son for over a decade. And he saw nothing wrong with this. In those days parents played a much larger role than love in their child's marriage, and the parents were more interested in the impact of the new in-law on the family than in the romantic love life of their child. To this day many marriage ceremonies retain a trace of parental control in the ritual whereby the father of the bride "gives her away" to the man she is about to marry, implying she could not go to him, even if she loved him, without her father's permission.

And we consider sexual love a much more important part of human dignity than did our cultural ancestors. They tended to separate body and soul and to see sex as an appetite of the body and a threat to the life of the soul. Today we do not think sexuality is a merely animal appetite or a disorder caused by the original sin of Adam; we understand it rather as an integral aspect of intimate human love when caring, commitment, and trust are present. And once the important role of sexuality in human love is appreciated, the traditional idea that every sexual act is morally acceptable only if it is susceptible to pregnancy loses much of its cogency.

Second, we now live in a time when overpopulation is undermining human life in many areas of the world. What is now clear to us, and what was never dreamed of by our ancestors, is that without some form of birth control, the human population will one day overwhelm the planet. There is no serious disagreement about the need for birth control; the disagreement is whether natural family planning will be sufficiently effective or whether artificial methods of birth control will be needed to prevent the human misery and famine exacerbated by overpopulation. At this point in history there is no evidence that abstinence or natural family planning will work, especially in those parts of the world where the population problems are most serious.

Third, contraception is not, considered in itself, something good. Contraceptive behavior, even natural family planning, is always a disorder, a bad feature, in sexual intimacy. Thus, the argument is not between those who say contraception is always wrong and those who say contraception is good. It is, rather, between those who say contraception is always a moral evil and those who say it is always bad but not a moral evil whenever there are sufficient reasons for introducing it into the interpersonal relationship.

Fourth, it is well to remember that contraception can be a moral evil, that is, unethical. This is so when it is motivated not by a seeking of the human good but by selfishness. It becomes a moral evil when it enables one to pursue more comfortably irresponsible and promiscuous sexual activity or when it encourages people to make sex trivial or reduces intercourse to lust without any caring.

Fifth, the morality of contraception can best be determined by considering the question as but one aspect of the entire interpersonal relationship. Ethical reflection will therefore focus on the people in the relationship, on their history and circumstances, on their children, and on their present and future needs. It will also consider the good of society, a good that can change with the times. Today, for example, overpopulation threatens many parts of the world, whereas for most of human history underpopulation was the problem. Underpopulation suggests the reasonableness of prohibitions against artificial contraception; overpopulation suggests the opposite.

Sixth, any consideration of the ethics of contraception cannot ignore our present knowledge about human sexual biology, something our predecessors did not have. We are now aware of the high degree of randomness involved in the beginning of a new human life. We know hundreds of thousands of spermatozoa advance toward an egg that will normally accept only one spermatozoon if any. If a different spermatozoon fertilizes that egg, the baby born nine months later will be a totally different person. The immense statistical odds against any specific person being conceived and born means the interventions to regulate conception will not appear as unreasonable to us as they would to many of our ancestors, who thought contraception prevented a specific predestined child from being conceived. It was their ignorance of how human life begins that led some of them to draw an analogy between contraception and abortion, or between contraception and homicide.

Seventh, any moral deliberation about contraception cannot ignore how unexpected pregnancy can undermine the emancipation of women in society. As more and more women see their role in life expanding beyond that of wife and mother, the control of pregnancy becomes more important and more reasonable.

Finally, we are increasingly aware that longer life spans are making pregnancy and parenthood an ever-smaller chapter in a marriage. Reproduction is an important chapter in most marriages, but not the most important one. Most parents now live long after the children are gone, and this longevity reminds us that the primary players in marriage are not the children but the couple. The strength of the marriage bond is not primarily the children but the depth of the spouses' love and affection for each other, a love and affection embodied in sexual love. The intimacy of sexual love in the relationship is always for the partners and only sometimes for pregnancy.

Although contraception is a moral issue and is sometimes contrary to the good of those practicing it and of society, no blanket condemnation of it is consistent with an ethics of right reason, where right reason denotes prudential reasoning oriented toward what will achieve the person's good. In our culture the only remaining major condemnation of all directly intended sterilization and artificial birth control comes from a few religious leaders. For some believers, this is enough. For nonbelievers, and for many believers, it is not.

The intent in this section was to raise consciousness about the moral seriousness of contraception and sterilization and to enable us to situate the necessary moral deliberation in a historical context. This may help us reflect in a morally serious way on the paradigm case of contraception—the couple wishing to limit or avoid pregnancies in their relationship—as well as on numerous subsidiary issues. Some of these subsidiary issues are the following.

1. Some public schools are now dispensing contraceptives. The most common types are condoms and birth control pills, but some high schools have begun offering surgically implanted Norplant capsules for girls who want them. Distribution of contraceptives in high schools upsets many people and needs more reflection and dialogue.

2. A few courts are suggesting or ordering sterilization in criminal cases involving violent sex offenders. This demands serious ethical deliberation.

3. There is some public pressure for sterilization. Some, for example, think women supported by public funds who continue to have children by unknown fathers, thus adding people to the welfare rolls, should be asked to accept sterilization as a condition of future welfare support.

4. Many hospitals sponsored by a religious organization opposed to contraception refuse to allow any sterilizations intended to prevent pregnancy or any other contraceptive interventions. When the hospital is the only one available to people in the area, this refusal puts a serious burden on patients and physicians who are convinced these interventions are medically and morally justified in particular situations. In some cases, it results in needless surgical interventions. For example, when a woman in poor health with a large family requests in good faith a tubal ligation during a cesarean section and the hospital rules will not allow it, she has to undergo another surgery for the ligation a few weeks later at another hospital.

5. Some advocate the sterilization of mentally challenged women who enjoy some degree of social freedom. The idea is to prevent their becoming pregnant by men who are taking advantage of them because they are not mentally and emotionally mature enough to avoid intercourse.

Issues such as these are the subjects of intense debate in some quarters. In the ethical approach we have been suggesting in this text, the morality or immorality of contraception will be determined by whether or not the intervention with its inherent disorder, risks, and side effects is justified by moral reasons showing that the alternatives to contraception will do even more harm to the good life of the moral agents involved.

We turn next to the other side of the reproductive issue, and we address the new techniques and technologies designed not to prevent, but to cause pregnancy.

ARTIFICIAL REPRODUCTIVE TECHNIQUES

We now consider the most popular methods of artificial reproductive technologies and some of the ethical issues they raise.

Artificial Insemination or Intrauterine Insemination

Artificial insemination or intrauterine insemination (IUI) was the first major success in assisted reproduction. Over two hundred years ago, the Italian priest Lazaro Spallanzani began artificially inseminating frogs and dogs. In 1790 a surgeon in Scotland successfully inseminated a woman with her husband's sperm, and the practice slowly began to spread.

It was not until the 1960s, however, that artificial insemination, IUI, became popular. It began as a treatment designed to correct infertility in married women when intercourse was impossible or when the husband had a low sperm count. Before long, sperm from other men was also used. Sometimes a sperm sample was added to the sperm of a husband with low sperm count; at other times it was the only sperm used.

Eventually, heterosexual women without a partner and lesbian women with no desire for a male sexual partner sought and received IUI. This created a new kind of situation because the medical intervention in these cases cannot be considered a treatment for infertility—most of these woman are quite fertile. For this reason as well as for concern for children deliberately conceived outside of marriage, some medical facilities decline to provide IUI in these circumstances.

The man providing the sperm for IUI is called a donor. If he is not the husband, however, the word is often misleading. Most sperm provided by third parties is not donated but sold to the physician or to a sperm bank. Usually the man remains anonymous so the mother and child do not know, and often can never know, the identity of the father. The father's genetic characteristics, however, are usually available to the woman using the commercial sperm.

IUI is the most widely used reproductive assistance at the present time, playing a role in more than thirty thousand pregnancies a year in the United States alone. Some IUI is done within marriage, but there are about seventy commercial sperm banks supplying more than three hundred IUI clinics in the United States. The sperm banks advertise for sperm in various publications, including college newspapers. A recent advertisement in the *Harvard Crimson*, for example, promised $105 per week ($35 per sample) to qualified students providing sperm for artificial insemination.

IUI is a relatively simple and inexpensive procedure. Sperm is obtained, usually by masturbation, and then inserted into the uterus during ovulation. To prevent transmission of disease, sperm from donors is tested for HIV and other problems. Some sperm banks now freeze the sperm for six months and test the sellers' blood, semen, and urine monthly during this time for disease and drug use.

When the practice of IUI using sperm bought from third parties or strangers became popular thirty years ago, little attention was paid to its ethical implications. People proceeded as if no moral issues were involved. Now there is increasing awareness that the procedure is not morally neutral, and the possibility that it can be the source of serious harms must be considered.

First, there is the matter of selling sperm by anonymous men who accept no legal or personal responsibility for their genetic offspring. Although this does not seem to harm most men providing the sperm, there are indications that children born of IUI can be distressed about their origins in the world. They come to know that half of their genetic material came from a father who provided it not in an act of sexual intimacy but as a commercial transaction, that the man has no interest in knowing or caring about them, and that he in all probability has so masked his identity that they will never know who he is.

Moreover, children of IUI by an anonymous seller of sperm can face potential problems when they begin to mate. Years ago some men donated sperm numerous times in the same geographical area, and it is therefore possible that people with the same father could unknowingly marry a half-sister or a half-brother. Other unhappy combinations are also possible. For example, a woman might someday marry the anonymous donor who provided the sperm used in the insemination of her mother and thus find herself married to her father.

Some have suggested that the anonymity of the father in IUI is akin to adoption, and most people accept adoption as a morally respectable procedure. But there is an important difference between IUI with purchased sperm and adoption. In adoption, the child already exists and the adoption is an attempt to compensate for the breakdown of the family structure. The whole motivation behind the moral acceptance of adoption is that, in some difficult situations, it is good for the child who is already here. In IUI with commercial sperm, on the contrary, there is no child whose best interests are at stake. Rather, there is a deliberate effort to father a child by a man not related to the mother in any way, and most often that man will deliberately remain anonymous and uninterested in his genetic offspring. Adoption is an attempt to help a child born into a less than ideal situation; IUI with purchased sperm is a deliberate attempt to produce a child with an unknown and disinterested genetic father.

Second, additional ethical issues arise with IUI when the woman is not married. A woman without a partner may intensely desire pregnancy, but the long-term effects on children intentionally born to a single parent are not yet known. Most people do think, however, that children are better off and that the society is stronger if children have traditional family support, although many different versions of "family" have existed in history and continue to exist today. Children born of a lesbian woman may face additional problems in a society still uncomfortable with homosexuality when the sexual orientation of the mother becomes known by other children. Children are not always without cruelty when it comes to isolating their peers who may have an idiosyncratic feature in their lives.

For IUI within marriage that uses the husband's sperm few ethical problems exist. Here the couple is simply trying to overcome a fertility problem and have a family. Even under these circumstances, however, some see an ethical issue in the procedure used to obtain the husband's sperm. The Roman Catholic Church, for example, has a long-standing position that masturbation is a serious moral wrong even when done for the purpose of producing a pregnancy. To avoid the sin of masturbation some theologians suggest that the couple have intercourse using a condom with holes in it. By using a perforated condom during intercourse, the husband is not masturbating, nor is he practicing birth control because a sufficient quantity of sperm will escape from the condom into the vagina. After the sperm trapped in the condom is retrieved, the woman takes it to her physician, who then inseminates her as with any IUI procedure. Other Catholic theologians do not agree with this position and argue that Catholic husbands could masturbate to obtain sperm for reasons such as fertility treatments or medical diagnosis.

In Vitro Fertilization

In 1978, after years of research, the first "test tube" baby, Louise Brown, was born in England. The first baby conceived by IVF in the United States was born in Norfolk, Virginia, late in 1981. The latest CDC figures indicate that in 2006 more than forty-one thousand successful IVF births resulting in more than fifty-six thousand infants (many IVF births are multiple births) occurred in the United States.

There are four major steps in the IVF process:

1. *Ovulation induction.* Before the procedure, hormonal products are injected into the woman to stimulate follicle growth and to prepare the eggs for retrieval at the proper time. This progress is monitored by ultrasound and blood tests to determine when ovulation is about to occur.

2. *Egg retrieval.* Two major options exist for the retrieval of the eggs: laparoscopy and vaginal ultrasound. In laparoscopy several small incisions under a light general anesthesia are made in the abdominal wall so that three instruments can be inserted. The first is a scope so that the physician can see inside the abdominal cavity, the second is a device to grasp the ovary, and the third is a hollow needle to suck up the ripened eggs from the ovarian follicles. In vaginal ultrasound, either a local or spinal anesthesia is given, and an ultrasound probe with a sheathed hollow needle is inserted into the vagina. The physician, guided by the ultrasound picture on the monitor, then passes the needle through the vaginal wall to reach the ovary and suck out the ripened eggs. After the laparoscopy or the vaginal ultrasound, the retrieved eggs are immediately transferred to an adjoining laboratory, treated, and placed in a special fluid for several hours. The patient leaves the IVF center when the retrieval is completed.

3. *Fertilization.* The semen obtained from the husband (or from a commercial sperm supplier) is brought to the laboratory, washed, and prepared for fertilization. Then concentrated sperm

is added to the eggs in each petri dish, and, if all goes well, a spermatozoon fertilizes the egg in the petri dish or "test tube." Once fertilized, the eggs are allowed to develop for about forty-eight hours. Then the woman returns to the hospital or clinic for the fourth step.

4. *Embryo transfer.* A number of fertilized ova, usually four, are inserted through the cervix into the uterus that has been prepared by yet another injection to ripen it for implantation of the embryo. Most of the time none of the embryos will implant, but there is a chance of about one in five that one will. Occasionally several will implant, and then multiple births result. At the time of the embryo transfer (ET) the embryo has about eight cells, considerably fewer than a normal embryo has when it arrives in the uterus.

Among the ethical concerns about IVF are the following.

1. Some people, most notably some religious leaders, have moral objections to obtaining sperm for IVF procedures by masturbation.

2. Some people, again most notably some religious leaders, have moral objections to a human fertilization process that occurs apart from sexual intercourse and outside the human body. In December 2008, for example, the Vatican released an Instruction titled *Dignitas personae* that stated once again the opposition of the Catholic Church to all forms of IVF. Opponents of IVF often find the idea of a new human life beginning in a laboratory morally objectionable because they believe it degrades human dignity. Some of them argue that it violates a human right, the right of every child to be conceived naturally. This rights-based argument is problematic—it is difficult to argue that someone has a right before he becomes a someone; that is, it is difficult to argue that a child has a right (and therefore must already exist) to a natural conception before the conception that led to the child occurred.

3. Many people think that IVF for married couples is ethical, but they have moral objections to using the fertility treatments for unmarried women. This is especially true if there is no fertility problem and if the IVF is used simply because the woman does not have (or does not want) a partner to father her child. They object for two reasons: (1) they see no cogent reason to use a fertility treatment when there is no infertility, and (2) they do not think it is good to cause a pregnancy deliberately outside the traditional family relationship of husband and wife. In IVF, it is possible to use purchased sperm and purchased eggs, and to transfer the embryo to a third party with no genetic or social relationship to the child. Thus, in a worst case scenario, adults may deliberately arrange for a future child to have many parents, perhaps as many as five: the man and woman raising the child, the man selling his sperm (the genetic father), the woman selling her egg (the genetic mother), and the woman receiving money for carrying the child in pregnancy (the gestational mother). The confusion of parenthood when IVF is extended beyond married couples using their own sperm and ova is a serious ethical concern.

Another twist to using ova from third parties surfaced in 1993 when it was reported that eggs could be retrieved from aborted fetuses, nourished so they would mature quickly, then fertilized by an IVF procedure to produce an embryo for transfer to a woman hoping to become pregnant. Using IVF in this way would produce a child whose mother was never born; in fact, it would produce a child whose mother was a dead fetus, and probably a dead fetus deliberately destroyed by her mother, the child's grandmother. There is no reason to believe that a child whose mother was a fetus destroyed by her grandmother would benefit from this arrangement, and there are many reasons to believe that she would suffer from it.

4. As IVF grew in popularity another ethical concern emerged—the problem of multiple pregnancies. In IVF, physicians often transfer four or five embryos from the lab to the woman in an effort to increase the chances of pregnancy. Unfortunately, placing so many embryos into women results in an abnormally high number of multiple fetuses when pregnancy does occur. According to CDC figures for 2006 (available at cdc.gov), 48 percent (25,967) of the 54,656 IVF babies born that year in the United States were multiple births. IVF babies represent only about 1 percent of babies born in the United States yet account for about 18 percent of the multiple births.

The multiple birth rate for natural pregnancy is less than 3 percent. Despite these figures the CDC found in 2006 that transferring more than two embryos in IVF remained a common practice.

Pregnancies with multiple fetuses are risky for mothers and children. According to the CDC 57 percent of IVF twins have low birth weight, and 65 percent are premature. The figures for IVF triplets are even worse: 96 percent have low birth weight, and 97 percent are premature. Low birth weight and premature birth introduce many current and future problems for the children. Thus, abortion often becomes a moral issue, since many women seek to reduce the number of IVF fetuses they carry by destroying some of them.

Even IVF single births produce added risks: an IVF singleton is 50 percent more likely to have low birth weight (9 percent versus 6 percent) and 100 percent more likely to have very low birth weight (2 percent versus 1 percent). In late 2008 the CDC reported that birth defects may be two to four times more common in IVF single births than in the general population of single births. Among the birth defects it noted were septal heart defects, cleft lip or palate, esophageal atresia, and anorectal atresia. Moreover, some problems might not show up at birth. For example, one study shows that Type 2 diabetes increases in inverse proportion to premature delivery; the more premature the birth the greater the chance of diabetes.

IVF clinics in the United States that are driven to attract clients by high numbers of pregnancies have not been morally sensitive to these issues. In fact, they present something of a conflict of interest for them. Both commercial and nonprofit IVF clinics invariably make money. Competition for clients is keen, so clinics want a high pregnancy rate to attract clients. And the way to get a high pregnancy rate is to insert many embryos, which is the very thing that causes the much higher than normal rates of twins, triplets, quadruplets, and other multiple births.

By the end of the 1990s the abnormally high rate of multiple pregnancies following IVF or the use of fertility drugs finally began to attract attention and concern. Fortunately two developments occurred that reduced some of the pressure to implant many embryos. Delaying insertion of the embryos for five days after fertilization instead of the usual two or three has resulted in a higher rate of pregnancies, allowing doctors to transfer fewer embryos. And a published study showed that IVF pregnancies were related more to the number of eggs fertilized in a given cycle than to the number of fertilized eggs inserted into the woman. If a woman produced many eggs that could be successfully fertilized, her chances of pregnancy were not diminished if only two embryos were inserted. If more than two were inserted it only increased her chances of a multiple pregnancy.

Despite the promise of these advances, the continuing high rate of multiple pregnancies in IVF remains a moral concern for a virtue-based ethic. Many countries have regulations preventing transfer of more than two or three embryos, but most IVF physicians in the United States resist such limitations despite the harms caused by high multiple pregnancy rates. Unfortunately, the media often present multiple births as a wonderful event, a tactic that undermines critical thinking about the burdens for parents and children associated with multiple pregnancies.

Nowhere was this more clear than in the media circus surrounding the birth of the McCaughey septuplets in 1997 as the result of fertility drugs. Producing the birth of seven babies with fertility drug treatments is a medical failure and a moral disaster. Although all seven babies survived, apparently without serious problems, the more likely outcome of pregnancies with five or more fetuses is fetal demise for some and serious neonatal problems for others, as well as difficulties and risks for the pregnant woman. A sevenfold pregnancy is a terrible mistake, something every reasonable person would wish to avoid.

The media circus happened again in January 2009 when a California woman named Nadya Suleman, a single mother of six young children, asked her doctor to transfer six of her embryos in an IVF procedure. He complied with her request. Two of the embryos divided, and she subsequently delivered by C-section eight very premature babies, another avoidable obstetrical disaster.

5. Efforts to increase the chances of pregnancy led to another development in the 1990s: intracytoplasmic sperm injection, known as ICSI. In this IVF procedure the sperm and ova are not placed in a petri dish so spermatozoa can fertilize the ova. Rather, the biologist captures a spermatozoon with a hollow needle and then injects it directly into an ovum. The spermatozoon is thus forced into the egg.

ICSI increases the chances of pregnancy, especially when the infertility problem is caused by low sperm count, poor sperm motility, or other male fertility problems. Sometimes it is the only way a couple can create an embryo. But ICSI also raises a new set of ethical concerns. It is often used when the sperm count is low or spermatozoa are not capable of penetrating ova in the normal way, a sign the sperm is immature or abnormal. Forcing a spermatozoon into an ovum when something relevant to the sperm is abnormal runs an increased risk of producing an embryo with a poor set of paternal genes.

Moreover, the normal process of fertilization involves a series of changes in both the spermatozoon and the ovum as the spermatozoon first attaches to and then penetrates into the egg, a process that takes hours. Direct injection takes only moments, and little is known about how bypassing the normal cellular alterations during fertilization will affect the subsequent child. Also, the injection aspirates some material from the ovum and temporarily deforms its shape. Finally, many ICSI embryos are subjected to "assisted hatching," a process whereby the outer covering of the embryo is nicked in an effort to make it more likely to implant in the uterus.

The risks of the aspiration and of the temporary deformity of the ovum and of nicking the surface of the embryo are not well understood. Although preliminary follow-up studies showed no increase in the expected number of congenital malformations, they did suggest higher rates of chromosomal abnormalities and delays in neurological development for children reproduced this way. By 2002 we knew there were problems. A study published in the *New England Journal of Medicine* showed that women undergoing IVF who allowed ICSI exposed their babies to double the risk of a major birth defect compared with children conceived naturally. Although this is a significant increase in risk, we need to keep in mind that the risk of a major birth defect itself is relatively low, so we are doubling a low number.

ICSI became an infertility treatment without extensive research to establish its safety for future children, and this was morally careless. ICSI is still in many ways a research protocol being marketed as a treatment to couples desperately seeking to bear a child. Prudential reasoning suggests that ICSI should have been tested in significant research studies before it was offered as a clinical treatment, but the intense desire for pregnancy on the part of couples as well as physicians blinded both groups to the potential harms that could be produced by the new technique. Prudential reasoning also suggests that IVF personnel employing ICSI should fully inform the women that the procedure is doubling the risk of a major birth defect for their child or children compared with natural conception.

6. Another major moral concern relevant to IVF centers on the moral status of the embryo. In many IVF procedures more eggs are fertilized than are needed at the time, so there is a question of what to do with the embryos that will not be transferred. Discarding a developing human embryo is obviously a moral issue since it is the deliberate destruction of new human life.

Sometimes the embryos are frozen so they will be available for the woman in the future if she needs them, but this also raises moral issues. The freezing process destroys some embryos, and, if those successfully frozen are not needed, they will have to be destroyed as well.

Several highly publicized cases have alerted the general public to the problems caused by freezing embryos. In 1983 Mario and Elsa Rios were killed in a plane crash, leaving frozen embryos in an Australian fertility clinic and an estate worth more than a million dollars. Questions about what to do with the embryos arose. If they were brought to term, they would inherit the estate; if not, others would receive it. A special panel suggested that the embryos should be destroyed, but the Parliament of the state of Victoria passed a special law protecting the embryos. At present, they remain frozen, and eventually will probably deteriorate beyond any chance for survival.

Another case arose in Tennessee when Mary Sue Davis and Junior Davis underwent IVF fertility treatments. Their excess embryos were frozen. After their marriage broke up, Mary Sue wanted to become pregnant with the frozen embryos, but Junior was now strongly opposed to her bearing his children. She considered the embryos her babies and insisted she had a right to bring them to term. In September 1989 a judge gave custody of the embryos to Mary Sue because they are "children," and it is in the interests of children to be born. Mary Sue then married another man and changed her mind about wanting to use the frozen embryos. A year later the court of appeals overruled the circuit judge and granted joint custody of the frozen embryos to Mary Sue and Junior. Then in 1992 the Tennessee Supreme Court held that Junior could not be forced into fatherhood against his will. Finally, in June 1993, Junior announced that the embryos no longer existed.

A more recent New York case underscores how these problems continue. Maureen and Steven Kass decided to divorce after numerous IVF attempts had failed to result in a viable pregnancy. Maureen wanted sole custody of their remaining frozen embryos so she could try again, but Steven no longer wanted to be the father of any of her children. The trial court gave the embryos to Maureen, but the decision was reversed by an appeals court. The case then went to the highest court in New York, the Court of Appeals, where Maureen lost her appeal in 1998. The court was lucky—both parents had happened to sign a consent form agreeing that any frozen embryos could be used for research if the couple were unable to make a decision about them. The court thus had a "hook" on which to hang its decision, but if no such agreement existed, one wonders how the court would have decided the issue.

What is troubling in these American cases is the tendency to treat human embryos as if they were pieces of property or products instead of new human beings. The courts decide these cases on the basis of contract law, but human embryos do not easily fit into traditional categories governed by existing contract law. Obviously regulation and perhaps even legislation restricting possible abuse of human embryos, something the courts cannot provide, is needed for the good of society.

The production of more embryos than will be immediately transferred into the woman is not the only problem in IVF; sometimes too few embryos are produced, thus reducing the opportunity for pregnancy. This has led some researchers to try splitting the human embryos produced by IVF in order to increase the number available for pregnancy. In 1993 several human embryos were actually split, and, although no efforts were made to implant them, they did begin to develop normally after they were split. The procedures were widely reported in the media as "cloning" human beings, but it would be more accurate to say that the early embryos were simply split, much as they sometimes split spontaneously in the first few days of life, a phenomenon we explained in chapter 6.

The American Fertility Society, now known as the American Society for Reproductive Medicine, has determined that embryos in the first fourteen days of development, although deserving of respect because they are human life, may be frozen for future use, discarded if not needed, or used for research with the parents' permission. Other national commissions and committees—most notably in England, Australia, and Canada—have taken similar positions. But not all ethicists agree; some claim that respect for the human embryo requires fertilizing at the time of retrieval only the number of eggs to be transferred. This may cause additional inconvenience and expense for the couple, but these ethicists feel that the practice of fertilizing only what will be immediately implanted protects the origin of new human life and acknowledges the value of the human embryo in a way that discarding or freezing them does not. Although their position is a minority view at the present time, there are good reasons for it.

The moral status of the embryo is the fundamental issue in IVF, and it is difficult to resolve. At one extreme are those who consider the embryo an unborn baby, and at the other extreme are those who think of it simply as human tissue. Both extremes are unreasonable. Most people fall somewhere in the middle in their evaluation and think that some special respect is appropriate for embryonic human life.

What, then, might be a reasonable moral position at this time in regard to IVF? Perhaps a position that seeks a middle ground between outright condemnation and casual acceptance. That prudential position might find IVF reasonable for married couples of child-bearing age when all else has failed and when the number of fertilized ova is restricted to the number that will be immediately returned to the woman's body. This is a starting point.

With more experience and ethical reflection on the process, a wider scope for IVF may be morally justified. It seems reasonable for couples who are carriers of serious genetic disease to resort to IVF in order to select only unaffected embryos for transfer. And it may be possible to give adequate reasons for splitting or freezing a couple's embryos, for example, despite the risks and damage to human life that these procedures entail.

An ethics of prudence requires us to consider all the relevant circumstances and consequences of our behavior, and we simply do not yet know the consequences that will ensue from many of the different ways IVF can be used. Thus, our moral judgments must be tentative and conservative lest we thoughtlessly harm ourselves and our chances for happiness.

We have been slow to recognize the ethical issues associated with the new reproductive technologies in the United States. Other countries have been more sensitive to the moral and social dimensions of the procedures and are not so willing to allow IVF or other fertility treatments in every kind of situation. In late 1993, for example, Canada's Royal Commission on the new reproductive technologies issued its long-awaited report recommending, among other things, that IVF be limited to women with blocked fallopian tubes and that men selling their sperm be limited to fathering no more than ten children. In many European countries there are also growing movements to introduce restrictions on the use of the new reproductive technologies.

It is ironic in a way that the moral vacuum surrounding IVF in the United States was generated, at least in part, by moral concerns. During the Reagan–Bush years (1980–1992) the government, committed to an antiabortion position, withheld practically all federal support for IVF research. Although this move did protect embryonic life, it also created an unfortunate situation, as we discuss in chapter 14. Without federal funding, IVF researchers sought private capital. Thus, the IVF research in this country was supported by commercial interests, and commercial interests are driven largely by financial motives.

Fertility treatments are very profitable, and it matters little to some people involved in the new reproductive technologies whether the woman is married or not, whether the eggs are hers or have been purchased from another woman, whether the sperm comes from her husband or is bought from a sperm bank, whether the woman is heterosexual or homosexual. What does matter is whether the client has access to funding and whether the chances of pregnancy are sufficiently high to make the procedures worthwhile.

As we will see in chapter 14 on research, if federal funding had been allowed for IVF research, the research would have been subjected to local review boards and could have been subjected to a national ethics committee as well. The reviews by local and national committees designed to protect the human subjects in research would have made the ethical issues associated with IVF far more prominent than they have been in the commercially funded research.

The morality of IVF cannot be determined by an ethics of rights. It is not enough for a woman or a couple to say "I have a right to have a baby" and conclude that IVF is morally justified. Nor is it enough for opponents to say "every child has a right to begin life in the body of the woman whose egg is fertilized." The morality of IVF is a morality of responsibility; we determine the morality of what we do by how it affects the human good. It is not difficult to recognize that infertility is a problem for couples desiring to reproduce their genetic children and that some medical interventions to alleviate this problem are morally reasonable.

The ethics of IVF becomes much more shaky, however, when we go beyond what we have to do to overcome infertility in a couple and begin to buy and use eggs and sperm from third parties or begin to cause pregnancies that will result in children whose fathers are anonymous and disinterested. Using IVF to help infertile couples have their own children is one thing many ethicists can readily accept; discarding and freezing human embryos are more difficult to justify; and the buying and selling of human sperm and eggs for purposes of reproduction are even more difficult to see as something good and noble.

Gamete Intrafallopian Transfer

In 1984 the reproductive technique of gamete intrafallopian transfer (GIFT) was developed. The most important difference between IVF and GIFT is that the fertilization with IVF occurs outside the body, whereas the fertilization with GIFT takes place inside the body in a fallopian tube. GIFT is the procedure whereby gametes (sperm and eggs) are placed in the fallopian tubes before the egg is fertilized. The first two steps of the procedure are the same as they were for IVF, although the egg retrieval for GIFT is more frequently by laparoscopy. In the third step some eggs are transferred by laparoscopy into the fallopian tubes along with the sperm. The entire procedure takes about an hour. Sometimes, of course, GIFT cannot help a couple because it requires at least one healthy tube, whereas the IVF procedure does not depend on healthy fallopian tubes.

GIFT avoids many of the moral issues found in IVF. First, the fertilization occurs in the body, not in a laboratory petri dish, and thus GIFT reduces the intrusion of medical manipulation into the beginning of human life. Second, GIFT avoids the sensitive questions about the moral status of the embryo in the laboratory or in the freezer. There are no extra embryos in GIFT to discard, freeze, or use for research; all the embryos are in the body, not the laboratory. There may be extra eggs, but discarding eggs does not present the same moral issues as does discarding embryos. Thus, many people uncomfortable with IVF from a moral point of view find it possible to consider GIFT a morally acceptable option.

Zygote Intrafallopian Transfer

Yet another process is zygote intrafallopian transfer (ZIFT), which is similar to IVF. Ovaries are prepared; eggs are retrieved (usually by laparoscopy) and then fertilized in a petri dish. The zygotes (very early embryos) are then transferred, usually the day after they are retrieved, into the fallopian tubes rather than into the uterus as with IVF. The moral issues for ZIFT are, in general, the same as they are for IVF.

Ovum Transfer

In this procedure, one woman sells or donates her eggs for insertion into another woman whose ovaries are not producing healthy eggs either because of abnormalities or because she has passed menopause. Sperm is then inserted, either by IUI or by intercourse. In late 1993 it was reported that a fifty-nine-year-old postmenopausal woman had become pregnant this way and delivered a child.

One moral issue with such a procedure is the use of eggs from a third party. This means the baby is not the genetic child of the woman gestating it. Moreover, the procedure can be used for questionable purposes not associated with infertility. It was also reported in 1993, for example, that a black woman married to a white man wanted a white child. She arranged for the insertion of an egg from a white woman; then her husband's spermatozoon fertilized this egg, producing a white baby. Among the several ethical issues in such a procedure is the issue of racism; good ethics requires that the intention of a racially mixed couple to avoid a child with any chromosomes from one race is not tainted with racism—the notion that one racial group is superior to others.

CLONING

In February 1997 a sheep named Dolly suddenly caught everyone's attention. A Scottish scientist named Ian Wilmut succeeded in reproducing sheep a new way. Instead of combining two germ cells (an ovum and a spermatozoon) each with a nucleus contributing half the chromosomes of the offspring, he fused the nucleus of a cell taken from the udder of a six-year-old sheep with the ovum from another sheep after the ovum's nucleus had been removed. As a consequence, all the nuclear chromosomes of the ovum came from one sheep and the resultant lamb thus received its chromosomes from one parent, not two. Dolly was born a clone, an almost-identical twin to her six-year-old genetic parent.

People could not help but wonder: What about us? What will happen if the technique is used to reproduce human beings? Human clones, once the fantasies of science fiction, suddenly became real possibilities.

As you would expect with any new development, many people had a poor understanding of cloning and its implications. The word cloning actually refers to several different procedures, and most of them would not result in a new individual of the species. Stretches of DNA are cloned to make copies of a healthy gene. Cells can also be cloned. Cloning DNA or cells, however, does not present the serious social or ethical problems that would arise if we cloned an entire human being.

The technical description of cloning an entire individual used by the National Bioethics Advisory Commission (NBAC) is somatic cell nuclear transfer (SCNT). A somatic cell is any cell in our bodies except our germ cells—ova and spermatozoa. What happens in SCNT is this: A somatic cell from one individual is transferred into an ovum of a second individual after its nucleus has been removed. The nucleus from the transferred cell replaces the nucleus in the ovum, and the ovum with the new nucleus develops into an individual whose total nuclear genetic code is derived from the somatic cell. The offspring receives its entire nuclear genetic code from the originating somatic cell, and almost no genes from the ovum of its "mother."

Somatic cell transfer can use cells from embryos, fetuses, or individuals. Actually, Dolly is not really the first lamb clone. Scientists first cloned a lamb using a somatic cell from an *embryo* in 1986. And they did the same with monkeys in 1995. This kind of cloning—embryo somatic cell nuclear transfer—received little attention probably because cloning an embryo did not strike people as really cloning another individual being. But, of course, it is, and the successful cloning of lambs from embryo cells in 1986 indicated that humans could be cloned long before Dolly appeared.

Lambs have also been cloned from fetal somatic cells; in fact, the same experiment that produced Dolly produced three other lambs through fetal somatic cell nuclear transfer. Again, this kind of cloning received little attention, probably because it was overshadowed by Dolly and partly because many people do not consider fetuses as individual human beings.

The cloning of Dolly, however, did catch everyone's attention. This was a case of adult SCNT; that is, the being contributing the nucleus of its cells was not an embryo or a fetus but a postnatal adult. Now the public could see the implications of cloning. They could imagine scientists taking a cell from a person and putting it into a human ovum whose nucleus was removed. That ovum would then develop into a baby with its thirty thousand or so genes almost identical to those of the person contributing the nucleus. Cloning with cells taken from embryos or fetuses was one thing; cloning with cells taken from human beings after birth was quite another.

Many think a cloned human being would be identical to the human being whose somatic cell was used in the cloning process. This is a false impression for several reasons. First, removing the nucleus of the ovum does not remove all its genes—a few genes exist outside the nucleus in the cytoplasm of the ovum. These mitochondrial genes in the host ovum will be passed on to the child. Hence, a clone would not be an identical genetic copy of the person providing the somatic cell—a few of its genes would come from the host ovum. This is enough to give it a different genetic identity. Second, genes mutate randomly in the cells of a body, so even the identical genes in the clone will divide and multiply in a slightly different way in the clone's body than they will in the source body. Finally, genes are not the whole story in personal identity. Genes interact with each other and with the environment, and these interactions shape the personal identity of genetically close human beings, as we know from studies of identical twins derived from a single fertilized ovum. There is no question then that a human clone would be significantly different from its source; he or she would truly be a "new one of us" who happened to have a very close genetic match with another person, just as an identical twin is with its sibling.

Shortly after the news of Dolly was announced in February 1997, President Clinton banned the use of federal funds for research on ways to clone human beings. He also asked NBAC to study the ethical and legal issues and to issue a report within ninety days, a very short time to evaluate a new and complex issue. The NBAC was an eighteen-member interdisciplinary commission that was formed in 1995 and began meeting in late 1996. Its charter expired in October 2001. Its two original priorities were the protection of human subjects in medical research and ethical issues involving genetic information. The NBAC had a relatively low profile until President Clinton asked it in early 1997 to produce the report on cloning. It responded well, given the limited time to study a complicated area, and issued its helpful report entitled *Cloning Human Beings* in June 1997, only four months after the announcement about Dolly. It made five major recommendations about human SCNT.

- Human SCNT is morally unacceptable at this time because it is not safe at this point.
- Federal legislation should prohibit SCNT for three to five years.
- No new restrictions on cloning DNA, cells lines, or animals are needed.

- Given the conflicting religious and ethical positions on cloning humans, the federal government should encourage widespread deliberation.
- Federal agencies should educate the public about cloning and genetics.

Several things are noteworthy about the commission's work and recommendations. First, the commissioners sought religious perspectives on cloning. The beginning of human life and new forms of creating human beings have always been of interest in religious traditions, and these voices need to be heard in a country where many people practice a religious faith. Representatives of many religious faiths provided testimony. As expected, there was substantial disagreement about human cloning, although there was general agreement that a cloned human being would still be created in the image and likeness of God and hence be fully human, that is, one of us.

Second, the commissioners focused only on cloning to produce children; they did not consider cloning to produce embryos for research. Cloning for research became a major issue only after the 1998 discovery of the potential therapeutic value of embryonic stem cells. This discovery immediately suggested cloning human embryos in order to obtain their stem cells.

Finally, the ethical reasoning of the commission focused on the obligation to prevent harm to children (the principle of nonmaleficence) and on the duty to recognize reproductive rights. Preventing harm and recognizing reproductive rights, although important, are not the main focus in virtue ethics, which focuses on the good. This ethic will focus on whether cloned children, who will suffer some health deficits as a result of the cloning (Dolly was not a healthy animal with a normal life span), will be able to flourish and on whether having a cohort of cloned people in the world will enrich society and the common good or undermine it.

Questions about how new reproductive techniques will be good for the child reproduced and for future human society have been notoriously absent in questionable reproductive matters such as surrogate motherhood, IVF treatments for women without fertility problems or for post-menopausal women, using ova from aborted fetuses, buying and selling ova and sperm resulting in anonymous genetic fathers and mothers, and so forth.

Unfortunately the NBAC, by sticking with a principle-based and rights-based moral approach, continued the American minimalist tradition of reproductive ethics. A richer ethic would have asked: What good is likely to come for the individuals cloned and for society if we clone human beings? If the answer is "not much good is likely," then pursuing research in cloning human individuals is not a reasonable venture. The fundamental moral challenge in cloning human individuals does not center on avoiding harm and respecting a person's right to reproduce but on putting forth reasons showing that cloning new individuals is likely to lead to a good life for those cloned and for societies peopled by human clones. Those arguments have yet to be made.

In 1998 the cloning controversy took a new turn when embryonic stem cells were isolated and when some scientists suggested cloning human embryos to produce these pluripotent stem cells for a whole new area of genetic research. Then, in November 2001 American researchers claimed to have successfully produced the first cloned human embryo. In January 2002 the National Academy of Sciences (NAS) issued a report titled *Scientific and Medical Aspects of Human Reproductive Cloning*, which agreed with the NBAC report that cloning to produce a child should not be done "at this time" because the risk of harm is too great. The NAS report acknowledged that cloning to produce a child might one day be medically safe for offspring, and hence, it encouraged a broad ethical debate so we would be ready for that day if it ever comes.

The President's Council on Bioethics (PCB), formed by President Bush in 2001, took up that ethical debate in its 2002 report titled *Human Cloning and Human Dignity: An Ethical Inquiry*. The report focused on both cloning children and cloning embryos to provide stem cells for research. The report noted the importance of accurate terminology when discussing the ethics of cloning and made an important suggestion. Instead of using the usual terms reproductive cloning (when the purpose is producing children) and therapeutic cloning (when the purpose is producing embryos for research), it suggested cloning-to-produce-children and cloning-for-biomedical-research. This is a positive step. As was noted in chapter 3, clear language is indispensable for good moral deliberation, and it is certainly misleading to speak of "therapeutic cloning" when no cloning therapies exist or will exist for years, if ever. Unfortunately, most of the literature still speaks of "therapeutic cloning." This makes it difficult to oppose because no one wants to oppose a therapy that could help someone. Research cloning is not a therapy, although it could lead to therapy in the future.

The PCB went a step beyond the NBAC and the NAS, which had said cloning-to-produce-children should not be attempted "at this time." The PCB ignored the qualification and concluded simply that cloning-to-produce-children is "morally unacceptable, and ought not to be attempted." It is interesting to note in passing that the 2004 Canadian Assisted Human Reproduction Act bans both cloning for children and cloning for research.

An interesting feature of the PCB report is that it did not rely heavily on the classic American principles of bioethics. Its ethical analysis looked at arguments that are both for and against cloning-to-produce-children and often explained them in terms of how cloning children might advance or undermine personal and social goods as well as the good of the cloned child. Such an approach has much in common with virtue ethics with its emphasis on achieving what is good.

SURROGATE MOTHERHOOD

Advances in the mastery of human reproduction have introduced still another phenomenon: surrogate motherhood. The general idea of surrogacy is that a woman unable or unwilling to become pregnant engages another woman to become pregnant in her place, with the understanding that this woman will give her the newborn child at birth. The conception of the child can happen in a number of ways. The most common is artificial insemination of the surrogate woman by the husband's sperm. This will make the husband and surrogate woman the genetic parents and the wife an adoptive parent. If the wife is willing to undergo egg retrieval, it is also possible that her egg could be used in a process such as IVF, GIFT, or ZIFT to begin pregnancy in the surrogate. This will make wife and husband the genetic parents, and the pregnant woman is simply the gestational mother carrying a child genetically unrelated to her.

The idea that a couple experiencing infertility can enlist the aid of a fertile woman to bear a child for them is an ancient one. The Hebrew Bible (Genesis 16:17) records the story of childless Sarah telling Abraham to sleep with her maid Hagar so he could have a child. Abraham and Sarah were living in Egypt at the time. Abraham complied with Sarah's request, slept with her maid, and she became pregnant. The Bible gives no indication that using a maid for a surrogate mother by the childless couple was immoral. In fact, the customs of ancient Babylonia (modern Iraq), where Abraham and Sarah dwelled, allowed the practice.

We should note that the notion of surrogate motherhood in these situations suffers from some linguistic confusion. Hagar, not Sarah, was the real mother of Abraham's first son, Ishmael. Hagar was both the genetic parent and the gestational mother. Today the "other" woman is called the "surrogate" mother. She does not become pregnant by intercourse with the husband, of course (that would now be considered adultery, although it was not so considered by the people of Abraham's time), but by artificial insemination. But if a woman becomes pregnant by intercourse or by artificial insemination and then delivers a child, she is not really the surrogate mother; she is, as was Hagar, the real mother.

If another reproductive technology such as IVF or GIFT is employed in the modern surrogacy arrangement, and the eggs of the wife are used, then it is true that the surrogate mother is not the genetic mother of the child. But there is still good reason to consider her the mother because she is the gestational mother—the one who conceives, carries, labors, delivers, and perhaps nurses the child. Merely contributing the egg to be fertilized does not make one a mother. We do not consider the women who sell their eggs the mothers of the children whom other women will conceive with these eggs. The woman with the strongest claim of motherhood is the woman who actually becomes pregnant and gives birth. Another woman may raise the child, and this makes her the mother in a real sense, but she does not thereby become the biological or natural mother. And another woman may have donated the egg, making her the genetic mother of the child, but she is not the natural mother whose body supported the fetus for nine months and then delivered the baby.

We stress this because there is a value in beginning with our traditional ways of viewing motherhood and then considering the new reproductive possibilities in light of them. Calling the artificially inseminated woman giving birth the surrogate mother implies that the woman who will adopt the baby after birth and raise the child is the only authentic mother. But this too easily demeans the woman who was pregnant and gave birth. It also sets the stage for a failure to appreciate the difficulty some women have in giving up a child after birth despite their agreement to do so nine months earlier.

We should also recognize at the outset two very different settings for what is called surrogate motherhood. The more common kind of surrogacy is commercial. It involves a contract and the exchange of money. The woman is recruited by some kind of broker or agency and then becomes pregnant, usually by artificial insemination. Her medical bills are paid, she signs a contract to give up the child, and she is paid a significant sum (around $10,000) when she does.

The second setting involves personal relationships and no money. By way of example, a woman may carry a child out of love for her sister who is unable to do so. The gestational mother may have contributed her own egg, which is fertilized by the artificially inseminated sperm of her sister's husband, or accepted an IVF embryo resulting from the medically assisted fertilization of her sister's egg by the sister's husband. This kind of family surrogacy presents far fewer moral issues than the surrogacy involving strangers and money. In the case of the sisters, the child remains in the family, as it were, and the natural mother remains bonded in the role of aunt. Of course, the surrogate need not be a sister. In 1987 a forty-eight-year-old grandmother in South Africa gave birth to triplets who originated from an IVF procedure using her daughter's eggs and the sperm of her daughter's husband. She is thus the gestational mother of her grandchildren and the grand-mother of her own children, which will make her the great-grandmother of her grandchildren.

The effort to show that family surrogacy is reasonable and good has a better chance of succeeding than does any form of commercialized childbearing. After all, surrogacy for another member of the family is rooted in love, not money. But there is a subtle shadow of immorality lurking beneath the surface of this selfless love. The sister, or mother, or other female relative offers her body in a spirit of altruism that many find morally appealing but others question. The pregnant woman becomes the altruistic woman giving and nurturing and providing for the needs of another who cannot become pregnant.

Extolling the maternal role of women for the sake of another, however, has a dark side—pregnancy and child rearing have often been used to turn women away from their own needs. As we become more sensitive to the ways women can be exploited and how victims of exploitation often willingly embrace the structures that exploit them, there will be doubts about the moral goodness of even family surrogacy where the woman undergoes pregnancy not for herself and her husband, but for the sake of a relative.

The moral analysis of surrogate motherhood must embrace all the relevant circumstances. It is not enough to say that the family surrogate is acting out of love, not money, and the action therefore is morally justified. We must also show how the action accords with the achievement of the human good. If family surrogacy places the women who do it in a position of exploitation, then the human good is undermined.

The fact that the woman chooses to be a surrogate is not enough to neutralize the moral questions. Migrant workers or illegal aliens may choose to work for below-minimum wage, but that does not mean they are not being exploited. Although it is possible to volunteer to work for substandard wages, or even to work for nothing, more often than not the "volunteer" is in a psycho-logical or social position where she just cannot say no. In other words, the choice is really the illusion of choice. And the same situation is an ever-present danger in family surrogacy, where the choice to become pregnant for one's sister may not be much of a choice at all because the potential surrogate would feel so bad, perhaps even guilty, if she did not perform this service for her sister.

Despite this objection, some ethicists do not object to family surrogacy. What they widely criticize, however, is commercial surrogacy—that is, entering into a child-bearing contract involving money with a stranger who was provided by a broker for a fee. The moral arguments supporting this practice are shallow; they usually rely on a gratuitous claim to reproductive freedom and on the supposed right of people to have a child. Often they introduce the idea of how noble it is for a woman to help another woman have a child by becoming pregnant for her and then experiencing the great joy of presenting her with the baby that will fulfill the other woman's life and needs.

We turn now to what is perhaps the most publicized case of commercial surrogate motherhood, the story of Baby M. It is a story where almost everything that could go wrong did go wrong. Thus, it does not represent most contractual arrangements, but it is a good case to consider because we often learn more about things when they break down than when they function well.

The Case of Baby M

The Story

In 1984 William and Elizabeth Stern decided to have a child. Later testimony revealed that William was very interested in having a genetic child, but there were no indications that Elizabeth felt strongly about becoming pregnant. There were also some indications that, despite lack of definitive medical diagnosis at the time, she had multiple sclerosis, which discouraged her from wanting to become pregnant. There is no evidence that she was infertile. Both the Sterns were well educated and well employed—she is a physician.

They were soon to meet Mary Beth Whitehead. Mary Beth had dropped out of high school, was married with two children, and was in serious financial difficulty. She and her husband had filed for bankruptcy after both mortgages on their home lapsed into default. In 1984 she applied to the Surrogate Mother Program in New York, but she was rejected. Then she applied to a program with less rigorous screening, the Infertility Center of New York, and was accepted. The center brought the Sterns and Mary Beth together in January 1985.

They made a contract. It stipulated that Mary Beth would not smoke, drink, or use drugs during pregnancy; that she would seek prenatal care; that she would not abort the baby unless it endangered her health; that she would undergo amniocentesis or similar tests to detect defects; and that she would have an abortion at the request of William if the fetus were defective. If she had the abortion she would receive $1000; if the baby was defective and she refused an abortion at William's request, then he had no obligation to accept the child. When the child was born and handed over to the Sterns, Mary Beth was to receive $10,000; if the child was stillborn she was to receive $1000.

After nine attempts at artificial insemination, Mary Beth became pregnant. Her obstetrician advised against amniocentesis because she was in her twenties and at low risk for an abnormal fetus. William insisted, however, so she had the test, thus needlessly risking damage to the fetus. Everything was normal.

The baby was born on March 27, 1986. Those assisting at the birth were unaware of the surrogacy arrangement. Mary Beth's husband was listed as the father on the birth certificate, and Mary Beth began nursing the child. She named her Sara Elizabeth Whitehead. Several days later, the Whiteheads took Sara home and reluctantly surrendered her to the Sterns. Mary Beth became very upset and asked to have the baby back for a few days. The Sterns agreed. Once Mary Beth had her baby back, she left with the five-day-old infant for her mother's home in Florida.

She soon returned to New Jersey but kept the baby, so William Stern got a court order directing her to surrender the baby to him. She refused. With the order and five police officers, he then went to the Whiteheads' house, but Mary Beth passed the baby out a rear window before they could retrieve her. William and the police left empty handed. The next day the Whiteheads fled to Florida, where they disappeared for almost three months. Florida police finally recovered the baby, and she was returned to the Sterns. They named her Melissa Stern. The Whiteheads returned to New Jersey and began legal action to recover Sara/Melissa.

The Court Decisions

In April 1987 a judge ruled that a contract is a contract, and thus "Baby M" belonged with the Sterns. Mary Beth appealed, asking the courts to declare any contracts signed by a surrogate mother void and unenforceable because no contract can force a mother to give up her child. In February 1988 the New Jersey Supreme Court, in a unanimous decision, agreed with her. It pointed out that laws forbid payments to induce women to give up their children; that a woman can give up her child for adoption only after birth; and that children cannot be taken from their mothers unless the mothers are shown to be unfit. The supreme court considered the child a baby conceived out of wedlock—the daughter of Mary Beth Whitehead fathered by a married man, William Stern. It then had to decide which parent—Mr. Stern or Mrs. Whitehead—should have custody of the child.

By the time of the state supreme court deliberations, Mary Beth had become pregnant by a person other than her husband (he had had a vasectomy). She then separated from her husband and married the father of her newest child in November 1987. Knowing this, the court gave custody of Sara/Melissa to William Stern in view of his more stable home life. And to Mary Beth, the child's mother, it gave visitation rights. It refused to allow Elizabeth Stern to adopt Sara/Melissa because Sara/Melissa's real mother, Mary Beth, did not want to give her up for adoption. For most of the year, Baby M was known as Melissa and lived in New Jersey with the Sterns, but every other weekend and during two weeks in the summer, she was known as Sara and lived in New York with her mother—now Mrs. Mary Beth Gould—and her mother's four other children.

The court wisely noted that this kind of surrogate motherhood comes close to selling babies. In a stinging comment, it said that a surrogate contract "guarantees separation of a child from its mother; it looks to adoption regardless of suitability; it totally ignores the child; it takes the child from the mother regardless of her wishes and her maternal fitness; and it does all this, it accomplishes all of its goals, through the use of money."

When Melissa turned eighteen in 2004 she was able to give her consent for the Sterns, who had raised her, to adopt her, which they did. The family has guarded its privacy carefully, but Melissa was quoted as saying in 2007: "I'm very happy I ended up with them. I love them, they're my best friends in the whole world, and that's all I have to say about it."

Ethical Reflection

In the minds of most ethicists commercial surrogacy is not an ethical dilemma because the bad features totally overwhelm any possible good features, and hence we will not do an ethical analysis of the story. Simply put, the bad features in this case are many and obvious; the good features are few or absent. Among the bad features are the following.

1. Deliberate and planned damage to the fullness of parenthood by separating maternal rearing from the maternal genetic and gestational aspects of motherhood.

2. Deliberate and planned distancing of a child from its genetic and gestational mother.

3. The undermining of human dignity by reducing human reproduction to a commercial contract, thus reducing the birth of a child to a legal arrangement akin to the sale of goods and services.

4. Payment of money for a child. Mary Beth was to receive $10,000 for the baby born live, but only $1000 if the baby were stillborn, thus showing that the major part of the payment was for a live baby and not simply for the inconvenience of pregnancy, as some claimed. Children are not property, and buying and selling them treats them as property.

5. Potential future harms to a child who may one day discover her mother became pregnant with the idea of rejecting her at birth. There is, of course, no hard evidence that children born in these circumstances will he hurt by the discovery that their mothers planned to reject them as soon as they were born, but it is an ethical issue we cannot ignore until we are sure it would not happen. It is difficult to see how a person would not be hurt by such a discovery.

6. Potential future distress to a woman who may easily one day regret deliberately becoming pregnant with the intention of handing over her baby to strangers for money.

7. Potential custody battles over who gets a child deliberately conceived outside of marriage.

8. Potential degradation of the gestational mother, whose actions have some analogy with prostitution. In prostitution, a woman allows the use of her reproductive system to fulfill the needs of a stranger in return for money. If his needs are sexual gratification without reproduction, we call the agent who arranges it a pimp or procurer and the activity prostitution. If his needs are reproduction without sexual gratification, we call the agent who arranges it a broker and the arrangement surrogate motherhood. Despite the more polite language of surrogacy, neither commercial arrangement is morally noble.

9. Payment for a live baby sets up exploitation of the gestational mother. It is not readily conceivable that a woman would become pregnant for a stranger unless she needed the money. Some say this is not exploitation if the woman freely chooses to do it. After all, they say, she has the right to use her body as she sees fit. But most would say the needy person choosing to become pregnant for a stranger is trapped into making a decision people would not make if they had enough money. Deciding to become pregnant by a stranger with a baby one intends to abandon at birth bespeaks a desperation that makes people vulnerable to exploitation. Desperate financial circumstances can undermine the ability to give truly voluntary consent. Surrogacy for money sets up a social phenomenon whereby the financially well off can pay to use the reproductive systems of the less well off, and this is a form of exploitation difficult to admire morally.

10. Potential harm to the surrogate's other children when they learn that their mother has babies and then gives them away for money, an unpleasant thought for children with their normal fears that their parents might abandon them.

Most ethicists can find no adequate reasons to justify commercial surrogacy, and thus there is widespread, albeit not total, consensus that it is immoral. Surrogacy within a family for altruistic reasons where no contract or money is involved fares better, yet many still have ethical objections to those arrangements. The reality of human existence is that some people of reproductive age want to have children but cannot. There are many techniques and technologies to help them, but it is naive to think all reproductive procedures and arrangements are morally noble. Surrogacy, especially commercial surrogacy, is most difficult to justify morally. Wanting a child very badly is not enough to make every means to have one morally reasonable.

ETHICAL REFLECTIONS

We have considered reproductive issues at some length because most medical interventions to prevent pregnancy as well as to cause it involve both good and bad features (that is, moral issues). Although most texts on health care ethics now take reproductive interventions for pregnancy seriously, that was not always the case. Both IUI and IVF became established medical practices before there was adequate moral reflection and dialogue. And few texts consider the moral issues involved in the medical interventions to prevent pregnancy.

What interventions designed to prevent or to cause pregnancy are moral, and under what circumstances, are frequently matters of moral dispute. We cannot settle these disputes, but the ethical approach we have been using suggests prudential reasoning will unfold within the following framework.

1. Sexuality is best lived in a stable and faithful relationship of love, caring, and trust.

2. Contraceptive interventions always introduce bad features in a sexual relationship; the interventions become moral evils whenever they are not reasonable and truly constitutive of the good of the couple and of society.

3. Reproductive interventions are also bad features in a sexual relationship; they become moral evils whenever they are not reasonable and truly constitutive of the good of the couple and society. The easiest reproductive interventions to justify are those involving infertile committed

couples using their own gametes and producing no surplus embryos. Introducing sperm and eggs produced by third parties for money, or trying to cause pregnancy outside socially acceptable family structures, seriously complicates the procedure and makes it all the more difficult to justify the interventions as morally reasonable. And surrogate motherhood for money has so many bad features that it is difficult to see how it could ever contribute to the human good of the adults involved, or of a child reproduced in such a way, or of society itself.

In the years since the birth of the first IVF child in 1978, the techniques for medically assisted pregnancy have improved and expanded tremendously. The whole field, however, still suffers from a lack of serious moral reflection and regulatory or legal guidance. As a result, virtue has taken a back seat.

The conceptual framework guiding artificial reproductive technology (ART) in the United States has almost exclusively centered on the rights of would-be parents—reproductive rights and the rights to privacy and self-determination—and free market principles. Almost totally forgotten in the new reproductive techniques and technologies are the children. The focus of IVF clinics is almost entirely on their "clients" who desire pregnancy and on the money that can be generated by providing fertility services for them. Too few people who are providing medically assisted reproduction are asking whether all possible scenarios of medical reproduction are good for the children and for society. The American Society of Reproductive Medicine has an ethics committee but serious concern for the children reproduced is notably lacking from its many statements, including its protocol for retrieving spermatozoa from corpses for fertilization.

We cannot live good lives by ignoring the welfare of the children we create. It is difficult to see how it is good to create children who will be denied knowledge of their genetic parents or who may discover that half their genes came from a female aborted fetus or from a male corpse or who will have spent the first nine months of their human life in the body of a woman who does not intend to be their mother and who, in most cases, carried and delivered them for money. And it is unlikely that children will benefit when they learn that they were once ready-made frozen embryos that would be allowed to develop if needed and, if not needed, would have been discarded, used for research, or sold to other couples looking for a child. Few IVF physicians and prospective parents are deliberating carefully about the possible harms for children and for society when children are deliberately conceived for birth into single or nonheterosexual parental environments.

Some thoughtful ethicists and national committees in other countries (the Human Fertilization and Embryology Authority in England is an example) do express moral discomfort with some of the ways the new reproductive techniques are being used. They argue for a child-centered moral analysis based on what is likely good for future children rather than an analysis based on parental rights and the principle of self-determination. They worry about likely harms to children deliberately denied in advance the chance to know their genetic parents and siblings, to children who might be cloned, to children produced from germ cells taken from dead bodies or fetuses, to children given away by their surrogate mother who carried them, and to children whose health and well-being are compromised by their origin in a high-risk multiple pregnancy caused by IVF or fertility drugs. In the United States the PCB addressed many of these concerns in its 2004 report titled *Reproduction and Responsibility: The Regulation of the New Biotechnologies*, but ART remains largely unregulated in the United States.

Some advocates for the right to reproduce and for unrestricted procreative liberty advance a curious argument against these worries about possible harms to future children. Their argument is that possible harms to children is not a good reason for restricting procreative liberty and reproductive choice because it will always be better for a child to exist than not to exist. In other words, although they acknowledge that some medical reproductive techniques may cause the child harm, the child will still be better off existing than not existing. As a well-known version of the argument goes, "being born is always a benefit despite the harms you know you might cause in the reproduction of that life."

The argument is logically questionable because we really cannot say existence itself is a benefit for the one reproduced. Benefits and burdens accrue to a human being only after it exists. It is misleading to suggest that reproduction is a benefit for a child because the child does not exist, and hence cannot benefit, before it is reproduced. Reproduction is not really a benefit for the one reproduced but rather the necessary precondition that makes all benefits and burdens possible.

SUGGESTED READINGS

The brief account of the history of contraception is drawn from John Noonan, 1986, *Contraception: A History of Its Treatment by the Catholic Theologians and Canonists*, enlarged ed., Cambridge, MA: Harvard University Press. The quotations from Augustine are taken from here. Also helpful is James Brundage, 1987, *Law, Sex, and Christian Society in Medieval Europe*, Chicago: University of Chicago Press. For a brief summary of the good and bad features of various contraceptive interventions, see Daniel Mishell, "Contraception," *New England Journal of Medicine* 1989, *320*, 777–86.

The idea that the leaders of the Catholic Church are needed to explain the natural law is found in Gerald Kelly, 1958, *Medico-Moral Problems*, St. Louis: Catholic Health Association, pp. 131–32. Kelly also wrote: "it follows, therefore, that the teaching of the Church is a practical necessity for an adequate knowledge of the natural law; and we should not be surprised when those who lack the benefit of this teaching are in error as to the existence or extent of some obligations. . . . In our age, this guidance seems to be particularly necessary in the matter of artificial birth prevention" (p. 153).

John Noonan has proposed a provocative and seldom noted strategy for reconciling artificial contraception with the current papal teaching that artificial contraception is against the natural law. Since nature restricts a woman's fertility to the few days surrounding ovulation, natural law proscribes using contraceptives only during these few days. In other words, Noonan claims that the official Roman Catholic position against all artificial birth control permits a couple with good reasons to use contraceptives (condoms and diaphragms, for example) any time except on the few days each month when fertility is thought to occur. See his "Natural Law, the Teaching of the Church, and the Rhythm of Natural Fecundity," *American Journal of Jurisprudence* 1980, *25*, 16–37, reprinted as an appendix in *Contraception*, pp. 535–54. For one of the few reactions to this innovative proposal see Joseph Boyle, "Human Action, Natural Rhythms, and Contraception: A Response to Noonan," *American Journal of Jurisprudence* 1981, *26*, 32–46. For Noonan's reply, see "A Prohibition without a Purpose? Laws That Are Not Norms?" *American Journal of Jurisprudence* 1982, *27*, 14–16. Noonan's ingenious effort to reconcile his church's position against artificial birth control with the practical need for contraception in some marriages is not necessary for Catholics who understand morality as primarily a matter of doing what achieves the human good in particular circumstances and not primarily a matter of observing laws, principles, rules, or dictates.

The key cases in the legal history of contraception in the United States are *Poe v. Ullman*, 367 U.S. 498 (1961); *Griswold v. Connecticut*, 381 U.S. 479 (1965); *Eisenstadt v. Baird*, 405 U.S. 438 (1972); and *Carey v. Population Services International*, 431 U.S. 678 (1977).

Sterilization is widely recognized as an ethical issue when the person is a minor, retarded, or directed by a court or other agency to have the surgery. In 1927 the U.S. Supreme Court, remarking that "three generations of imbeciles are enough," ruled that state statutes providing for compulsory sterilization of retarded people were constitutional (*Buck v. Bell*, 274 U.S. 200 [1927]). Punishing criminals by sterilization, however, was declared unconstitutional in *Skinner v. Oklahoma*, 316 U.S. 535 (1942). Nonetheless, interesting legal and ethical cases continue to arise. In 1988, for example, Indianapolis newspapers reported that an unmarried pregnant woman was charged with murdering her four-year-old son. She was allowed to plead guilty to a lesser charge. Before sentencing, the judge indicated he would impose a reduced prison term if she agreed to sterilization after the child she was now carrying, conceived while awaiting the murder trial, was born. She had her baby, immediately surrendered him for adoption, and consented to the sterilization. This kind of case sets up a major ethical conflict. A psychiatrist had testified that she was sane and not a threat to anybody except her children, so the judge thought it was reasonable to shorten her prison term if she agreed to sterilization. But it is also reasonable to suggest that a person cannot give consent freely for a surgical procedure when the only alternative is spending time in prison, and therefore that the surgery was unethical.

An excellent (and free) starting point for reading about artificial reproductive technology (ART) is the 2004 report of the President's Council on Bioethics titled *Reproduction and Responsibility*, available online at bioethics.gov. For the personal and social ethics of artificial reproduction, see also Thomas Shannon, ed., 2002, *Reproductive Technologies: A Reader*, New York: Rowman and Littlefield; Kenneth Alpern, ed., 1992, *The Ethics of Reproductive Technology*, New York: Oxford University Press; Richard

Hull, ed., 1990, *Ethical Issues in the New Reproductive Technologies*. Belmont: Wadsworth Publishing Company; Andrea Bonnicksen, 1989, *In Vitro Fertilization: Building Policy from Laboratories to Legislatures*, New York: Columbia University Press; Peter Singer and Deane Wells, 1985, *Making Babies: The New Science and Ethics of Conception*, New York: Charles Scribner & Sons; Bonnie Steinbock, 1992, *Life Before Birth*, New York: Oxford University Press, chapter 6; Machelle Seibel, "A New Era in Reproductive Technology: In Vitro Fertilization, Gamete Intrafallopian Transfer, and Donated Gametes and Embryos," *New England Journal of Medicine* 1988, *318*, 828–34; Marcia Angell, "New Ways To Get Pregnant," *New England Journal of Medicine* 1990, *323*, 1200–1202; Arthur Caplan, "The Ethics of In Vitro Fertilization," *Primary Care* 1986, *13*, 241–53; Edward Hill, "Your Morality or Mine? An Inquiry into the Ethics of Human Reproduction," *American Journal of Obstetrics and Gynecology* 1986, *154*, 1173–80; Hans Tiefel, "Human In Vitro Fertilization: A Conservative View," *JAMA* 1982, *247*, 3235–42; Lori Andrews, "Legal and Ethical Aspects of New Reproductive Technologies," *Clinical Obstetrics and Gynecology* 1986, *29*, 190–204; John Robertson, 1994, *Children of Choice: Freedom and the New Reproductive Technologies*, Princeton: Princeton University Press; Lori Andrews, 1999, *The Clone Age: Adventures in the Now World of Reproductive Technology*. New York: Henry Holt and Co.; John Harris and Søren Holm, eds., 1998, *The Future of Human Reproduction: Ethics, Choice, and Regulation*, New York: Oxford University Press; Diane Kondratowicz, "Approaches Responsive to Reproductive Technologies: A Need for Critical Assessment and Directions for Further Study," *Cambridge Quarterly of Healthcare Ethics* 1997, *6*, 148–56; and Thomas Murray, "What Are Families For? Getting to an Ethics of Reproductive Technology," *Hastings Center Report* 2002, *32* (May–June), 41–45, reprinted in Shannon's *Reproductive Technologies* cited above, pp. 113–21. Murray is critical of the approach to artificial reproductive technologies based on the framework of procreative liberty and argues instead for what he calls a "flourishing-centered approach"; that is, on what makes good lives and enhances the values of children, parents, and the families they form.

Many organizations have issued position papers on the new techniques of assisting pregnancy. Some of the more important examples are the reports and statements by the Ethics Committee of the American Society for Reproductive Medicine (ASRM, formerly called the American Fertility Society), available at asrm.org/media/ethics. See also *A Question of Life: The Warnock Report on Human Fertilization and Embryology* issued by the Department of Health and Social Security in Great Britain in 1985; the Instructions on *Respect for Human Life in Its Origin and the Dignity of Procreation: Reply to Certain Questions of the Day* (*Donum Vitae*, 1986) and *Dignity of the Person* (*Dignitas Personae*, 2008) issued by the Vatican and available at usccb.org. Despite strict Vatican statements to the contrary, some Catholic university hospitals have active programs in reproductive technologies and preimplantation genetic diagnosis, especially in Belgium and the Netherlands. See, for background, I. Brosens, ed., 2006, *The Challenge of Reproductive Medicine at Catholic Universities: Time to Leave the Catacombs*, Leuven, Belgium: Peeters Publishers. *Infertility: Medical and Social Choices* released by the Office of Technology Assessment in 1988, available at fas.org/ota/reports, is still of interest. For an excellent summary of the major committee statements in the early years of ART see LeRoy Walters, "Ethics and the New Reproductive Technologies: An International Review of Committee Statements," *Hastings Center Report* 1987, *17* (June), suppl., 3–9.

The New Jersey Supreme Court decision in the Baby M case is *In the Matter of Baby M*, 537 A.2d 1227 (1988). See also Phyllis Chesler, 1988, *Sacred Bond: The Legacy of Baby M*, New York: Times Books; Dianne Bartels, ed., 1990, *Beyond Baby M: Ethical issues in New Reproductive Techniques*. Clifton, NJ.: Humana Press; George Annas, "Baby M: Babies (and Justice) for Sale," *Hastings Center Report* 1987, *17* (June), 13–15, and "Death without Dignity for Commercial Surrogacy: The Case of Baby M," *Hastings Center Report* 1988, *18* (April–May), 21–24; Angela Holder, "Surrogate Motherhood and the Best Interests of Children," *Law, Medicine & Health Care* 1988, *16*, 51–56; Ruth Macklin, "Is There Anything Wrong with Surrogate Motherhood? An Ethical Analysis," *Law, Medicine & Health Care* 1988, *16*, 57–64; and Lisa Cahill, "The Ethics of Surrogate Motherhood: Biology, Freedom and Moral Obligation," *Law, Medicine & Health Care* 1988, *16*, 65–71. Also helpful is New York State Task Force on Life and the Law, 1988, *Surrogate Parenting: Analysis and Recommendations for Public Policy*, Albany: Health Education Services. The quotation of Melissa Stern (Baby M) is taken from the *New Jersey Monthly* for March 2007, available at njmonthly.com.

On the hidden undesirable features of altruistic surrogacy (that is, the offer of a woman to bear another's child for love, not money), see Janice Raymond, "Reproductive Gifts and Gift Giving: The Altruistic Woman," *Hastings Center Report* 1990, *29* (November–December), 7–11. Raymond notes: "altruism has been one of the most effective blocks to woman's self-awareness, and demand for self-determination. . . . The social relations set up by altruism and the giving of self have been among the most powerful forces that bind woman to cultural roles and expectations" (p. 9).

The New York State Task Force on Life and the Law has produced a fine public report, the first in the United States, on individual and social concerns triggered by infertility treatments, *The Assisted Reproductive Technologies: Analysis and Recommendations for Public Policy*, 1998, Albany: Health Education Services (the executive summary is available at health.state.ny.us). The report offers many recommendations for professional guidelines, state regulation, and state legislation. Most important, however, is the way it frames the questions of reproductive technologies: The central issue is not reproductive freedom and rights but the welfare of children. The report is very much child-centered—the wishes of adults wanting children and of providers wanting to market their services are considered less compelling than the best interests of children.

The study showing an increase in major birth defects for IVF with ICSI is Michele Hansen et al., "The Risk of Major Birth Defects after Intracytoplasmic Sperm Injection and In Vitro Fertilization," *New England Journal of Medicine* 2002, *346*, 725–30; and the study showing the increase in premature birth after ART is Laura Schieve et al., "Low and Very Low Birth Weight in Infants Conceived with Use of Assisted Reproductive Technology," *New England Journal of Medicine* 2002, *346*, 731–37. The study showing the increased ratio of risk between Type 2 diabetes and premature birth is Peter Whincup et al., "Birth Weight and Risk of Type 2 Diabetes: A Systematic Review," *JAMA* 2008, *300*, 2886–97. For new developments in IVF that may reduce the problem of multiple pregnancies, see Alan Templeton et al., "Reducing the Risk of Multiple Births by Transfer of Two Embryos after In Vitro Fertilization" and David Meldrum et al., "Two-Embryo Transfer: The Future Looks Bright," *New England Journal of Medicine* 1998, *339*, 573–77 and 624. A good summary of ICSI with an awareness of its potential for harming children is Gerald Schatten et al., "Cell and Molecular Biological Challenges of ISCI: ART before Science?" *Journal of Law, Medicine & Ethics* 1998, *26*, 29–37. An excellent starting point for learning about medical reproductive techniques is the series of articles in the *Encyclopedia of Bioethics*, rev. ed., volume V, 1995, 2207–48. The entry "Ethical Issues" by Cynthia Cohen (2233–41) is especially helpful. See also Cynthia Cohen, "Give Me Children or I Shall Die": New Reproductive Technologies and Harm to Children," *Hastings Center Report* 1996, *26* (March–April), 19–33.

The case of Mary Sue and Junior Davis is *Davis v. Davis*, 842 S.W.2d 588 (1992), and the case of Maureen and Steven Kass is *Kass v. Kass*, 91 N.Y.2d. 554 (1998). For commentary on *Kass* and another recent case, see George Annas, "The Shadowlands—Secrets, Lies, and Assisted Reproduction," *New England Journal of Medicine* 1998, *339*, 935–39.

Also see Carson Strong, 1997, *Ethics in Reproductive and Perinatal Medicine: A New Framework*, New Haven: Yale University Press. His "new framework" moves away from polar extremes based on nonnegotiable rights to an approach that recognizes the need to resolve conflicts between a woman's reproductive freedom and the interests of her fetus by carefully working through paradigm cases illustrating these conflicts. His case-based approach is both casuistic and prudential as he goes beyond cases to include, as did Aristotle, current political and moral opinions and also to acknowledge the priority of some values or goods over others.

For a good overview of the growing practice of using commercial ova for IVF, see Cynthia Cohen, ed., 1996, *New Ways of Making Babies: The Case of Egg Donation*, Bloomington: Indiana University Press. The essays were originally written for the National Advisory Board for Ethics in Reproduction (NABER) and include chapters by supporters of four IVF centers using commercial eggs followed by nine chapters written by more cautionary ethicists. NABER's recommendations for legislation and policy conclude the book.

The NBAC report *Cloning Human Beings* (1997) is available at bioethics.georgetown.edu/nbac, and the PCB report *Human Cloning and Human Dignity: An Ethical Inquiry* (2002) is available at bioethics.gov. The executive summary of the NBAC report on cloning can be found in the *Hastings Center Report* 1997, *27* (September—October), 7–9. The same issue includes several very helpful commentaries on the NBAC report by James Childress, Susan Wolf, Courtney Campbell, Daniel Callahan, and Erik Parens. A special section on cloning in the *Cambridge Quarterly of Healthcare Ethics* 1998, *7*, 115–205 contains eleven articles as well as an interesting interview with Ian Wilmut and other scientists and a bibliography. Two articles framing the debate for and against cloning humans are John Robertson, "Human Cloning and the Challenge of Regulation" and George Annas, "Why We Should Ban Cloning," pp. 119–22 and 122–25. See also Jerome Kassirer, "Should Human Cloning Research Be Off Limits?" *New*

England Journal of Medicine 1998, *338*, 905–6; Andrea Bonnicksen, "Procreation by Cloning: Crafting Anticipatory Guidelines," *Journal of Law, Medicine & Ethics* 1997, *25*, 273–82; and Patrick Hopkins, "Bad Copies: How Popular Media Represent Cloning as an Ethical Problem," *Hastings Center Report* 1998, *28* (March–April), 6–13. A very readable account of cloning is Gina Kolata, 1998, *Clone: The Road to Dolly and the Path Ahead*, New York: William Morrow. Also helpful is Lee Silver, 1997, *Remaking Eden: Cloning and Beyond in a Brave New World*, New York: Avon Books. The National Academy of Sciences report *Scientific and Medical Aspects of Human Reproductive Cloning*, Washington, DC: National Academy Press, was published in 2002. Chapter 5 of the 2002 PCB report *Human Cloning and Human Destiny: An Ethical Inquiry* is highly recommended for a clear overview of arguments pro and con regarding cloning to produce children.

ELEVEN

Prenatal Life

B Y PRENATAL LIFE we mean the period of human life extending from implantation until the birth or the extraction of the fetus. The developing human life is usually called an embryo through the eighth week of development and then a fetus until birth. For the sake of simplicity, we will use the words "fetus" and "fetal" to describe prenatal human life from implantation until viability. Once a fetus has developed sufficiently to live outside the uterus it seems more reasonable to consider it a baby within the mother rather than a fetus. Viability—the expectation that the fetus can survive outside the uterus—normally occurs toward the end of the second trimester. Although some object to using the language of "baby" for any of the unborn, we actually do speak this way in many contexts. For example, if a woman seven months pregnant suffers a miscarriage, we usually do not say she lost her fetus; we say she lost her baby. When she feels movement, she usually does not say she is feeling the fetus move; she says she is feeling the baby move. And if she in a serious accident, the media usually do not report that doctors are trying to save her fetus; they report that doctors are trying to save her baby.

A heated controversy rages over just when a fetus becomes a "person." It is a controversy worth avoiding. The debate about the personhood of the fetus is endless and not resolvable. "Person" is one of those terms people define arbitrarily. Some say a newly fertilized egg is a person, whereas others insist we cannot speak of a person until a later stage of embryonic, fetal, or even neonatal development.

A more promising approach is to ask when the developing fetal body becomes "one of us." As was pointed out in chapter 6, not every living human body is one of us. A human being that meets the criteria for whole brain death, for example, is no longer one of us, yet his human body may live for weeks or months, thanks to life-support equipment. And a fetus without the ability to perceive is not yet one of us because it is not yet a sentient or psychic body. It makes little sense to say that a human body without the capacity for even the most rudimentary perception, either because it has irreversibly lost it or has not yet developed it, is at this moment actually one of us. Human existence is never simply vegetative; it is always an "existence-in-the-world" with aware-ness, or at least with the actual capacity for awareness, of its environment. Human existence does not mean something human "is"; it means something human "is-in-the-world." When the devel-oping fetal body becomes psychic, it becomes one of us because its existence is now in-the-world by virtue of its sentience.

It is important to remember, however, that a fetus is human life before it becomes one of us. All human life is valuable, and thus an ethics of the good calls for special respect toward prenatal life from the beginning, not simply from the time it becomes a psychic or sentient body. Virtue ethics is a life-affirming ethics. It cherishes life and flourishing; it does not advocate deliberately harming or destroying human life unless there are proportionate and compelling compensating reasons. What constitutes an adequate reason for damaging or destroying a fetus, however, varies with its stage of development. Once the fetus becomes a psychic or sentient body, only very serious reasons justify intentionally damaging it, and once the fetus is viable, the reasons justifying delib-erate damage become even more serious, almost as serious as those justifying deliberate damage to a newborn.

In this chapter we consider two situations: interventions to destroy fetuses (abortion) and efforts to save fetuses that are contrary to the wishes of the pregnant woman. Before taking up these issues, it will be helpful to acknowledge two major features of prenatal life.

First, pregnancy makes a major impact on the life of the woman, and it may cause considerable discomfort. Pregnancy is sometimes accompanied by physical and psychological problems, and the physical risks are occasionally life-threatening. In view of a fetus's impact on her life, a woman obviously needs some control over whether and when she will become pregnant. It is, after all, her body that becomes pregnant, and each of us has an important interest in determining what happens to our bodies. Every discussion about pregnancy, therefore, is a discussion about a woman's life.

Second, an embryo is a new human life. It is a living human being with a new genetic identity. Although the fetus cleaves within another body for its existence until birth, it is genetically distinct from its human host. Every discussion about pregnancy, therefore, is also a discussion about a new human life.

Prenatal life, then, raises questions about two important human goods: (1) the woman's personal choices and responsibility for her life, and (2) the important reality of a distinctively new human life. It is precisely this dual nature of prenatal life, of course, that creates the major moral dilemmas.

ABORTION

The most conspicuous clash of these human goods occurs when abortion is the issue. The Centers for Disease Control and Prevention (CDC) reported in 2004 that legal abortions increased gradually from 1973 (the year of *Roe v. Wade*) until 1990, when that number started to decline. In 2002, 854,122 abortions were reported to the CDC, a ratio of about 246 abortions for every one thousand births. New York City had the highest number (almost 92,000) followed by the states of Florida (almost 88,000) and Texas (almost 80,000). About 87 percent of the abortions were performed in the first trimester (less than thirteen weeks). The Guttmacher Institute has given somewhat different figures. After surveying abortion providers in 2005 it reported that the annual number of abortions had dropped to 1.2 million, down from 1.6 million in 1990. The Institute also found that the number of pregnancies ending in abortion dropped to 22.5 percent in 2005, down from 24.5 percent in 2000.

More than a million abortions a year in the United States raises an obvious moral question: is the destruction of so much human life good or bad for people? Does it enhance or does it undermine our respect for living things? At a time when people are becoming more aware of a moral responsibility for animals and for the environment itself, what is the appropriate ethical attitude toward this extensive destruction of prenatal human life?

Much of the debate about abortion in our country is couched in terms of rights—the right to life and the right to choose. And the public debate is also characterized by extreme positions— many people defending either the right to life or the right of choice allow no exceptions to their positions. The result is a noisy and often ugly stalemate. Careless rhetoric has replaced careful thought, ill will has replaced good will, ideology has replaced reason, and simplistic self-righteousness has replaced awareness of just how complex the whole question really is. The ideological right-to-life position tramples on a woman's prerogative to make choices about her body, and the ideological right-to-choose position fails to appreciate the human life of the fetus.

The intractable stalemate about the morality of abortion argued from uncompromising positions suggests we must look elsewhere for moral insight. A moral reasoning that first acknowledges the complexity of the issue and then seeks a solution according to right reason may be helpful. The abortion issue is complex because it involves, among other things, two human lives, so many relevant circumstances, and such long-term effects.

Any adequate consideration of the ethics of abortion will include (1) something of the history of the dilemma; (2) acknowledgment of the bad features present in every abortion; and (3) recognition of the widespread agreement that some elective abortions are morally justified, that is, consistent with the human good, despite the destruction of human life they entail.

Abortion in History

Abortion is not a new moral concern. People have been having and performing abortions for a long time, and physicians and ethicists have been debating the ethics of the interventions over many centuries. Some ancient commentators, as the Hippocratic Oath so vividly reminds us, thought abortion was always immoral. Others thought it could be justified in certain situations. The conditions most frequently proposed to justify abortion were these: the pregnancy was endangering the health of the woman, population control was needed, or the pregnancy would cause extreme difficulty for the woman. An example of extreme difficulty would be the situation in which society punished a woman's adultery by death, and abortion was the only way to conceal adulterous behavior.

Although neither the Hebrew Bible nor the Christian scriptures mention abortion, the influential translation of the book of Exodus from Hebrew into Greek (third century B.C.E.) revised the original biblical text to say that the destruction of a "formed" fetus was equivalent to homicide. (We have discussed this textual revision by translators in chapter 6.) Several centuries later the influential Jewish philosopher Philo of Alexandria associated abortion with infanticide, a practice he deplored. To consider abortion equivalent to homicide or infanticide is, of course, to consider the act seriously immoral.

The Christian stand against abortion was strong from the beginning. An influential summary of Christian prohibitions composed in Syria around the year 100 explicitly listed the sin of abortion alongside sins of killing, stealing, adultery, and fornication. All the early fathers of the Christian church condemned abortion. After the Roman Empire, which covered much of Europe, adopted Christianity as its official religion in the fourth century, the Christian position against abortion became normative, and its moral position was almost unquestioned in Europe for a thousand years.

The rise of medical education in the new universities that were springing up in the thirteenth and fourteenth centuries stimulated renewed interest in the ethics of abortion. At the beginning of the fourteenth century John of Naples, who taught at the universities of Paris and of Naples, argued that it is morally justified for a physician to perform an abortion of an early pregnancy to save the woman's life. Most moralists of the time declined to support his views.

By the end of the sixteenth century, however, the important Jesuit moralist Tomas Sanchez was arguing that abortion of an early fetus could be supported by plausible arguments in three cases: (1) serious danger to the woman's health, (2) fear of family reprisals for an extramarital pregnancy, and (3) avoidance of the injustice an adulterous pregnancy would cause a husband who would have to support a child he did not father. Sanchez thought the arguments for abortion in these circumstances were not simply "probable" but "more probable." "More probable" is a technical term in moral theology indicating arguments stronger than merely probable arguments but weaker than arguments providing us with moral certitude.

The work of Sanchez prompted other Christian moralists to question the absolute prohibition against abortion more openly. They were aware that Christian morality had embraced the biblical commandments against killing and stealing yet had allowed exceptions to these laws of God in extenuating circumstances. They suggested the same approach could be used for abortion.

Although some Christian moralists began proposing exceptions to the traditional Christian prohibition against abortion at this time, papal authority and the leaders of the other Christian churches springing up in the sixteenth century were moving in the opposite direction. In 1588, for example, Pope Sixtus V issued an official document (called a papal bull) condemning all abortion at any stage of prenatal development without exception and, as we saw in the last chapter, all contraception as well. Lest there be any doubt about how serious the sin of abortion was in his mind, he ordered the heaviest penalties of church and civil law imposed on those performing any abortion, even an abortion necessary to save the woman's life. This meant the abortionist would be excommunicated and, if he or she lived in the territories where the church had civil jurisdiction, as it did in central Italy, would be executed. (History does not record anyone being executed for abortion or for contraception; the penalties were never strictly enforced, and the successor of Pope Sixtus cancelled most of them.)

By the end of the nineteenth century most Christian churches still considered all abortion immoral. Christianity, however, has not been the only historical factor shaping the American consciousness about abortion; there is also a legal history. During the nineteenth century most of the opposition to abortion in the United States came from legal and medical sources, not from religious movements. Connecticut enacted the first state law against abortion in 1821. It was a limited law, forbidding only drugs used to induce abortions of "quickened" fetuses (that is, abortions after fetal movement is experienced).

By 1840 seven more states had placed restrictions on abortions after quickening. During this time the abortion rate continued to climb in the United States. It reached, according to some estimates, 250 abortions for every thousand live births. This represents about 20 percent of all pregnancies, a rate about the same as that of today.

Abortions in the nineteenth century were often painful, unsafe, and botched. People performing them were not well trained medically, and they operated on the fringes of the medical profession. Most people performing them were not physicians. It is not surprising, then, that reputable physicians became concerned, especially when women harmed by abortionists came to them for help. Many physicians, therefore, began to take a stand against the practice of abortion.

A turning point was reached when the newly established American Medical Association (AMA) adopted an antiabortion stance at its annual convention in 1859. The physicians' position against abortion was influential, and it stimulated political action. As a result, by the end of the century, state laws against abortion were widespread in our country. They usually allowed one exception: an abortion necessary to preserve the life of a woman.

It is somewhat ironic how the struggle by physicians against abortion at this time was actually setting the stage for the current practice whereby physicians now have the exclusive authorization to perform abortions. By making all abortions illegal except those to save the woman's life, the only legal abortions were those performed by physicians trying to save a patient's life. For decades these abortions were few because abortion is seldom necessary to save the life of the woman. But when abortions for other reasons became legal in the twentieth century, society simply assumed physicians should continue to perform them, and thus elective abortion became a medical intervention only physicians could provide. This is what makes abortion a topic in medical ethics and not merely a matter of choice or a legal question.

As time went on some physicians used a very broad interpretation of abortions needed to "preserve the life of a woman." For a few this phrase meant that any abortion was justified if there were reason to believe that the woman would seek an illegal abortion if she could not obtain a legal one, thereby exposing herself to life-threatening injuries and perhaps death.

By the 1950s a movement was well under way in the United States to reverse the laws against abortions, especially in one or more of these situations: (1) the pregnancy was dangerous for the woman, (2) the fetus was seriously defective, and (3) the pregnancy resulted from rape or incest. Soon the state laws began to change. By the early 1970s, nineteen states had relaxed their abortion laws to some extent, and four states (Hawaii, New York, Washington, and Alaska) allowed early abortions at the request of the woman without any justifying reason. Pressure for change was mounting, and many state legislatures were responding by liberalizing the abortion laws. Then, in one stroke, the Supreme Court dramatically undermined the legislative process with the famous 1973 decision known as *Roe v. Wade*.

Abortion and the Supreme Court

In *Roe v. Wade* the Supreme Court decided (by a 7–2 vote) that most laws restricting abortion were unconstitutional because they violated a woman's "privacy," something not explicitly mentioned in the Constitution but nonetheless guaranteed by it.

The name "Jane Roe" was used to designate the woman whose attorney challenged the abortion laws in Texas. This was her story. In the summer of 1969 she was walking home from work late in the evening when she was jumped and gang raped. She did not report the crime to the police. When she realized she was pregnant a few weeks later, she wanted an abortion, but abortion was illegal in Texas except in order to protect the life of the woman. Roe's lawyer, Sarah

Weddington, challenged the Texas law, and a three-judge panel, after listening to her story, ruled that she could have a legal abortion. Henry Wade, the district attorney of Dallas County, did not agree, and he appealed the ruling to the U.S. Supreme Court. The famous case is known as *Roe v. Wade*.

The U.S. Supreme Court ruled in 1973 that the Texas abortion law was unconstitutional. In *Roe v. Wade* it decided that

- In the first trimester, states cannot make any laws regulating abortions.
- In the second trimester, states cannot make any laws regulating abortions unless they are related to the health of the woman.
- In the third trimester, states may make laws regulating abortions, and even forbid them, unless the abortion is necessary to preserve the life or the health of the mother.

The real name of Jane Roe is Norma McCorvey. Her story was a lie—she was not raped. She had already given up custody of her first baby and released the second one for adoption at birth. Now she simply wanted to end her third pregnancy. Her subsequent admission that she had lied about how she became pregnant and why she wanted the abortion does not, of course, affect the Supreme Court ruling. And she never had the abortion; she gave her baby up for adoption, and the little girl is now a middle-aged woman.

The history of abortion since *Roe v. Wade* has been marked by intense controversy. The tedious but valuable process that had begun to work its way through state legislatures was destroyed as seven men (the decision was 7–2) made, in effect, a new law for the land on a very important and controversial issue. They based their decision on a right, the right of personal privacy. They acknowledged that this right is not explicitly mentioned in the Constitution but insisted its roots are found in the "penumbras" (or shadows) of the Bill of Rights and in the concept of liberty guaranteed by the Fourteenth Amendment to the Constitution. They also ruled that the right of privacy covering abortion is not unqualified; it "must be considered against important state interests in regulation."

The *Roe v. Wade* decision is extremely liberal. It does not allow states to restrict abortion at all in the first trimester and allows restrictions in the second trimester only on how the abortions will be performed. In the second trimester, for example, states may insist on regulations governing abortionists and abortion clinics, as long as these standards do not unduly restrict a woman's access to an abortion. In effect, then, the Supreme Court decision allows abortion on demand during the first six months of pregnancy. No reason is needed to justify the decision.

We can see how extreme this decision is by comparing it to the positions other countries take on abortion. Abortion is now legal in every other Western country except Ireland, but the legal restrictions are more conservative. Most of the countries do not allow abortion on demand but only for reasons judged adequate to justify it. Those few that do allow abortion on demand (examples are Norway, Sweden, Denmark, Austria, and Greece) generally restrict it to the first trimester. Sweden is the most liberal of the abortion-on-demand countries, allowing it through the eighteenth week, but this is still more conservative than what the law allows in the United States.

Roe v. Wade does not provide much protection for prenatal life. The fetus is not protected at all until the third trimester, and then it is not protected unless the individual states choose to restrict or forbid abortions, and most states do not so choose.

The failure of the Supreme Court to offer any protection to prenatal life in the first two trimesters and its claim that abortion was somehow an almost unlimited "right" during these trimesters have caused intense political distress from the very beginning. The ruling sent the wrong message to many people. Many Americans could have accepted laws allowing early abortions in difficult situations as the lesser of two evils, but they almost instinctively react to a position that gives no indication that prenatal life is of any importance in the first two trimesters and that views the choice to destroy a fetus as a constitutional right. In hindsight we can see the great political mistake of *Roe v. Wade*: regardless of its merit in acknowledging and protecting a woman's choice about her pregnancy, it failed to acknowledge that prenatal human life in the first two trimesters is also something important and valuable.

The history of the abortion debate in the United States since *Roe v. Wade* has been largely the story of reactions to that Supreme Court decision. Many of the battles have gone to the Supreme Court as some people have tried to narrow the application of *Roe v. Wade* by passing state laws restricting abortion.

At first the Supreme Court took a dim view of the efforts of any state to restrict abortions and struck down most of the new laws as unconstitutional in light of the *Roe v. Wade* decision. As the years went on, however, new justices with more conservative ideas about abortion were appointed to the Court, and its recent decisions tend to give states more room to make some regulations about elective abortions, as long as the laws do not impose an undue burden on the woman seeking an abortion. The following are some of the more notable positions on abortion taken by the Supreme Court after *Roe v. Wade*.

- *Planned Parenthood v. Danforth* (1976)
- *Maher v. Roe* (1977)
- *Harris v. McRae* (1980)
- *City of Akron v. Akron Center for Reproductive Health* (1983)
- *Thornburgh v. American College of Obstetricians and Gynecologists* (1986)
- *William Webster v. Reproductive Health Services* (1989)
- *Planned Parenthood Association of Southeastern Pennsylvania v. Casey* (1992)
- *Carhart v. Stenberg* (2000)
- *Gonzales v. Carhart* (2007)

Planned Parenthood v. Danforth (1976)

Missouri tried to limit abortions by adding numerous restrictions, among them parental consent if the woman is a minor and spousal consent if she is married. The law also required doctors to make efforts to preserve the life of the aborted fetus. The *Danforth* decision struck down these restrictions, but it did let stand a description of viability that included survival outside the uterus made possible only by life support equipment.

Maher v. Roe (1977)

Some people claimed that *Roe v. Wade* gave women on welfare the right to have free abortions. This would mean that federal and state governments, using tax dollars, would be paying for abortions. In fact in the first three years after *Roe v. Wade*, about a third of all abortions (almost 300,000 annually) were actually funded by Medicaid, a federal and state welfare program for poor people. Some states, however, refused to use tax dollars for abortions. Connecticut was one such state, and its refusal to use Medicaid funds for elective abortions was challenged. Its refusal was upheld, however, by the Court in *Maher v. Roe*, but the majority on the Court supporting *Roe* dropped to 6–3. The decision means states may refuse to pay for abortions for women on welfare, and many states do refuse. The decision also implies that women do not have an unrestricted "right" to abortion—they have to find a willing provider and a way to pay for it.

Harris v. McRae (1980)

At about this time, some members of Congress were trying to prevent the use of federal funds for abortions. In 1976 Congress passed an amendment to the federal Medicaid Act first proposed by Representative Henry Hyde that prohibited the use of federal funding for abortion unless the woman's life was endangered. The day after the first Hyde Amendment was passed in 1976, it was challenged in federal court by Cora McRae. She lost her case when the Supreme Court upheld the constitutionality of the Hyde Amendments in *Harris v. McRae*.

The annual amendments restricting federal funding for abortion are still known as the Hyde Amendments. In 1993 Congress relaxed the Hyde Amendments' federal ban somewhat by requiring Medicaid (the state-run program partially supported by federal funds) to pay for abortions after rape or incest beginning April 1, 1994.

In view of *Danforth, Maher*, and the Hyde Amendments, states need not, and the federal government cannot, fund abortions unless the pregnancy threatens the woman's life or is the result of rape or incest. In other words the right of privacy that the Supreme Court invoked to allow a woman to choose abortion in the first two trimesters does not mean that federal or state funds have to pay for it if she cannot afford to pay for it herself.

In this sense, *Roe v. Wade* does not give every woman the right to abortion on demand; it does not guarantee that she can have an abortion. Its position is more modest; it simply says that states cannot make laws preventing a woman from having an abortion in the first two trimesters. It does not say that the state or the federal government has to provide the abortion for her—unless her life is endangered or, since 1994, the pregnancy was caused by incest or rape. A pregnant woman cannot argue: "*Roe v. Wade* gives women the right to an abortion; hence, if I cannot pay for my abortion, my medical care under a welfare program must provide it." A few states do pay for elective abortions, but they have gone beyond what *Roe v. Wade* requires.

City of Akron v. Akron Center for Reproductive Health (1983)

A city ordinance in Akron, Ohio, had placed numerous restrictions on obtaining abortion, among them parental consent or judicial approval for girls under fifteen; the need to provide women with information about fetal development, possible emotional complications after abortion, and adoption agencies; a twenty-four-hour waiting period; and disposal of the fetus in a "humane" way. The Court struck down these restrictions. It ruled that minors of any age who have good reasons for not seeking parental consent need not obtain it. States may, however, require that they appear before a judge in a confidential hearing to show that they are mature enough to make the abortion decision for themselves. The *Akron* decision upheld *Roe v. Wade*, but the majority on the Court supporting *Roe* dropped to 6–3.

The dissenting opinion in *Akron* written by Justice Sandra Day O'Connor underlined two important issues that would become more prominent in the abortion controversy. First, she opined that states should be able to make laws restricting abortion at any stage of the pregnancy provided the restrictions do not "unduly burden" the right to seek a legal abortion (Roe had greatly limited the ability of states to restrict abortions in the first two trimesters), and she famously commented that Roe's three-semester approach to abortion "is clearly on a collision course with itself." This is so because medical improvements have raised the time for safe abortions beyond the end of the first trimester and have also lowered viability into a period before the third trimester begins. Hence, "there is no justification in law or logic for the trimester framework adopted in Roe."

Thornburgh v. American College of Obstetricians and Gynecologists (1986)

Pennsylvania's 1982 Abortion Control Act had stipulated that a woman considering abortion had to be given certain information that included the gestational age of the fetus, the physical and psychological risks of the abortion procedure, the assistance she could receive for having the baby and then giving it up for adoption, the financial liability of the father for the support of the child, and an offer to review literature that showed "the probable anatomical and physiological characteristics of the unborn child at two-week gestational increments from fertilization to full term, including any relevant information on the possibility of the unborn child's survival."

In *Thornburgh* the Court found these restrictions were "overinclusive" and "not medical information that is always relevant to the woman's decision, and . . . may serve only to confuse and punish and to heighten her anxiety, contrary to accepted medical practice." The Court found that all this information went beyond what was needed for informed consent to abortion and thus struck down the Pennsylvania Abortion Control Act. *Thornburgh* continued to uphold the central position of *Roe v. Wade*, but the majority on the Court supporting Roe dropped to 5–4.

The *Thornburgh* decision is not without a certain irony. On one hand, the ruling protects the woman from being manipulated during the informed consent process by people trying to make her change her mind about the abortion allowed under *Roe v. Wade*. On the other hand, the ruling undermines the pregnant woman's ability to give truly informed consent by allowing abortionists to withhold information about side effects and acceptable alternatives to abortion. As we saw in chapter 4, truly informed consent means that the physician discusses all reasonable alternatives with the patient.

Withholding information about the side effects and alternatives to abortion might make it more probable that the woman will continue with her decision to have the procedure, but it also undermines her ability to make a truly informed choice. Our choices are not informed unless we have all the available relevant information. Thus—and this is the irony—the *Thornburgh* decision makes it easier for women to choose an abortion but undermines an authentic pro-choice position. It strengthens the right to abortion on demand, but it undermines the informed consent process necessary for sound choices about any invasive medical procedure. Justice Burger made this very point in his dissenting opinion in *Thornburgh*. His remarks are all the more significant because he was one of the seven justices who originally had voted for *Roe v. Wade*.

William Webster v. Reproductive Health Services (1989)

Missouri had inaugurated a number of regulations aimed at restricting abortion. These included that physicians employed by the state may not perform abortions, that state facilities may not provide abortions, and that physicians performing abortions must try to determine whether the fetus is viable whenever there is question of an abortion at or beyond twenty weeks. These regulations were challenged, and in *Webster* the Court ruled that the state of Missouri could make these regulations. In effect, *Maher v. Roe* had already established that states could not be forced to fund elective abortions, and this easily allowed the Court to uphold state laws prohibiting nontherapeutic abortions in state hospitals and prohibiting physicians on the state payroll from performing abortions.

The Missouri regulation requiring physicians to determine viability of fetuses beyond twenty weeks of gestation, however, was not so easy for the Court to resolve. *Roe v. Wade* had said that states cannot make regulations affecting fetal life before the third trimester, which at that time was thought to begin about the twenty-fourth week. The Missouri twenty-week test thus contradicted the trimester framework of *Roe v. Wade* and would seem to be unconstitutional.

The Court responded by saying the trimester framework of *Roe* is outmoded. Moreover, it saw no reason why a state's interest in protecting prenatal life "should come into existence only at the point of viability." In other words, in contrast to *Roe v. Wade*, the Court now acknowledged that fetal life has some value before viability and that states might have an interest in protecting it. In *Webster*, the Court does not see why "there should therefore be a rigid line allowing state regulation after viability but prohibiting it before viability." Once the Court accepted the view that states have an interest in protecting prenatal life before the third trimester, it could easily conclude that the testing of fetuses at twenty weeks, which is in the second trimester, is constitutional.

Planned Parenthood Association of Southeastern Pennsylvania v. Casey (1992)

After the 1986 *Thornburgh* decision Pennsylvania enacted a new and more carefully crafted Abortion Control Act in 1989. It included the following restrictions: (1) The woman seeking an abortion must notify her husband in writing; (2) the physician must inform the woman of fetal age and the risks of abortion, pregnancy, and childbirth; and a counselor must provide information about fetal development, alternatives to abortion, and possible state aid available if pregnancy continues; (3) a twenty-four-hour waiting period between consent and the abortion procedure; and (4) if the woman is a minor, at least one parent must also give consent, unless a judge waives this requirement.

The restrictions of this Abortion Control Act were challenged, but in *Casey* the Court upheld all of them except the requirement of notifying the husband. This decision pleased neither the defenders nor the opponents of *Roe v. Wade*. Defenders thought that the court should have found all the restrictions in the Pennsylvania law unconstitutional; opponents were disappointed that the court did not simply overturn *Roe v. Wade*.

The *Casey* decision is important for what it said about the value of prenatal life. Whereas it insisted that a woman has the right to choose abortion before viability without undue interference from the state, it also said that the state has legitimate interests in protecting both the woman's health and the "life of the fetus that may become a child" before viability. The decision allows states to regulate abortions before viability, provided the regulation is not an "undue burden" on the woman's right to have the abortion. The Court defined a burden as undue "if its purpose or effect is to place a substantial obstacle in the path of a woman seeking an abortion before the fetus attains viability." The Court concluded that the twenty-four-hour waiting period and the requirements for information about the risks, fetal development, and alternatives to abortion were not "undue burdens."

Carhart v. Stenberg (2000)

After the *Casey* decision concluded that "the essential holding of *Roe v. Wade* should be retained and once again reaffirmed," some opponents of *Roe*, perhaps taking a cue from the language in the *Casey* decision itself, adopted a new approach. In a joint opinion in *Casey*, several justices had argued that overruling Roe's essential holding would cause "profound and unnecessary damage" to "the Nation's commitment to the rule of law." This suggested to some that the road to banning abortion lay with the nation's law-making branches of government—Congress and state legislatures, which could outlaw certain types of abortion. They focused first on a procedure known as an "intact D&X" that is sometimes used for abortions beginning in the late second trimester. The intact D&X procedure involves dilating the cervix, moving the fetus so the legs and trunk are in the vagina, and then suctioning out the contents of the skull so it can be compressed and the newly dead but otherwise intact fetus can be removed. To win public support for their efforts to have a law outlawing intact D&X they renamed the procedure "partial birth abortion." Actually, "partial birth abortions" are relatively rare. At the turn of the century one published report reported that they averaged about 2,200 a year or about one-sixth of one percent (0.17 percent) of the abortions in the United States.

In March 1996 Congress passed a ban on partial birth abortions, but President Clinton vetoed it, and the effort to override the veto failed. In October 1997 Congress passed a second ban on partial birth abortion, but President Clinton again vetoed it, and the effort to override the veto again failed. By the late 1990s, however, thirty-one states had banned partial birth abortions, but federal appeals courts found these laws unconstitutional whenever they were challenged. There were two main sticking points. First, the laws criminalized partial birth abortions in the second trimester before viability, and this conflicted with *Roe v. Wade*, which held that states could only regulate abortion in the second trimester "in ways that are reasonably related to maternal health." Partial birth abortion does not add any risk to a woman's health; in fact, it is a medically accepted procedure for late abortions. Second, most of the state laws criminalized all abortion after viability except in one case: when the abortion is necessary to preserve the life of the mother. This clause also conflicted with *Roe v. Wade*, which held that states could not criminalize abortion after viability "where it is necessary, in appropriate medical judgment, for the preservation of the life *or health* of the mother." (emphasis added).

After a Nebraska state law banning partial birth abortion was declared unconstitutional by both a federal district court and a federal appeals court, a partial birth abortion appeal finally reached the U.S. Supreme Court in April 1999 as *Carhart v. Stenberg*. The Nebraska law described partial birth abortion as "an abortion procedure in which the person performing the abortion partially delivers vaginally a living unborn child before killing the unborn child and completing the delivery."

The federal appeals court in *Carhart* had distinguished two procedures for the second trimester abortions that Dr. Carhart was performing before the Nebraska law banning partial birth abortion became effective. One was *dilation and evacuation* (D&E), which is not partial birth abortion because the fetus is dead before its remains are evacuated from the uterus. The second procedure was *dilation and extraction* (D&X), also known as *"intact dilation and evacuation"* or *intact D&E*, which is a partial birth abortion because what the Nebraska law calls a "substantial portion" of a "living unborn child" is extracted from the uterus into the vagina while the fetus is still living, and then physician ends the life of the fetus before extracting the fetal body.

The federal appeals court based its description of D&X on a medical definition from the American College of Obstetricians and Gynecologists (ACOG): "all the body except the head is removed from the uterus, the skull is punctured so its contents can be extracted, and then the now dead but otherwise intact fetal remains are removed from the woman's body." Of course, after viability, if a living fetus were removed from the woman it would actually be a birth, and the destruction of the newborn would no longer legally be abortion but homicide. Hence, the person performing the abortion has to be sure the heart is stopped before completely removing the body from the uterus.

Both the federal district court and the appeals court had found that the Nebraska law was unconstitutional for several reasons: It did not allow the health exception mandated by *Roe* after viability, and it placed an "undue burden," contrary to *Casey*, on women for abortions before viability because the general language of the "substantial portion" of the fetal body could easily be used to ban not only the D&X procedure in the late second trimester but also the D&E procedure. This is so because sometimes an arm or a leg is pulled out of the uterus in the course of a D&E procedure. Although Nebraska argued that the law was intended to criminalize only the D&X procedure, both federal courts found the "substantial portion" phrase so vague that it might apply to some D&E procedures as well and therefore be clearly in conflict with *Roe v. Wade*.

In 2000 the Supreme Court essentially agreed with the lower federal courts and ruled 5–4 in *Stenberg v. Carhart* that the Nebraska law banning partial birth abortion was indeed unconstitutional. It based its decision on the two main points raised by the lower courts. First, the language of the law is so broad that it could be used to prohibit D&E procedures as well as D&X (otherwise known as intact D&E) procedures. And since D&E is widely used in perfectly legal second trimester abortions, the law did impose, contrary to *Casey*, an "undue burden" on women. Second, the law did not allow, contrary to *Roe*, any exceptions for D&X abortions after viability that are necessary for the preservation of the mother's health. The decision, written by Justice Stephen Breyer, contained a seldom noted suggestive remark. He wrote that a law with more precise language and with an exception allowing abortion in the third trimester for the preservation of the woman's health might be constitutional. He left the door open: A carefully crafted law proscribing partial birth abortion could be constitutional.

Gonzales v. Carhart (2007)

In 2003 Congress passed its third ban on partial birth abortion, and this time the president, who was then George W. Bush, signed it into law with great fanfare on November 5, 2003. The Partial Birth Abortion Act threatens physicians found guilty of violating it with up to two years in prison and fines. The language of the Act does describe more precisely than the Nebraska law what is meant by partial birth abortion or D&X. However, the Act also allows partial birth abortion after viability only "when it is *necessary to save the life of a mother* whose life is endangered" (emphasis in original). This is the only exception; abortion after viability to preserve the health of the mother, as *Roe v. Wade* required, is not allowed.

As expected, the Act was immediately challenged in federal courts as unconstitutional because of its conflict with *Roe v. Wade*. Three federal district courts and three federal appeals courts quickly found the Act unconstitutional chiefly because it retained some vague language and still did not allow the D&X procedure if it were necessary to preserve the *health* (and not just the life) of a woman. Supporters of the Act then appealed to the U.S. Supreme Court.

In April 2007 the Supreme Court overturned the three federal appeals court decisions and ruled in *Gonzales v. Carhart* that the 2003 Partial Birth Abortion Ban Act was indeed constitutional. With votes from two new members of the Court, Chief Justice John Roberts and Justice Samuel Alito, the Court moved away from the position it had taken in the 2000 *Stenberg v. Carhart* decision. The procedure known as D&X is now a criminal offense punishable by jail unless it is necessary to save the life of the mother.

The decision was written by Justice Kennedy who had written a dissent in *Stenberg v. Carhart*. He argued that the language of the federal Act is not vague because it clearly distinguishes what he calls "intact D&E" from standard "D&E" abortions. Intact D&E involves delivery of an intact fetus, whereas standard D&E is "the removal of fetal parts that are ripped from the fetus as they are pulled through the cervix." In other words, ripping the fetus apart before pulling it out (standard D&E) is legal; pulling it out while intact (intact D&E) is not.

Justice Kennedy also argued that criminalizing intact D&E or partial birth abortion (except to save the life of a woman) is consistent with *Casey* and not an undue burden on women because the intact D&E is never really needed. Justice Kennedy pointed out that the Act only prohibits the intact delivery of a *living* fetus; it does not prohibit killing a fetus and then removing it. "If the intact D&E procedure is truly necessary in some circumstances, it appears likely an injection that kills the fetus is an alternative under the Act that allows the doctor to perform the procedure."

This argument strikes some as curious: If Justice Kennedy is right, banning partial birth abortion does not save any of the unborn because, as he himself points out, other ways to abort third-trimester fetuses remain legal under the Act. What the Act does do, he argued, is to outlaw abortions where the "fetus is killed just inches before completion of the birth process," a procedure that undermines "respect for the dignity of human life" and also could be damaging to women who might later experience "severe depression and loss of esteem" when they realize how their partially delivered intact living child was destroyed. What the Act does not do, he himself pointed out, is reduce the number of late abortions.

These sections have given us some idea of the religious and legal history behind the abortion controversy. In the next section, we consider the moral issues of abortion. Every abortion destroys human life, and that is *prima facie* a bad thing to do. The bad features of abortion remind us that deliberate abortion, just as deliberate killing, will be contrary to human flourishing unless there are adequate reasons justifying the destruction of human life.

Moral Issues of Abortion

As we have noted, most of the debate about abortion in the United States has been couched in the language of rights. What follows is an approach based on prudential reasoning.

Abortion Is Always Something Bad

Some argue that the rights of privacy and choice imply a right to destroy prenatal life regardless of the reason; others argue that the right to life implies that few, if any, reasons are sufficient to justify destroying prenatal life. Some say the fetus's right to life trumps the woman's right to make decisions about what happens in her body; others say the woman's right to choose trumps the fetus's right to life. The debate reveals a fundamental weakness in arguments that use rights as trump cards—when more than one right is in play, no resolution is possible because each side considers its right the trump card.

An alternative approach is needed. Ethics is ultimately not about rights but about what is good. Life, even prenatal life, is a very basic good. Ethics encourages us to cherish life, especially human life. Prenatal human life has a value, and this value is lost if we destroy it. Destroying any form of life—the environment, an animal, a fetus, a person—is bad, and ethics requires us to consider it immoral unless we have an adequate reason to justify the destruction.

We begin the ethical consideration of abortion, then, by considering it as something bad because it is a destruction of human life. Abortion is always a moral decision and a serious one because it is the taking of human life. Our society has struggled hard to inculcate a presumption in favor of life, including the lives of the frail, the elderly, and the dying, and the lives of fetuses as well. Society has an interest in preserving that presumption, and so do we.

Since abortion is bad, we need serious reasons to justify it, or it will be immoral; that is, it will undermine our good. People will disagree, of course, over just what reasons are adequate to justify an abortion, but that is a separate issue. The important thing is to begin every discussion of abortion not with a claim based on rights—the right of a woman to choose it or the right of a fetus to live—but on the recognition that destroying human life—even prenatal human life—is a very serious action, and it should never be done without compelling reasons.

This ethical approach to abortion is nothing new. We have used it for centuries in questions about killing postnatal life. Our culture has always said "Do not kill . . . unless there are good reasons for killing." "Thou shalt not kill" has always been understood to mean that killing is bad, but some exceptions can be justified. What we say about killing postnatal life can also be said about destroying prenatal life. As we will argue in the next section, the presumption in favor of fetal life can sometimes be overridden by the woman's choice to have it destroyed, but that choice is an ethically sound choice only if the reasons supporting it are strong enough to justify the destruction of human life.

Areas of Widespread Agreement about Abortion

Despite the intense rhetoric on both sides in the debates about the ethics of abortion, many people share a common position: although all abortions are regrettable, some are morally reasonable, and some are not. What follows are examples that show how abortion could be morally reasonable in some situations but morally unreasonable in others. The examples are admittedly "easy" ones, but they show how an ethic of prudence avoids extremes such as "abortion is always immoral" or "abortion is primarily a matter of the woman's choice." Examples where one can argue that abortion would be morally reasonable include ectopic pregnancies, pregnancies with too many fetuses, and severely defective fetuses.

Ectopic Pregnancy

Some embryos implant outside the uterus, usually in a fallopian tube, although sometimes an embryo attaches to an ovary or to the cervix. If the pregnancy continues, the growing fetus will threaten the life of the woman before it becomes viable. The accepted medical response, once an ectopic pregnancy is diagnosed, is to abort it. The abortion will be a first trimester abortion, and few physicians or women, even those otherwise opposed to abortion, think it is immoral to perform these abortions.

These abortions are easy to accept in an ethics of right reason. The destruction of fetal human life is unfortunate, but it is the only reasonable action in the situation. Nothing can be done to save the fetus, which is not yet one of us, and if the pregnancy continues, it will cause the deaths of both the woman and the fetus. Once an ectopic pregnancy is diagnosed, the best we can do is to abort it as simply as possible.

In passing, however, we should note that one important religious denomination, the Roman Catholic Church, still opposes the direct intended abortion of an ectopic pregnancy. The Vatican condemned ectopic abortions in 1902. Some women with ectopic pregnancies adhered to the church teaching and, unfortunately, died as the result of their ectopic pregnancies.

By the 1930s, however, Catholic theologians found a way to save the lives of these women and yet avoid the ban on aborting ectopic pregnancies. They applied the "principle of the double effect," a principle explained in chapter 3, to the problem of ectopic pregnancies. If the site of the ectopic pregnancy is considered pathological (as the result of an embryo growing in or on it) and a threat to the woman's life, surgical removal of the site would have two effects, one good and one bad. The good effect is the removal of the pathological site threatening the woman's life; the bad effect is the destruction of the fetus. Since the intervention is directed toward the site, however, and not the fetus, it is not a direct abortion. The principle of double effect permits surgery to remove a life-threatening pathological organ even if a fetus dies in the process.

Unfortunately this theological response to the problem of ectopic pregnancies is not a reasonable solution. Although it saves the woman's life, it also causes her unnecessary harm in most cases. Surgically removing the site of the ectopic pregnancy permanently damages the woman's reproductive system. In fact, terminating an ectopic pregnancy by removing the site when there is no medical need to do so is simply bad medicine. It is hard to see how it would not be medical malpractice; it is also hard to see how it is a morally reasonable response to the ectopic pregnancy.

Selective Abortion

Sometimes, possibly as the result of fertility drugs or a fertility procedure such as IVF, a woman may become pregnant with more than one fetus, perhaps as many as six or more. The risks to the woman and to the fetuses increase with the number of fetuses in the pregnancy. Most people think that five or more fetuses pose a matter of serious risk for the woman and for the fetuses themselves. One persistent problem in multiple pregnancies is premature birth and the many problems associated with it.

An ethics that cherishes life, especially human life, will do everything possible to prevent multiple pregnancies with five or more fetuses. But when it does occur, the woman and the physicians are presented with a moral dilemma. The dilemma is compounded by the fact that it happens so rarely that we do not have good information about outcomes involving five or more fetuses. Thus, our analysis has to be speculative.

Let us consider the rare pregnancy of five or more fetuses. We want to salvage as much human life as possible. We certainly want to preserve the woman's life, and we also want to take reasonable care of the fetuses. As soon as we begin to think that the many fetuses in the uterus are leading to a situation in which great damage will be done to the woman and to the fetuses themselves, we have to ask how we might reduce this damage. One obvious option is to abort some of the fetuses. This can be achieved by injecting potassium chloride or some other agent into some of the fetuses at about the twelfth week of gestation. They will die, and the remains will be absorbed by the mother's body. The abortion of selected fetuses is intended to give the other fetuses and the mother a more realistic chance of survival and health.

In these situations, the intent is not really to terminate a pregnancy (the woman remains pregnant) but to increase the chances of a healthy pregnancy and the birth of healthy babies. To accomplish this, some fetuses have to be destroyed. It is truly a conflict situation, but an ethics of right reason or prudence indicates that life can be better cherished in such a situation by selective abortion. The deliberate abortion of some fetuses is tragic, but less tragic than (1) losing all of them or losing some and leaving the others terribly impaired and (2) undermining the health and well-being of the mother and perhaps losing her life itself.

Although many people, including those ordinarily opposed to abortion, would agree that reducing multiple pregnancies with five or more fetuses is the best we can do in the unfortunate situation, the moral perplexity increases when the number decreases. What are we to think when a woman with triplets wants the pregnancy reduced? Certainly, triplets are a burdensome pregnancy, and carrying triplets often does more damage to a woman's body than a pregnancy of one or two babies. But are the burdens of carrying triplets sufficient to justify the destruction of one of them? In an ethics of prudence that cherishes human life, such a reduction, assuming there are no other complications with the pregnancy, is suspect because the reasons for destroying human life in the case of triplets are weaker than they are in pregnancies with a higher number of fetuses.

Seriously Defective Fetuses

Once we discover early in a pregnancy that a fetus is seriously defective, the question of abortion arises, and with good reason. Terminating an early pregnancy when the fetus is expected to die later in the pregnancy or shortly after birth, especially if it is known that the fetus or newborn will suffer significantly in its brief life, can be defended as reasonable. There is little point in continuing a pregnancy for months once we know that little more than suffering and an early death await the fetus. We can give good reasons why we should not kill a mature fetus or a newborn infant, no matter how short the life expectancy, but it is much more difficult to say that the abortion of a grossly defective human fetus in the early stages of development undermines the human good.

How defective must a fetus be before an ethics that cherishes life can acknowledge the cogency of the reasons for aborting it? Obviously, the defects must be serious. Anencephaly is one such serious defect. The afflicted child, who lacks a brain, or most of it, has a high chance of being born dead; even if he or she is born alive, death usually follows within a matter of hours. The defect is so devastating that everyone agrees most life-sustaining treatments are not appropriate for the unfortunate neonate. Other examples of seriously defective fetuses include those with the genetic defects known as trisomy 13 or trisomy 18. If born, these babies will suffer significantly both from the genetic defects and from the interventions often employed to sustain their lives, yet they seldom survive beyond the first year of life. It is at least arguable that the reasons supporting early abortion of these defective fetuses are plausible.

It is not possible to say exactly which prenatal defects are serious enough to justify an early abortion. In an ethics dedicated to the affirmation of life, they would be few. An ethics that cherishes life will generally find abortion unreasonable, and the more mature the fetus, the stronger the objections. Exceptions occur when the failure to abort will do more harm to the human good than the abortion. Before an exception can be made, however, moral reasoning must clearly establish the justification for destroying the prenatal life. Human life, even prenatal human life, is a fundamental good deserving of great protection, and its destruction should always be an exception. Good reasons exist for making such exceptions when the pregnancy is ectopic or involves five or more fetuses. It can be reasonably argued that good reasons exist in other tragic situations as well.

Very Premature Rupture of Membranes

Sometimes a pregnant woman experiences a rupture of the amniotic sac, sometimes called breaking her water, long before her delivery date, perhaps as early as seventeen or eighteen weeks into her pregnancy. This presents a serious problem because of the high possibility of infection if she tries to continue the pregnancy for several months until she gets to about thirty-two weeks, when obstetricians can induce labor and deliver a baby who will still be about two months premature. In this instance there is a high likelihood that the baby will not make it to thirty-two weeks because of infection, and there is also a risk that the mother will also suffer from infection that could become life threatening to her. Many obstetricians in the Boston area are aware of a tragic story of a young woman pregnant with twins who suffered ruptured membranes weeks before viability and decided to continue the pregnancy despite being offered the option of abortion. Infection soon set in, and she was rushed to a major teaching hospital where physicians induced labor and delivered her stillborn twins shortly before she died despite a massive effort to save her life.

In cases of very premature rupture of membranes the chances of a successful birth are so slim and the possibility of lethal maternal infection so real that a woman relying on prudential reasoning could well conclude that abortion would be a wise option for her in her situation. She would consider many things, including how many children she might leave motherless, her medical history in dealing with infections, what the latest medical literature says about extremely premature rupture of membranes, what her husband thinks, the advice of her obstetricians, the tragedy of destroying fetuses she hoped to welcome into her family, the risks of late second-term abortion, and so forth.

RU-486

In the late 1950s researchers developed contraceptive pills. These pills introduce enough estrogen—a hormone associated with pregnancy—into a woman's body to block ovulation. Over the years the pills were refined, and today they are widely accepted as a reliable and relatively safe means of birth control.

More recently researchers have developed what some now call "the abortion pill." These pills introduce an agent into the woman's body that blocks progesterone, another hormone associated with pregnancy. Progesterone prepares the lining of the uterus to receive a fertilized ovum during each menstrual cycle. If that function can be thwarted, the fertilized ovum or embryo will not implant, or, if it is implanted, it will be dislodged.

In 1980 scientists working at the French firm of Roussel Uclaf synthesized an antagonist of progesterone called mifepristone or, as it is more widely known, RU-486 or "miffy." Tests in women soon showed that this antiprogestin drug could both prevent implantation and dislodge an implanted fetus. The abortive function of RU-486 is highly effective when its ingestion is followed in forty-eight hours by a low dose of a prostaglandin analogue. The prostaglandin causes the uterus to contract, and the contractions expel the dislodged fetus. RU-486 abortions are usually called "medical" abortions.

By the end of 1998 it was estimated that over 500,000 women had used RU-486 for abortions, mostly in France, China, Great Britain, and Sweden. Over 100,000 women had used RU-486 in France alone since its approval there in 1988. It was also widely used in Great Britain and China. At first Great Britain restricted its use to residents. Beginning in 1994, however, it allowed visitors to receive RU-486, and women began traveling to England for medical abortions.

In the United States the process of approval progressed slowly. The Food and Drug Administration (FDA) must approve all new drugs, and this requires research and testing in accord with FDA standards. Roussel Uclaf was in no hurry to seek FDA approval. The reason was at least partly political. Opponents of legalized abortion, alarmed by the possibility that abortion could be made so simple and private, mounted a strong campaign in this country against the drug, and they found a sympathetic ear in the first Bush administration. In 1988 the FDA took the rather unusual step of issuing an "import alert" prohibiting people from bringing the drug into the country.

This led to a well-publicized case in July 1992. Leona Benten, claiming she was pregnant, announced that she was bringing some RU-486 back from Europe. Since the pills violated the FDA import ban, U.S. Customs confiscated the pills in New York. Ms. Benten's lawyers took the case to federal district court and won—the court ordered immediate release of her RU-486 pills. But the order of the federal district court was stayed by the federal court of appeals, and this prevented release of the drug. Her lawyers filed an application with the U.S. Supreme Court, asking it to lift the stay, but the Supreme Court declined in a 7-2 opinion. Thus, Ms. Benten's pills were not released.

Actually, the FDA "import alert" was not as ominous as it sounds; it applied only to the importation of unapproved drugs into the country for personal use. Roussel Uclaf, the company with the worldwide patent for RU-486, could have imported RU-486 for purposes of testing but decided not to because it feared any efforts to test and market the drug would result in antiabortion protests. The potential profits from RU-486 are slight—only one pill is needed for an abortion—and Roussel Uclaf was concerned that opponents of abortion would encourage the boycott of all their products in the United States if they moved to introduce RU-486. When the Clinton administration took office in 1993 Roussel Uclaf made preliminary agreements for clinical trials in the United States.

After various twists and turns, clinical trials did occur for women between ages eighteen and forty-five, and the FDA approved RU-486 in 2000 for abortions through the forth-ninth day of pregnancy. The FDA-approved regimen calls for mifepristone (Mifeprex) on the first day to dislodge the fetus, misoprostol (Cytotec) on the third day to cause uterine contractions and expulsion, and a checkup on the fourteenth day to confirm a successful pregnancy termination. Danco Laboratories, the company that provides the drug directly to doctors (not pharmacies), has reported that more than 840,000 women in the United States used RU-486 in the first seven years after FDA approval. The 2005 Guttmacher survery reported that the number of medical abortions using RU-486 was rising and accounted for 13 percent of them that year.

Drugs inducing abortions thus introduced a new kind of abortion for consideration, medical abortion. Unlike the surgical abortion where a physician aborts the fetus, the woman who takes RU-486 performs the abortion herself. Medical abortions are also more private than surgical abortions, more difficult for antiabortion groups to protest, and more difficult for the law to control. The medical abortions may also become more simple, and some states allow some health care providers to dispense RU-486 under a physician's supervision.

Although use of RU-486 makes available a new kind of abortion, it does not introduce any new dimensions to the moral reasoning about abortion. It matters little from the ethical point of view whether fetal life is destroyed by a drug or a vacuum device that dislodges it from the endometrial lining of the uterus. In both procedures fetal human life is being destroyed, and in the ethical framework we have been using, the morality of that action depends on whether or not there are adequate reasons for doing it.

MATERNAL-FETAL TREATMENT CONFLICTS

For a very long time physicians did not care for pregnant women unless they were sick, and they did not assist at births. Most births did not occur in hospitals. Pregnancy and birth, after all, are not illnesses, and doctors and hospitals are for sick people. There was little prenatal care, and most deliveries were assisted by midwives.

All that began to change a century or so ago. Physicians took over the delivery of babies, and midwifery all but disappeared. Physicians soon realized that prenatal medical care was important, so they began to offer this as well. In this way both birth and pregnancy became medical concerns, and the hospital became the place where most babies came to be born.

Until recently prenatal care was directed almost exclusively toward the woman. Not much could be directly known about the fetus. The physician's knowledge could only come from such practices as palpating the fetus and by inference from laboratory analyses of the woman's urine and blood. In short, prenatal medical care was the care of one patient—the woman who was pregnant.

The development of techniques and technology to diagnose fetal health changed this. Ultrasound, alpha-fetoprotein screening, chorionic villi sampling, and amniocentesis are now often used, along with other diagnostic interventions, to detect fetal abnormalities. Once problems are diagnosed, the obvious next step is to see whether they can be treated. In recent years, for example, physicians have begun operating on fetuses during the pregnancy. Although still in its infancy fetal surgery has been used to correct urinary obstructions, diaphragmatic hernias, and hydrocephalus. Results range from poor to modest; surgery for hydrocephalus has had poor results, whereas surgery to repair the hernias and urinary problems has been more promising.

Once the fetus is viewed as a human subject worthy of medical intervention for its own sake, a drastic change occurs in the physician–pregnant woman relationship. The pregnant woman is now no longer the only patient—the fetus also becomes a patient needing treatment, perhaps even surgery. This raises complex ethical issues because (1) we have to consider whether the treatment is reasonable not simply for the fetus, but also for the woman who will be affected by an intervention of no direct biological benefit to her, and (2) we have to consider what is the right thing to do when the fetus needs treatment, but the woman declines to give informed consent for the intervention into her body. Although society can take custody of a child whose parents refuse to provide proper medical care, it cannot take custody of a fetus or unborn child when the woman refuses medical care for it.

Some, however, suggest that interventions to aid the fetus without the woman's permission are justified in some situations. Perhaps the most dramatic examples of this are the few cases where physicians successfully have convinced courts to allow invasive medical interventions, usually cesarean sections, against the woman's wishes. In 1987 a nineteen-year-old Washington, DC, woman named Ayesha Madyun arrived at the hospital after two days of labor. Eighteen hours later she still had not delivered, and there were signs of fetal distress. Physicians recommended a cesarean section, but she refused consent. Protected by a court order, they forced the surgery on her and saved the baby.

However, not all courts have responded this way. In New York a judge refused to order a cesarean section on a thirty-five-year-old woman with ten children despite the physicians' predictions that the cord wrapped around the baby's neck would strangle the baby if a vaginal birth were attempted. The judge, herself a woman, said no one can be forced to have surgery for the benefit of another person, even if the other person is her child. More recently, other courts have followed this reasoning.

These cases highlight a new kind of moral dilemma that arises for physicians when a fetal problem is diagnosed and a treatment is available. What does a physician do when a pregnant woman refuses medical treatment for her fetus or unborn child? The more the fetus is viewed as a patient, the more difficult it is for the physician to be comfortable doing nothing when something medically helpful can be reasonably done. It is somewhat ironic that at about the same time that *Roe v. Wade* viewed abortion in terms of a right to privacy and neglected to consider the value of prenatal life, medicine was elevating the hitherto inaccessible fetus to the status of a patient worthy of diagnosis and treatment.

To illustrate the complexity of maternal-fetal conflicts, we turn to a well-publicized case that involved a possibly viable fetus and a dying pregnant woman.

The Case of Angie

The Story

Angela Carder was approximately twenty-six weeks into her pregnancy when a routine checkup uncovered a large malignant tumor in her lung. She had already battled bone cancer for almost ten years and had been in remission for the previous two years. She was admitted to George Washington University Hospital in the District of Columbia, and her condition rapidly deteriorated. It soon became clear that she was dying. She was heavily sedated, and her physician thought it was likely she would die within twenty-four hours. A priest administered the last rites, as her family prayed with her.

She had consented to treatments that might prolong her life in order to give her fetus a better chance at survival, but her primary concern, which was echoed by her husband and parents and supported by her physicians, was the comfort care she needed in her dying. She had previously agreed that a cesarean could be performed if her life could be extended another two weeks, but she did not want a cesarean section before twenty-eight weeks because she thought that the risks to the child resulting from a delivery before that time were too great.

Hospital administrators questioned her decision, and they sought legal advice. The attorneys, in turn, sought a judicial opinion. In other words, they wanted a judge to tell the hospital whether or not the physicians should intervene to save the fetus. A neonatologist who supported immediate intervention predicted a 50 to 60 percent chance of survival for the child, and a better than 80 percent chance that a surviving baby would not be handicapped. At this point, Angie's mother reported that her daughter remained opposed to the delivery at twenty-six weeks. Her only wish was "I only want to die, just give me something to get me out of this pain."

Ethical Analysis

Situational awareness.   We are aware of the following facts in Angie's story.

1. Angie was imminently dying and in need of comfort care.
2. If a cesarean section were performed, the premature baby would have about 50 to 60 percent chance of surviving; if it did survive, there would be about one chance in five it would be handicapped.
3. Angie had refused consent for a cesarean section before the twenty-eighth week of her pregnancy.

We are also aware of these bad features:

1. The cesarean section would add more pain and suffering to a dying woman.
2. Given her current position, any surgical intervention would be without informed consent; indeed, it would be forced on her against her wishes.
3. Angie was not expected to live until the twenty-eighth week. If she died while pregnant, the unborn child would almost certainly die also. If the surgery was done at once, there would be about an even chance a new life could be saved.

Prudential Reasoning in the Story of Angie

Patient's perspective. Note, first, that we are concerned with two patients here, Angie and her twenty-six-week possibly viable fetus. This complicates things immensely, especially since Angie's life is ending. We begin by considering the moral question from Angie's perspective. The surgery is of no benefit to her, will cause her significant additional pain, and could actually contribute to her death. Of course, the surgery could well save her fetus or unborn child, and this is a circumstance the pregnant woman has to consider if her refusal of surgery is to be morally justified. This is so because her refusal of the surgery means almost certain death for a possibly viable twenty-six-week fetus.

What the patient has to weigh in a situation such as this is her pain and suffering against the possible life of her fetus. Was she reasonable in declining surgery at this point? It certainly seems so. She had determined that she did not want to give birth before twenty-eight weeks. Before that point, she felt the chances of a good outcome for the fetus did not outweigh the risks to the fetus and the pain and suffering she would experience. That is a reasonable position. On the other hand, had she decided to take a chance and have the cesarean delivery, that choice also seems morally justifiable.

Suppose her fetus were not at twenty-six weeks but at thirty-six weeks—would she still be morally justified in refusing surgery? This would be much harder to justify in an ethics of reason that cherishes life. Many, of course, would argue that a woman's choice over her fetus is absolute, and thus, if she chose to decline the surgery at thirty-six weeks, then that is her choice. Indeed it is, and if that is her choice then it should be respected because the alternative—forcing surgery on an unwilling human being—is wrong. But the real question here is whether the decision to decline surgery to save a thirty-six-week fetus would be a morally justified decision.

Providers' perspective. The second stage of the ethical problem began when Angie declined the surgery. In such a case, should the hospital, judge, obstetrician, neonatologists, and attorneys try to force the surgery in order to save the other patient, the twenty-six-week fetus that could be viable? Certainly the death of the fetus is a bad thing that the hospital should try to avoid, although in this case there is about a 40 or 50 percent chance death would occur even if the surgery were done.

Is it reasonable for providers to force treatment on a woman in order to save, or in this case to try and save, her fetus? It seems not. Forcing surgery on someone who does not want it is itself a terrible evil. It is an assault that violates the dignity and bodily integrity of the human being who becomes no longer a patient but a victim. Certainly the intention—to save the fetus—is good, but good intentions by themselves do not justify the morality of our actions, or, in more traditional language, the end does not justify the means. Even if one is convinced a woman is acting immorally toward her fetus, that still does not justify another immoral action—operating on her against her will. Forced interventions are not ethical interventions; they are not reasonable treatments, but immoral assaults.

The Court Decisions

Judge Emmett Sullivan of the District of Columbia Superior Court rushed to the hospital with a police escort on the morning of June 16, 1987. He was to spend most of the day there conducting hearings to decide what medical care should be provided for the fetus. Those advocating the surgery argued that Angie's death was imminent, so we might as well try to save the fetus. Angie's family and the lawyer representing her argued that we could not do the surgery against her will and that the surgery would in effect kill her since she was so weak at this point. During the rushed hearings the hospital started prepping Angie for the cesarean section.

The judge heard the arguments of both sides and then concluded: "It's not an easy decision to make, but given the choices, the court is of the view the fetus should be given an opportunity to live."

It was a little after four o'clock in the afternoon when the obstetrician told Angie of the judge's decision. Although she was on a respirator, she indicated her agreement with it. Then, a little later, the chief of obstetrics reminded her that Dr. Hamner, her obstetrician, would do the cesarean section only if she consented to it. Then she very clearly mouthed "I don't want it" several times. The chief of obstetrics immediately reported her refusal of consent to the judge. An attorney pressing for the surgery argued that her refusal made no difference because the assumption of the entire hearing was that she was refusing consent. He pointed out that if she had given consent, there would have been no need for the judicial intervention.

The surgery was scheduled for half past six that evening. Meanwhile, the attorney for Angie had appealed the judge's decision, and the surgery was delayed while a hastily assembled panel of three judges heard the appeal over the telephone. The arguments were of necessity brief. After a short consultation the three-judge panel declined to stay the first judge's order. In effect, this gave the green light for the surgery.

Angie was taken to the operating room and, since her obstetrician refused to operate without her consent, another physician willing to perform the cesarean had to be found. The cesarean section was done, and a premature infant of twenty-six weeks was delivered. Despite extensive treatment in the neonatal intensive care unit of the university hospital, the baby died in two hours. Two days later, Angie died. Her death certificate listed several causes of death—one of them was the surgery.

In November 1987 the panel of three judges who had heard the appeal over the telephone issued their written opinion giving the reasons for the decision they had made the previous June. Their arguments were weak. One argument, for example, was that, although Angie could have aborted her third trimester fetus under *Roe v. Wade* if it was threatening her life, this did not give her the right to deny the fetus proper care once she decided not to abort it. Hence, they claimed that she should have consented to the cesarean section. Another argument centered on an analogy: just as a parent cannot refuse treatment necessary to save a child, so a woman cannot refuse treatment necessary to save her fetus.

The opinion of the three-judge panel upholding the order for the surgery was then remanded for further consideration by the full court of appeals. Finally in April 1990, almost three years after the incident, the District of Columbia Court of Appeals in a decision known as *In Re: A. C.*, reversed the 1987 decisions: "We hold that in virtually all cases the question of what is to be done is to be decided by the patient—the pregnant woman—on behalf of herself and the fetus." The court of appeals recognized that the previous judges should not have ordered the surgery against Angie's will.

In an interesting footnote the court noted that judges should not be called into hospitals to decide issues of life and death: "We observe nevertheless that it would be far better if judges were not called to patients' bedsides and required to make quick decisions on issues of life and death."

Ethical Reflection

There are two major ethical questions in this case. First, was Angie's decision to decline surgery designed to save her child before the twenty-eighth week morally reasonable, and, second, were the decisions of the judges, attorneys, and physicians to force the surgery on her against her will in order to save the unborn child morally reasonable? We have already tried to show that Angie's decision, given the burden to her and the uncertain outcome, was reasonable. That leaves the second question, the prudential judgment of those who advocated for the surgery. Can this be justified? It seems not. We have no convincing reason for forcing surgery on a dying person to save a possibly viable fetus.

Part of the temptation to see the surgery as morally justified comes from a failure to distinguish the unborn from the born. The crucial distinction between the fetus an hour before birth and an hour after birth does not hinge on the physical structure of the fetus—the body of a newborn is pretty much the same as it was an hour before birth—but on the circumstances. The fetus is inside another human being, and we cannot claim custody of the unborn child without invading her body. All that changes at birth. If a mother refuses proper medical care for her neonate, we can take custody of the child without invading her body against her wishes, and that is the crucial difference.

The debate over the conflict between respecting the woman's control of her body during pregnancy and providing appropriate care for her fetus is far from over. The final court of appeals decision in Angie's case is more easily justified morally than was the attempt by the hospital to force surgery on a dying woman in an effort to save a premature unborn baby. Nonetheless, this decision left the door open for exceptions. What might they be? It is difficult to say, but surveys of obstetricians point to the following situations where some argue that interventions to save an unborn baby near term could be undertaken against the woman's wishes: (1) the head is clearly too large for the birth canal, (2) the placenta has detached from the uterine wall, and (3) the placenta is blocking the birth canal.

Professional organizations have tried to resolve these difficult dilemmas. In 1987 ACOG issued an ethical statement titled "Patient's Choice: Maternal-Fetal Conflict," and the American Academy of Pediatrics (AAP) followed in 1988 with an ethical statement titled "Fetal Therapy: Ethical Considerations." As the titles suggest, the ACOG statement tends to support the wishes of the woman, whereas the AAP statement underlines the potential benefits to the fetus.

Both statements, however, try to overcome the woman's refusal of treatment that could be beneficial to her fetus by education and persuasion rather than by coercion. Both statements discourage appeals to the judicial system in an effort to force treatment on unwilling patients, but neither rules it out altogether. Finally, both statements reflect a wide ethical consensus that everything possible should be done to prevent providers from making the patient an adversary. Providers do not make the patient, or the proxy, an adversary when they disagree with the patient or proxy on a moral issue and communicate the reasons for that disagreement. But providers do make patients adversaries when they try to coerce them by using the power of the law to force invasive medical interventions on them against their wishes. The woman's choice may not be morally reasonable, but usually it is not morally reasonable to force invasive medical interventions on unwilling patients.

ETHICAL REFLECTIONS

Underlying this entire chapter is the awareness that prenatal life is human life and that an ethics of the good tries to enhance life whenever possible and never damages or destroys human life without a sufficiently strong reason to balance the bad inherent in every destruction of life. Medical interventions now extend to the fetal patient. Whether these interventions are designed to destroy fetuses or to treat fetuses, they raise important moral issues, and we have considered but a few of them.

SUGGESTED READINGS

Abortion statistics are from cdc.gov/mmwr and guttmacher.org. For the history of abortion, see John Noonan, 1979, "An Almost Absolute Value in History" in *The Morality of Abortion: Legal and Historical Perspectives*, John Noonan, ed., Cambridge, MA: Harvard University Press, pp. 1–59. For the history of the abortion controversy in America, see Laurence Tribe, 1990, *Abortion: The Clash of Absolutes*, New York: W. W. Norton & Company; John Noonan, 1979, *A Private Choice: Abortion in America in the Seventies*, New York: The Free Press; Gilbert Steiner, ed., 1983, *The Abortion Dispute and the American System*, Washington, DC: Brookings Institution; Sidney Callahan and Daniel Callahan, eds., 1984, *Abortion: Understanding the Differences*, New York: Plenum Press.

Two more recent histories are Rickie Solinger, ed., 1997, *Abortion Wars: A Half Century of Struggle, 1950– 2000*, Berkeley: University of California Press; and James Risen and Judy Thomas, 1997, *Wrath of Angels: The American Abortion War*, New York: Basic Books. The latter book is particularly good for tracing the rise of antiabortion activism.

The major legal turning point in the United States came on January 22, 1973, in *Roe v. Wade*, 410 U.S. 113 (1973). The court decided a second abortion case the same day—*Doe v. Bolton*, 410 U.S. 179 (1973). Mary Doe, a pseudonym, was a twenty-two-year-old married woman living in Georgia and pregnant with her fourth child. A former mental patient in a state hospital, she was impoverished and unable to care for her children. The two older ones were in a foster home, and the third had been placed for adoption. Her husband had abandoned her, forcing her to live with her indigent parents and their eight children, but she and her husband had recently reconciled. Unlike the Texas law at issue in *Roe v. Wade*, a law dating back to the middle of the nineteenth century that forbade all abortions except those to save the life of the mother, the nineteenth-century Georgia laws had been revised in 1968 to allow abortions of pregnancies that would seriously and permanently injure the woman's health or that involved a seriously defective fetus or that were the result of rape. In *Doe v. Bolton*, the court, consistent with its findings in *Roe v. Wade*, found that limiting abortions to these situations was unconstitutional. The Supreme Court did, however, let stand some parts of the Georgia law, among them an important provision that allows physicians and nurses to refuse participation in abortions and protects them from any retaliation if they do refuse. This is the legal basis, later codified in the Church amendments, that protects physicians and nurses who work in organizations such as a hospital or a health maintenance organization (HMO) and decline to participate in abortions.

For an extensive historical and legal account of the cultural and legal developments leading to *Roe v. Wade*, see David Garrow, 1994, *Liberty and Sexuality: The Right to Privacy and the Making of Roe v. Wade*, New York: Macmillan. For the sad and difficult real life of "Jane Roe," see Norma McCorvey with Andy Meisler, 1994, *My Life, Roe v. Wade, and Freedom of Choice*, New York: HarperCollins. After an abusive marriage and giving up her three children by three different fathers, Norma was then supporting herself by cleaning houses in Dallas.

Citations for the other Supreme Court cases relevant to abortion and mentioned in the text are *Maher v. Roe*, 432 U.S. 464 (1977); *Harris v. McRae* 448 U.S. 297 (1980); *Planned Parenthood v. Danforth*, 428 U.S. 52 (1976); *City of Akron v. Akron Center for Reproductive Health*, 462 U.S. 416 (1983); *Thornburgh v. American College of Obstetricians and Gynecologists*, 476 U.S. 747 (1986); *Webster v. Reproductive Health Services*, 492 U.S. 490 (1989); *Planned Parenthood Association of Southeastern Pennsylvania v. Casey*, 505 U.S. 833 (1992); *Carhart v. Stenberg*, 530 U.S. 914 (2000); and *Gonzales v. Carhart* 550 U.S. 124 (2007).

For an excellent summary of the early Supreme Court's abortion decisions, see the Introduction in Leon Friedman, ed., 1993, *The Supreme Court Confronts Abortion: The Briefs, Argument, and Decision in Planned Parenthood v. Casey*, New York: Farrar, Straus & Giroux.

For commentaries on the Supreme Court decisions, see George Annas, "The Supreme Court, Privacy, and Abortion," *New England Journal of Medicine* 1989, *321*, 1200–03; and "The Supreme Court, Liberty, and Abortion," *New England Journal of Medicine* 1992, *327*, 651–54; Claudia Mangel, "Legal Abortion: The Impending Obsolescence of the Trimester Framework," *American Journal of Law and Medicine* 1988, *14*, 69–108; Tara Koslov, "Abortion on the Supreme Court Agenda: *Planned Parenthood v. Casey* and Its Possible Consequences," *Law, Medicine & Health Care* 1992, *20*, 243–48; and Patricia Martin, "The Role of Women in Abortion Jurisprudence: From Roe to Casey and Beyond," *Cambridge Quarterly of Healthcare Ethics* 1993, *2*, 309–19. This issue (pp. 327–30) also contains a helpful bibliography on the ethical issues surrounding prenatal and neonatal life. Also helpful is *Roe v. Wade*, annotated by Bo Schambelan, 1992, Philadelphia: Running Press, which has the complete texts of *Roe v. Wade* and *Doe v. Bolton* as well as a postscript summarizing the relevant Supreme Court decisions since *Roe v. Wade*.

Although the Supreme Court has been the prime mover in the effort to liberalize the restrictive abortion laws inherited in most states from the nineteenth century, it need not have happened this way. All the Western European countries but one (Ireland) also abandoned their strict abortion laws in the latter half of the twentieth century, but in a different way. Instead of judicial fiat, they changed their laws in a process of parliamentary debate. Moreover, the new laws allowing abortion often begin by affirming the value of fetal life and the responsibility to protect it and only then allow exceptions for grave reasons. This differs greatly from the decisions of our Supreme Court, which begin by affirming the right of the woman to destroy fetal life and then restrict this right for the sake of the fetus only in the third trimester. For an important essay on this difference between the American and European liberalization of abortion laws, see Mary Glendon, 1987, *Abortion and Divorce in Western Law*, Cambridge, MA: Harvard University Press, chapters 1 and 3.

The Catholic moral position on terminating ectopic pregnancy by the often medically unnecessary procedure of removing the fallopian tube or other affected site was summed up in the *Ethical and Religious Directives for Catholic Health Facilities*, 1971, Washington, DC: United States Catholic Conference. Directive 19 reads:

> In extrauterine pregnancy the dangerously affected part of the mother (e.g., cervix, ovary, or fallopian tube) may be removed, even though fetal death is foreseen, provided that: a.

the affected part is presumed already to be so damaged and dangerously affected as to warrant its removal, and that b. the operation is not just a separation of the embryo or fetus from its site within the part (which would be a direct abortion from a uterine appendage); and that c. the operation cannot be postponed without notably increasing the danger to the mother.

This directive represented the "solution" to the problem of ectopic pregnancy advanced by T. Lincoln Bouscaren in 1933. The Catholic Church had forbidden ectopic abortions, and the women who obeyed the proscription were dying. Bouscaren found a clever way around the Vatican condemnation—he said physicians could operate to remove the site, not the fetus, and hence the surgery would not be a direct abortion. See T. Lincoln Bouscaren, 1933, *Ethics of Ectopic Pregnancy*, Chicago: Loyola University Press. Today some theologians find Bouscaren's approach to ectopic pregnancies inadequate. See, for example, James Keenan, "The Function of the Principle of Double Effect," *Theological Studies* 1993, *54*, 294–315.

Nonetheless, the latest *Ethical and Religious Directives* approved in June 2001, although it drops the paragraph quoted above, still forbids (directive 48) the direct abortion of an ectopic fetus: "In cases of extrauterine pregnancy, no intervention is morally licit which constitutes a direct abortion." A direct abortion is intentionally using any intervention to dislodge a nonviable fetus from its site. The latest edition of the *Directives* is available at usccb.org/bishops/directives.

For a discussion of selective abortion, see Richard Berkowitz, "Selective Reduction of Multifetal Pregnancy in the First Trimester," *New England Journal of Medicine* 1988, *318*, 1043–47; and Richard Layzer, "Selective Reduction—A Perinatal Necessity." *New England Journal of Medicine* 1988, *318*, 1062–63. Another kind of case where selective abortion is an issue is the rare situation where one twin is so defective it cannot live outside the uterus and its continued presence in the uterus constitutes a threat to the healthy twin. If nothing is done while the seriously deformed twin is living, the healthy twin may also be lost; if the deformed twin is removed, then an abortion occurs. In such a situation, the deformed twin is threatening not the life of the mother but the life of the healthy twin. See George Robie, "Selective Delivery of an Acardiac, Acephalic Twin," *New England Journal of Medicine* 1989, *320*, 512–13.

For late-term abortions see George Annas, "Partial-birth Abortion, Congress, and the Constitution," *New England Journal of Medicine* 1998, *339*, 279–83; Janet Epner et al., "Late-Term Abortion," Leroy Sprang and Mark Neerhof, "Rationale for Banning Abortions Late in Pregnancy," and David Grimes, "The Continuing Need for Late Abortions," *JAMA* 1998, *280*, 724–29, 744–47, and 747–50. In a brief editorial comment on these three articles the editor of JAMA at that time, George Lundberg, noted that Americans are constitutionally guaranteed religious freedom and then wrote: "This editor considers abortion to be a religious issue." Although abortion is a religious issue for many, it is not necessarily so, and it certainly is not a religious issue for those who are not religious. Destroying viable human life in late-term abortions is better thought of as a moral concern for all people, those who are religious and those who are not. Considering late-term abortion a religious or strictly personal issue unfortunately removes it from the important public debate about its ethical status.

An excellent review of *Gonzales v. Carhart* is George Annas, "The Supreme Court and Abortion Rights," *New England Journal of Medicine* 2007, *356*, 2201–07. See also R. Alta Charo, "The Partial Death of Abortion Rights," *New England Journal of Medicine* 2007, *356*, 2125–28; Lawrence Gostin, "Abortion Politics: Clinical Freedom, Trust in the Judiciary, and the Autonomy of Women," *JAMA* 2007, *298*, 1562–64; Rebecca Dresser, "Protecting Women from Their Abortion Choices," *Hastings Center Report* 2007, *37* (November–December), 13–14.

A good source of information about RU-486 is fda.gov/cder/drug. For the medical aspects of RU-486 see Beatrice Couzinet et al., "Termination of Early Pregnancy by the Progesterone Antagonist RU-486 (Mifepristone)," *New England Journal of Medicine* 1986, *315*, 1565–79; Etienne-Emile Baulieu, "RU-486 as an Antiprogesterone Steroid: From Receptor to Contragestion and Beyond," *JAMA* 1989, *262*, 1808–14, and "Updating RU-486 Development," *Law, Medicine & Health Care* 1992, *20*, 154–56. Baulieu also published, with M. Rosenblum, 1991, *The "Abortion Pill"; RU-486: A Woman's Choice*, New York: Simon & Schuster. Etienne-Emile Baulieu played a major role in the development of RU-486. Volume 20 (1992) of *Law, Medicine & Health Care* is devoted to articles on the ethical, legal, and medical issues associated with the drug. See especially Judith Senderowitz, "Are Adolescents Good Candidates for RU-486 as an Abortion Method?" pp.

209–14; and Ruth Macklin, "Antiprogestin Drugs: Ethical Issues," pp. 215–19. See also Lisa Cahill, "'Abortion Pill' RU-486: Ethics, Rhetoric, and Social Practice," *Hastings Center Report* 1987, *17* (October–November), 5–8. For the political pressures operating until recently against efforts to license the drug in this country, see Lawrence Lader, 1991, *RU-486: The Pill That Could End the Abortion Wars and Why American Women Don't Have It*, New York: Addison-Wesley. Lader is the founder of Abortion Rights Mobilization (ARM) and a prime mover behind the ARM Research Council that was the only U.S. supplier of RU-486 in the 1990s. For the results of a study of over two thousand women using RU-486, see Irving Spitz et al., "Early Pregnancy Termination with Mifepristone and Misoprostol in the United States," *New England Journal of Medicine* 1998, *338*, 1241–47. Mifepristone is the same as RU-486, and misoprostol is a prostaglandin used to expel the fetus from the uterus. This study showed that medical abortions with RU-486 were about 99 percent effective up to seven weeks, but the number dropped to 91 percent by nine weeks. About 3 percent of the women needed hospitalization and subsequent surgical intervention.

The case of Angie is taken from *In re A.C.*, 573 A-2d 1235 (1990). For commentaries on this and similar cases see William Curran, "Court-Ordered Cesarean Sections Receive Judicial Defeat," *New England Journal of Medicine* 1990, *323*, 489–92; George Annas, "She's Going to Die: The Case of Angela C." *Hastings Center Report* 1988, *18* (February–March), 23–25, and "Foreclosing the Use of Force: A.C. Reversed," *Hastings Center Report* 1990, *20* (July–August), 27–29. See also Martha Field, "Controlling the Woman to Protect the Fetus," *Law, Medicine & Health Care* 1989, *17*, 14–29; Lawrence Nelson and Nancy Milliken, "Compelled Medical Treatment of Pregnant Women," *JAMA* 1988, *259*, 1060–66; Veronika Kolder et al., "Court Ordered Obstetrical Interventions," *New England Journal of Medicine* 1987, *316*, 1192–96; Thomas Elkins et al., "Maternal-Fetal Conflict: A Survey of Physicians' Concerns in Court-Ordered Cesarean Sections," *Journal of Clinical Ethics* 1990, *1*, 316–19; and Deborah Homstra, "A Realistic Approach to Maternal-Fetal Conflict," *Hastings Center Report* 1998, *28* (September–October), 7–12.

TWELVE

Infants and Children

THERE IS A MYTH ABOUT BABIES, and, like most myths, it is not totally realistic. The myth is that all babies are healthy and beautiful; the reality is that some babies are born diseased, seriously defective, or too early. Deciding how to treat these babies is one of the more difficult challenges parents and physicians face in health care ethics.

Until a half-century ago there was not much to decide. Neither neonatologists nor neonatal intensive care units (NICUs) existed. Their absence meant fewer ethical dilemmas because many impaired infants did not survive with the simple treatments that were available. Today we can save many neonates who would have died a few decades ago, but the interventions can be painful, and they often provide only limited lives marked by significant suffering. And so we have to ask about the morality of invasive treatments: When are they prudent and when are they unreasonable? Or, to phrase it another way, when do the medical interventions contribute to the infant's overall well-being despite the discomfort they cause, and when do they cause so much pain for so little benefit that it would be unreasonable to use them? These questions are especially important when, as the result of a terrible genetic defect or other problem, we know the infant is doomed to a short life of considerable suffering.

In this chapter we proceed as follows. First, we make a few remarks about the history of neonatal medical care; second, we review some of the more common problems affecting neonates; third, we consider two special difficulties in making moral decisions about neonatal treatment; fourth, we examine what are called the Baby Doe rules; and fifth, we examine three cases including the famous Baby Doe case.

HISTORICAL BACKGROUND

Today most pregnant women seek medical care during their pregnancy, plan on delivering their babies in a hospital with the help of physicians or midwives and nurses, and expect to receive some postnatal care for themselves and their babies. Moreover, if the baby is impaired in any way, most parents expect the physicians and nurses to provide treatment.

These are relatively new expectations. For most of human history physicians did not provide prenatal care, most women did not deliver in a hospital, and little or nothing was done—because there was little that could be done—for infants who did not thrive. In the United States only 5 percent of babies were born in hospitals at the beginning of the twentieth century. Forty years later this had climbed to a national average of 50 percent and to 75 percent in urban areas, where hospitals were more accessible. Today almost all births in the United States occur under medical supervision.

Moving births into the hospital and under the care of physicians meant all babies automatically became hospital patients and received medical treatment if they required it. As a result more and more children survived the early days, months, and years of life, and more and more parents came to expect that medicine could save their children despite impairments.

Parents of earlier generations had no such expectation. They expected to lose some of their children in the early years and often did. In the first half of the eighteenth century in London, for example, three out of every four babies died before the age of five. The frequent deaths of babies and young children led to a kind of fatalism about infant mortality. People simply took it for granted that many newborns and infants would die in the early years of life.

Coupled with the great natural loss of babies and infants was the practice of infanticide, the killing of unwanted babies. It is difficult to know just how widespread this practice was in the societies that preceded us in our cultural tradition. Ethicists supporting the euthanasia of defective infants tend to see infanticide as quite widespread in our history, whereas those opposed to the killing of defective babies suggest the practice was more rare and, when it did occur, was tolerated rather than praised as a noble and good thing to do.

The general Hebrew, Christian, and Stoic attitudes against abortion would have set the stage in the ancient Judaic-Christian and Greek-Roman worlds for a stand against infanticide. Moreover, the ancient practice of "exposure" of unwanted infants, usually defective ones, was not always a death sentence. Babies being abandoned by "exposure" were often left where others would likely find them. Some were picked up and raised by adoptive parents, as the famous and tragic drama of Oedipus reminds us. Abandoned by his parents Jocasta and Laius, he was raised by another couple, thus setting the stage for him to kill, unknowingly, the man who was his father, and then to marry, again unknowingly, the woman who was his mother.

On the other hand, Plato (*Republic* 460c) wanted defective babies set aside to die in hidden places, and Aristotle (*Politics* 1335b20) advocated laws against raising them. The famous Twelve Tablets of Roman law ordered defective babies to be killed quickly, and Seneca, a Roman philosopher and political leader of the first century, clearly condoned infanticide (*De Ira* 1.15).

The killing and abandonment of impaired infants has now been condemned for centuries. The current emphasis is on saving these infants, an attitude reinforced by the medical setting where most infants are born. Some survivors, however, cannot live long or fare well even with the miracles of modern medicine, and this creates the moral dilemmas. Parents and physicians wonder whether great effort should always be made to keep severely handicapped babies alive when the most that can be expected is a short life of frequent surgeries and hospital admissions or a longer life of significant suffering and little chance of engaging in simple human activities.

In October 1973 an English physician named John Lorber published a landmark article describing how aggressive treatment was withheld from some infants with spina bifida. In his cohort of thirty-seven babies over a twenty-one-month period, twelve were selected for aggressive treatment, and the remaining twenty-five were considered so compromised by paralysis, large lesions, reverse spine curvature, multiple congenital defects, or a grossly enlarged head that they received comfort treatment but no oxygen, tubal nourishment, antibiotics, or cardiopulmonary resuscitation. Nor were they subjected to any invasive medical tests. All twenty-five died within nine months, as did one of the twelve selected for aggressive treatment. Only three of the twelve aggressively treated babies fully recovered, seven of the twelve survived with slight paralysis, but some of these were incontinent, and one survived with severe paralysis, kidney problems, lateral spine curvature, and incontinence. The article forced many people to question the prevailing expectation that every neonate should be given maximum treatment.

At almost the same time, Raymond Duff and A. G. M. Campbell reported on a thirty-month period in which 1,615 babies entered the Yale–New Haven Hospital by birth and another 556 were accepted in transfer. Of the 299 who died, 256 had been treated aggressively; parents and physicians had made decisions to forgo life-sustaining treatment for the remaining forty-three. Again, the article forced readers to face the question of when to treat, and when not to treat, seriously deformed and critically ill infants.

Unlike John Lorber, who took a strong stand against euthanasia and infanticide, Duff and Campbell recognized in their article "a growing tendency to seek early death as a management option, to avoid that cruel choice of gradual, often slow, but progressive deterioration of the child who was required under these circumstances in effect to kill himself."

Seeking "early death as a management option" suggests, of course, infanticide or the euthanasia of seriously impaired infants. Today a number of ethicists support this option. The important thing, they argue, is good comfort care; once we decide unreasonable life-sustaining medical treatment will be withheld or withdrawn, then we should recognize that killing these infants is better than allowing them to die slowly. Others oppose it, arguing that euthanasia of children lacks a key element every serious proposal for euthanasia contains—the patient does not voluntarily request it. Euthanasia of infants is always involuntary euthanasia.

The articles by Lorber and by Duff and Campbell, along with a host of others that rapidly followed in the next decade, set the stage for the moral debate about the treating of infants. The ethical issue is simple: When is it better for an infant to bear the many burdens of interventions such as the long-term use of ventilators, multiple surgeries, and frequent cardiopulmonary resuscitations when the most that can be hoped for is a shortened life of considerable suffering? Before considering some of the moral aspects of this question, we will look at a few of the major problems afflicting newborns.

A SAMPLING OF NEONATAL ABNORMALITIES

This section addresses a number of abnormalities that can affect infants at birth.

Low Birth Weight

Babies weighing less than 2,500 grams (about five-and-one-half pounds) are considered low-birth-weight (LBW) infants. Most of them are premature, and many weighing close to 2,500 grams do well with some supportive care. Others, especially those closer to the 500-gram mark, do poorly if they survive. About 75 percent of babies weighing under 1,000 grams (about 2 pounds, 3 ounces) will experience bleeding in the brain, and one in four of these will suffer severe impairments such as mental retardation with an IQ below seventy or cerebral palsy.

Most LBW babies are premature and suffer from the common problems of prematurity. Often their lungs are not sufficiently developed, and resuscitation and ventilators are frequently needed. Unfortunately, these interventions can cause additional harm to the delicate premature lungs. Moreover, extremely premature infants often have feeding problems. Their gastrointestinal tracts cannot handle adequate nutritional intake, and both sucking and swallowing reflexes are not fully developed. Nourishment by IV lines can help, but it is often difficult to find sites for insertion, and sometimes the kidneys are not yet able to handle the fluids being provided. Finally, premature infants are susceptible to infections because their immune systems are immature.

Spina Bifida

This congenital problem results from the failure of the spine to fuse properly, leaving a section of the spinal cord exposed. Sometimes the membrane with its spinal fluid and nerve tissue bulges outward, creating a more serious problem.

Although the severity of spina bifida varies greatly from patient to patient, most victims suffer additional damage. They are at risk for infection, and they frequently suffer some paralysis and nerve damage in the lower extremities, causing loss of bowel and bladder control. Many also have fluid in the brain because the cerebrospinal fluid cannot circulate well in the spinal column. A surgically implanted shunt can drain the fluid into the abdomen where it can be absorbed, but the operation is delicate and carries some risk both of physical and mental damage.

The history of treating infants with spina bifida has been one of changing attitudes. During some periods it was thought that aggressive surgical, medical, and rehabilitative interventions should be employed for every infant; at other times less aggressive treatment, more in line with the approach of Dr. Lorber, was thought best.

Anencephaly

This condition is a more severe problem of the neural tube—the neocortex or cerebral hemispheres of the brain simply do not develop. Although anencephaly admits of some variation, the basic diagnosis is the absence of almost all the brain except the brain stem. Some anencephalic infants can breathe on their own. Today, the number of anencephalic infants is dropping because many women elect to abort once prenatal diagnosis confirms the problem. Of those not aborted, many are stillborn, and the remainder die within hours because they are seldom fed or treated. If fed, a few anencephalics can live for months or even a year or more, but they can never develop normally because they have little or no brain tissue within their skulls.

In some ways, an anencephalic infant resembles what some call neocortically dead persons, and, as was mentioned in chapter 6, some people would like to equate the two. But the neocortically dead and the anencephalic infant differ in several crucial ways. First, the neocortically dead person once had a living neocortex and the brain tissue then died, whereas the anencephalic infant never had a living neocortex, and therefore no brain tissues ever died. The anencephalic infant suffers from the lack of a brain, not the death of the brain. Death implies something was living and then ceased to live, but the anencephalic child never had a brain. This difference undermines the efforts to draw an analogy between neocortical death and anencephaly.

Second, the best evidence available today indicates that older children and adults suffering from neocortical death have lost all capability of awareness. They cannot, and will never again, feel anything. There is some evidence, however, that anencephalic infants can feel at birth. Whereas destruction of the neocortex in an older child or, in an adult precludes awareness, this is not so certain in the case of infants, where the brain stem may support primitive awareness. We cannot call a human being neocortically dead as long as the possibility of awareness is present.

The traditional therapeutic response of the obstetrical team to an anencephalic infant was to do nothing except provide basic comfort care until the infant died. Nobody seriously considered treatment because treatment cannot restore a missing brain. If the anencephalic neonate did have awareness, it would soon be lost, and infants with irreversible loss of awareness have no interests. It cannot be said, then, that treatment would be in their best interests. For most people, withholding treatment from anencephalic infants was morally incontrovertible.

More recently, however, several ethical controversies have arisen concerning anencephalic infants. First, some ethicists suggest that aggressive interventions to keep them alive are justified to preserve their organs for transplantation. In such cases, the life-support equipment will keep the baby alive until the recipients are ready, then the life support will be withdrawn, the baby will die, and the fresh organs will be immediately harvested.

Second, some suggest these infants should be considered brain dead. The rationale behind this argument is the desire to harvest their organs while the donor is still breathing, much as organs can be harvested from a brain-dead patient breathing on a ventilator. A few years ago some physicians in Germany were actually taking organs from anencephalic infants, but legal authorities put an end to the practice.

Third, some are beginning to suggest that infants with anencephaly should be given sedatives to ease their dying, even though even the smallest dose of a sedative carries a high risk of being lethal. These people are not arguing for euthanasia; they advocate only the lightest dose of sedation to relieve distress, although they do recognize that sedation might also be lethal.

Fourth, some do advocate euthanasia for anencephalic infants. They argue that the baby is dying anyway and that treatments are not going to be provided, so the most humane course to follow would be to kill these infants with a lethal injection, especially if there are signs of suffering.

Fifth, some parents are now insisting that physicians treat their anencephalic baby with medical nutrition and life-sustaining treatments. In 1993 one such case involving a child known as "Baby K" received widespread publicity; we will describe the circumstances later in the chapter.

Trisomy

Normally the chromosomes of a human being are found in twenty-three pairs, but occasionally one of the pairs is really a triplet—it carries an extra chromosome. The condition is known as trisomy. Trisomy 21 means the twenty-first chromosome is not a pair but a triplet, trisomy 18 means the eighteenth chromosome is a triplet, and so on. Some of the more important abnormalities involving trisomy are the following.

1. *Trisomy 13*. This chromosomal abnormality causes facial distortions, including widely spaced small eyes with abnormal retinas, low-set ears, and poorly formed lower jaw. The infants

are severely retarded, and they often suffer congenital heart disease and central nervous system disorders. Life expectancy is short; almost half die during the first month, and the fewer than 20 percent that do survive the first year suffer from mental defects, seizures, and failure to thrive. Physicians and parents often wonder whether it is reasonable to use aggressive life-sustaining treatment since the long-term prognosis is so poor.

2. *Trisomy 18.* This abnormality also causes physical deformities and mental retardation. The skull is narrow and elongated with poorly formed ears placed lower than normal, hands are clenched with overlapping fingers and malformed thumbs, and the feet bulge outward on the bottom. Most of the infants have congenital heart disease and significant gastrointestinal and renal problems. About half the infants will die in the first two months; only 10 percent survive the first year. With aggressive treatment and institutionalization, about 1 percent will reach the age of ten. Again, people naturally wonder whether the burdens of treatment to the child are justified in light of such a poor prognosis.

3. *Trisomy 21.* This is perhaps the best known trisomy problem. The more familiar name is Down syndrome. It is marked by a sloping forehead and low-set ears. The eyes are almond-shaped and have gray or yellow spots. Mental retardation ranges from moderate to severe, and life expectancy can often be measured in decades. Babies with Down syndrome do not normally present moral dilemmas because they are not suffering and do not need special medical attention. With supportive care they can easily enjoy limited thriving, and some suggest their mental retardation is such that they are not fully aware of their condition and may actually live rather happy lives.

Many babies with Down syndrome, however, have some additional physical problems. Blockages (atresias) in the intestine or the esophagus are common, as are openings (fistulas) between the esophagus and the trachea. Attempting to feed babies with these problems, of course, is out of the question. Luckily the blockages and the openings can usually be corrected with relatively simple surgery, and the infants can then be fed normally.

However, several notable cases have arisen where the parents refused consent for the surgeons to correct these physical problems. Without informed consent the surgeons could not operate, and without the operation, the babies could not be fed. We will consider the story of one of these babies, the baby known as "Baby Doe," and we will review the history of the "Baby Doe" regulations this famous case produced.

Significant Intestinal Loss

Some infants develop problems before or after birth that destroy large segments of their intestines. Perhaps the intestines became so twisted that the blood supply was cut off and the tissue died, or perhaps an infection caused the damage. The loss is life-threatening if the remaining functioning intestine is so short that the absorption of food necessary for life cannot occur. Tubal feeding is of no help because the intestines cannot absorb the nutrients.

Recently, the total parenteral nutrition (TPN) feeding techniques we explained earlier have been used with some success. Nutrition by central IV lines has its problems, however, because infection often sets in, and finding sites on a baby's body for the insertion of IV lines is a challenge. An ethical dilemma, therefore, centers on whether to start these infants on TPN, knowing that they will probably never be able to eat or drink and will probably need TPN for the rest of their lives. This dilemma may disappear in the future, however, if the transplantation of intestines from infant cadavers (now being tried) ever becomes a reliable surgical response to the problem.

Conjoined Twins

Some babies born joined together can be surgically separated so both can live individual lives despite the handicaps resulting from the conjoining. Others cannot be separated, but they can live joined lives. Still others cannot be separated and cannot live joined lives. If they remain joined, both will soon die, but if they are separated, the stronger might live. This last situation presents a formidable ethical dilemma that, mercifully, happens only rarely.

Consider, for example, conjoined twins sharing the same heart mass, and the cardiac mass cannot be divided so each will have enough of a heart to survive. If the twins are not surgically separated, both will soon die because the heart mass cannot support two growing bodies. If the twins are separated, the surgery will, in effect, kill the weaker twin but enable the other to live longer with the heart that will now provide for only one body. Sometimes most of the heart mass is located more in the weaker twin's chest. In this case the surgical separation becomes a kind of heart transplant—the heart mass located mostly in the weaker twin is removed and placed in the chest of the stronger. A heart is thus transplanted from a living human being so that the sibling can live. One brother or sister is killed so that the other brother or sister can survive.

In August 1993 there was widespread publicity about just such a case. Surgeons at the Children's Hospital in Philadelphia separated the Lakeberg twins of Wheatfield, Indiana, after they were flown in from a hospital in Chicago where they had been born. The parents and surgeons knew the operation would kill one twin, but they hoped to save the other. Although the chances of survival were slim, one baby, Angela, did survive the operation.

Angela never left the ICU and needed continuous ventilation most of the time. Ten months after the separation she developed a bacterial infection and died in June 1994. Dr. Russell Raphaely, a physician at the hospital, reported that a medical team had resuscitated her two or three times in the three hours preceding her death. Her parents were not with her when she died.

As often happens, the ethical issues in this case are many. The surgery that saved Angela killed her sister, was unlikely to benefit her significantly, caused her pain and suffering during the ten months it prolonged her mostly ventilator-dependent life in the ICU, and cost over a million dollars, some of which Indiana Medicaid agreed to pay. Moreover, physicians responded with CPR several times when she suffered cardiopulmonary arrests in the last few hours of her life.

Although these cases of conjoined twins are rare, the problem is worth noting because it creates such an important ethical dilemma: Doing nothing means both babies will die, but saving one will kill the other. If the prohibition against directly killing the innocent allows no exceptions, nothing can be done. In an ethics of right reason, however, there is a way to justify the surgery. This ethics recognizes that the situation is truly tragic: Either both will shortly die, or one will die, and the other will have a chance at life. It is at least arguable that letting both die is less reasonable than taking the drastic step of separating the twins in a desperate effort to save one. Such a move, however, challenges the important claim made by many people that directly killing an innocent person is always wrong. It shows once again how difficult it is to formulate an ethics in terms of absolute prohibitions that admit of no exceptions.

Of course, other ethical issues surround this kind of case, not the least of which are the slim chance that the survivor would live well for more than a few months or years and the immense costs of treatment. In the minds of many ethicists, these factors indicate that the surgery is rarely reasonable and should not have been attempted in the Lakeberg case.

Diaphragmatic Hernias

As a fetus develops, the diaphragm normally closes the opening between the abdominal and chest cavities. When it does not, the intestines migrate into the chest cavity and prevent lung development. About one in four thousand babies suffers from this defect, and many need ventilator support until surgery to repair the hernia. For some babies, however, ventilator support is not enough; they need extracorporeal membrane oxygenation (ECMO) if they are to survive. ECMO is a machine that draws blood from the baby's jugular vein, enriches it with oxygen, then returns the oxygenated blood to the carotid artery. It provides what the lungs cannot provide even when assisted by mechanical ventilation.

The babies needing ECMO can be roughly divided into two groups. Half of them are so sick that only 10 percent will survive after corrective surgery; the remaining half are strong enough that 80 percent of them will survive. The ethical dilemmas center on the group with only a 10 percent survival rate. We have to ask whether it is reasonable to subject the newborn infants in this group to the discomforts of the ECMO technology and of the multiple surgeries that are usually required when 90 percent of the time these burdens result in little but suffering for a dying infant.

For each success story in this group, nine other infants were aggressively and painfully treated when it was of no benefit to them. The problem, of course, is that we do not know beforehand which baby will, and which nine will not, benefit from ECMO and the surgery.

SPECIAL DIFFICULTIES IN DECIDING FOR NEONATES AND SMALL CHILDREN

Two special difficulties occur in making decisions about treatment for very young children. First, the best interests standard is enormously complicated and at times not relevant for infants, and, second, the baby's parents are not always able to function as reliable proxies for their children.

Problems with the Best Interests Standard

Babies and young children clearly cannot make their own decisions—they need a proxy. And proxies clearly cannot make the decisions for the infants based on the preferred standard, substituted judgment, because the infants never had the opportunity to form their own wishes and preferences. Hence, the proxy for an infant has to rely on the best interests standard.

But making decisions on the basis of best interests is more difficult for babies than it is for adults. The proxy has some information about an adult's attitudes and interests in life, and this can be a big help in figuring out what is in the adult patient's best interest. But babies have not yet developed any life of their own, so the proxy is working in a kind of vacuum.

Moreover, it is difficult to assess how the burdens caused by congenital impairments and by treatments affect babies. In general, many impairments seem less burdensome for children than they would be for comprehending adults, and many treatments seem more burdensome.

Congenital impairments may be less burdensome for some infants because their perspective is different. We may not think it is in our best interests to live with the impairments of some infants, but the person born in such a condition may well have a different view. If we imagine, for example, an infant born blind, deaf, and missing a limb, we might be tempted to think that his life is not worth living and to withdraw treatment. But we are thinking from our point of view, as someone who knows what it is to have sight, hearing, and a whole body, and then to lose them. A child who never enjoyed these might not think the same way. What we would consider a terrible loss may not be experienced as such a loss by him because he never had what he now lacks.

On the other hand, treatments may be more burdensome for babies because the neonatal body is so small and fragile. Of course, we can only guess at the suffering medical interventions cause infants. We can get a pretty good idea of how much discomfort medical interventions cause adults from their reactions, but babies do not react to pain as do adults. And we cannot simply extrapolate from the discomfort a ventilator, an IV, a feeding tube, CPR efforts, or surgery causes adults to the discomfort these same interventions cause babies. Nonetheless, it does seem that an IV in the arm, for example, would be less of a burden to a one-hundred-pound patient than it would be to a four-pound premature infant.

The best interests standard in relation to infants is further undermined by the high level of prognostic uncertainty endemic to neonatology. In the Baby Jane Doe case (1984) that we will consider, for example, the experts at a renowned facility predicted early death without surgery to correct a spina bifida problem. However, the surgery was not performed, and the infant has lived for years and attended a school for the developmentally disabled.

Finally, in some situations the best interests standard for infants becomes suspect because it leads to unreasonable conclusions. Best interest centers on an analysis of benefits and burdens—a decision is in someone's best interest if the benefits outweigh the burdens; that is, if the good outweighs the bad. Life itself is an important good, and sometimes it can be sustained with little or no burden to the infant. Ventilation, for example, can prolong the life of some newborn anencephalic infants who may have some awareness and be of little burden for them. Thus, the best interests standard suggests using these treatments, yet most everyone agrees that ventilators are unreasonable for anencephalic infants.

Before leaving our consideration of the difficulties in using the best interests standard for infants, we should mention an additional factor that some people believe is relevant to an infant's best interests. They say that best interests embrace the kind of social life that the baby will have if he or she survives. If the impaired baby happens to be born in unfortunate circumstances, then they suggest it might not be in the child's best interests to be treated aggressively because follow-up care at home would not be available. For example, if an impaired baby is delivered by a woman with a long history of dysfunctional mothering, then saving the baby now might be doing little more than setting the child up for more suffering in an unsuitable home situation, a terrible burden for any child. According to this argument, treatment might be in the infant's best interests if the child was part of a loving, mature, and supportive family, but it would not be in the child's best interests if the child is a member of a dysfunctional family that obviously could not, and perhaps would not, provide needed support for the impaired child.

There are good reasons for thinking this approach is profoundly discriminatory and therefore immoral. Moreover, interpreting the best interests standard this way undermines the efforts of society to care for sick people of any age who do not happen to have family support. We do not become good and noble people by declining treatment because babies lack family support. Socially induced burdens are truly burdens for a child, especially one suffering from serious impairments, and some home situations are definitely not beneficial for children. But these social burdens are peripheral to our consideration of the benefits and burdens of the child's treatment, and this is what we evaluate in the best interests standard. The ethical response to unfortunate social burdens faced by the infant is not to withhold treatment but to provide whatever treatment is medically appropriate and then to make efforts toward correcting the wider social problem.

Problems with Parental Proxies

The second special difficulty associated with making treatment decisions for infants is that the customary proxies for infants, the parents, may not always make good judgments about what is truly in their child's best interests. This can be so for two reasons: some parents find it so difficult to accept the birth of a defective child that they decline reasonable treatment, and some parents find it so difficult to accept the death of a child that they insist on unreasonable treatment. The actual cases at the end of this chapter illustrate both of these positions.

Parental distress on the discovery of a seriously impaired or deformed infant is understandable, especially if it comes as a surprise. The distress increases as the future impact on their lives, and on the lives of the children they may already have, begins to sink in. If parental consent for life-sustaining treatment is needed, parents are sometimes tempted to see withholding consent as a way to resolve the tragedy that could affect them and their other children for many years. Once this thought begins to take hold, the parental proxies are enmeshed in a conflict of interest that can easily undermine their ability to make decisions based on the child's best interests. Many see the Baby Doe case as an example of this.

Some parents tend to be unreasonable in the other direction; that is, they insist that everything possible be done for their baby, even when the burdens of "everything" obviously outweigh whatever slim and dubious benefits the infant might gain. Parents sometimes demand treatments that, because of circumstances, amount to little more than child abuse, although they do not see it that way. They sometimes insist on invasive and painful therapies that do little more than prolong a life of misery because they believe life, no matter how painful, limited, and short, is always in the child's best interest. Parents unable to decline unreasonable life-sustaining treatment for their child are not really able to act well as proxies, and their insistence on treatment can do more harm than good. Many see the stories of Danielle and Baby K as examples of this tendency.

THE *BABY DOE* REGULATIONS

In 1982 what was to become one of the most highly publicized cases involving medical treatment for infants unfolded in Bloomington, Indiana. The baby was known as Baby Doe, and in the next section we provide an ethical analysis of the case. In this section, however, we want to review the regulations and legal requirements generated by the case. In a modified form, these regulations, often called the *Baby Doe* regulations, are still in effect. Many people find some aspects of them morally suspect, so it is well to know something about them and their history.

History of the Baby Doe Regulations

In April 1982 parents in Bloomington, Indiana, refused consent for relatively simple life-saving surgery on their baby. The baby suffered from Down syndrome and an additional life-threatening disorder. Without the surgery the baby could not be fed, and the child soon died despite the efforts of providers to obtain court authorization for the surgery.

In May 1982, acting on President Reagan's instructions, the Department of Health and Human Services (HHS) responded by issuing a notice affecting every hospital receiving federal funds. It clearly stated the following: "Under section 504 it is unlawful for a recipient of federal assistance to withhold from a handicapped infant nutritional sustenance or medical or surgical treatment required to correct a life-threatening condition if: (1) the withholding is based on the fact that the infant is handicapped; (2) the handicap does not render the treatment or nutritional sustenance medically contraindicated."

Section 504 of the 1973 Rehabilitation Act outlaws discrimination against people on the basis of handicap. The notice from HHS was an attempt to extend the Rehabilitation Act to the medical treatment of defective infants.

In March 1983 HHS published an interim rule requiring hospitals to display posters informing everyone that treatment cannot be withheld from infants with handicaps. Any person having knowledge "that a handicapped infant is being discriminatorily denied food or customary medical care" was urged to call the Handicapped Infant Hotline (1–800–368–1019) at HHS to report violations. Callers could remain anonymous, and reports of serious infractions would trigger investigations.

In April 1983 a federal court struck down this interim rule on the grounds that it was "arbitrary and capricious" and that the usual opportunity for public comment about a proposed rule had been waived by HHS without justification. The hotline, however, stayed open, and calls continued to come in. The government investigated over forty complaints in the next six months. Some people called the teams of government investigators "Baby Doe Squads."

Here are two examples of what happened. On the morning of March 29, 1983, an anonymous caller reported a case in the Strong Memorial Hospital in Rochester, New York, involving conjoined twins. Two investigators from the New York Office of Civil Rights rushed to Rochester, arriving by late afternoon. They were joined by a third investigator who had flown in from Washington, DC. They met for three hours with a hospital administrator and the attending physician and reviewed the medical records. The physician informed the investigators that the parents were worried about publicity.

The investigators met with the neonatologist whom the government had hired as a consultant when he arrived in Rochester after nine o'clock in the evening. When this physician discovered the parents had not consented to the investigation, he declined to review the records or visit the hospital.

The next morning the hospital administrator asked the federal investigators to stay away from the hospital because the case was receiving publicity in the media and the parents were upset. Unwelcome at the hospital and lacking the cooperation of its medical consultant, the team left Rochester without further action. More than nine months later, HHS acknowledged it had not yet completed its review. After nothing ever came of the investigation, people were left wondering why the investigators from New York and Washington had rushed to Rochester to investigate the treatment of the babies.

Another investigation occurred at Vanderbilt University Hospital in Nashville. Just before noon on March 23, 1983, the hotline received a call reporting that ten infants were not receiving proper treatment or nourishment. Less than ten hours later, two investigators from the Atlanta Office of Civil Rights and one from Washington, DC were on the scene, along with a medical consultant the government had retained. They worked at the hospital until after midnight and then returned the next morning at eight o'clock to continue their investigations until late afternoon. They then left without telling the worried physicians and nurses what they had found. Only some time later did the Office of Civil Rights inform the hospital that it had found no violations of the HHS regulations.

Between March and the end of November that year, the Office of Civil Rights received over fifteen hundred calls on the hotline and investigated forty-nine of them. HHS acknowledged in January 1984 that none of the forty-nine investigations resulted "in a finding of discriminatory withholding of medical care." The federal investigations, of course, were upsetting for the already distressed parents and for the physicians as well.

In July 1983 HHS issued a more carefully crafted proposed interim rule to replace the one the federal judge had struck down in April. Notice of this rule did allow for public comment, and almost seventeen thousand reactions were received, most of them in favor of the rule as the result of an intense campaign by groups convinced that most cases of withholding treatment from impaired infants violates their right to life. HHS made some modifications in light of these comments and published its final rules in January 1984.

In June 1984 a federal court struck down these rules on the grounds that section 504 of the Rehabilitation Act was never intended by Congress to apply to health care decisions for impaired infants. The court also said that the investigations by the Office of Civil Rights must stop. HHS appealed this ruling, and the case went all the way to the U.S. Supreme Court. In June 1986 the Supreme Court upheld the lower court ruling, thus affirming that section 504 of the 1973 Rehabilitation Act does not apply to health care for impaired infants. This ended the government's efforts to mandate the medical care of infants under the Rehabilitation Act.

Meanwhile, proponents of the *Baby Doe* regulations had initiated another approach. They successfully lobbied Congress to include laws requiring treatment of impaired infants in amendments to the Child Abuse Prevention and Treatment Act. This act authorizes federal grants to help states prevent and treat child abuse. The amendments expand the definition of medical neglect to include the "withholding of medically indicated treatment." The amendments further mandated that, in order to qualify for federal grants under the act, states must have programs or procedures in place to respond to reports of such medical neglect. The amendments to the Child Abuse Act were signed into law by President Reagan on October 9, 1984.

This means that the legal basis for the *Baby Doe* rules now in effect is amendments to a public law enacted by Congress. The public law, however, does not contain provisions for a hotline or for any "Baby Doe Squads" to investigate reported noncompliance. In fact the *Congressional Record* for July 26, 1984, reveals that one of the six senate sponsors of the *Baby Doe* amendments, Senator Nancy Kassebaum, said for the record that she was deeply troubled by the aggressive enforcement actions HHS had taken in this matter.

The Substance of the Current Baby Doe *Regulations*

The amendments to the Child Abuse Prevention and Treatment Act define "medical neglect" to include "withholding of medically indicated treatment." The key issue, then, is: What constitutes "medically indicated treatment"? In response, the amendments define three interventions as *always* "medically indicated." These are: nutrition, hydration, and medication. In addition, all other interventions "most likely to be effective in ameliorating or correcting" the infant's life-threatening conditions are also "medically indicated," except in three situations designated by A, B, and C in the following section. The most important paragraph in the regulations reads as follows:

> The term "withholding of medically indicated treatment" means the failure to respond to the infant's life-threatening conditions by providing treatment (including appropriate nutrition, hydration, and medication) which, in the treating physician's or physicians' reasonable medical judgment, will be most likely to be effective in ameliorating or correcting all such conditions, except that the term does not include the failure to provide treatment (other than appropriate nutrition, hydration, or medication) to an infant when, in the treating physician's or physicians' reasonable medical judgment, (A) the infant is chronically and irreversibly

comatose; (B) the provision of such treatment would merely (*i*) prolong dying, (*ii*) not be effective in ameliorating or correcting all of the infant's life-threatening conditions, or (*iii*) otherwise be futile in terms of the survival of the infant; or (C) the provision of such treatment would be virtually futile in terms of the survival of the infant and the treatment itself under such circumstances would be inhumane.

What can be said about these regulations that require nutrition, hydration, and medication in all cases, and all other treatment thought to ameliorate or correct life-threatening conditions in all but three narrowly defined exceptional circumstances? A great deal may be said, but we will confine our commentary to several remarks.

First, as we can see, the definition of medically indicated treatment is not presented very clearly in these regulations, and people still disagree on what the regulations mean by it.

Second, the regulations seem to require medical nutrition for babies in a persistent vegetative state (PVS). These babies are not comatose and hence do not fall under the first exception. This leaves us in a strange situation because it does not make much sense to allow withdrawal of feeding tubes from comatose infants but not from those in PVS.

Third, if the infant is not irreversibly comatose and is not dying, and if the treatment is effective in ameliorating or correcting the life-threatening conditions and not futile in terms of survival, then the regulations seem to require that treatment must be given unless it is "virtually futile . . . *and* . . . inhumane" (emphasis added). Now, suppose the treatment is not actually or virtually futile but is nonetheless inhumane because it is painful and will leave the baby in great pain. For example if it is possible to keep a badly burned baby who might survive alive for months with life support, the treatment is not virtually futile. In some cases, however, because of great suffering and a poor prognosis, it could be considered inhumane to subject the burn victim to this life-sustaining treatment. Yet the treatment is required by the *Baby Doe* regulations because, although inhumane, it would not also be virtually futile.

Many ethicists understandably have a strong objection to federal rules that require physicians and nurses to provide any inhumane treatments. If the rule said an exception could be made for treatment that was virtually futile or inhumane, this problem would not exist. But the regulations allow treatment to be withheld only if it would be *both* virtually futile *and* inhumane. Thus, inhumane treatments that are not virtually futile, and there are some, must be given according to the current *Baby Doe* regulations.

Fourth, the *Baby Doe* rules require medication at all times without exception. Although some medication is for pain relief, and this should always be given where appropriate, other medications are directed toward curing illness, and there are times when it makes no sense to give these medications. Consider a suffering, dying child who develops pneumonia. Since the *Baby Doe* regulations require medication for illness at all times, the physician must treat the pneumonia with antibiotics. Insisting that the pneumonia of every suffering, dying child must be treated strikes many people as morally unreasonable.

Reaction to the Baby Doe *Regulations*

Many people disagree with the *Baby Doe* regulations. They argue that the regulations undermine the parents' prerogative to decide what is in the best interests of their baby and in some cases actually mandate treatment that is at least arguably not in the best interests of the child.

A survey that received 494 responses from members of the Perinatal Pediatrics Section of the American Academy of Pediatrics showed that 76 percent believed the regulations were unnecessary, 66 percent believed they interfered with parents' ability to determine what is in the best interests of their children, and 60 percent believed the regulations did not adequately consider the suffering caused by treatments prompted by the regulations. The survey article summarized many of the arguments against the *Baby Doe* regulations, including the following points.

1. The regulations are not needed. The U.S. Supreme Court had found that no evidence supported the HHS claim that such regulations were needed when it struck down the *Baby Doe* regulations that HHS had tried to impose under section 504 of the Rehabilitation Act.

2. The regulations ignore what the Supreme Court had called "the decisional responsibility" of the parents.

3. The regulations cause a misuse of scarce resources.

4. The regulations exert undue pressure on state agencies and physicians.

5. The regulations are not clear; the survey showed many perinatal physicians disagreed about what was required in specific cases. The lack of clarity is obvious in the paragraph quoted above.

6. The regulations sometimes require treatment so burdensome that it is not in the child's best interests and is therefore unethical.

Enforcement of the Baby Doe *Regulations*

As burdensome as the *Baby Doe* regulations seem, their actual impact on parents and physicians is not, or should not be, as great as some would have us believe. What happens to someone who ignores the rules and is caught? The short answer is: nothing that would not have happened under the state laws already in existence before the *Baby Doe* rules were passed by Congress. The only federal penalty for violation of the federal *Baby Doe* rules affects the states, not individuals. And the penalty is not for any violation of the treatment regulations but for the state's failure to have programs and procedures in place for investigating complaints about violations of the regulations. And the penalty for this failure does not affect any person directly—if a state does not have programs and procedures to investigate violations of the *Baby Doe* regulations, the only consequence is that it may suffer the loss of future federal grant money for its child protection agency. Violations of the *Baby Doe* rules do not subject any parent, physician, or nurse to any penalty; the only penalty is a loss to the state of federal grant money.

We should note that some states (Alaska, Arizona, Indiana, Oregon, and Pennsylvania) choose not to apply for these federal grants and thus are not directly affected by the *Baby Doe* rules at all. Other states have elected to establish procedures to enforce the *Baby Doe* regulations in order to maintain eligibility for federal grants. Massachusetts is one such state, and a look at its procedures for investigating *Baby Doe* complaints will be helpful in understanding how reported violations of the *Baby Doe* regulations are handled.

In Massachusetts, responsibility for protecting children rests with the Department of Children and Families (DCF), which was known as the Department of Social Services (DSS) until 2008. The DCF is the Commonwealth's child protection agency. If it receives a report that the *Baby Doe* regulations are being violated, it assigns a social worker to investigate the complaint. The social worker must then obtain signed consent from the parents permitting the hospital to discuss the medical record of its patient and permitting the social worker to review a patient's medical record. Among other things, the social worker will ascertain whether there was a consensus about treatment among physicians and nurses and whether the case was already reviewed by a committee at the hospital. (An ethics committee is helpful here.)

If the parents decline to give consent for the social worker to look at their child's medical records, or if the hospital declines to let the social worker talk to people or see the infant, the social worker reports this to DCF authorities, who will attempt to resolve the issue of access. If necessary, they can seek court action.

If the parents do give consent, the social worker investigates the complaint and makes a report. The report is reviewed by the social worker's supervisor, the area or regional director, and, if appropriate, a DCF attorney. Should these people determine that the parents gave informed consent for the treatment of their child that is consistent with the definition of "medically indicated treatment," then they will dismiss the complaint. If they think the treatment is not consistent with "medically indicated treatment," then "a decision is made as to how to proceed with the case." What precisely does this mean? The Massachusetts policy and procedures say only that the DCF will inform the parents and hospital of its decision and, if necessary, seek temporary custody of the infant to obtain the "medically indicated treatment." The DCF policy also states: "Department staff are not expected to make decisions about the care or treatment of a child or to 'second guess reasonable medical judgment.'".

From this account we can see that the *Baby Doe* regulations do not become an issue in Massachusetts until somebody complains to the state child protection agency, the DCF. If this agency finds the regulations are being violated, it can seek temporary custody of the infant to ensure that medically indicated treatment is provided. The important point is that the DCF has no authority to assess any penalties against physicians or parents for violations of the federal *Baby Doe* rules. If the DCF discovers that parents are not giving proper medical care to a child, it simply seeks legal custody of the child under state law so a guardian can give consent for appropriate treatment.

This is not a very threatening situation for a physician. Yet as the survey of physicians indicated, many perinatologists feel forced to treat excessively as a result of the *Baby Doe* regulations. In view of the very limited state and federal reactions, if an investigation does show that the regulations were not followed, the fears of parents and physicians about exposure to serious penalties for making decisions outside the scope of the *Baby Doe* regulations seem more imaginative than realistic.

The Case of Baby Doe

The Story

The story behind the *Baby Doe* regulations is a brief and tragic one. The infant who was to become known as the famous Baby Doe was born with both Down syndrome and a life-threatening defect on April 9, 1982, at the Bloomington Hospital. The esophagus was not open to the stomach and had a fistula allowing nourishment to pass into the lungs, where it would cause pneumonia and other problems. Physicians wanted to correct the problem with surgery. When the parents refused to give informed consent, the hospital sought a court order for the surgery. A judge held a hearing at the hospital with the baby's father and with the physicians involved with the delivery and pediatric care of the infant. Some physicians thought the child should have the surgery; others did not. The father, who had worked with children suffering from Down syndrome in his job as a schoolteacher, and the mother decided not to give consent for the surgery.

The judge ruled that Mr. and Mrs. Doe had the right to choose a medically recommended course of treatment for their child in the present circumstances; that is, they could follow the recommendation of those physicians who thought it would be appropriate to withhold surgery. The hospital appealed the judge's decision, but the order was upheld by the Supreme Court of Indiana. Lawyers representing the hospital were on the way to Washington to seek a review by the U.S. Supreme Court when the baby died. Later efforts to have the U.S. Supreme Court review the case failed.

The complete story of Baby Doe will never be known because the courts have sealed the records to protect the family. Press reports indicate that the family lawyer said the baby had additional problems and would have needed multiple surgeries with only a 50 percent chance of survival. A consulting pediatrician, on the other hand, was reported as saying that there were no other problems and gave the infant a 90 percent chance of survival. The autopsy report did not mention any life-threatening defects except those connected with the esophagus.

The death of Baby Doe caused a national reaction. Critical editorials appeared in the *New York Times* and *Washington Post*. George Will, the parent of a child with Down syndrome, wrote: "The baby was killed because it was retarded."

Ethical Analysis

Situational awareness.   We are aware of the following facts in the Baby Doe story.

1. Baby Doe had Down syndrome. In addition, the baby had a tracheoesophageal fistula and may have had other problems as well.

2. Down syndrome is not physically painful and, despite the handicaps obvious to observers, seems not to be a serious emotional burden for the victims of this genetic disorder. Most people with Down syndrome manifest a contentment that we find somewhat baffling.

3. The esophageal problems can be successfully corrected by surgery most of the time, and parents would be expected to give consent for the necessary operation if the child were otherwise normal.

4. The parents refused consent for the life-saving surgery, and the child died in several days because it could not be fed.

We are also aware of these good and bad possibilities in the case.

1. The life of a person with Down syndrome is a good; the person does not have the longevity of other people, but the Down syndrome individual can live for decades without evident emotional distress.

2. The surgery will cause some discomfort but save the infant's life.

3. Withholding surgery will result in the loss of the infant's life.

4. Raising a child with Down syndrome is a significant burden for the parents and usually becomes something of a burden for the community as well.

Prudential Reasoning in the *Baby Doe* Story

We are handicapped in this case because the court records containing the facts were sealed, but let us suppose the situation is one that happens with some frequency: A baby is born with Down syndrome and also suffers from a life-threatening but correctable defect. What response does prudential reasoning suggest for the parents and for the physicians?

Proxies' perspective. The answer in most cases is clear: Unless there are other, more serious, complications, we have every reason to think the surgery to correct the life-threatening problem is in the baby's best interest. The surgery will be a minor burden for the baby but provide a great benefit—it will save a life that can be lived without undue suffering and with a considerable degree of contentment. The fact that the child happens to suffer also from Down syndrome is not a reason to decline medical care, especially life-saving surgery with a high degree of success.

The reasonableness of this view becomes clearer if we imaginatively vary the story a little. Think of a ten-year-old child with Down syndrome and also life-threatening appendicitis, and imagine that the parents, not wanting such a child, refuse consent for the surgery and the child dies. Most people could easily see that it is not reasonable to let a ten-year-old child with Down syndrome die when surgery could correct the life-threatening problem. Yet, except for the difference in years, the case of Baby Doe is not significantly different from that of an older child with Down syndrome who needs an appendectomy.

Providers' perspective. News stories indicated that physicians were divided about what to do when the parents declined consent for the surgery. Reports indicate that the obstetrician thought forgoing surgery was an acceptable option, whereas those caring for the baby thought that providing it was a moral responsibility. The Indiana courts, perhaps overemphasizing parental autonomy and rights in the matter of health care decisions for children, sided with the parents.

It is impossible to see how any physician or court could support the parents' position in this case. Certainly, parents are the proper proxies for their children, but simply because they decide on something does not make it right for the providers to go along with it. Neither the self-determination of a patient nor the determination of a proxy for a patient is ever sufficient to establish the moral reasonableness of what is decided; we always have to ask whether the decision of the patient or proxy, especially if it is to decline life-saving treatment, is morally justified. In this case there is no reason strong enough to justify withholding the surgery from the infant who will die without it. No provider would hesitate to recommend this surgery for an older child or adult with Down syndrome, and none should hesitate to recommend it for an infant with the same condition. On the other hand, those providers fighting to treat the infant had good reason for doing so—the surgery would significantly benefit the child with very little burden.

Ethical Reflection

No parent wants to cope with a baby suffering from Down syndrome, but this is not a reason to refuse normal medical care to keep the baby alive. The primary criterion for moral judgment centers on what is in the baby's best interest. There is almost universal agreement among ethicists that a baby with Down syndrome suffering from a rather common life-threatening problem with his esophagus or intestines should be treated so he can live.

A year before Baby Doe was born, a similar case involving a baby with Down syndrome and also a life-threatening intestinal problem came before the courts in England. There the Lord Justice concluded, correctly I believe, that parents' wishes are very important, but they are not necessarily the views that must prevail in treatment decisions for their children. The Lord Justice decided that, since a Down syndrome person is not living a life full of pain and suffering, the surgery that would be performed without question on anyone else with this intestinal problem must be performed on infants with Down syndrome as well.

Despite the moral lapse that occurred in the *Baby Doe* case, the reactions of the Reagan administration and of HHS are very difficult to justify morally. It is not helpful to have a federal department or even a public law setting forth rules and regulations for the medical treatment of impaired infants. These situations are often very ambiguous and call for a very nuanced prudential reasoning. When there are clear cases of providing treatment, such as surgery for infants with Down syndrome to correct life-threatening defects, laws and procedures already exist whereby the parents' unreasonable refusals can be overridden. Long before the *Baby Doe* regulations were formalized as amendments to the federal Child Abuse Act, state courts had the authority to remove children, temporarily or permanently, from the custody of their parents in order to arrange for their proper medical care.

Unquestionably, life-and-death decisions affecting vulnerable persons are not simply matters of private decision—they fall under public morality and eventually the law itself. But laws protecting children have existed for a long time—the child abuse and neglect statutes in every state make parental failure to provide adequate medical care for their children a criminal offense. Courts have consistently held that normal treatment for children must be provided over the objections of the parents, if necessary. No new *Baby Doe* regulations, let alone on-site investigations by teams from the office of Civil Rights, were needed.

The Reagan administration and HHS were on solid moral ground when they said Baby Doe should have been treated. But they were not on solid moral ground when they tried to regulate health care for infants under section 504 of the Rehabilitation Act. And Congress was not on solid moral ground when it incorporated the *Baby Doe* regulations in amendments to the child abuse law. Trying to regulate medical and surgical care by federal regulations or law creates more burdens than benefits. The *Baby Doe* regulations have caused unnecessary upset in many people's lives, intruded on the parent-physician relationship, wasted tax money, caused some infants to be overtreated and to suffer unnecessarily from medical interventions that good ethics would not require, and they have brought little, if any, benefit to impaired infants.

The Handicapped Infant Hotline is gone, as are the "Baby Doe Squads," but the *Baby Doe* regulations still linger. In reality they are not a serious threat because enforcement is left to the states, and no penalty is levied against parents or providers for lack of compliance. Nonetheless, the shadow of these regulations still looms large over many who care for infants and, unfortunately, still has a chilling effect that undermines good medical and moral reasoning.

The Case of Baby Jane Doe

The Story

Baby Jane Doe was born on October 11, 1983, at St. Charles Hospital in Port Jefferson on Long Island and then transferred for intensive care to the NICU of the State University of New York Hospital at Stony Brook. She suffered from spina bifida, hydrocephalus (excessive cerebrospinal fluid in the brain), and microcephaly (a small head). She could not close her eyes, was unable to suck effectively, had a malformed brain stem and hand, and was prone to spasticity in her upper extremities. Her parents were told she needed surgery to close the opening on her back and to drain the fluid from her brain. With surgery, she was expected to survive twenty years but would be severely retarded, paralyzed, bedridden, epileptic, and susceptible to constant urinary tract and bladder infections. Without surgery, she was expected to live anywhere from a few weeks to two years.

After discussing the situation at length with physicians, nurses, social workers, and a priest, the parents decided against surgery on her back. They did, however, consent to other treatments, including antibiotics to fight the inevitable infections.

Ethical Analysis

Situational awareness. We are aware of the following facts in the Baby Jane Doe case.

1. Baby Jane had a serious problem with spina bifida. Surgeries to close the opening on her back and to drain fluid from her skull could help, but, if she lived, her life would probably last less than twenty years, and she would have serious and chronic medical problems. She would also suffer significant mental retardation. Yet prognosis is very difficult in these cases, so great uncertainty existed about just what kind of a life she would have. Her pediatrician at Stony Brook did predict, however, that it would not be very good and that she would not live long without the surgeries.

2. Her parents declined the surgery to close the lesion on her back, but they readily gave consent for other treatments. Baby Jane Doe was all too typical of the dilemmas parents and physicians face in the NICU—she needed surgery to live, but the most that it was expected to provide would be a limited life of considerable suffering and discomfort.

We are also aware of these good and bad features in the Baby Jane case.

1. Her life was a good, and her death would be unfortunate.

2. The pain and suffering from the surgery and from the chronic medical problems that would haunt her life were bad.

3. A child with spina bifida is a serious burden for parents to bear. Seriously impaired infants require a great deal of care and support.

Prudential Reasoning in the Baby Jane Doe Story

Proxies' perspective. The parents were in a real dilemma because it is impossible to know just how much the child would suffer with the spina bifida and the associated problems. No loving parent wants to give consent for several surgeries if the outcome is only a short life of misery for the child. And no loving parent wants to decline surgeries that would, all things considered, bring more benefits than burdens to their child.

The parents' decision making was made more complicated by the conflicting views they received from the pediatricians. One physician thought the surgeries should be done; another thought the problems were so serious it made little sense to try to keep Baby Jane alive. Dr. George Newman, a pediatrician who did not think the surgeries were indicated, testified that the parents made their decision "on the basis of the combination of malformations that are present in this child," which are such that "she is not likely to ever achieve any meaningful interaction with her environment, nor ever achieve any interpersonal relationships." Another physician at Stony Brook, Dr. Albert Butler, also later testified he thought the parents were making a reasonable choice.

People can make decisions only on what they know and believe at the time. If the parents thought Baby Jane could never interact with her environment, then her life would have been of little benefit to her. No "meaningful interaction" means a life without meaning, and it is at least arguable that an ethics based on right reason does not require proxies to give consent for painful interventions and surgeries that do no more than keep a meaningless and painful life going. The proxies may well have thought this at the time after discussion with Dr. Newman, although the encouragement of other providers to treat the infant should have suggested that Newman's opinion was just that—an opinion.

Providers' perspective. The providers advocating treatment were on the stronger moral ground here. They felt this baby's life was worth saving with the surgery despite the unresolved chronic problems. Undoubtedly Baby Jane would bear exceptional burdens in life, as would her parents, but they did not think those burdens clearly indicated that people should refuse to treat her at this point.

Ethical Reflection

Prudence often suggests we should provide most treatments when we think they might be helpful. This gives us a chance to see how the situation evolves. If the treatments bring little benefit and cause significantly disproportionate burdens, then they can be stopped. Because the prognosis for spina bifida infants is so uncertain, the prudent response might be to give most infants suffering from spina bifida a chance by treating them and then reevaluating the interventions as time goes on, with the knowledge that clearly unreasonable treatments can always be stopped.

There are exceptions. It does not make sense to use medical treatments to prolong an infant's life when there is no possibility of its human interaction with the world. And it would be cruel to use medical interventions to maintain an infant whose life is and will continue to be afflicted with chronic and intense pain and suffering. But things have to be exceptionally bad before we can justify forgoing life-sustaining treatment for infants expected to live through childhood, as was the case with Baby Jane Doe. Many spina bifida children do have meaningful interactions with people, and their pain can be made tolerable.

From the perspective of an ethics based on prudential reasoning, the right course would have been to operate on this infant's back to close the spina bifida lesion and to insert a shunt to drain the excess fluid from the brain and thereby minimize brain damage. Then, as future problems developed, the reasonableness of any additional treatments would have to be weighed anew.

Baby Jane Doe and the Courts

Although the matter would probably have ended if the medical staff had simply gone along with the parents' decision to decline the surgery, it did not. A lawyer long active in the right-to-life movement, Lawrence Washburn, a resident of Vermont but affiliated with firms in New York, was informed by someone in the hospital about the parents' decision to decline surgery. Without seeing Baby Jane or her medical records or talking with her parents, he brought a suit against the parents in a New York state court. At the initial hearing on October 20, Judge Melvyn Tanenbaum presided. In the previous year this judge had run for public office as a nominee of the New York Right-to-Life Party.

When Washburn's right to intervene in the case was challenged in court, Judge Tanenbaum appointed a local attorney, William Weber, to be the guardian *ad litem* for Baby Jane. After his report and two days of hearings, the judge ruled that Baby Jane needed surgery and authorized Weber to give consent for it.

When Weber had first talked with the parents and Dr. Newman, he was inclined to agree with them that surgery was not indicated. But when he read the medical record, he noticed things were not as bleak as Dr. Newman was telling the parents. Thus, he felt it was right for him to give consent for the surgery.

The attorney for Baby Jane's parents appealed Judge Tanenbaum's finding and Weber's consent for surgery. The New York Appellate Division reversed the Tanenbaum ruling and supported the parents' right to make the decision declining the surgical intervention. Now it was the guardian's turn to appeal, and he took the case to the highest court in New York, the Court of Appeals.

In a unanimous decision on October 28, 1983, this court affirmed the right of the parents to make the decision about surgery for their child. The court noted that the proper agency to bring court proceedings in cases of the mistreatment or neglect of children is not an individual citizen but the state child welfare agency and that this agency had investigated and found no cause for complaint. The court was critical of those who would displace parental responsibilities and engage in "unusual, and sometimes offensive, activities and proceedings." These remarks were obviously directed against attorney Washburn, the stranger whose action brought everyone into court.

Guardian Weber, however, still thought the surgery should be done, and he appealed the decision of the New York Court of Appeals to the U.S. Supreme Court. On December 12, 1983, the U.S. Supreme Court refused to review the case, thereby allowing the ruling of the New York high court to stand.

Meanwhile the case got into the federal court system in two separate actions. First, after the New York Court of Appeals ruling, Lawrence Washburn asked the federal district court in New York to appoint another guardian for Baby Jane. The court's response of January 20, 1984, must have startled him. Not only did the federal court refuse his request, but it fined him $500 under a federal law allowing penalties against lawyers who "harass, cause unnecessary delay or needlessly increase the cost of litigation." The federal judge also called Washburn an "interloper" and said that the State of New York could make a legal effort to recover its legal costs in the case from Washburn.

The other federal court involvement actually began earlier. Investigators from the Office of Civil Rights, a "Baby Doe Squad," were sent to Stony Brook on October 19 to see whether discrimination against the handicapped under Section 504 of the 1973 Rehabilitation Act was involved. When investigators asked to see the medical records, the hospital refused on the grounds of patient confidentiality. HHS asked the Department of Justice to intervene, and Attorney General Edwin Meese gave approval for the government to sue the hospital in federal court to obtain the medical records. The Justice Department filed suit on November 2, arguing that government investigators should have access to the records to see whether Baby Jane's civil rights were being violated under the *Baby Doe* regulations.

Since the New York courts had already resolved the case in favor of the parents, the Attorney General of New York now represented the hospital against the U.S. Department of Justice. He, together with the lawyers for the parents, argued that section 504 of the Rehabilitation Act (the law forbidding discrimination on the basis of handicap) was never intended by Congress to apply to treatment decisions for impaired children and, therefore, did not give the federal investigators authorization to inspect a patient's medical records. He also argued that the investigators were violating the family's constitutional right of privacy.

On November 16 the federal district court judge denied the request of the Department of Justice to allow federal investigators access to the medical records. The Department of Justice appealed this decision. On February 23, 1984, the federal court of appeals upheld the district court. The Department of Justice then appealed this decision, this time to the U.S. Supreme Court. The Supreme Court upheld the decision of the federal court of appeals in June 1986. This is the U.S. Supreme Court case that finally stopped the government's attempt to base *Baby Doe* regulations on section 504 of the Rehabilitation Act.

From this review, we can see how complicated these cases can become and how tragic they are for the family. It is somewhat ironic that William Weber and Lawrence Washburn were probably right to think the surgery was morally indicated. Baby Jane Doe, whose real name is Keri-Lynn, was not as ill as her physicians thought. While the court proceedings were under way, her parents had quietly given consent for the shunt to drain fluid from her skull and for other treatment, but not for the surgery on the spine. The spinal lesion healed by itself, and Keri-Lynn has been living at home and has done better than many of her doctors expected. She interacts in a meaningful way with her environment, she talks, and she attended a school for the handicapped. She cannot walk, but she has some mobility in a wheelchair.

The story of Baby Jane shows how hard it is to predict just how well an infant with spina bifida will manage and suggests the prudent response is treatment unless the treatment is clearly unreasonable.

The story of the original Baby Doe involved a case of parents' refusing life-sustaining treatment for their child. There are other stories that run in the opposite direction: Some parents insist on unreasonable treatment for their children. The tragic stories of Danielle and Baby K are two such stories.

The Case of Danielle

The Story

Danielle was born prematurely on March 26, 1985, at Brigham and Women's Hospital in Boston. She weighed less than four-and-a-half pounds and had some serious problems: anoxic encephalopathy (lack of oxygen to the brain), severe retardation with seizures, a strong possibility of developing pneumonia and pulmonary edema (fluid in the lungs), and spastic quadriplegia (paralysis with spasms of all four extremities and extending into the trunk). Physicians discussed various treatment options with Barbara, her mother. She told them she wanted everything possible done for her child.

Danielle was transferred to neighboring Children's Hospital for a week, then moved back to the NICU at Brigham and Women's, then to a long-term care rehabilitative facility. In July she was transferred back to Children's Hospital, where she remained through the following winter. It looked as if Danielle would be spending her life in an institution, but Barbara had other ideas. She persuaded the staff at Children's Hospital to train her so she could care for Danielle at home.

At the end of February, Danielle suffered a serious setback and again needed hospital care, including a ventilator. Physicians and nurses at Children's Hospital began to think that the burdens of all the medical interventions were outweighing any benefits a baby with such a poor prognosis could ever hope to receive. Barbara disagreed. Treatment continued; Danielle did improve somewhat, and in April 1986, thirteen months after she was born, she was able to return home, breathing on her own.

Two weeks later, she was back at Children's Hospital with pneumonia. The infection was quickly controlled, and she returned home once more. In early May she was back in the hospital for six weeks, then home for a month. In the following seven months she was readmitted three more times, and in February 1987 she was again admitted, this time with serious respiratory problems that would require a ventilator.

At this point, a large group that included eight physicians, five nurses, a social worker, and a hospital attorney discussed Danielle's deteriorating condition. Some of the people were members of the hospital ethics committee, and questions about the ethics of using a ventilator on such a sick infant were raised. The group unanimously agreed that such invasive treatment was not in the best interests of the child and that they could not in good conscience provide it. Barbara did not agree. The hospital stabilized Danielle without ventilation and then began seeking a facility that would accept Barbara's decision to use a ventilator that would likely be needed. Meanwhile, Barbara contacted an attorney at the Disability Law Center. This began a legal process that we will return to later.

Barbara's insistence on ventilation despite the physicians' belief that it was not in the best interest of Danielle created a concrete moral dilemma at the hospital. The hospital ethics committee convened a meeting on short notice to consider the problem. With but one exception, members of the ethics committee thought that it would be ethical to withhold further advanced life-support interventions because they would cause too much suffering with too little benefit. The handwritten notes of its meeting included the following points:

- Mechanical ventilation would be inhumane in view of the pain and suffering it would cause Danielle, with no expectation it would reverse her acute deterioration.
- Mechanical ventilation was so unreasonable that it would, in effect, be medical abuse.
- The desired benefit from ventilation is so doubtful and limited that the invasive and painful life-support procedures cannot be justified. Hence, providers felt that their position against using mechanical ventilation "could be supported by moral arguments."

The next day, Massachusetts General Hospital accepted Danielle as a patient. Less than a month later, she was well enough to go home again. Since that time she has stabilized and has needed fewer days in the hospital. Court findings in 1993 indicate that Danielle "is blind, deaf, profoundly retarded, unable to eat or swallow, has almost no use of her arms or legs, cannot speak or communicate in any clear way and needs round-the-clock acute nursing care." She is nourished by a gastrostomy tube and suctioned frequently to keep her breathing passage opened. She has constant seizures. Her pulmonary status has improved, but she still requires supplementary oxygen. Her mental status will remain that of a three-month-old infant.

Estimates for the costs of Danielle's care range between $1 and $2 million for the first two years of her life. When Danielle was about seven, a jury returned a verdict of negligence against several obstetricians attending Barbara during her delivery and awarded $20 million, of which $11.5 million was designated for Danielle's future medical expenses over the next twenty-five years she is expected to live. The total cost for treatments prolonging the life of this profoundly retarded, blind, deaf, almost immobile human being needing constant acute nursing care, therefore, could easily exceed $15 million.

Ethical Analysis

Situational awareness. We are aware of the following facts in the story of Danielle.

1. Danielle was severely retarded and paralyzed. Her ability to interact with her environment was extremely limited, and she had no potential for significant improvement.

2. She had required a ventilator several times in the past and may well need it in future if respiratory crises develop.

3. Her life expectancy was, as is so often the case with handicapped infants, uncertain. Physicians at Children's Hospital were convinced Danielle was inexorably sliding toward death when they objected to starting the ventilator in March 1987, but the pediatricians at Massachusetts General Hospital were not so sure, and they were right when they said she was not necessarily dying at that time. Court findings when she was about seven indicated she could live another twenty-five years.

4. Her mother wanted everything done; some providers thought future attempts at resuscitation and use of a ventilator had become unreasonable in view of her condition and the suffering the interventions caused.

We are also aware of these good and bad features in the case.

1. The preservation of Danielle's life is a good; human life is always a good, even if the quality of that life is minimal.

2. The pain and discomfort caused by the continual treatment, some of it invasive, are unfortunate.

3. The burden of care on Danielle's mother was also great, although interviews with her imply she has no second thoughts or regrets about her decision to have everything done for Danielle. Private nurses usually cover two shifts a day, and Danielle's mother provides care at other

times. Barbara stated in an interview: "I no longer play tennis. I don't go to movies or dinner. I'm in this house twenty-four hours a day. But look at what my staying in has accomplished."

4. The financial burden, already immense and continuing as long as Danielle lives, is also significant. Although it is covered by a health insurance plan, the millions of dollars needed for treatment that cannot cure but merely preserve the status quo obviously burden others in the plan.

Prudential Reasoning in the Story of Danielle

Proxy's perspective.   Barbara deserves the greatest empathy. Every parent naturally wants to save his or her child's life. Her sincerity is unquestioned—she has sacrificed much to care for her daughter. Her dedication to her child, and the sacrifices she has made, attest to the generosity of her spirit.

The difficulty, of course, is for parents to adjust to the new era of advanced life-support systems. In principle everyone knows their use is sometimes unreasonable and even inhumane. Unless a parent is ready to admit that advanced and invasive medical interventions are sometimes not in the infant's best interest, no real moral reasoning can occur. The imperative "Do everything to keep my baby alive" is not always morally justified because "everything" can sometimes be unreasonable or even cruel for the child.

An ethics of right reason would certainly support a parent who decided at some point that resuscitation and ventilation were not in the best interests of a child in this condition. It is more difficult, however, to determine when providing these interventions becomes unreasonable and therefore unethical. Yet reasons are not easily found that justify the extensive, and sometimes painful, treatments for such a damaged child. It simply is not always good to keep some human beings alive as long as possible with modern techniques and technology, and this may well be one of those cases where the better parental decision would have favored a more modest treatment protocol.

We should also note that the wishes of Danielle's father, Frank Hall, are conspicuously absent from the published report of this case. His silence is as noteworthy as Barbara's intense involvement. Normally, both parents would be functioning as proxies for their child, but there is no evidence of that in this case. It would be very helpful to know what Danielle's other proxy, her father, thought was in his child's best interests.

Providers' perspective.   Once providers are convinced the treatment has degenerated into what is tantamount to bad medicine or even child abuse, they have little choice but to refuse to perform it and to seek a transfer of the patient. Sound morality does not allow anyone to do what he thinks is not right, and neither does the law. In a 1986 case involving withdrawal of medical nutrition and hydration from a PVS patient named Paul Brophy, the Massachusetts Supreme Court reminded providers that the law does not compel medical professionals to "take active measures which are contrary to their view of their ethical duty toward their patients." And more than a decade ago the President's Commission report *Deciding to Forego Life-Sustaining Treatment* stated: "Health care professionals or institutions may decline to provide a particular option because that choice would violate their conscience or professional judgment though, in doing so, they may not abandon a patient."

The fact that the physicians at Children's Hospital incorrectly thought that Danielle would not overcome the crisis that hit her in February 1987, when she was about two years old, is not relevant to an ethical evaluation of their position. People can only respond as they honestly see the situation at the time, and that is what this patient's medical team did. They thought her decline had become inevitable even if ventilation were used, and therefore, they thought it unreasonable to subject their patient to the ventilator. As it turned out, Danielle was not as sick as they had thought, but that is irrelevant when we evaluate the morality of their decision. People can only decide on what they truly think will happen, and given their diagnosis and prognosis at that time, their decision was ethical.

Physicians at Massachusetts General arrived at a different prognosis and, on the basis of this more optimistic prediction, had a slightly better reason to treat Danielle. However, the fact that they managed to keep Danielle alive and get her home does not automatically mean that they made the right moral decision. For an infant such as Danielle, the primary moral challenge is to know when the aggressive treatment is not in her best interests. This, of course, is not an easy thing to do, and thus the decision by physicians at Massachusetts General was not necessarily unethical, especially in view of the fact that the baby's mother was convinced aggressive treatment should be given.

Ethical Reflection

The case of Danielle presented a truly ambiguous situation—and one without an ethically definitive answer. There are many reasons for thinking the burdens caused by the lengthy and aggressive treatments that included ventilator support and several emergency resuscitations could not be justified in view of the little benefit the life they saved could offer Danielle. On the other hand not everyone involved in the case agreed with this. Barbara Hall certainly did not, but neither did everyone on the ethics committee at Children's Hospital, and neither did some pediatricians at Massachusetts General Hospital. For some providers, the ventilator did seem ethically justified. Perhaps what can be said is this:

1. It is fairly easy to justify morally the decision of a proxy to forgo a ventilator in a situation such as this; it is much more difficult, but not impossible, to justify the decision of a proxy to insist on the ventilator.
2. It is also fairly easy to justify morally the decision of providers not to provide such extensive treatment; it is much more difficult, but not impossible, to justify the decision of providers to treat, especially if that is what both parents want, and if the child's suffering is not intense and unremitting.

The reason for leaving the door for treatment open a crack is based on a wider consideration than the simple best interests of the child. Prudential reasoning makes an effort to consider seriously a wide range of circumstances, and one salient circumstance in the treatment of infants is the wishes of the parents. Now this is not a *carte blanche*—parents certainly cannot demand what are unquestionably unreasonable and clearly abusive treatments. But, given the difficulty of prognosis in the care of handicapped infants, it is seldom easy to know what constitutes unreasonable treatments.

One very important feature of this case is that the mother wanted this treatment, and some people at both hospitals, as well as a judge who examined the situation, were not convinced that her request was unreasonable. In cases such as these, where providers and others involved in the situation disagree about what is the right thing to do, the parents' desire that their child be treated counts for something in resolving the issue. Certainly, providers who believe the parents' request is unquestionably immoral should not violate their ethical integrity and provide it. But their conscientious objection to treatment is not necessarily the only morally justifiable answer.

Thus, one could argue that forgoing aggressive treatment such as ventilators and CPR is the right thing to do in this case; one could also argue that, given the mother's insistence and deep personal involvement, following her request was also not unreasonable. Unless we are prepared to condemn Barbara's decision as patently immoral, then we could not absolutely exclude a moral ground for providing treatment at her request. And although the reasonableness of her decision was not apparent to many, her demand for treatment was an informed one, and there was no reason to question her love for Danielle.

Often the bond between parent and child is not totally captured in the medical and moral judgments of best interests. Parents who are not actually neglecting or abusing their infants need a little extra margin of leeway that we might not grant to any other proxy decision maker. If they truly care for their children, they are in the best position to know what is right for their infants. They might make the wrong decision, as anybody acting in good conscience might do, but unless we are willing to accuse them of neglect and child abuse, the less worse position might be that we have to allow this parental responsibility for infants to play itself out in the decisions the parents make, provided it is not obvious that these decisions are causing unjustified suffering for the children.

The immense costs of the treatments and the little benefit they produce beyond the prolongation of a terribly impaired life are additional important ethical issues in this case. But these are issues on another level, a social level. If Frank and Barbara Hall had to bankrupt their family and deprive their other children of life's necessities, then Barbara's decision would be more difficult to defend. But this was not the case, and it is not the case that welfare funds were being used, so the cost of the treatment was not a major issue for the parents or the hospitals in this instance.

Cost is, however, a major ethical issue for society and third-party payers. We do have to ask how many millions of dollars should be spent to provide aggressive treatment for a severely paralyzed child who is unable to eat, subject to respiratory arrest and seizures, and whose mental development will remain about that of a three-month-old infant. Maybe several million is indeed a reasonable sum, but at some point the sheer cost of such treatment for such a damaged life becomes unreasonable in a society where so many other children lack adequate primary care.

The Legal Proceedings

The attorney whom Barbara contacted on March 5, 1987 obtained a probate court hearing that very day. Judge Mary Muse immediately issued a temporary restraining order preventing the hospital from entering a DNR order. Then she appointed a guardian *ad litem* to discover the facts in the case for the court and a second guardian to represent Danielle. After his discovery process, the guardian *ad litem*, fearing Danielle was getting worse, asked the judge to hold an immediate hearing in a hospital conference room. The judge agreed, and the hearing got under way at about ten o'clock that night.

Dr. Robert Crone of Harvard Medical School and Children's Hospital explained the providers' position: Putting Danielle back on the ventilator would not reverse her deteriorating condition and yet would cause more pain and suffering since, in addition to the mechanical ventilation through the tracheotomy, new monitoring catheters would have to be inserted in her veins. The lawyers for Barbara Hall and the guardians appointed by the court argued for treatment. It was well past midnight when the judge suspended the hearing until the next morning.

The next day the guardian *ad litem* arranged for a pediatrician from Massachusetts General Hospital to examine Danielle and make a recommendation to the court. Dr. Eileen Ouellette examined Danielle and reported to Judge Muse in the afternoon. Dr. Ouellette testified that Danielle was capable of experiencing pain and so sick she might not survive even with mechanical ventilation. Nonetheless, she said her hospital, Massachusetts General, would provide treatment at the mother's request. The transfer was arranged that very day. When Danielle left Children's Hospital the legal dispute ended.

Judge Muse, however, realized that the case was extremely complex and difficult. She suggested that it might be worthwhile for the parties to appeal it to the appellate level, perhaps even to the Massachusetts Supreme Judicial Court, so a precedent-setting ruling could be made that might prevent such unfortunate conflicts in the future. The lawyers for Barbara Hall agreed. So did the court-appointed guardians who were also attorneys. But the attorneys for Children's Hospital were not interested in pursuing the matter further, so an appeal was never made.

Given the helpful contributions of many court decisions, including major Massachusetts decisions involving DNR orders and withdrawing medical nutrition from PVS patients, it is unfortunate the issue was not argued further in court. This is so because it is absurd to force physicians always to do "everything possible" whenever parents or families request it, since "everything possible" can be very bad medicine indeed. It is also a very difficult and touchy situation to forgo life-sustaining treatment when the parents are requesting it. Because both the legal and ethical responses in this kind of case are unclear, some legal direction from a state supreme court would have been helpful to physicians and hospitals.

Although it does not directly concern our ethical analysis of how Danielle should have been treated, there is a legal footnote worth noting in this case. Attorneys for the Halls brought a medical malpractice suit against three physicians involved in Danielle's delivery. They claimed that the physicians had been negligent and had failed to inform Barbara adequately about Danielle's fetal distress and the risks of a vaginal delivery. The jury agreed and awarded the $20 million mentioned above. The exceptionally high award was $1.6 million more than attorneys for the Halls had sought. The jury's decision was appealed, but in 1993 a state superior court ruled that the $20 million was not excessive and noted that juries are allowed some latitude in the calculation of damage awards.

The Case of Baby K

The Story

Ms. H delivered Baby K by cesarean section on October 13, 1992, at Fairfax Hospital in Falls Church, Virginia. During the pregnancy Ms. H was told her fetus was anencephalic and that abortion was an option, but she decided to continue the pregnancy. Immediately after delivery, Baby K experienced respiratory distress and was placed on a ventilator. After several days physicians informed Ms. H that no treatment could help her anencephalic infant and that the ventilator should be withdrawn because it was medically inappropriate. Ms. H insisted on retaining the ventilator. A three-person subcommittee from the hospital ethics committee was consulted; they concluded that the ventilator should be discontinued because it was "futile" and recommended legal recourse if the mother refused to allow its withdrawal. By this time it was clear that Baby K was permanently unconscious.

By the end of November 1992, Baby K was able to breathe without the ventilator. The hospital transferred her to a nursing home with the understanding that it would accept her again as a patient if ventilator support were needed in the future. Baby K was back in the hospital on January 15, 1993, for ventilation, but she returned to the nursing home on February 12. Then she was admitted again for ventilation on March 3 and remained a patient until April 13.

The hospital sought a ruling in federal court allowing it to withhold ventilation if Baby K were brought back to the emergency department in respiratory distress. It argued that the ventilation was medically and ethically inappropriate for permanently unconscious anencephalic infants. The court appointed a guardian *ad litem* to represent Baby K; the guardian agreed that the ventilator was truly inappropriate treatment for Baby K. Baby K's father also believed that his baby should not receive ventilator support.

Ms. H, however, insisted her baby should be placed on a ventilator whenever she required it. According to court documents, her position stemmed from her "firm Christian faith" that all life should be protected. She believed "that God will work a miracle if that is his will." Otherwise, she believed, "God, and not other humans, should decide the moment of [my] daughter's death."

Ethical Analysis

Situational awareness. We are aware of the following facts in the story of Baby K.

1. Baby K is an irreversibly unconscious anencephalic infant. There is no chance of improvement—she has no brain. She will live in a vegetative state until she dies.

2. She has required a ventilator several times in the past and may well need it again.

3. Her father, her physicians, and the guardian *ad litem* do not think a ventilator is an appropriate medical treatment in her situation. Ms. H, her mother, insists on using it. Her position is based on her religious faith—she believes it would be contrary to her Christian beliefs to withhold a ventilator from her baby.

4. The hospital is so disturbed over the mother's demand for what it perceives as unreasonable medical treatment that it has petitioned the federal district court for relief.

We are also aware of these good and bad features in the story.

1. If Baby K does not receive ventilation when she needs it, she will die, and death is always bad. The death of a persistently vegetative body, however, is not nearly as bad as the death of a psychic body (that is, a body with the capacity for awareness). The vegetative body has already suffered almost total neurological damage. The end of the vegetative life will simply be the last stage in the loss of human life that has already occurred.

2. Not using the ventilator will cause distress to Ms. H; using the ventilator will cause distress to the father, and to the caregivers forced to provide a treatment they believe is not medically indicated.

3. Although ventilation provides nothing beneficial for Baby K, nor harms her in any way, it does require considerable financial support. Someone is paying for expensive medical support that is of no benefit to the baby, and this is bad.

Prudential Reasoning in the Story of Baby K

Patient's perspective. Baby K obviously had no prior wishes about anything. She is not a moral agent in the story. Nor does she have any interests. Since nothing matters to her, not even whether she lives or dies, neither providing nor withholding treatment can be said to be in her "best interests."

Proxies' perspectives. Her parents are her proxies, and they are unable to use either the substituted judgment or the best interests standards of proxy decision making. They can only rely on our third standard in cases such as this, the reasonable treatment standard. Since a ventilator is of no benefit to a permanently unconscious anencephalic infant, there is no reason to provide it except to fulfill Ms. H's desires. And there are several reasons for not providing the unreasonable treatment, among them irrational expenditure of money and the distress to caregivers asked to provide medically inappropriate treatments.

Ms. H's position, however, is not grounded in reason but on her religious faith. As we pointed out in the Wanglie case (chapter 7), religious beliefs are notoriously hard to critique. Although some important religious thinkers—the thirteenth-century theologian Thomas Aquinas was one of them—insist that no moral position derived from the Christian faith could ever conflict with reason, not every Christian believer embraces this position. Many claim that what is unreasonable or foolish in the eyes of the moral philosopher is not always foolish in the eyes of God. For these believers, the religious belief becomes a trump card; once played, no reasoning can undermine it. The religious belief, no matter how unreasonable, becomes, in the mind of the believer, the reason for the decision.

Providers' perspective. Providers and the guardian *ad litem* agree with the father that the ventilator should not be used. Their position is the only reasonable one when the status of the patient is considered.

But the providers have another problem, a problem similar to the one that the providers faced in the Wanglie story. A proxy is demanding treatment for a patient on religious grounds. Refusal of the life-support therapy will be viewed by the mother as contrary to her religious beliefs.

If the medically inappropriate use of the ventilator were causing the baby any burden, then the providers' primary responsibility to protect the patient from unreasonable medical treatment would lead them to reject the proxy's demands. But the ventilator does not cause any burden to Baby K; she is irreversibly unconscious. This suggests, as it did in the Wanglie case, that it could be reasonable, given the mother's religious position that cannot be touched by any reasoning, to continue to provide ventilation when needed. The treatment makes no sense, but it causes no harm to the patient. And, as was pointed out in the Wanglie case, the idea that vegetative life is valuable is recognized in our culture. As evidence of this, we need only remind ourselves that a person coming into the ICU and shooting Baby K would be legally charged with murder, something that reminds us of the importance placed on vegetative life in law.

In a pluralistic society, respect has to be given to the religious beliefs of others whenever possible. Since the ventilator causes no harm to the patient, a case can be made that the unreasonable medical treatment can be provided by the physicians and nurses out of respect for the mother's religious convictions.

However, the unreasonable medical treatment does cause other harms, and these have to be considered. Providing treatment to a patient who can experience no benefit can be distressing. Those paying for the useless life-sustaining treatments are also being harmed. They might well argue that the burdens they are forced to undergo as the result of the inappropriate treatment outweigh the mother's unreasonable demands and decline to finance it. In other words, whereas the providers, once they realize that the treatment does not harm the patient, may decide to stop short of opposing the mother's wishes, those paying for the treatment might well feel that it is their responsibility to decline payment for expensive and unreasonable treatment. In practice, however, this is difficult to accomplish in the current political climate and unlikely to help in this particular case.

The Court Decision

On July 7, 1993, Judge Claude Hilton of the federal district court issued his opinion. He noted that the parents disagreed on what should be done but accepted Ms. H's contention that she has the right to decide what is in her child's best interests since she was more involved in her care than the baby's father. Moreover, he asserted: "When one parent asserts the child's explicit constitutional right to life as the basis for continuing medical treatment and the other is asserting the nebulous liberty interest in refusing life-saving treatment on behalf of the minor child, the explicit right to life must prevail."

This sentence captures the essence, and the inherent weakness, of rights-based arguments in complex moral dilemmas. In the extreme form exemplified in this case, the mother's right-to-life position is coupled with her right-to-decide position; and both are then used to demand that all requested life-sustaining medical treatments must be provided for her irreversibly unconscious anencephalic infant, regardless of how unreasonable they are or how much burden they cause others. Extreme rights-based positions, whether they advocate the right to life or the right to choose, simply fail to function well in complex situations involving life and death.

The judge also noted that Ms. H appealed not only to the right to life, but to a religious argument, and that this has constitutional implications, specifically those under the First Amendment, which allows people the free exercise of their religion. Obviously, we cannot harm others in the name of religion—human sacrifice, once accepted by many religions, would not be tolerated by the First Amendment—but here the ventilation causes the patient no harm. Whenever it is a matter of practicing religion, the government needs "clear and compelling" interests to violate a person's First Amendment religious rights, and the court did not think such compelling interests were present in this case. The judge also noted, correctly, that providing ventilation for Baby K whenever it was needed "is not so unreasonably harmful as to constitute child abuse or neglect." Thus, in its own way, the court recognized the religious trump card that we mentioned above and acknowledged that the mother's religious convictions played a role in its decision, something it could allow especially since the treatment caused no harm to the unconscious baby.

The decision of the federal district court was appealed. On February 10, 1994, a three-judge panel of the Fourth Circuit upheld, by a 2–1 decision, Judge Hilton's ruling. Unlike Judge Hilton, who argued on the basis of several conclusions of law, among them the Emergency Medical Treatment and Active Labor Act (EMTALA), section 504 of the Rehabilitation Act, section 302 of the Americans with Disabilities Act, and the 1984 amendments to the Child Abuse Act, as well as other constitutional and common law issues, the appeals court considered only the provisions of EMTALA.

This legislation is designed to prevent "patient-dumping," a practice whereby patients without financial resources were turned away from emergency departments despite being in serious trouble or in active labor. The law requires the hospitals to accept the patients or at least to stabilize them before transfer. Attorneys for Ms. H argued that the EMTALA requires ventilation for Baby K if she arrives at the hospital in respiratory distress. And once she is on ventilation, the hospital will have to continue her care (no one else is anxious to accept her in transfer) until she can once again breathe on her own.

Efforts to argue that the EMTALA was never intended for treatment of anencephalic infants in PVS convinced only the dissenting judge. The other two judges found no such exception in the wording of the law and therefore concluded that everybody coming to the hospital and needing emergency life-sustaining interventions must be treated. They noted that the only recourse is for Congress to amend the law. They also acknowledged "the dilemma facing physicians who are requested to provide treatment they consider morally and ethically inappropriate," but they insisted a court cannot ignore the plain language of a statute and stated it was "beyond the limits of our judicial function to address the moral or ethical propriety of providing emergency stabilizing medical treatment to anencephalic infants."

A petition was made requesting a review of the case by the full panel of judges on the federal appellate court, but the petition for a rehearing was denied by the court in March 1994. In October 1994 the U.S. Supreme Court refused to review the ruling of the Fourth Circuit, so its decision stands.

Baby K, now identified as Stephanie Keene, attained her second birthday in October 1994. She still existed in PVS, totally unaware of her self and of her surroundings. Her mother's insurance company had paid almost $250,000 for her medical care, and Medicaid was paying the nursing home for the care of her vegetative body. Physicians told her mother, Contrenia Harrell, that she would never recover any awareness but she did not believe them. "I believe in God for a total miracle . . . that she'll be a living testimony to the world" (*USA Today*, October 13, 1994). Six months later Stephanie was brought back to the hospital for yet another intervention to keep her vegetative body alive. This time it failed; she died on April 5, 1995.

The Case of Ashley

The final case we consider is the tragic and complicated story of Ashley because it presents such a challenge to prudential reasoning.

The Story

Not too long after her birth in 1997, Ashley showed signs of poor neurological development. Eventually she was diagnosed with static encephalopathy (SE), a rare but devastating brain pathology that left her as helpless as a three- to six-month-old infant with practically no possibility of improvement. She could not sit up or roll over and, of course, she could never walk or talk. She was nourished by a PEG feeding tube. Her body continued to grow and develop despite the brain damage.

In early 2004, when she was not yet seven, she began developing signs of puberty. Her parents became concerned about several things. First, if Ashley continued to develop sexually, she would begin experiencing menstrual discomfort and be at risk for pregnancy if she were ever sexually abused, a concern if she ever needed to be placed in a long-term care facility. Also, if she continued to grow physically, as was expected, her size would make it much more difficult to care for her. Finally, if her breasts developed, it could present a number of problems because women in her family tend to have large breasts and this would interfere with the supportive harness that enabled her to sit up, there is a family history of breast cancer and fibrocystic breast disease, and breast development would sexualize her body, thus increasing the possibility of sexual abuse if she were ever institutionalized.

Ashley's parents sought the advice of Daniel Gunther, a pediatric endocrinologist at Children's Hospital in Seattle. With his help they devised a three-stage treatment plan: removal of Ashley's uterus (leaving the ovaries in place but removing her appendix), removal of her breast buds (leaving the areolas in place), and high doses of estrogen that would reduce bone growth and leave her shorter and lighter than a normal adult. These procedures would prevent menstruation, avoid problems associated with breast development, and keep her height and weight to approximately four foot six and seventy pounds (rather than an expected five foot six and 120 pounds). Her parents thought these interventions would be an overall benefit for Ashley and make it easier for them to care for her. On the other hand, removing healthy parts of a disabled child's body and stunting her growth raise some important ethical issues.

Before proceeding, Dr. Gunther consulted with the ethics committee at Children's Hospital. Dr. Douglas Diekema, who coincidentally happened to be a member of the National Committee on Bioethics of the American Academy of Pediatrics, was also a member of that ethics committee, and he played an active role in its deliberations. Dr. Diekema later became the Director of Education at the Treuman Katz Center for Pediatric Bioethics at Children's Hospital in Seattle. Before looking at the rest of the story, we will consider the ethical aspects of the proposed interventions.

Ethical Analysis

Situational awareness. We are aware of the following facts in the story of Ashley:

1. Ashley is locked into the psychological development of an infant, but the rest of her body continues to grow toward adolescence and adulthood. She is as dependent on her caregivers as any infant aged three to six months would be, but her body will soon be that of an adult. She could live for decades.

2. Her parents are providing a high level of care for her and have integrated her into the family that includes two other children born after her. They are finding it very difficult to move and lift her as her weight increases, yet they want to be able to continue caring for her and taking her on family outings, and they want to keep her out of a long-term care facility for as long as possible.

3. The medical and surgical ways to prevent her body from maturing can facilitate her care in the hands of her parents and reduce some of the discomforts experienced by postpubescent women, but they are not standard care; in fact, they have not been done before, and they carry some risk. Surgery has its risks, as does high-dose estrogen, which can cause deep vein thrombosis and blood clots.

4. Although Ashley will remain small for her age, she will not remain physically a child. When she is nineteen, she will look like a short nineteen-year-old child, and when she is fifty, she will look like a short fifty-year-old woman.

5. The ethics committee at Children's Hospital happens to have a member well known for his work in ethics—Dr. Douglas Diekema, a member of the American Academy of Pediatrics Committee on Bioethics since 2001. Dr. Diekema, the author of *Christian Faith, Health, and Medical Practice* (1989) and a number of articles on bioethics, had been a member of the hospital ethics committee since 1991, and he was also chair of the hospital's Institutional Review Board at that time.

Prudential Reasoning in the Ashley Story

Proxies' perspective. Ashley's parents have been caring for her for years and want to continue for as long as possible, but Ashley's ever increasing height and weight are making care more difficult for them.

Moreover, Ashley gets upset easily. When she sneezes, for example, it often startles her and causes her to cry, perhaps because the sneeze of a six-year-old child is being experienced by a three-month-old baby! Her parents wonder how her infant awareness will cope with monthly periods and, years down the road, with menopause. They also know that significant breast development, which tends to run in the family, will make using her support harness more difficult (Ashley cannot sit up on her own).

All things considered, Ashley's parents think that the interventions to slow her growth and the surgical removal of her uterus and breast buds will be the most reasonable approach for both Ashley and themselves.

Provider's perspective. Dr. Daniel Gunther, the endocrinologist caring for Ashley, agreed that these interventions would be in the best interests of Ashley but sought the opinion of the ethics committee at the hospital.

Ethics committee perspective. Thanks to an interview with Dr. Diekema on CNN (January 8, 2007), we have some access to the deliberations of the ethics committee. Members looked at two main issues: whether stopping Ashley's growth at about age nine and removing her uterus would make her life better and whether these interventions would likely cause her harm. A consensus emerged that the interventions would make her life better and that the discomforts and risks were relatively small in view of the gain in her welfare. Many members felt that a person with the awareness of a three- to six-month-old infant would not be troubled by being twelve inches shorter than her peers or by not having a sexually mature body. Ashley, Dr. Diekema said, would not care if she were short, flat-chested, and unable to have children; no infant cares about such matters.

Members of the ethics committee acknowledged that the interventions would also be in her parents' best interests because it would make it easier for them to care for Ashley. And the committee did recommend that the family obtain a judicial review before they gave consent for the removal of her uterus. However, after a letter from the family's attorney arguing that a court order was not necessary, the committee no longer thought the judicial review was necessary.

The Decision

After much deliberation and discussion physicians took steps to stop Ashley's growth and removed her uterus and breast buds in July 2004 when she was about six-and-a-half years old. The two doctors who played the major role in the case, Gunther and Diekema, published an account of the interventions in the *Archives of Pediatric Adolescent Medicine* in October 2006. Their report was accompanied by an editorial commentary raising questions about the procedures.

Ashley's parents set up a website, and soon a lively national debate about the ethics of what became known as the "Ashley Treatment" erupted online and in the media. Objections to the interventions fell into several major categories. Some asserted that Ashley's right to develop as normally as possible was violated; some argued that the interventions were not natural and therefore wrong; some argued that the interventions should not have been done because they place us on a slippery slope leading to the physical mutilation of children with disabilities for the convenience of parents; some argued that Ashley's inherent dignity as a human being was undermined by preventing normal growth and sterilizing her; and some argued that the interventions were the wrong response to what is really a social problem—the failure of social systems to provide the help parents need to manage severely disabled children as they grow larger and their bodies mature.

Ethical Reflection

Ashley's static encephalopathy is a tragedy for her and for her parents. The main argument supporting the interventions centers on improving Ashley's quality of life by reducing the likelihood that she would have to be institutionalized, by eliminating the monthly discomfort she would experience for decades if her body reached puberty, by removing the possibility of pregnancy if she were ever raped, by making it more comfortable for her to wear her supportive harness, and by making it easier for her parents to care for her.

How might one reason prudentially in a case such as this where a person is locked into the psychological level of an infant but whose body will develop as a sexualized adult thanks to a feeding tube and supportive care? What parental and medical responses would be reasonable? It is not immediately obvious that it is morally reasonable to intervene as was done with Ashley. Pursuing this innovative option presupposes some careful moral deliberation. This is a new kind of dilemma.

An important preliminary step in deliberation is to use language carefully, something that both proponents of the interventions and opponents do not always keep in mind. For example, supporters refer to the interventions as the "Ashley Treatment," whereas in fact the interventions still are not recognized as approved treatments or therapies for children. Once we say "treatment" we are assuming established therapeutic value and are leaning in the direction of providing it. Supporters also frequently refer to Ashley and others like her as "Pillow Angels" because they are usually pictured resting on pillows. Yet Ashley and others like her are not angels but tragically disabled human beings. Angels, if they exist, do not have physical bodies, and it is precisely the bodies of children in Ashley's condition that constitute the center of controversy; namely, whether it is moral to modify their bodies in a drastic way. Another well-meaning phrase that often appears in the literature about Ashley and children like her is that they are a "gift from God," an unfortunate phrase because it implies that the creator God of the Jewish, Christian, and Muslim religious traditions deliberately creates deformed children and is thus some kind of sadist.

On the other hand, opponents of the "Ashley interventions" sometimes used inflammatory language such as "maiming" Ashley, spoke of "lopping off her breasts" (which is actually factually inaccurate), of "infantilizing" her (her body was not returned to an infant state, and her psychological development was already and will always be that of an infant), of calling the surgery the "mutilation" of a child, and so forth. We cannot engage in mature moral deliberation as we try to figure out what is the less worse response for Ashley and her parents if we use prejudicial and misleading language.

One might begin prudential deliberation by recognizing the value of bodily integrity. Sterilizing a child and stunting her growth are not things we would do without very persuasive reasons. We would also recognize that the case is not simply about Ashley but about her family; their needs are a factor, as is their desire to care for her as long as they can.

We also need to be aware of the slippery slope in cases like this; it is important to be careful about setting a precedent that would allow widespread retardation of growth and sexual development for children with disabilities that might be far less severe than those of Ashley. Both Ashley's parents and physicians were aware of this and opined that the interventions would be reasonable only for a very small number of seriously disabled children, perhaps about 1 percent. Nonetheless, there is always a tendency to expand the number of children who would qualify, especially if parents pushed for it. Yet the response to slippery slope arguments is often not to avoid the first step on the slope but to tread carefully. Ethics has a long history of drawing lines on slippery slopes. Sometimes they hold, and sometimes they give way, but often human flourishing is better protected by working to hold the line rather than by declining to take the first step.

One could also recognize that making children smaller than they otherwise would be and sterilizing them introduces a level of moral discomfort. It calls into question our deepening sense of respect for persons and the inherent dignity we do well to accord every human being in a morally mature community. Yet making people shorter and sterilizing them does not always undermine human dignity. We amputate legs for medical reasons and sterilize adults with their consent, which suggests that the real issue is not undermining inherent dignity by growth attenuation or sterilization but rather doing it without medical reasons for someone who cannot give consent. The crucial point is not whether or not the interventions are medically indicated for Ashley who cannot give consent but whether or not they will likely help Ashley and her family live better despite her irreversible disability.

Perhaps we can make some progress in our deliberations if we reframe the interventions and consider them more akin to research than to treatment. We could think of the use of estrogen to limit growth and the surgical removal of the uterus and breast buds not as a treatment but as an experiment with an untried and unproven intervention. In other words, because we have some reasons to think this innovation might be better than letting her develop physically with the mind of a six-month-old infant, we could consider the intervention a trial and then monitor it to see how it goes. If we approach it this way, we gain several advantages.

First, we acknowledge the therapeutic uncertainty of the interventions, and this avoids some of the debate between those who claim that the interventions are an ethical treatment and those who claim that they are not. Research is not treatment; it is a trial to see whether an intervention is safe and beneficial and can be accepted as a treatment. Second, we gain review by an Institutional Review Board (IRB), which is better equipped to handle innovative interventions than the typical hospital ethics committee. Third, we put in place a mechanism for review that an IRB typically puts in place. This means there will be periodic, or at least annual, review of the trial. Fourth, if the interventions cause unexpected troubles or fail to contribute to the well-being of the child, we will have a strong basis for speaking out against them in the future. Conversely, if the interventions are shown to contribute to the well-being of the child, we will have a strong basis for accepting them as therapies in the future.

Federal regulations (45 CFR 46.405) governing research on children allow research of more than minimal risk to children if the procedure holds out the prospect of direct benefit for the individual child as long as (1) the risk is justified by the anticipated benefit, (2) the risk-benefit proportion of the intervention is at least as favorable as that presented by available alternatives, and (3) provisions are made for the permission of parents and, if possible, the assent of the children.

The research on Ashley would seem to meet the federal criteria. There is reason to think that the risks of the high-dose estrogen for a short time and the surgeries are reasonable in view of the expected benefit and that the risk-benefit proportion is at least as favorable as the alternative, which is doing nothing. If nothing is done Ashley is at risk for a number of things including distress associated with sexual maturity, increased difficulties with home care as a result of her normal weight gain and quite possibly earlier institutionalization as she develops an adult body, and a statistically higher risk of possible sexual abuse if she is institutionalized.

Prudential reason might suggest, then, that parents of seriously disabled children who will develop adult bodies despite being locked into the psychological level of an infant might reasonably consent to have their child's growth attenuated and, if the child is a girl, her body surgically blocked from developing sexual maturity, by interventions considered research rather than treatment. As we learn from experience, we will be better able to discern whether or not these interventions on such severely disabled children will provide an overall benefit for them and their families.

Fortunately we can learn something about how Ashley, who was the first child known to undergo these interventions, was affected by them. On March 12, 2008, more than three-and-a-half years after the surgeries, Ashley's parents, who continue to remain anonymous, gave an exclusive interview on CNN. They reported: "Thankfully, the 'Ashley treatment' went smoothly, and it has been successful in every expected way. Her recovery from surgery was quick and uneventful, the scars are barely visible. There have been no side effects to the estrogen therapy. Ashley did not grow in height or weight in the last year; she will always be flat-chested, and she will never suffer any menstrual pain, cramps, or bleeding."

There is a tragic footnote to the story—Dr. Gunther had taken his own life several months before the interview. When Ashley's parents were asked about his death, they replied that his care of Ashley had energized and motivated him, but that he was also frustrated about being blocked in his efforts to provide these interventions for other children in need.

The hospital later acknowledged, after criticism from the Washington Protection and Advocacy System, a nonprofit organization that protects the rights of people with disabilities, that it would have been better to obtain a court order before Ashley's hysterectomy. The hospital also agreed that it would seek a court order before performing these interventions on other severely developmentally challenged children in the future. From a legal perspective this might make some sense—the courts have a responsibility to protect vulnerable human life—but it does not change the ethical perspective. The decision making in the case is fundamentally a medical and ethical issue, and the courts are not the best places to make these decisions for children, especially when challenging ethical issues are involved. Caring parents and physicians are in the best position to decide for children. If, for example, parents and physicians decide that the most reasonable response is a DNR order or the withdrawal of life-prolonging treatment, few think they need a court order to pursue this course of action. So too, if parents and physicians decide that the most reasonable response for the well-being of a child in Ashley's condition is surgery and other interventions understood as a kind of exploratory research that could contribute to the well-being of their child, it is difficult to think that they should be required to seek a court order before proceeding.

Infant Euthanasia in the Netherlands

We noted at the beginning of the chapter that Duff and Campbell, in their landmark 1973 article, reported "a growing tendency to seek death as a management option" rather than let a dying child die a slow death. Thus far few in the United States have advocated seeking euthanasia for dying infants, but the move toward infant euthanasia has become a reality in the Netherlands.

In 1996 two cases of infant euthanasia became public; one physician ended the life of a baby with a severe form of spina bifida, and another ended the life of a baby with trisomy 13, a lethal chromosomal disorder. When the doctors were put on trial, they argued that they were practicing good medicine by preventing meaningless suffering, and they were acquitted.

From 1997 through 2004 another twenty-two cases of infanticide were reported to authorities, but no prosecutions ensued. National surveys during this time indicate that physicians in the Netherlands actually ended the life of ten to fifteen neonates annually.

Fearing that the growing practice of ending the life of infants would lead to abuse if it continued without oversight, two pediatricians at the university medical center in Groningen, Eduard Verhagen and Pieter Sauer, began working with the local prosecutor to develop a protocol that would provide guidelines for physicians and prosecutors and ensure legal oversight of the practice. Since its publication in 2005, the Groningen Protocol, as it is called, has been at the center of significant moral controversy. Physicians who follow the Protocol are not guaranteed legal immunity—nonvoluntary euthanasia remains illegal in the Netherlands—but to date (2008) no prosecutions have taken place when the Protocol was followed.

It is important to situate the Groningen Protocol in the Dutch context; the Protocol exists in a country where voluntary euthanasia is legal for adults. The Netherlands have legally tolerated euthanasia since the 1980s and then made it fully legal, under certain conditions, on April 1, 2002. The Groningen Protocol echoes many of the requirements set forth in the law that legalized euthanasia. It requires, among other things, informed consent from both parents, hopeless and unbearable suffering, a second opinion from a physician not involved in the case, and a formal detailed report of the death by euthanasia to legal authorities.

Verhagen and Sauer identify three groups of infants where the decision to end life would be an option. Group 1 consists of neonates who are dying despite aggressive life-sustaining treatments. Often physicians withdraw life support from these infants, and they die quickly, but sometimes they linger and suffer. Group 2 consists of babies who can survive with aggressive life-sustaining treatments but whose prognosis is grim. Often these infants have extensive brain damage that does not allow for improvement. Group 3, the most controversial group, consists of infants who do not need aggressive life support but who have serious conditions such as extensive paralysis or the inability to communicate in any way.

How widespread is the euthanasia of infants in the Netherlands? A 2007 study (published online in *Pediatrics*) of infant deaths between January and July 2005 in the NICU at Groningen and at one other hospital suggest that it is rare. The study noted thirty neonatal deaths in the two NICUs during this period. All the infants were in groups 1 or 2. In twenty-eight cases the infants died after life-sustaining treatment was withdrawn or withheld. The other two deaths occurred despite aggressive life-sustaining treatment. In other words there were no cases of infant euthanasia in these two NICUs during the six-month period of the study.

Nonetheless, the protocol remains in place, infant euthanasia does occur, and thus the ethical issues of practicing nonvoluntary euthanasia remain. Published reports indicate that many neonatologists in France and Belgium believe that deliberately ending the life of a neonate is acceptable in some cases. From the perspective of virtue-based ethics, however, there are cogent reasons for insisting that it is not good for us to allow the killing of human beings except as a last resort. The main idea behind ending the lives of seriously ill infants is the prevention of suffering and distress. Once this can be accomplished without using lethal drugs to end the life of the infant, the moral reasoning behind allowing physicians to do this loses its force.

As chapter 15 points out, one of the arguments against legalizing euthanasia and physician-assisted suicide is the slippery-slope argument. Opponents claim that once we legalize voluntary euthanasia, it will only be a matter of time before we extend the practice to involuntary euthanasia, to adults without decision-making capacity, and to children and babies. Indeed, this has been the trend in the Netherlands.

After opponents of the Groningen Protocol pointed this out, Verhagen and Sauer, who did not hesitate to describe the Protocol as euthanasia in their 2005 articles in the *New England Journal of Medicine* and *Pediatrics*, eschewed the term by 2007 because, they say, euthanasia under Dutch law presupposes voluntary informed consent. They now recommend speaking of "ending life," not euthanasia. Hence, their opponents can no longer accuse them of sliding down the slippery slope from voluntary euthanasia to nonvoluntary euthanasia because intentionally taking steps to end the life of an infant is no longer considered euthanasia at all.

Good moral reasoning, however, will go beyond linguistic modifications and focus on describing the actions in question. What is at stake is whether allowing doctors to put some infants to death will be good for us when widely accepted care plans—withdrawal of life-sustaining treatments and aggressive palliative measures including palliative (terminal) sedation—that can prevent suffering are available.

SUGGESTED READINGS

For a brief introduction to infanticide, see Stephen Post, "History, Infanticide, and Imperiled Newborns," *Hastings Center Report* 1988, *18* (August–September), 14–17. John Lorber's article on withholding treatment from infants with spina bifida appeared as "Early Results of Selective Treatment of Spina Bifida Cystica," *British Medical Journal* 1973, *4*, 201–4. Raymond Duff and A. G. M. Campbell's article appeared as "Moral and Ethical Dilemmas in the Special-Care Nursery," *New England Journal of Medicine* 1973, *289*, 890–94. See also John Lorber, "Results of Treatment of Myelomeningocele: An Analysis of 524 Unselected Cases with Special References to Special Selection for Treatment," *Developmental Medicine and Child Neurology* 1971, *13*, 279–303; John Freeman, "The Shortsighted Treatment of Myelomeningocele: A Long-Term Case Report," *Pediatrics* 1974, *53*, 311–13, and "To Treat or Not to Treat: Ethical Dilemmas of the Infant with a Myelomeningocele, *Clinical Neurosurgery* 1973, *20*, 134–46.

The harvesting of organs from living anencephalic infants in Germany was reported in Wolfgang Holzgreve et al., "Kidney Transplantation from Anencephalic Donors," *New England Journal of Medicine* 1987, *316*, 1069–70.

For a reflection on separating conjoined twins when the separation will be lethal for one of them, see David Thomasma et al., "The Ethics of Caring for Conjoined Twins: The Lakeberg Twins," *Hastings Center Report* 1996, *26* (July–August), 4–12.

For ethical reflections on defective newborns in general, see Earl Shelp, 1986, *Born to Die? Deciding the Fate of Critically Ill Newborns*, New York: Free Press; Robert Weir, 1984, *Selective Nontreatment of Handicapped Newborns: Moral Dilemmas in Neonatal Medicine*, New York: Oxford University Press; Allan Buchanan and Dan Brock, 1989, *Deciding for Others: The Ethics of Surrogate Decision Making*, Cambridge, UK: Cambridge University Press, chapter 5; Helga Kuhse and Peter Singer, 1985, *Should the Baby Live? The Problem of Handicapped Infants*, New York: Oxford University Press; Thomas Murray and Arthur Caplan, eds., 1985, *Which Babies Shall Live? Humanistic Dimensions of the Care of Imperiled Newborns*, Clifton, NJ: Humana Press; Richard McCormick, "To Save or Let Die: The Dilemma of Modern Medicine," *JAMA* 1974, *229*, 172–76; Anthony Shaw, "Dilemmas of 'Informed Consent' in Children," *New England Journal of Medicine* 1973, *289*, 885–90; Albert Jonsen et al., "Critical Issues in Newborn Intensive Care: A Conference and Policy Proposal," *Pediatrics* 1975, *55*, 756–68; Nancy King, "Transparency in Neonatal Intensive Care," *Hastings Center Report* 1992, *22* (May–June), 18–25; Andrew Whitelaw, "Death as an Option in Neonatal Intensive Care," *Lancet* 1986, *2*, 328–31; John Arras, "Toward an Ethic of Ambiguity," *Hastings Center Report* 1984, *14* (April), 25–33; Nancy Rhoden, "Treating Baby Doe: The Ethics of Uncertainty," *Hastings Center Report* 1986, *16* (August), 35–42; William Silverman, "Overtreatment of Neonates? A Personal Retrospective," *Pediatrics* 1992, *90*, 971–76; Carson Strong, 1997, *Ethics in Reproductive and Perinatal Medicine*, New Haven: Yale University Press; Jonathan Muraskas et al., "Neonatal Care in the 1990s: Held Hostage by Technology," *Cambridge Quarterly of Healthcare Ethics* 1999, *8*, 160–70; David Stevenson and Amnon Goldworth, "Ethical Dilemmas in the Delivery Room," *Seminars in Perinatology* 1998, *22*, 198–206. The rapid development of many new genetic screening tests for newborns has raised a host of ethical questions, especially when the screening uncovers risks for poorly understood diseases that we are unable to treat effectively at this time. For an overview of this relatively new issue, see the 2008 White Paper *The Changing Moral Focus of Newborn Screening: An Ethical Inquiry by the President's Council on Bioethics,* available at bioethics.gov. Several of these authors advocate involuntary euthanasia for severely impaired infants (Weir, Shelp, Singer, and Kuhse, for example), as does H. Tristram Engelhardt, 1986, *The Foundations of Bioethics,* New York: Oxford University Press, pp. 228–36. On the question of euthanasia for infants, see also Richard McMillan et al., eds., 1986, *Euthanasia and the Newborn,* Dordrecht: Reidel.

The current Baby Doe regulations were published in the *Federal Register* 50 (April 15, 1985), 14878–901. The account includes brief summaries of the on-site investigations triggered in response to calls received on the hotline. The Massachusetts response to the Baby Doe regulations is found in the Department of Social Services Policy #86–010 titled "Policy and Procedures for the Receipt and Investigation of Reports of Medical Neglect Alleging That Medically Indicated Treatment Is Being Withheld from Disabled Infants with Life-Threatening Conditions," revised 7/1/89.

Among the many commentaries on the Baby Doe case itself and on its associated legal and political controversies are Dixie Huefner, "Severely Handicapped Infants with Life-Threatening Conditions: Federal Intrusions into the Decision Not to Treat," *American Journal of Law & Medicine* 1986, *12,* 171–205; Nelson Lund, "Infanticide, Physicians, and the Law: The 'Baby Doe' Amendments to the Child Abuse Prevention and Treatment Act," *American Journal of Law & Medicine* 1985, *11,* 1–29; Stephen Newman, "Baby Doe, Congress and the States: Challenging the Federal Treatment Standards for Impaired Infants," *American Journal of Law & Medicine* 1989, *15,* 1–60; Thomas Murray, "The Final, Anticlimactic Rule on Baby Doe," *Hastings Center Report* 1985, *15* (June), 5–9; John Moskop and Rita Saldanha, "The Baby Doe Rule: Still a Threat," *Hastings Center Report* 1986, *16* (April), 8–14; and John Lantos, "Baby Doe Five Years Later: Implications for Child Health," *New England Journal of Medicine* 1987, *317,* 444–47.

For the survey of the members of the Perinatal Pediatrics Section of the American Academy of Pediatrics mentioned in the text, see Loretta Kopelman et al., "Neonatologists Judge the 'Baby Doe' Regulations," *New England Journal of Medicine* 1988, *318,* 677–83. For the remark of George Will and the decision of the English court favoring treatment for a baby with Down syndrome and also a life-threatening defect, see Richard McCormick, 1981, "Saving Defective Infants: Options for Life or Death," in *How Brave a New World?* Washington, DC: Georgetown University Press, chapter 18.

The Baby Jane Doe story is taken from Kathleen Kerr, "An Issue of Law and Ethics," *Newsday,* October 26, 1983. Ms. Kerr was the lead reporter on the team that won a Pulitzer Prize for the reporting of the Baby Jane Doe story. See also Kathleen Kerr, "Reporting the Case of Baby Jane Doe," *Hastings Center Report* 1984, *14* (August), 7–9; Bonnie Steinbock, "Baby Jane Doe in the Court," *Hastings Center Report* 1984, *14* (February), 13–19; and Gregory Pence, 2004, "The Baby Jane Doe Case" in *Classic Cases in Medical Ethics, 4th ed.,* New York: McGraw-Hill, chapter 7. The story of Danielle is based on Seth Rolbein, "A Matter of Life and Death," *Boston Magazine,* October 1987; and John Paris, Robert Crone, and Frank Reardon, "Physicians' Refusal of Requested Treatment: The Case of Baby L," *New England Journal of Medicine* 1990, *322,* 1012–15.

The story of Baby K is taken from *In the Matter of Baby K,* 16 F3d. 590 (4th Cir 1994). For a commentary see George Annas, "Asking the Courts to Set the Standard of Emergency Care—the Case of *Baby K,*" *New England Journal of Medicine* 1994, *330,* 1542–45. An interesting survey of physicians revealed almost universal agreement that treating Baby K in her vegetative state was inappropriate, yet almost all also agreed they would treat such a baby if parents insisted. Unfortunately, when parental insistence on inappropriate treatment is successful, it establishes a precedent that strengthens the case for other parents demanding inappropriate treatment. See Lawrence Schneiderman and Sharyn Manning, "The *Baby K* Case: A Search for the Elusive Standard of Medical Care," *Cambridge Quarterly of Healthcare Ethics* 1997, *6,* 9–18. For a review of the legal arguments in favor of treating Baby K by one of the attorneys representing her mother, see Ellen Flannery, "One Advocate's Viewpoint: Conflicts and Tensions in the *Baby K* Case," *Journal of Law, Medicine & Ethics* 1995, *23,* 7–12. Ellen Clayton's critique of Flannery's arguments and of the courts' decisions follows the article.

Ashley's parents launched an informative blog in January 2007 at ashleystreatment.spaces.live.com. By March 2008 the site had received more than 2,500,000 hits. The article describing the "Ashley Treatment" by doctors Daniel Gunther and Douglas Diekema is "Attenuating Growth in Children with Profound Developmental Disability," *Archives of Pediatrics and Adolescent Medicine* 2006, *160,* 1013–17. For an example of the criticism that found the ethical deliberations supporting the interventions "faulty and slipshod," see Gerald Coleman, "The Irreversible Disabling of a Child," *The National Catholic*

Bioethics Quarterly 2007, *7*, 711–28. For a more balanced position, which holds that the estrogen intervention may well have been in Ashley's best interests but that the surgeries were more questionable, see S.
Matthew Liao et al., "The Ashley Treatment: Best Interests, Convenience, and Parental Decision-
Making," *Hastings Center Report* 2007, *37* (March–April), 16–20. An example of an article supporting
the interventions is Benjamin Wilfond, "The Ashley Case: The Public Response and Policy Implications," *Hastings Center Report* 2007, *37* (September–October), 12f.

For the euthanasia of infants in the Netherlands see Eduard Verhagen and Pieter Sauer, "The Groningen
Protocol—Euthanasia in Severely Ill Newborns," *New England Journal of Medicine* 2005, *352*, 959–62;
Eduard Verhagen and Pieter Sauer, "End of Life Decisions in Newborns: An Approach from the
Netherlands," *Pediatrics* 2005, *116*, 736–39; Eduard Verhagen et al., "Physician Medical Decision-
Making at the End of Life in Newborns: Insight into Implementation at Two Dutch Centers," *Pediat-
rics* 2007, *120*, e20–28. In the last article Verhagen suggests not using the term "euthanasia" for ending
the life of newborns because, under Dutch law, euthanasia always presupposes voluntary consent. For
criticisms of the Groningen Protocol see Alan Jotkowitz and S. Glick, "The Groningen Protocol:
Another Perspective," *Journal of Medical Ethics* 2006, *32*, 157–58; Kate Costeloe, "Euthanasia in Neonates: Should It Be Available?" *British Medical Journal* 2007, *334*, 912f; Frank Chervenak et al., "Why
the Groningen Protocol Should Be Rejected," *Hastings Center Report* 2006, *36* (September–October),
30–33. For a supportive article see Hilde Lindemann and Marian Verkerk, "Ending the Life of a Newborn: The Groningen Protocol," *Hastings Center Report*, 2008, *38* (January–February), 42–51.

THIRTEEN

Euthanasia and Physician-Assisted Suicide

THE WORD EUTHANASIA means "good death." If that were all it meant, euthanasia would not be controversial. We all hope for a good death, a death without pain and suffering. In some religious traditions people pray for a "happy death" and call it a "blessing" when someone dies after a painful terminal illness. In current usage, however, euthanasia means something more than a good death or dying well. When people speak of euthanasia today, they mean causing a patient's quick and painless death, usually by lethal injection or drug overdose. Euthanasia is the intentional killing of a patient in response to her informed and voluntary request. Physician-assisted suicide is also the killing of a patient—a patient killing himself with the assistance of a physician.

Euthanasia and physician-assisted suicide are major issues in health care ethics for two reasons. First, those seeking to so die are patients, usually very ill patients, and second, the people currently giving the lethal injections or prescribing the lethal drugs are physicians. Thus, euthanasia and assisted suicide have become issues in the ethics of patient-physician relationships.

Euthanasia and physician-assisted suicide have also become the center of intense public controversy in our country and in other countries as well. This was perhaps an inevitable development. In the 1970s the great debate was whether it would be moral for physicians to withdraw life-sustaining treatments—most notably respirators. In the 1980s the debate had shifted to whether it would be moral for physicians to withdraw medical nutrition and hydration—most notably feeding tubes. Then, in the 1990s, major debates began about whether it would be moral, and should be legal, for physicians to help patients commit suicide or for physicians to put such patients to death.

HISTORICAL OVERVIEW

In recent centuries most people, including physicians, were unalterably opposed to physicians killing their patients or helping them kill themselves. So strong was this opposition that euthanasia and suicide were not even considered topics for serious moral discussion. This is no longer true; these topics are now the subject of serious debate and, in some places, political action.

The debate is really an ancient one. In the classical world of Greece and Rome (ca. 500 B.C.E. to 350 C.E.), many thought euthanasia and suicide were morally acceptable in appropriate circumstances. One group of people was a notable exception—the Pythagoreans. They developed a strong tradition in medicine, one devoted to the ethical formation as well as to the medical education of their physicians. Hippocrates was a physician in the Pythagorean tradition, and many people still appeal to the Hippocratic Oath for moral guidance in medicine.

The Pythagoreans in general, and the Hippocratic medical tradition in particular, were opposed to euthanasia. The reason is not hard to discern. Pythagorean religious beliefs included two important doctrines—the kinship of all life and the transmigration of souls. Pythagoras believed that life was somehow a single reality shared by all living things; there was no such entity as "my" life or "your" life, but simply life. Our souls recycle through life in different forms many times over until they finally attain some form of purified reincarnation. The Pythagoreans thought great care must be taken not to disrupt or destroy this cycle of life. Deliberately bringing about any death, even the death of animals, was considered wrong.

Most other people in classical Greece, however, accepted euthanasia and suicide in extenuating circumstances. Aristotle, for example, thought it ethical to end the life of defective infants. His view on suicide was somewhat complex. He argued against it whenever it violated any of the virtues. For example, a person committing suicide to escape from the troubles and sufferings of life acts cowardly and thus fails the virtue of courage. And a person committing suicide in a city-state where it was prohibited by law, as it was in Athens, violates the virtue of justice by breaking the law. But there is no blanket condemnation of suicide in Aristotle's teaching. If a suicide did not conflict with any virtues, there would be no reason to consider it immoral. In fact, it might even be an act of courage and love, as would be a suicide for the sake of saving the lives of others.

Other Greek philosophers actually advocated suicide. Epicurus encouraged hedonism and made seeking pleasure and avoiding pain the norm of living. Once the pain of living overwhelms the pleasures one can hope for, he thought suicide was an appropriate moral response. Stoicism, the philosophy that dominated the Greek and Roman classical worlds for centuries after 300 B.C.E., also advocated suicide at the end of life. Stoic philosophy advocated living "according to nature," and many Stoics did not hesitate to kill themselves when the struggle to live became an unreasonable effort to prevent death. For them death was natural, and so helping it to come at the end was reasonable and virtuous. And, since they thought that exercising the virtues constituted a good life, suicide becomes reasonable whenever illness, poverty, or pain so overwhelms a person that living virtuously is no longer possible.

The Hebrew culture, another great tradition shaping our moral consciousness, was more conservative than the Stoics about suicide. Undoubtedly this stemmed in great measure from the biblical belief that human life was created by Yahweh or God, a belief that implies we should be careful about destroying what God has created. Because of this belief in divine creation, and the later Christian acceptance of it, the Mosaic commandment "Thou shalt not kill" has played a powerful role in our culture's prohibition of suicide.

For centuries the biblical commandment "Thou shalt not kill" has been understood to forbid all intentional taking of innocent life, including one's own life, and therefore to prohibit euthanasia and suicide. A careful reading of the Hebrew Bible, however, reveals that this conclusion is a misunderstanding. Although the Bible does show a strong respect for life, it does not set forth absolute prohibitions against killing the innocent or committing suicide. The killing of the first-born child in every Egyptian family during the night of the original Passover is not seen as immoral (Exodus 11). In fact the killing of the Egyptian children during the exodus from Egypt, as well as the terrible damage to the crops and marine life inflicted by the plagues, were remembered by the Hebrews as great deeds of the Lord (Deuteronomy 11).

The Bible also commands the Israelites to kill innocent people in military campaigns. It depicts God as commanding his people to kill all the children and women, as well as the men, whenever their army has conquered a nearby enemy city (Deuteronomy 20). The deliberate killing of all the inhabitants in the captured cities is particularly disturbing from a moral point of view because the Bible depicts the Hebrews as the invaders; they were moving in from the desert to take the already-occupied land and cities for themselves.

The Bible does not restrict the killing of children to the enemies' children; it commands the Israelite parents of a stubborn and rebellious son to have him apprehended and brought to the elders so the parents can testify against him. If their testimony is convincing, the townspeople will then gather round and stone the young man to death (Deuteronomy 21).

It is, of course, impossible to know how often the biblical commandments authorizing such killings were actually carried out. Records dating back to the Mosaic era are practically nonexistent, and it may be that many of the killings sanctioned by the early biblical texts seldom occurred in practice.

We also read about suicide in the Bible. King Saul killed himself. Badly wounded, he had asked his armor bearer to kill him, but the man refused, so Saul killed himself with his own sword. Later, a member of Saul's camp told David that Saul had asked to be killed and claimed he had killed him. Far from being shocked at the report of King Saul's request for euthanasia, David laments him as an honorable and illustrious man (1 Samuel 31 and 2 Samuel 1).

The biblical story of Samson's suicide is also well known. His enemies bribed his mistress, Delilah, to find out the secret of his great strength. Three times he lied to her, but finally admitted it was his long hair. While he was sleeping, she cut off his hair. Now powerless, he was captured, blinded, and forced to work as a slave. Some time later he was dragged before his captors during a celebration in some sort of large building, and they mocked him. By this time, enough of his hair had grown back to restore his incredible strength. In anger, he managed to pull down the two main columns supporting the roof, killing himself and thousands of his enemies. His last words were: "Let me die with the Philistines!" (Judges 16:30).

The fact that Samson killed himself did not prevent St. Paul from considering him one of the heroes of the Hebrew faith, along with David, Samuel, and the prophets (Hebrews 12:32). And there is no doubt Samson's action was understood as a suicide. With his strength restored, he could have escaped, but he chose to die. So clearly is this a suicide that St. Augustine thought it necessary to claim that God himself must have made an exception to the moral law forbidding all suicide and secretly ordered Samson to pull the building down on himself (*City of God*, 1:21).

Given the commandments both for and against killing in the Hebrew Bible, it is unwise to use biblical texts as arguments for or against killing, even killing the innocent. Biblical quotations are not good arguments for or against abortion or killing the innocent or euthanasia or suicide or capital punishment. The texts are not consistent and therefore not conclusive. What does seem clear, however, is that the people of the biblical tradition, as time went on, tended more and more to kill less and less, and that this tendency to avoid killing is a major factor behind our culture's traditional stand against euthanasia and suicide.

Another strong cultural factor against euthanasia and suicide is Christianity. Christians were deeply moved by the example of their founder, who refused to allow the use of weapons to defend his life, and who accepted his rigged trial and execution without a struggle. Christians took a strong stand against killing, and most of them considered late abortions, infanticide, capital punishment, warfare, and suicide immoral homicides.

At the end of the fourth century, when the Romans made Christianity the official religion of the empire, political realities intruded and forced the Christians to reconsider their earlier doctrines of nonviolence. Soon they began allowing exceptions to their prohibition against killing. The most notable exception was in response to the need to defend the empire, chiefly from the barbarians coming down from northern Europe. Christian theologians set forth what became known as the "just war" doctrine. This doctrine, developed originally by Cicero and then in great detail by St. Augustine, allowed unjustly attacked people to defend their empire or country with lethal force if necessary.

Christians accepted the morality of capital punishment at about the same time. The empire had to be protected against criminals, and the death penalty was seen as a powerful deterrent to criminal activity. The list of crimes subject to the death penalty varied from time to time and place to place. In the Middle Ages Christians expanded it to include the ecclesiastical crime of heresy. People who refused to give up theological doctrines condemned by the Roman Catholic authorities were killed, usually by being burned alive.

These exceptions to the prohibition "Thou shalt not kill" were all "official" killings, that is, killings sanctioned by civil or religious authorities. The authorities sent soldiers into battle, and the civil or religious courts and tribunals condemned the criminals and heretics to death. But medieval Christians introduced another exception for killing, one that did not need official approval; they allowed killing in self-defense. In self-defense, the person attacked, a private citizen, is the one deciding to use lethal force, not the public authorities. Some Christians found it rather difficult to justify killing in self-defense because it contradicted the example of Jesus—when his enemies came to kill him he made no defense—but eventually killing in self-defense became as morally acceptable as killing in war and killing those condemned by civil or religious tribunals.

All the killings that the Christians considered exceptions to the prohibition against killing shared a common theme: The person killed was somehow not innocent. According to the just war theory, the enemy was not justified in attacking, so the enemy soldiers are not innocent. And criminals and heretics are not innocent, nor is the person assaulting someone. All these people are guilty of serious crimes and can be killed if necessary.

Thus, what began for Christians as a universal prohibition against all killing became in time a more narrow prohibition: Do not deliberately kill innocent people. This remains a central Christian position today. We should note, however, that a few Christians continue to reject the exceptions to the original prohibition against killing and remain convinced that any killing is contrary to Christian morality. They are called pacifists. They oppose all capital punishment and killing in self-defense and adopt a pacifist stance on questions of war. Although these Christians are a small minority of Christians in the world today, their doctrine was the one embraced by the majority of early Christians and is actually more easily reconciled with the teachings of Christ and the Gospels than the later Christian moralities of war, capital punishment, and self-defense.

The religious prohibition against killing the innocent has received strong philosophical support in the past few centuries. When the political theories that centered on natural rights blossomed in the seventeenth century, the primary right, the right to life, was obviously a move to protect every human being against being killed. The development of the right to life in political and moral philosophy provided a strong basis for protecting the lives of the innocent.

Yet, in a somewhat ironic way, the rights movement that originally protected human life is now used to justify destroying it. This happens in one of two ways. First, if life is understood as a right of mine, it can be argued that I should be able to waive that right and kill myself or ask someone to kill me. Second, if I have rights other than the right to life—the right to die and the right to choose, for example—then I should be able to kill myself or have someone kill me. Both of these rights-based arguments are now used to defend euthanasia and physician-assisted suicide.

Immanuel Kant developed another seminal modern philosophy with a strong prohibition against killing the innocent, and his moral philosophy remains very influential today. He wrote that suicide is a horrible violation of our duty toward ourselves and "nothing more terrible can be imagined." We are "horrified at the very thought of suicide; by it man sinks lower than the beasts." He went on to say that "moral philosophers must, therefore, first and foremost show that suicide is abominable."

In another work, however, Kant raised questions about specific cases that cannot but make us wonder whether or not he would allow exceptions to his apparently absolute prohibition of suicide. Kant knew that his king, Frederick the Great, carried lethal poison into battle so he could kill himself rather than be captured and held for a ransom that would financially ruin his country. Kant hesitated to condemn the king's plan as immoral. And he also wondered whether it would really be unethical for a person, suffering from an incurable disease that would cause him to go mad, to commit suicide lest his madness cause harm to others.

From this brief overview we can see an almost unanimous long-standing religious and philosophical position against private decisions to kill. The one exception was lethal force as a last resort in self-defense. In the past few decades, however, the movement to expand acceptable killings to include "rational" suicide and active euthanasia has been growing stronger in an ever-intensifying movement to legalize euthanasia and physician-assisted suicide.

Recent Developments

In 1988 the *Journal of the American Medical Association* published an anonymous account of a doctor, still in residency, who killed a young woman suffering from cancer. The piece, titled "It's All Over, Debbie," aroused widespread and heated reactions. In 1989 *The New England Journal of Medicine* published an article by twelve respected physicians on caring for hopelessly ill patients. Ten of them concluded that it was not immoral for a physician to assist in the rational suicide of a terminally ill patient. Less than a year later, a physician in Michigan, Dr. Jack Kevorkian, designed a "suicide machine." A woman in the early stages of Alzheimer disease used it, with his help, to kill herself. That suicide, and dozens of others that he also helped arrange, received widespread publicity and resulted in several arrests. Eventually Kevorkian was found guilty, not of physician-assisted suicide but of an act of euthanasia because he actually physically intervened in a death, and he was sentenced to a prison term.

In 1991 Dr. Timothy Quill of New York wrote an article in the *New England Journal of Medicine* describing how he had helped a patient with incurable leukemia to kill herself with an overdose of barbiturates. And that same year, Derek Humphrey's book, *Final Exit: The Practicalities of Self-Deliverance and Assisted Suicide for the Living*, appeared. It advocated assisted suicide and euthanasia for dying patients who wanted this option. The book sold well despite its lack of thoughtful reasoning and misleading statements about the rights people already have under present law to stop treatments.

Advocacy for euthanasia has increased on political and legal fronts as well, especially in Holland, where euthanasia has been practiced for decades. Although the Dutch Penal Code had made euthanasia a crime, prosecutors had agreed not to prosecute physicians if they followed guidelines published by the Dutch Medical Association. This agreement lasted until 2002 when the Euthanasia Act made both physician-assisted suicide and euthanasia legal and hence regulated in the Netherlands. That same year Belgium, after a debate of several years, adopted a euthanasia law that is similar to the Dutch law, although the Belgian law does not regulate physician-assisted suicide. Both countries require physicians to limit euthanasia in general to cases where these three conditions exist: (1) voluntary and persistent request by the patient, (2) unbearable suffering, and (3) the physician has consulted with a colleague about the patient's condition and about the appropriateness of the patient's request to be killed and must report the euthanasia to civil authorities. Both countries also require the physicians to file a detailed report of the euthanasia with authorities. If they do not, the euthanasia is deemed illegal; in fact, it is considered murder in Belgium and a homicide in the Netherlands. Neither country requires the patient to be terminally ill. There also has been renewed debate about euthanasia in Switzerland, where euthanasia remains illegal but helping someone to commit suicide is not considered illegal if the assistance is given for altruistic reasons.

The situation in Belgium is noteworthy for three reasons. First, unlike the Netherlands, the Belgian euthanasia law regulates only euthanasia, not physician-assisted suicide. Suicide assistance is not prohibited in Belgian law, so physician-assisted suicide is technically legal, but by not being included in the euthanasia law, it remains unregulated and unmonitored.

Second, the Belgian law permits euthanasia for persons suffering from irreversible unconsciousness if there is an advance directive for euthanasia. Thus, physicians can end the life of people in a persistent vegetative state (PVS), which means that the condition of "unbearable suffering" need not always be met before euthanasia occurs because patients in PVS are not experiencing any suffering.

Third, despite a long history of official Catholic teaching condemning euthanasia, some Catholic hospitals in Belgium have policies permitting euthanasia. This rather surprising and highly controversial reality came about in the following way. By the beginning of 2000 when it became clear that Belgium would eventually legalize euthanasia, the ethics committee of the Association of Care Institutions, which covers fifty-two Catholic hospitals and almost four hundred nursing homes, began developing updated guidelines for end-of-life care. The day after Belgium legalized euthanasia in May 2002, Caritas Catholica Vlaanderen, an umbrella organization that includes the Association and other charitable institutions, approved the recommendations of the Association's ethics committee titled *Caring for a Dignified End of Life in a Christian Health-Care Institution*.

The document sets forth respect for the human person as a fundamental moral value but criticizes the one-sided emphasis on autonomy and encourages aggressive palliative care for everyone. However, in rare and exceptional cases where palliation does not work and the voluntary request by a competent patient already in the terminal phase of actually dying persists, the document states: "Caritas Vlaanderen respects a decision made in good conscience by the physician and members of the support team to initiate euthanasia." Following the Caritas Catholica Vlaanderen recommendation, a number of Catholic hospitals and nursing homes in Belgium have developed policies allowing euthanasia in exceptional and rare circumstances, a move that has stirred considerable controversy within the Roman Catholic medical and theological communities.

PHYSICIAN-ASSISTED SUICIDE AND STATE LAWS

Efforts to make euthanasia and physician-assisted suicide legal sprang up in several states in the United States toward the end of the twentieth century. Many states permit voters to change state laws by voting for initiative petitions, so one strategy for change consists of putting the issue on the ballot as a referendum question. In 1991 the Hemlock Society proposed a series of amendments to Washington State's 1979 living-will law that would have allowed euthanasia and physician-assisted suicide. The proposal, known as Initiative 119, failed but received 46 percent of the state vote.

In November 1992 Proposition 161 appeared on the ballot in California. It would have allowed both euthanasia and physician-assisted suicide, but it was defeated, although it also received 46 percent of the vote.

In November 1994 the Hemlock Society sponsored Measure 16 on the Oregon ballot. It was narrowly drafted, allowing only physician-assisted suicide and not euthanasia, in an effort to attract more support. Moreover, the physicians would be able to help patients kill themselves only by prescribing lethal drugs and not by other means such as the carbon monoxide poisoning used by the now well-known Dr. Kevorkian. The measure included other restrictions as well. Two physicians must agree that death is expected within six months, the patient must be competent, two requests (at least fifteen days apart) for the lethal overdose must be made, and then a waiting period of forty-eight hours must pass before the prescription can be written. This ballot measure passed, and Oregon thus became the first state to vote for the legalization of physician-assisted suicide.

Almost immediately the constitutionality of the new law, scheduled to take effect on December 8, 1994, was challenged in federal court. The first set of court challenges continued until the U.S. Supreme Court effectively put an end to them in October 1997 by turning down without comment an appeal of a lower court decision that allowed the law to stand, thus clearing the way for physician-assisted suicide to begin in Oregon. In the fall of 1997 the citizens of Oregon were also asked to vote a second time on the measure. This time they passed the Death with Dignity Act (DWDA) by a 60–40 margin (the first vote was a 51–49 margin).

Two Republican lawmakers, Orrin Hatch, the chair of the Senate Judiciary Committee, and Henry Hyde, the chair of the House Judiciary Committee, mounted another major challenge to the Oregon DWDA. They prevailed on the administrator of the Drug Enforcement Administration (DEA) to warn doctors writing prescriptions for lethal drugs that they could be prosecuted for drug abuse under the Controlled Substances Act (CSA). The CSA allows physicians to write prescriptions of controlled substances only for "currently accepted medical use" and the senators argued that prescribing drugs for suicide was not an accepted medical use. The DEA warning did not stop some physicians, however, and in March 1998 *The Oregonian* reported the first two legal physician-assisted suicides in the state. In June 1998 Attorney General Janet Reno ruled that the DEA had overstepped its authority when it tried to determine "currently accepted medical use," something best left to state law and the medical profession itself to decide.

The first legal physician-assisted suicides in 1998 did not begin without moral concerns. One of the first two people to commit suicide, a woman in her eighties with breast cancer, had trouble finding a doctor to assist her. Finally, a physician who knew her for less than three weeks wrote the lethal prescription. Legally all was in order, but there are legitimate concerns about doctors helping people they hardly know commit suicide. And another weak point in the law soon emerged—it has no effective way of assuring compliance and preventing negligence or abuse.

In February 1999, the Oregon Health Division published its first report on the legalization of physician-assisted suicide. During the first year (1998), physicians reported giving twenty-three patients lethal drugs for suicide. Of the twenty-three, fifteen killed themselves, six died of natural causes, and two were alive on January 1, 1999. Most of the patients had terminal cancer. The report contained a comment worth noting: After acknowledging that the Health Division had the obligation to report cases of noncompliance to the Board of Medical Examiners, the report acknowledged that it is "difficult, if not impossible, to detect accurately and comment on underreporting," and hence, "we cannot determine whether physician-assisted suicide is being practiced outside the framework of the Death with Dignity Act."

Efforts to challenge the DWDA continued. In 2001 the newly appointed Attorney General John Ashcroft issued an Interpretative Rule of the CSA stating that prescription of controlled substances for physician-assisted suicide was not a legitimate medical purpose, and hence physicians prescribing these substances for that purpose could be subject to suspension or revocation of their DEA authorization to prescribe any controlled drugs. Ashcroft's rule was immediately challenged in federal court. The federal district court ordered its enforcement suspended and then, in 2004, the federal Appeals Court in the Ninth Circuit confirmed that Ashcroft's rule was invalid.

Attorney General Alberto Gonzales, who had replaced John Ashcroft, appealed the Ninth Circuit's decision to the Supreme Court, and in 2006 the Supreme Court decided 6–3 in *Gonzales v. Oregon* that the Attorney General had no authority under the CSA to prohibit doctors from prescribing controlled substances for physician-assisted suicide. The Court also ruled that the practice of medicine is an activity that is state regulated and not federally regulated. Justice Scalia, in a dissent jointed by Chief Justice Roberts and Justice Thomas, argued that Congress does have a legitimate interest in what constitutes legitimate medical practice and that physician-assisted suicide cannot be considered a legitimate medical practice because none of the other forty-nine states allows it and major medical associations such as the AMA have taken a stand against it.

The legal option of physician-assisted suicide has been continuously available in Oregon since 1998. The 2007 annual report of the Oregon DWDA showed that a total of 341 residents had committed suicide with the help of their physicians in those ten years. The figures for 2007 showed that forty-five physicians wrote a total of eighty-five prescriptions during that year, that forty-six of the patients with prescriptions had killed themselves along with three others whose prescriptions had been written earlier, that patients ranged in age from twenty-nine to ninety-three, that 90 percent had died at home, that 88 percent had been enrolled in hospice, that all had had health insurance, that 15 percent were college graduates, that most had had cancer, and that the time between taking the lethal drugs and death had ranged from six minutes to eighty-three hours, with a median time of twenty-five minutes.

For eleven years Oregon was the only state where physician-assisted suicide was legal. Then in November 2008 people in the neighboring state of Washington voted overwhelmingly (59 percent to 41 percent) for a physician-assisted suicide law similar to that of Oregon. The Washington Death with Dignity Act also restricts physician-assisted suicide to adult residents of the state, and its provisions are almost identical to the DWDA in Oregon. The Washington DWDA became effective early in 2009, and a sixty-six-year-old woman with pancreatic cancer became the first person to commit suicide under the law in May 2009.

PHYSICIAN-ASSISTED SUICIDE AND THE CONSTITUTION

The voting booth was not the only setting for debates on euthanasia and physician-assisted suicide; proponents also pursued, much as proponents of abortion did in the 1970s, a constitutional challenge to state laws against physician-assisted suicide. Proponents of physician-assisted suicide challenged as unconstitutional the laws forbidding suicide assistance in two states, Washington and New York. By 1996 these challenges reached the federal appellate level. The Washington case was heard by the Ninth Circuit Court of Appeals, and the New York case was heard by the Second Circuit Court of Appeals. Both federal appeals courts found that the state laws prohibiting physician-assisted suicide were indeed unconstitutional; in other words, patients have a constitutional right to physician-assisted suicide. Opponents of physician-assisted suicide appealed both of these decisions to the U.S. Supreme Court. The Supreme Court accepted the cases, and thus the stage was set for one of the most important Supreme Court decisions in health care ethics. Before looking at its decision of June 1997, we will look more closely at the two cases.

In Washington State a dying AIDS patient asked Dr. Harold Glucksberg for a prescription so he could obtain a lethal dosage of drugs to kill himself. Dr. Glucksberg refused to write the prescription lest he violate the state law against suicide assistance. His patient later committed suicide by jumping from a bridge. Dr. Glucksberg, three other physicians, and three dying patients then challenged the constitutionality of the Washington State law in federal district court. The judge found in their favor, but on appeal a three-judge panel of the Ninth Circuit Court ruled 2–1 against them. They appealed this ruling to the Ninth Circuit Court, which overruled its panel and upheld the district court decision. This case was first known as *Compassion in Dying v. Washington* but became *Washington v. Glucksberg* when it was heard by the Supreme Court.

In New York a dying cancer patient asked Dr. Timothy Quill for a prescription so she could obtain a lethal dosage of drugs to kill herself. Dr. Quill wrote the prescription despite the state law against physician-assisted suicide. His patient later committed suicide with the drugs. An analysis of this story appears at the end of this chapter as "The Case of Diane." After her death Dr. Quill and two other physicians, along with three dying patients, challenged the constitutionality of the New York law forbidding physician-assisted suicide. The Second Circuit Court ruled in their favor. This case was first known as *Quill v. Koppell* but became *Vacco v. Quill* when it was heard by the Supreme Court.

How did the two federal appellate courts conclude that the state laws against physician-assisted suicide were unconstitutional? They claimed that the state laws violated the Fourteenth Amendment, although they disagreed on which clause of that amendment was violated. The Ninth Circuit focused on what is called the due process clause, which reads: "No state can make laws that abridge any right, privilege, or protection of citizens . . . unless he has been found guilty of a crime in a court of law by *due process* of law" (emphasis added). Hence, the majority judges argued that it is unconstitutional for states to make laws abridging the right of dying patients to commit suicide since they have not been found guilty of any crime.

The Second Circuit focused on what is called the "equal protection clause" of the Fourteenth Amendment, which reads as follows: "No state may deny any person . . . *equal protection* of the law" (emphasis added). Hence, the majority judges argued that the state law is unconstitutional because it does not equally protect all dying patients—those on life support can receive physician assistance in dying by having their physicians remove the equipment, but those not on life support cannot receive physician assistance in dying because their physicians cannot write a prescription for lethal drugs.

If the arguments either of the Ninth Circuit or of the Second Circuit were valid, it would mean that a right to physician-assisted suicide exists in the Fourteenth Amendment of the Constitution. This was the heart of the issue before the Supreme Court.

On June 26, 1997, the Supreme Court overturned the decisions of both federal appeals courts and concluded that no constitutional right to physician-assisted suicide exists. The decision in both cases was a rare 9–0. The Supreme Court decision means that the laws in over thirty states forbidding assistance in suicide, including physician-assisted suicide, are not unconstitutional. Thus, states may enact laws forbidding physician-assisted suicide if they so desire. And, if they so desire, states may also make laws allowing physician-assisted suicide, as Oregon and Washington have done. The Supreme Court decision only says that state laws forbidding physician-assisted suicide are not unconstitutional; it makes no judgment about state laws allowing physician-assisted suicide.

The circuit court opinions and the Supreme Court decision ranged far beyond narrow legal matters and addressed several issues of fundamental ethical importance that are worth mentioning.

First, the opinion of the Ninth Circuit favoring assistance in suicide included a long treatise that contained a literary history of suicides. It found the suicide of Jocasta in Sophocles' *Oedipus Rex* "an honorable way out of an insufferable situation." Queen Jocasta, you may remember, was a tragic figure who discovered she had unknowingly married her son.

The opinion also cites Homer's *Iliad* on the suicide of the great warrior Ajax, who killed himself when the generals awarded the magnificent armor of the dead Achilles to Odysseus and not to him. The opinion also uses the historical suicides of Socrates and Judas to build the case for suicide. But it is not easy to consider these suicides as honorable. Socrates' suicide was an execution after what most consider an unfair trial. And Christians view Judas' suicide as unfortunate because he could have repented and received forgiveness for his treachery.

Second, the opinion of the Ninth Circuit favoring assistance in suicide argued that ending life by withdrawing life support or by administering palliative drugs for pain—something long accepted as legal—"is nothing more nor less than assisted suicide." In other words the court saw no significant difference between withdrawing a ventilator or feeding tube at the request of a patient and helping the patient kill himself. Once the court equated withdrawing treatment with suicide, it could advance its "equal protection" argument: since laws allow life-support withdrawal, they should also allow an "equivalent" action—suicide.

The Supreme Court rejected this view on two grounds: *intent* and *causality*. On the matter of *intent* it was on solid moral ground. Intentions are significant in ethics as well as law, and a clear distinction exists between the intention to withdraw unreasonable life support or to provide adequate palliation and the intention to kill or to assist in a suicide.

On the matter of *causality*, however, the Supreme Court remained on soggy ground by stating: "when a patient refuses life-sustaining medical treatment, he dies from an underlying fatal disease or pathology; but if a patient ingests lethal medication prescribed by a physician he is killed by that medication." In other words, the court claimed disease is the cause of death if physicians withdraw life support, but lethal drugs are the cause of death if physicians assist in suicide. The court cited dozens of earlier cases beginning with the *Quinlan* case where courts routinely "recognized, at least implicitly, the distinction between letting a patient die and making a patient die."

As we saw in chapter 3, however, the distinction between withdrawing life support to "let the patient die" and causing the patient's death is not based on the latter's being a cause while the former is not. The claim that removing needed life support plays no causal role in the person's death is untenable. Removing life support is one causal factor (the other is the disease) in a person's death. If an unauthorized person invaded an ICU and disconnected a patient's life-support equipment, we would have no trouble understanding that he played a causal role in that patient's death at that time. As far as causality is concerned, the situation is no different when a physician goes into an ICU and disconnects a patient's life-support equipment. The physical actions are the same, although, of course, the intent and the moral status of the physician's actions are quite different from those of the intruder. Withdrawing life support, assisting in suicide, and euthanasia all play causal roles, albeit of substantially different intensity, in the resulting deaths.

Third, the Supreme Court recognized the value of the *slippery-slope argument* against physician-assisted suicide and euthanasia. It feared that legalizing suicide assistance for suffering and dying patients with decision-making capacity will not stop there but spread to euthanasia, both voluntary and nonvoluntary; to suicide assistance for the sick but not dying if they request it; and to suicide assistance for those whose mental capacity may be compromised by depression, despair, or mental illness. The Supreme Court cited what we will see later in the chapter: evidence from the Netherlands shows that physicians in significant numbers do not adhere to the guidelines for euthanasia and physician-assisted suicide. The Court insisted that government has an interest in preventing a "slide down a slippery slope to voluntary and perhaps involuntary euthanasia."

Before we examine the ethical arguments for and against euthanasia and physician-assisted suicide, a review of some relevant distinctions will be helpful.

Relevant Distinctions

Most discussions of euthanasia and assisted suicide include at least some of the following distinctions.

Euthanasia and Assisted Suicide

This seems like a very clear and sharp distinction, most notably because the physician does the killing in euthanasia, and the patient does it in suicide. Yet the distinction between euthanasia and assisted suicide is weaker than it might first appear. In both cases the physician plays an important role in the killing. In euthanasia the physician alone causes the death, and in physician-assisted suicide both the physician and the patient cause the death. By providing the lethal overdose and the proper instructions for suicide, the physician is very much an active participant in the killing that occurs in the physician-assisted suicide. For this reason it may be helpful to think of physician-assisted suicide as "medical suicide" and euthanasia as "medical killing."

We can see the physician's role in physician-assisted suicide more clearly if we imagine that a man wanted to kill his wife, told his physician about it, and asked the physician to provide the lethal overdose and instructions on how to use it to kill. Here we have no trouble recognizing that the physician is very much an active participant in the subsequent killing. The physician's role is no less active if the man wanted the overdose to kill himself.

Thus, euthanasia and physician-assisted suicide are similar in a crucial way. In both the physician is a moral agent deeply involved in causing the death of a patient. In the case of suicide, of course, there is a second moral agent active in causing death, the patient himself, but the physician is still playing a major causal role. Teaching a person how to kill someone, whether that someone is the person to be killed or another, and providing that individual with the poison to do it, is morally simply not that different from actually injecting the lethal dose. Efforts to consider physicians helping people commit suicide as only "indirect" involvement in the killing are suspect; the law and common sense have always recognized that people who provide poisons for a planned killing are directly implicated in that killing.

Moral reasoning about euthanasia and physician-assisted suicide, as well as debates about whether these should be public policy and legally allowed for those who want to die this way, should recognize the strong similarity between euthanasia and physician-assisted suicide. Although there is some difference between them, the similarity is so strong that they stand or fall together. In euthanasia the physician alone causes the death; in physician-assisted suicide the physician and the patient form a team to cause the death.

Active and Passive Euthanasia

This widely used distinction echoes the distinction between causing death and "letting die" discussed earlier. Sometimes the distinction is clear. If a person is dying and I do absolutely nothing to prevent it, then I am letting the person die, and that is truly passive. Most often, however, people use the active-passive euthanasia distinction in a questionable way. They want to call removing life support or medical nutrition from a dying patient "passive" euthanasia. But "passive" is not the proper word here because the actual removals of life-sustaining treatments are certainly activities.

Even if the distinction between active and passive euthanasia, causing death and letting die, is used correctly, however, it is not really morally helpful. It does not tell us whether something is moral or immoral. Being passive in the face of a death does not necessarily absolve one of responsibility for that death. Parents neglecting their sick infant are passive in regard to the infant's death, but their behavior is still immoral. And necessary pain medications may actually cause death, but providing them in appropriate circumstances is still moral. It would be well if we could drop the phrase "passive euthanasia" and use the word euthanasia to designate the intentional killing of a patient (medical killing) and not treatment withdrawals or medications intended to mask pain. Unfortunately, "passive euthanasia" seems so firmly entrenched in people's minds that it will be with us for a long time.

Voluntary, Involuntary, and Nonvoluntary Euthanasia

Voluntary euthanasia occurs when the patient voluntarily asks to be killed. It presupposes that all the requirements for informed consent are met. These are the requirements: (1) the patient has the capacity to understand, reason, and communicate; (2) the patient has sufficient information about diagnosis, prognosis, treatment options, and so forth; and (3) the patient is not coerced or manipulated into giving consent. If these requirements are met and the patient wants to be killed, then it is a matter of voluntary euthanasia. Proponents of euthanasia usually begin by supporting only voluntary euthanasia.

Nonvoluntary euthanasia occurs when any of these requirements is missing. The patient may never have had the capacity to make such a decision or, if she had the capacity, never made the decision. Or, perhaps, the patient may not have all the information or was depressed by her suffering or was so distressed by the burden she was causing the family and providers that she felt obligated to request euthanasia.

Most moralists reject nonvoluntary euthanasia in their writings, but this rejection does not always follow in practice. As we shall see, there is now convincing evidence from Holland, where only voluntary euthanasia is permitted under the guidelines, that a considerable number of patients have been killed who could not have given voluntary consent. The extension of euthanasia from cases where the patient voluntarily requests it to those not requesting it is logical in one sense—if the rationale for euthanasia is relief of suffering, then it follows that we should relieve the suffering of all, even those without the capacity to request euthanasia. Thus, although in theory only voluntary euthanasia is advocated by supporters of euthanasia, in practice the Dutch experience reveals how easily voluntary euthanasia leads to nonvoluntary euthanasia and how, once voluntary euthanasia is legal, some physicians do begin killing people without their consent and feel justified in so doing.

Involuntary euthanasia occurs when a patient is opposed to being killed. No moralist of any stature sees any justification for this. Most, simply and correctly, consider it murder.

Terminal Sedation and Physician–Assisted Suicide

When the Supreme Court heard the oral arguments for *Quill* in January 1997, an attorney arguing for the legalization of physician-assisted suicide, Laurence Tribe, described a medical practice he called "terminal sedation." He argued that terminal sedation is a form of assisted suicide, and since it is legally permitted, so should physician-assisted suicide be legalized. The Supreme Court disagreed and distinguished physician-assisted suicide and terminal sedation in its 1997 *Vacco v. Quill* decision. In June 2008 the AMA Council on Ethical and Judicial Affairs issued a report entitled *Sedation to Unconsciousness in End-of-Life Care* that also distinguishes permanent palliative sedation from both euthanasia and physician-assisted suicide.

What is "terminal sedation," now sometimes called "palliative sedation?" It occurs as a last resort when physicians realize that the only way to prevent a dying patient from suffering is to keep him totally sedated until death occurs. Once the treatment plan calling for permanent sedation is in place, then a second step becomes reasonable—withdrawal of life-prolonging treatment. Death without suffering usually occurs within three days.

Superficially, terminal sedation and suicide assistance may appear the same, but they are not. Both the intentions and the causal dynamics differ. The intention of palliative sedation is to mask pain and not to kill, and the intention to stop life support is to forgo unreasonable treatment and not to kill. As explained in chapter 3, the actions of removing life support or medical nutrition do play a causal role in the subsequent death, and those doing it need offsetting reasons if their actions are to be virtuous because they know their actions will contribute to a death. But the motivating intention of these actions can be to stop unreasonable treatment rather than to kill. The intention to kill or to help a patient kill himself is one thing; the intentions to mask pain with permanent sedation as a last resort, and then to withdraw life support which no longer makes sense with permanent sedation constitute another act entirely. Intentions do play a role in evaluating moral actions along with a consideration of circumstances and expected consequences. The causal dynamics of terminal sedation also differ from suicide assistance and euthanasia: the drugs used in terminal sedation cause only coma, whereas the drugs in suicide assistance and euthanasia cause death.

Hence, terminal sedation is not equivalent to suicide assistance because both the agent's intentions and the causal factors in the two actions differ significantly. Terminal sedation remains a morally reasonable response as a last resort to mask pain. Far from being an argument for legalizing physician-assisted suicide, it is actually an argument against it by offering an alternative to the radical acts of killing or assisting in a suicide.

Some people distinguishing palliative or terminal sedation from euthanasia and physician-assisted suicide invoke the principle of double effect to justify their distinction. Unfortunately, this leaves their distinction open to a trenchant criticism because, as we explained in chapter 3, the principle of double effect has some serious problems, and applying it, as applying any principle in a principle-based ethics, can undermine prudential reasoning. Prudential reasoning in a virtue-based ethics simply tries to recognize the less worse scenario when there are really no good options, and the idea here is that it is more reasonable to relieve suffering without legalizing euthanasia or physician-assisted suicide if any alternative short of doing this is available. Admittedly there is a fine line here, but the law does distinguish terminal sedation from euthanasia, and there is good reason to make the same distinction in ethics.

Suicide and Physician-Assisted Death

There is a growing tendency by those favoring the legalization of physician-assisted suicide to make a distinction between suicide and physician-assisted death. One way to do this is to consider physician-assisted suicide not as a suicide but as an assisted death wherein a physician helps a person die. The word "suicide" is used for killing oneself without physician assistance, and the phrase "physician-assisted death" is used for killing oneself with physician assistance.

This distinction is suspect for several reasons. First, it disguises the central reality of what is going on—namely, a person is taking a lethal overdose to end her life. Second, the purpose of making the distinction is not to clarify the issues so one can engage in thoughtful deliberation and dialogue about a controversial topic where good people honestly disagree but to win support for a position that one has already definitively decided is correct—physician-assisted suicide should be legal—by linguistic manipulation, a technique well-known in sales and politics.

If the phrase "physician-assisted death" is allowed to replace "physician-assisted suicide," the debate about physician-assisted suicide will then center on whether or not physicians should offer assistance when their patients are dying. This is not a debate at all; of course physicians, as well as nurses, family, and friends, should help dying people die by providing medical and emotional comfort. The soothing language of physician-assisted death misleads us about the crucial ethical question: Do physicians ever behave in a good and noble way by killing their patients or helping them kill themselves? That is, is killing ever the less worse option for relieving suffering when other options are available?

Recourse to the misleading but soothing language of "physician-assisted death" actually undermines the arguments (but not the political spin) of those proposing the legalization of euthanasia or physician-assisted suicide because it suggests that their proposal cannot withstand debate if direct and realistic language is employed. The ethical problem we face is not selling physician-assisted suicide to physicians and the public so that it can be legalized but, rather, determining what is actually the less worse option for society—intentionally causing death or palliation, including total palliative sedation if necessary. Proponents of legalizing physician-assisted suicide actually do their position a disservice when they use misleading language.

Ethics and Public Policy

Sometimes it is argued that a distinction should be made between personal morality and public policy. The main idea driving this move is the recognition that irresolvable conflicts on some basic moral issues exist in our pluralistic society, so some matters are better ignored by public policy. Abortion is frequently given as one example of this. Some argue that public policy should recognize that abortion is a private matter between a woman and her physician. Thus, it should allow those believing abortion is morally justified to have an abortion and allow those believing it is not morally good to avoid involvement. In somewhat the same way some argue that euthanasia should be recognized as a private matter between a suffering patient and his physician, and thus public policy should allow those who believe euthanasia is morally justified to practice it and allow those who do not believe it is morally good to avoid involvement.

A second idea underlying the effort to distinguish personal ethics and public policy goes in the opposite direction. It envisions a public policy forbidding euthanasia in order to prevent abuse but making no effort to prosecute it when physicians follow published guidelines. This was the situation in Holland until euthanasia became legal in 2002; the law forbade euthanasia, but prosecutors did not bring charges as long as physicians followed the guidelines.

The distinction between ethics and public policy has its advantages. On some issues there are essential differences between public policy and the moral values one personally embraces. Yet there are serious dangers with such a distinction, especially when it is a matter of ending human life. Taking life is seldom a purely private matter; it almost always affects the common good, the good of the society.

Although the distinction between public policy and private ethics has some merit, it would only be a temporary stopgap. Sooner or later a society must reach some consensus on when human life can be destroyed, or the dissent festers and eventually surfaces. The history of the abortion controversy in the United States reminds us of this. In 1973 the Supreme Court ignored the efforts of state legislatures to reach consensus on a state-by-state basis and made it a matter of personal choice in the first two trimesters. This approach has not worked, and the socially disruptive controversy about abortion continues to this day.

MORAL REASONING AND EUTHANASIA

Before we turn to the arguments for and against euthanasia, six remarks will be helpful.

1. "Killing" and "kill" are the appropriate words to use in discussions of euthanasia and assisted suicide. Euthanasia and suicide are killings, and we should not conceal that reality by calling these actions by any other name. In euthanasia, physicians kill their patients; in assisted suicide, physicians help patients to kill themselves. The moral question is whether physicians and patients can morally justify these killings when they are voluntary and motivated by compassion and mercy.

2. In euthanasia and assisted suicide, the person killed is "innocent." This means euthanasia and assisted suicide are not akin to the usual exceptions we make for killing (namely, just war, capital punishment, and self-defense). In these cases, the person killed was an enemy, a criminal, or an attacker and therefore not considered "innocent."

3. In euthanasia and assisted suicide, the innocent person is not giving up his life to save the life of others. Therefore, we cannot use any argument based on heroic self-sacrifice to justify the loss of life.

4. It is impossible to deliberate morally about euthanasia if we begin by saying "intentionally killing the innocent" is "always and everywhere wrong" or "intrinsically evil" or "immoral without exception." In most cases, intentionally killing an innocent person is immoral, but there are exceptions. For example, suppose a well-armed severely ill mental patient is on a rampage killing people. He is, morally and legally, innocent. The police officer who can kill him to stop the rampage kills an innocent man, but few would say the killing is immoral: tragic yes, but not immoral. Again, suppose a captured spy commits suicide to avoid revealing under torture the identity of other spies; few would say his suicide is immoral, although he does kill a person he considers innocent—himself.

What is always and everywhere wrong is not intentionally killing the innocent, but intentionally killing without adequate reasons to justify the loss of human life. The issue is whether or not the killing of the innocent in euthanasia and assisted suicide is morally justified by sufficient reasons. If the reasons for the killing are not adequate, then the killing is not morally acceptable.

5. Voluntary euthanasia and assisted suicide are, in effect, team killings. Both the patient and the physician are deeply involved, and hence both are moral agents. The specific moral question is: When, if ever, is it morally good for physicians to kill patients who request it, or to help patients kill themselves? To morally justify euthanasia and physician-assisted suicide, both the physician and the patient must show how the killing makes their lives good, or at least less worse than other options. And it is never enough for the physician to justify his role in causing death by saying that it was done at the patient's request.

6. We should keep in mind that there are various degrees of causing death and that we consider some of these morally good in appropriate circumstances. In chapter 3 we listed the six major ways physicians' actions have a causal impact on the patient's death: active euthanasia,

assisted suicide, pain medication so heavy it shortens life, withdrawal of medical nutrition and hydration, and withdrawal of needed life-sustaining treatment and equipment.

As we discuss euthanasia and physician-assisted suicide, then, we have to acknowledge that the question is not whether it is ethical for physicians to play any causal role in patients' deaths; we already know that they do and that this is morally reasonable in appropriate circumstances. The question is whether we should limit the physicians' causal roles in death to treatment withdrawals and medications intended to mask pain or whether we should allow physicians to kill by lethal injections and to help patients kill themselves. The central issue in the euthanasia debate is whether we can morally justify extending the physician's causal impact on a patient's death from the already accepted cases of withdrawing life support and using necessary pain medication, even terminal sedation, to the stronger causal actions of assisting in suicide and administering lethal injections.

We turn now to this central moral question: Is the killing called euthanasia and physician-assisted suicide ever morally reasonable in our heath care environment? We will consider first the reasons advanced by proponents of euthanasia and assisted suicide, then some criticisms of those reasons, and finally the reasons advanced by opponents of these practices.

Reasons for Euthanasia and Physician-Assisted Suicide

Three main reasons have been advanced to justify the intentional killing of willing patients by physicians.

Respect for Patient Self-Determination

The idea that people should decide for themselves how they want to live and die is central to most arguments favoring euthanasia and suicide. In the early 1970s in one of the first major ethical documents in the young field of medical ethics, the National Commission for the Protection of Human Subjects proposed three ethical principles; one of them was autonomy for patients with decision-making capacity. A decade later the President's Commission for the Study of Ethical Problems in Medicine and Biomedical and Behavioral Research proposed three similar underlying values; one of them was patient self-determination. The reliance of these two landmark reports on the principles and values of autonomy and self-determination underlined the growing importance of decision making by patents in medical ethics.

At first, the notions of autonomy and self-determination were employed solely to justify withdrawal of unwanted life-sustaining treatments. Soon, however, autonomy and self-determination were being used in another way. Some patients began insisting that self-determination enabled them to have physicians kill them or at least help them to kill themselves. If autonomy and self-determination are accepted as moral norms, then voluntary requests for assistance in suicide or for lethal injections will seem morally justified to some.

Closely associated with the argument for euthanasia based on self-determination are arguments from rights. For centuries our culture has championed liberty, the right to choose, as a fundamental right. If liberty is a human right, there seems no reason why a person cannot freely choose to kill herself or ask someone else to do it for her. Some people also create an additional right, the right to die, and argue that this right justifies suicide and euthanasia. In a culture sensitive to rights, no one wants to violate a patient's rights, and this makes the rights-based arguments for euthanasia and suicide appear plausible.

People relying on rights-based ethics, of course, do advocate another fundamental natural or human right, the right to life. The right to life is obviously contrary both to the right to choose death and to the right to die. A chronic conflict haunts moralities based on rights as they try to harmonize a right to life with the right to choose death and the right to die. The paradox is most often solved by claiming that rights can be overridden or waived. In cases of suicide and euthanasia, the strategy is to say that the patient voluntarily waives the right to life. Once the right to life has been waived, the rights to choose and to die can prevail. These rights, it is claimed, justify the collaboration of the patient and the physician in the killing.

Relief of Suffering

Some people suffer terribly before they die. Advocates of euthanasia argue that the pain of dying is sometimes uncontrollable and that a quick merciful death is morally justified in these cases. Opponents of euthanasia claim that most if not all suffering can be controlled by medication, although sometimes this means so heavily sedating dying patients that they are "snowed"—that is, virtually unconscious. Advocates of euthanasia claim this makes no sense; if dying people are suffering terrible intractable pain and want to die, they say it is more humane to honor requests for euthanasia than to induce somnolence by drugs while the patient awaits inevitable death.

The argument here is a powerful one because it is based on two of the noblest human feelings: compassion and mercy in the face of another's suffering. The relief of suffering has long been one of the primary goals of medicine, and good physicians are always eager to alleviate pain. For some, this is reason enough to argue that physicians should respond to the pleas for euthanasia or assistance in suicide. If a suffering patient believes with good reason that he would be better off dead, then the physician refusing to help can appear to be lacking mercy and compassion if she refuses to kill him or help him commit suicide.

Proponents of this argument for euthanasia are usually quick to say that the suffering need not be physical; it could be psychological. The fear of losing control or dignity at the end as the result of diseases such as Huntington chorea, amyotrophic lateral sclerosis (ALS), Alzheimer disease, and others can cause great distress and can also be, some say, a valid reason for euthanasia or assistance in suicide when the final disintegration sets in.

Normal Medical Practice

The third argument for medical aid in euthanasia and assisted suicide is rooted in the claim that these actions are no more than a normal evolution in modern medicine faced with three changing circumstances. First, thanks to medical research and better diagnosis, we now know more about the inexorable and painful degeneration of certain diseases. The certainty of what will be a painful dying suggests to some that we might try to make the inevitable death easier for the patient. Second, although many people influenced by Christianity once saw meaning and value in suffering, fewer do today. They see no reason for enduring a miserable end and seek euthanasia to avoid it. Finally, now that a growing acceptance exists about withdrawing life-support treatments—what some call passive euthanasia—the move to active euthanasia seems to some a reasonable next step for medicine at the end of life.

It is true that medical practice evolves, and significant stages in this evolution are apparent. From a widespread conviction that death was an enemy that must be kept at bay because its victory would be a defeat for the physician and his craft, medicine has developed the more mature idea that the physician, with his equipment and remedies, should retreat in some cases and focus on comfort measures. In the medical ethos now developing, the physician often welcomes death and sometimes helps it arrive by withdrawing treatment.

For some, as we saw above, there is little difference between these withdrawals and lethal injections or between heavy sedation for pain and deliberate lethal overdoses. They view euthanasia and assistance in suicide as consistent with the legitimate medical desire to prevent the indignity of personal disintegration that accompanies some deaths, as an extension of normal caring for a patient who does not want the suffering and indignity of a terrible and messy death. Dying patients, after all, desire only what everyone wants: a good death. If a good death is a blessing, as so many have said for so long, then medical assistance in dying is an act of beneficence, a part of the total care a physician provides for her patient. In this way, euthanasia and physician-assisted suicide can appear compatible with the noble aims of medical practice.

Moreover, polls indicate that assistance in dying is now what many people want from their physicians. Recent efforts to place euthanasia and assisted suicide on state ballots have succeeded, and the ballot questions have drawn an impressive percentage of the vote. More and more people, it seems, are considering the options of euthanasia and assisted suicide normal parts of medical practice.

REASONS AGAINST EUTHANASIA AND PHYSICIAN-ASSISTED SUICIDE

Killing a human being is a momentous act, and our history reveals a tendency to limit the scope of morally acceptable killing. The killing of enemy prisoners, once practiced by such great European heroes as Charlemagne and the Crusaders, is now widely condemned. Public executions are also a thing of the past, and, in fact, most countries in our cultural tradition have abolished capital punishment. Infanticide is no longer tolerated, and people killing their own babies are now prosecuted as murderers, something unheard of in earlier times. Weapons of mass killing have been built and were used twice at the end of World War II, but many have raised strong moral objections to any future use of strategic nuclear weapons.

In all this we can see the effort to reduce killing, to narrow down the range of morally and legally acceptable killings to the point where killing is morally suspect unless authorized by political or judicial authorities (war and capital punishment or undertaken privately as a last resort to save a life). This suggests that a strong *prima facie* case exists against killing. The burden of proof in the question of euthanasia and assisted suicide, therefore, rests with the advocates of change, with those desiring to establish the legal and moral validity of these private killings.

The reasons for not killing patients and for not helping them kill themselves fall into two groups of arguments. The first group comprises attempts to refute the arguments used to justify euthanasia and physician-assisted suicide. If the reasons used to justify euthanasia and physician-assisted suicide are not sufficiently convincing to overcome the traditional cultural stance against the private killing of innocent people, then the traditional stance against euthanasia and physician-assisted suicide should prevail.

The second group of arguments against euthanasia and assisted suicide focus on the reasons why it is not good for physicians to kill patients, nor good for patients to kill themselves, nor good for society to have physicians killing patients or helping them kill themselves. In tragic situations where no option the patient chooses will promote a good life in any meaningful sense, these arguments focus on showing that there are less worse alternatives than euthanasia or physician-assisted suicide. In other words, the second class of arguments represents substantive arguments designed to show why euthanasia and physician-assisted suicide are not morally justified.

Critiques of the Arguments Favoring Euthanasia and Assisted Suicide

Critique of the Patient Self-Determination Argument

Arguments for euthanasia and physician-assisted suicide based on patient autonomy, patient self-determination, or the right to choose all contain a major limitation: they cannot by themselves establish what is morally right or wrong. Saying something is morally right simply because it is autonomously and freely chosen is missing the whole point of ethics. The task of ethics is to determine that what is freely chosen is morally good; that is, that it will truly contribute to the agent's good. The agent may think the killing is good, and freely choose it, but that is not enough. Ethical reasoning must show that the killing will be truly good, or the less worse, for those engaging in it.

Certainly patients should be responsible for their lives and make the important choices, but no choice becomes morally justified simply because it is chosen. Few people think those who freely choose to play Russian roulette or take part in a duel are doing something morally good. And few think that slavery is moral for those who freely choose to enslave themselves to slave owners. Self-determination, choice, and personal responsibility are important moral notions, but they are not moral reasonings. Unfortunately, the tendency in the United States to consider autonomy or patient self-determination a fundamental moral principle from which we can deduce moral judgments about particular actions has led some to think that whatever a patient chooses is morally justified.

Moreover, even if we accepted the argument from self-determination, it would justify euthanasia and assisted suicide only for those people with the capacity to request it. Just as not everyone has the capacity to give informed consent for treatment, so not everyone has the capacity to request voluntary euthanasia or assistance with suicide. The requirements for recognizing the validity of self-determination when euthanasia is the issue will have to be at least as stringent as the requirements for informed consent when accepting or rejecting life-sustaining treatment is the issue.

In fact, a good case can be made that informed consent requirements for euthanasia and suicide should be more stringent than for treatment refusals. We would hesitate, for example, to let suicidal persons make major decisions affecting their lives; how much the more should we hesitate to let them make a decision about being killed or killing themselves. People who are suicidal are not always in the best frame of mind to make good decisions about important issues of life and death. And we should keep in mind that we have very little knowledge about how illness, especially painful and lengthy illness, affects the reasonableness and voluntariness of decision making.

It should be a matter of concern that those proposing euthanasia and assisted suicide have not yet developed anything as advanced as the widely accepted doctrine of informed consent for accepting and declining treatment. This doctrine sets forth, as we saw in chapter 4, important requirements for determining the capacity of the patient to make decisions, for the extensive information that must be provided, and for avoiding any manipulation that would undermine the voluntary aspect of the decision. These requirements cannot be met in situations involving many severely sick and dying patients.

It is somewhat ironic that so many who invoke patient self-determination as a justification for euthanasia have thus far failed to insist on full-fledged informed consent for the lethal injection. One important aspect of informed consent, as we saw, is providing the person with information about all the alternative treatments that could be employed, but some supporters of euthanasia spend little time explaining the alternative approaches available to control their patients' suffering. Without the patient's having a good grasp of what alternatives such as hospice care can do, the patient's request for euthanasia or physician-assisted suicide is not a truly informed request.

Finally, ethicists supporting euthanasia invariably acknowledge that the argument from self-determination alone is not strong enough to justify suicide and euthanasia. Their argument is never that the simple desire to be killed is sufficient to justify the killing but that other realities such as actual or expected suffering, approaching death, or permanent loss of awareness must be present. Thus, self-determination is not really an adequate argument or a sufficient reason justifying euthanasia and physician-assisted suicide. It is, rather, a condition that most advocates of euthanasia insist must be met before the killing can be considered morally justified. Advocates of euthanasia or physician-assisted suicide do not claim it is right to kill people, or to help them kill themselves, simply because they want to be killed; they always give another reason to show why the killing is the right thing to do. And that other reason is rooted in compassion for the patient's suffering.

Critique of the Argument Based on Relief of Suffering

Long before autonomy or patient self-determination became a paramount concept in health care ethics, those advocating euthanasia relied on an argument based on relief from suffering, and it is a strong argument. Relief of suffering has always been a goal of morally good people and of medicine itself. The argument claims physicians should, in cases where the suffering is intractable and death inevitable, respond in a spirit of mercy and compassion to a patient's desire for euthanasia or assistance in suicide.

Stated this way, the argument prompted by mercy is clearly a limited one. Euthanasia and physician-assisted suicide are moral options only when patients are experiencing, or expect to experience, severe intractable suffering that cannot be otherwise controlled. This means patients in an indefinite coma or in PVS are not candidates for euthanasia, even if their advance directives indicate this is what they would want. They are not candidates for euthanasia because they are not suffering and no merciful act can benefit them.

The relief of suffering argument, however, is even more limited than this because suffering can almost always be relieved without killing the person. It is possible to medicate patients so heavily that they are beyond awareness. This, of course, creates a very unsatisfactory situation in that sometimes it means patients are so drugged that their existence is reduced to a vegetative state.

Nobody really wants to live in such a state, but this is not the point. The point is whether it is morally less worse to relieve suffering by killing when we can relieve it short of killing the person. In other words, medicating patients into oblivion as they are dying may well be the worst thing we can do to them except for the other alternative—killing them. If we can relieve pain and suffering with medications, then no matter how unsatisfactory the situation, it is at least arguable that this route is less worse than killing them. Given our cultural tradition against private killing, the only situation where euthanasia would be justified by the relief of suffering argument, then, is a situation where the suffering can be relieved by no other way than by killing the patient. There may be such situations (on the battlefield, for example), but they are almost inconceivable in a normal health care setting.

Ironically, the argument for euthanasia based on relief of suffering was much stronger before anesthesia and pain medication became so effective. Until recently the suffering of some patients was truly intense and intractable, but now massive doses of medication to reduce or even eliminate awareness are available. Knowing a heavy dose of pain medication might in fact kill the person does not make giving it an action akin to euthanasia because the intention is radically different. The intention—and intentions are important in ethics—in giving medication for pain is fundamentally different from the intention in giving a lethal injection. It is one kind of moral action to give drugs in order to mask pain; it is quite another kind of moral action to give drugs in order to kill.

Critique of the Argument Based on Normal Medical Practice

Arguments derived from the idea of normal practice are never persuasive in ethics. Although normal practice is a good starting point for moral reflection, the rightfulness of conduct is not established by it but by reasons. The moral philosopher must show not that something is considered normal but that what is considered normal will actually contribute to the good.

In ancient Greece the Sophists had argued that custom or personal preference established moral goodness. Socrates, Plato, Aristotle, and the Stoics all argued that something more was needed for virtue. In some societies cannibalism was normal practice; in others, polygamy, infanticide, torture, and slavery were normal practices. Few today claim these practices are morally right. It was once normal medical practice to operate and to do medical research without informed consent, to conceal a grim diagnosis and prognosis from patients, and to discard defective newborns, but few today claim these practices are morally sound.

Furthermore, it is not at all clear that responding to the desire to be killed with euthanasia or assistance in suicide is truly a part of medical practice. The decision of a person to be killed, or to kill herself, is much more than a medical decision—it is a fundamental decision about a person's whole life and how it should end. It is not a clinical decision involving treatment of disease or of pain but an existential decision involving the destruction of human life. Physicians and nurses have no special training or expertise whereby they can join in decisions about ending someone's life. This is not a professional or clinical decision. Killing people, and helping them kill themselves, are social issues of immense consequence. Killing innocent people has never been, and is not now, normal practice for any segment of our society.

Arguments against Euthanasia and Physician-Assisted Suicide

Because there is a cultural presumption against killing innocent people even when they request it, criticisms of the arguments favoring euthanasia constitute a good reason for not accepting euthanasia and physician-assisted suicide. Opponents of euthanasia and physician-assisted suicide, however, have also offered more positive arguments designed to show that euthanasia and assistance in suicide are immoral behaviors. What follows are some of the more popular arguments against euthanasia and physician-assisted suicide.

The Religious Argument against Euthanasia and Assisted Suicide

There is first the familiar biblical injunction "Thou shalt not kill." Despite the references indicating that the Bible sanctions various killings, including at times the killing of the enemy's women and children and of one's own unruly sons, a consensus has emerged that the Bible takes a strong stand against most intentional killing of innocent people. Thus, for those accepting a moral tradition rooted in the Bible, the prohibition "doctors must not kill" seems to be well grounded.

A second aspect of the religious argument against euthanasia and assisted suicide rests on the doctrine of creation. According to this doctrine, God created the world out of nothing and continues his creative involvement to this day. For believers, God is the lord and giver of life; that is, he gives life as a gift and remains lord of it. Killing, therefore, is a rejection of the gift of life and of God's sovereignty over it. By killing people assume a power over life and death that belongs not to them but to God. God decides who are to be born and when and how they are to die. People act immorally if they usurp God's sovereignty over life and begin "to play God." As Deuteronomy 32:39 says: "Learn that I, I alone, am God, and there is no God besides me. It is I who bring both death and life."

The religious argument has great appeal for many, especially those influenced by the biblical doctrine of creation. Its use is not confined to theologians. Kant, for example, was a philosopher who argued at great length that morality is an affair of reason not religious revelation, but he employed a religious argument against suicide. He believed we were placed in this world by God for specific purposes and that people who commit suicide desert their posts and are rebelling against God. John Locke, a major architect of the theory that every human being has natural rights, among them the rights to life and liberty, also argued against suicide by claiming that God sent us into the world to be about his business, and thus we are bound to preserve ourselves and not quit our station willfully.

Although the religious arguments against euthanasia and physician-assisted suicide will be important for many believers, they obviously presuppose certain beliefs about the biblical commandments and creation. For those not believing in divine laws or creation, these arguments can carry little weight. Moreover, some religious traditions strongly opposed to euthanasia are experiencing dissent in their institutions. Some Catholic hospitals in Belgium, for example, have put policies allowing euthanasia in place since euthanasia became legal in 2002. Thus, the religious arguments against suicide are limited because they are based on religious beliefs not shared by all.

The Argument from Nature against Euthanasia and Assisted Suicide

Some philosophers claim killing ourselves, or asking others to kill us, is immoral because it runs counter to the natural impulse for self-preservation and is thus against human nature. Certainly, asking someone to kill us, or doing it ourselves, does seem to go against the natural desire to live, but the argument from nature is actually a weak one. The natural desire for self-preservation can be overridden in two ways: by the experience of great and hopeless suffering and by the choice to sacrifice our lives for a cause, perhaps religious martyrdom or heroic self-sacrifice whereby we give up our lives that others may live.

The weakness of the argument from nature against euthanasia also arises from the ease with which it can be turned into a reason for euthanasia or suicide. The Stoics, for example, the original proponents of a morality based on "acting according to nature," were comfortable with suicide. They thought death is "according to nature," and thus we can bring it about at the proper time. And if one accepts Freud's analysis of human nature, then the natural instinct to survive and thrive is accompanied by an equally natural instinct for self-destruction. For the Freudian the drive to self-destruction is as natural, although normally not as powerful, as the drive for self-preservation. The often repeated story of how Freud asked his physician for a lethal overdose at the end of his own life adds an interesting footnote to his theory of the interplay of *eros* and *thanatos*, the natural instincts for life and death in all of us.

The Social Argument against Euthanasia and Assisted Suicide

As far back as Aristotle the argument was made that suicide was an act of injustice against society. Whatever might be the advantages of suicide from the individual's point of view, others will be hurt by it, most notably the society. Suicide is wrong when it undermines the common good, the good shared by the many now weakened by the death of one who killed herself or requested that she be killed. Certainly there are situations where this is true. The death of contributors to the common good will weaken that good, much as the death of a parent in a family of small children brings great distress to the family.

But this is also a weak argument against euthanasia and physician-assisted suicide. By far, the usual candidates for euthanasia or assisted suicide in medical settings are already beyond contributing much to the common good. Those closest to them, and others in the community as well, may already be praying for their happy death and will consider that death, when it comes, a blessing and not a detriment to society.

The Argument against a Public Policy of Euthanasia and Assisted Suicide

Proponents of this argument often sidestep the debate over whether or not euthanasia and assisted suicide are morally right or wrong and focus instead on the public policy level. Their position is that regardless of whether you think euthanasia is moral or immoral it would not be moral to institute a public policy of euthanasia and physician-assisted suicide because such a public policy would do more harm than good. They advance several reasons to show why this is so.

The possibility of mistakes.   Most proponents of euthanasia insist they are advocating only voluntary euthanasia. No one will be killed unless he requests it.

But the notion of voluntary is problematic here. We can never be sure the request to be killed, given the fact we consider most killings tragic, is truly voluntary. The more the patients are suffering, the more likely they will be candidates for euthanasia, and the less likely they will be free of depression, despair, exhaustion, and the influence of medications. Illness distorts judgment and can make us less able to act in a truly voluntary way. The last thing a physician wants to do is kill somebody as the result of a misunderstanding, but unless we can say for sure that the sick, suffering, medicated person's request for euthanasia or assistance in suicide is truly well informed and voluntary, then the risk of killing someone by mistake—that is, killing a patient who is not fully informed (including all alternatives) and freely choosing to be killed—remains such a strong possibility that no public policy should allow an environment where it might occur. It is a function of public policy to forbid situations where there is reason to believe inappropriate or accidental death might easily happen.

Morally sensitive physicians, of course, will make every effort to determine whether the person asking to be killed is suffering from any pain or depression that would affect judgment or undermine the ability to choose freely, but determining whether or not the decisions of sick, suffering, and dying patients are truly informed and voluntary is a most difficult task. The decision to be killed is a major decision, and major decisions are often not well made when people are besieged by pain and suffering. There is some merit, then, in a public policy that will not allow physicians to kill or help to kill patients.

Undesirable consequences of legalizing euthanasia.   Many fear that legalization of voluntary euthanasia and physician-assisted suicide will lead to various undesirable consequences for medical practice; among them are the following possibilities.

1. Legalization of euthanasia will, or at least could, undermine the trust that some suffering patients would have in their physician once they know the physician is willing to kill them if they give the word. And some of these patients may feel very vulnerable because they are not insured and are incapable of paying for care. In a society that accepts euthanasia, these patients cannot help but worry about the financial pressure their medical treatment and hospitalization places on physicians and institutions. And they know that once the deed is done, the person killed cannot complain that it was done without voluntary consent.

Physicians have awesome power. They have ready access to lethal drugs; many know how to kill quickly and quietly and how to enter the proper cause of death in the records. Unlike the rest of us, people die around them all the time, so no one suspects anything is amiss when another sick person dies. Medical examiners seldom look carefully at deaths of extremely sick people that occur in a hospital or nursing home. In a society that rejects euthanasia, abuses are few and far between because they amount to murder. At the present time our doctors are well aware that it is illegal to kill, and few want to risk prosecution for murder. But in a society that accepts euthanasia, this protection is lost. It will become much more difficult to prevent killing that is not within the guidelines, as the experience in Holland well shows. The physician-patient relationship is based on trust, and that trust will be eroded in the minds of some, perhaps many, if any killing by physicians is socially authorized.

2. Legalization of euthanasia will, or at least could, also undermine our commitment to provide the best of care to those dying patients who decline to choose suicide or euthanasia. In a society where other patients in similar circumstances generously exercise their "right to die," and thereby cease to be a drain on personnel and resources, it is easy to consider those refusing to step out of the way selfish and their demand for care inappropriate.

3. Legalization of euthanasia will, or at least could, put additional burdens on sick patients because it presents them with another choice—and a most serious one. At the present time, patients do not have to make any decision about euthanasia; if it becomes legal, then it will become an option for them. They may do nothing about it, but doing nothing will then be a choice not to accept the legal option of euthanasia or assistance in suicide.

4. Legalization of euthanasia will, or at least could, be divisive for physicians who still think of themselves in some ways as colleagues and who often call their organizations "colleges." With euthanasia as a social policy, a divide will inevitably exist between physicians who consider the killing immoral and those who do not, between those willing to kill their patients and those scandalized by the very thought of doing it. Hospitals and nursing homes will also be divided along these lines because in our country many of these institutions are operated by church-affiliated groups whose religious traditions consider suicide and euthanasia immoral, and they will steadfastly oppose it. And a divide will open up between some physicians and some institutions because hospitals and nursing homes opposed to euthanasia will hesitate to admit physicians known to practice it in an effort to avoid, on their premises, what they consider murder.

5. Legalization of euthanasia will, or at least could, change the face of medicine in a way that will be disconcerting to many. For centuries the primary goal of medicine has been to cure, not to kill. Medicine has also tried to comfort, but the idea that physicians should comfort some people by killing them has not been a major part of medicine's ethos. Physicians have been trained to diagnose illness and then to treat it if possible and to comfort where necessary, but they have not been trained to kill patients or to help them kill themselves. The goal of medicine has never been to destroy life. Introducing euthanasia and assisted suicide will change all that by introducing a third and conflicting goal in medicine. Medicine would now have three goals: most of the time its goal will be saving and improving life, some of the time it will be comforting the dying, and some of the time it will be killing. Instead of cherishing life always, the ideal will now include destroying life sometimes. The thought of such a change in the goals of medicine causes many people, including some physicians, great distress, because it is such a radical departure from the traditional view of what physicians do when they practice medicine.

6. Legalization of euthanasia will, or at least could, undermine the delicate relation between the law and medical decisions to forgo life-sustaining treatment. Prosecutors and judges have come to recognize that there is an area at the end or at the edge of life where decisions to forgo treatment supporting life, including medical nutrition, do not normally require judicial oversight. One reason why courts have been comfortable doing this, despite their traditional concern for the protection of innocent human life, has been the existence of the clear line between withdrawing life-sustaining treatment and giving lethal injections or overdoses to bring about death. Prosecutors and judges do not have to worry about whether doctors are killing patients inappropriately because all killing is now illegal. At the present time the central question is never whether a lethal injection or

overdose to end life should be given but whether treatment should be withdrawn. The courts have tended, with some notable exceptions, to leave treatment decisions to medical experts.

This respect for medical decisions at the end of life will change if we expand medical decision making to include euthanasia and assistance in suicide. If some deliberate killing (euthanasia and physician-assisted suicide) is legally allowed, we can expect intense scrutiny by prosecutors and judges because society has a great interest in monitoring killing. The prosecutors and courts that tended to leave treatment decisions to physicians will not feel the same about euthanasia and assisted suicide. These actions are not about withdrawing treatments but about killing, and any killing invites close legal scrutiny by law enforcement personnel.

The long struggle to have the courts leave medical decisions to forgo life-sustaining treatment to the patient and physician will thus become undermined if medical practice is expanded to include euthanasia. Once physicians begin to kill, the law will move to the bedside. There will have to be legal guidelines for euthanasia, and those charged with enforcement will want to be sure these guidelines are followed exactly. Put simply, physicians can expect prosecutors and courts in our country to be much more concerned about euthanasia than they have been about withdrawals of life-sustaining treatments and medical nutrition.

Legalization of euthanasia might well open an ethical "slippery slope."   Many argue that a public policy accepting voluntary euthanasia for the suffering and hopelessly ill patient can easily serve as a wedge to dislodge traditional barriers against other kinds of killing. If we legalize voluntary euthanasia, then involuntary euthanasia is likely to follow. Proxies, not knowing for sure what an incapacitated patient wants, will decide it is in the patient's best interest to be put to death quietly and quickly, and they will expect the decision to be carried out as any other health care decision made by a proxy. Parents and physicians will decide euthanasia is best for their defective children; children and physicians will decide euthanasia is best for aging parents who have lost decision-making capacity. People will argue that those human beings so mentally compromised that they were never capable of making health care decisions should not be deprived of compassion when they are suffering, and thus euthanasia should be available for them. Accepting voluntary euthanasia will thus quickly lead to the acceptance of nonvoluntary euthanasia.

And, if we legalize euthanasia for the terminally ill, euthanasia for those not terminally ill will likely follow. Some will see no reason why the self-determination of patients, which now enables them to refuse life-sustaining treatments even when they are not hopelessly ill, should not extend to requests for euthanasia and assistance in suicide. It will be argued that the refusal of treatment necessary for life is equivalent to a decision to die, and once patients have decided to die, they should be able to choose the manner of their death and to be helped by their compassionate physicians to achieve it.

And, if we legalize euthanasia to relieve suffering, then euthanasia for those not suffering will inevitably follow. Some already see no reason why people in a permanent coma or in PVS should not be killed; yet these patients are not suffering. Once we accept euthanasia for these permanently unconscious patients, it will likely spread to other cases where suffering is not an issue.

Thus, the argument runs, a public policy of voluntary euthanasia will likely lead to public acceptance of involuntary euthanasia, a public policy of euthanasia for the hopelessly ill will likely lead to public acceptance of euthanasia for those not hopelessly ill, and a public policy of euthanasia for people suffering severe pain will likely lead to public acceptance of euthanasia for people not suffering pain.

In short, once we legalize euthanasia and assisted suicide for the patient most often mentioned as appropriate—the person with a hopeless disease suffering unbearable pain who requests it—we can expect the practice to spread to other situations. Physicians will likely begin killing, or helping to kill, people who never said they wanted it or who are not suffering or who are not terminally ill.

All these considerations constitute what is widely known as the "slippery slope" argument against euthanasia and physician-assisted suicide. In essence it is an argument that concentrates on the undesirable consequences the legalization of euthanasia will likely generate. Some proponents of this slippery slope argument think euthanasia itself is immoral; other proponents think it could be morally justified, at least in some extreme cases. But both groups argue that legalizing euthanasia or physician-assisted suicide for any reason, no matter how sound, will lead to situations in which it is not morally defensible. They feel there is no way to control the killing once it starts and that it will expand to infanticide and other forms of killing people without their consent or for reasons other than those that might be prescribed by the legal guidelines.

Some presentations of the slippery slope argument against euthanasia invoke the chilling history of Nazi Germany, where euthanasia was accepted years before the death camps became a reality. The progression from euthanasia to wholesale killing in Nazi Germany is a powerful version of the slippery slope argument because many older Americans remember World War II and the great military effort to defeat Germany. That war was followed by the famous trials of Nazi leaders in Nuremberg, where shocking evidence of forced euthanasia and other medical abuses by German physicians emerged.

In the minds of many, the road to abuse in Germany began when a few physicians adopted the attitude that some people—those who were severely impaired or chronically ill—were living lives not worthy to be lived. Once this attitude set in, it was but a small step to accept ending such "worthless" lives. Then the category of people living unworthy lives was expanded to include those not contributing to society, and then to those not wanted in the society because of their religion, ideological views, or racial identity.

Eventually, some say inevitably, what began as a modest euthanasia movement in the 1920s became the Holocaust of the late 1930s and the 1940s, where at least eight million innocent people were murdered under this aegis. This shows, some argue, that once we begin killing innocent people, especially if it is physicians performing the act, terrible evils will follow. The only way to prevent the abuse is to draw a strong line against all killing, including euthanasia.

Today's proponents of euthanasia disagree with such a conclusion. They sometimes attack the validity of the slippery slope argument by saying enough protection can be built into the legalization of physician-assisted suicide and euthanasia that the slide into immoral killing will not occur. The defeated referendum known as Initiative 119 on the 1991 ballot in the state of Washington stipulated, for example, that the proposed legalization of euthanasia would apply only when the patient was (1) competent, (2) voluntarily requesting it, and (3) terminally ill with less than six months to live. The 1992 referendum in California, also defeated, added still more protections by including the qualifications that the voluntary request must be "enduring" and communicated in a revocable written directive signed by two unrelated witnesses and that the physicians carrying out the killing must report the euthanasia and the circumstances to appropriate authorities. The 1994 referendum in Oregon, which was successful, was even more restrictive, allowing only physician-assisted suicide. Putting such protections in place, it is argued, will prevent any slide down a slippery slope.

Moreover, proponents of euthanasia argue that the situation in Germany earlier in the century, especially during the Nazi years, bears so little resemblance to Europe and to the United States at this time that no significant comparisons can be drawn between that society and our own. And, in many ways, they are right.

There is, however, the more recent example of euthanasia in Holland that does strengthen the slippery slope argument. As we noted earlier, although the Netherlands did not legalize euthanasia until 2002, prosecutors in Holland had made it clear since 1984 that euthanasia in cases of necessity would not be prosecuted provided physicians followed the guidelines published by the Royal Dutch Medical Association, the State Commission on Euthanasia, and the Dutch government. The key points in the Dutch guidelines were as follows.

- The patient must have the capacity to make decisions, have an irreversible disease, be experiencing unbearable suffering, and be well informed about euthanasia and about alternative ways of controlling suffering.
- The patient's request must be voluntary and persistent; it must reflect an enduring longing for death.

- The physician must consult at least one colleague with experience in euthanasia and, after the killing, provide a written report to the coroner explaining the disease and how the guidelines were followed.

These requirements, designed to prevent the slide down a slippery slope by restricting euthanasia to situations of patient self-determination and physician compliance, have been in place for decades in Holland. Have they been successful in holding the line on euthanasia?

The simple answer is no. A 1991 Dutch report, authorized by the Committee on the Study of Medical Practice Concerning Euthanasia (also called the Remmelink Committee because its president was the attorney general of the Supreme Court, J. Remmelink), acknowledged that there have been hundreds of cases of nonvoluntary euthanasia and defended these cases even though they violated the published guidelines. The report analyzed the 129,000 deaths in Holland during 1990 and found that 2,300 of them were by euthanasia. In more than a third of these cases (about 1,000), a crucial guideline accepted by the Dutch Medical Association was violated: the patients killed had made no clear request for euthanasia. A few of those patients were children. Furthermore, only 486 (18 percent) of these euthanasia deaths were reported to the local medical examiner as required by the guidelines; hence, doctors failed to observe reporting requirements for 82 percent of the patients they put to death.

A second published survey of euthanasia in the Netherlands covered the 135,500 deaths in 1995. It showed that 3,200 of these deaths were reported as euthanasia and that 900 of these patients who were put to death had not made a clear request for euthanasia. It also showed that only 1,466 (41 percent) of these euthanasia deaths were reported to the medical examiner; hence, doctors were still failing to report the majority of euthanasia deaths more than ten years after the guidelines had been put in place.

The high number of outlaw cases of nonvoluntary euthanasia is disturbing as well as the failure to report many deaths caused by voluntary euthanasia. Obviously, some physicians would report a natural cause for the death whenever the euthanasia was not strictly in accord with the guidelines. Hence, the number of patients actually killed without compliance with the guidelines in these years was undoubtedly higher than the number actually reported.

However, a third study reporting euthanasia and physician-assisted suicide in 2005 found that the situation did change somewhat after the Netherlands legalized euthanasia and physician-assisted suicide in 2002. The number of physicians properly reporting euthanasia rose from 18 percent in 1990 and 41 percent in 1995 to 80 percent in 2005. However, this still leaves about one in five cases of euthanasia not being reported as required by law. Also, the number of deaths under terminal sedation rose from 5.6 percent of all deaths in 2001 to 7.1 percent in 2005, and the percentage of deaths from euthanasia and physician-assisted suicide actually dropped from 2.8 percent of all deaths in 2001 to 1.8 percent in 2005. This suggests a growing preference in recent years for aggressive palliative care rather than euthanasia. Finally, the percentage of people put to death by euthanasia without their explicit request (nonvoluntary euthanasia) dropped from 0.8 percent of all deaths in 1990 and from 0.7 percent in 1995 to 0.4 percent of all deaths in 2005.

Although this is an improvement, it still means that many physicians are not adhering to the legal guidelines and are performing hundreds of outlaw cases of nonvoluntary euthanasia in the Netherlands each year. One might think that physicians putting hundreds of people, some of them children, to death each year without their voluntary informed consent would be seen as a worrisome wrong and generate a serious scandal in the Netherlands, but for the most part it has not caused much of a reaction.

Advocates of euthanasia point out that those killed without having clearly requested it were in terrible condition and unable to request euthanasia. Although interviews suggest that this was undoubtedly true in many cases, it is not relevant to a very important question in the debate about the legalization of euthanasia. That question is this: Can we rely on physicians to adhere to the legal guidelines? The most recent (2005) evidence from Holland continues to show that we cannot. Moreover, one of the main arguments for euthanasia is based on patient autonomy and patient self-determination, and ending the lives of patients who were not fully informed or did not explicitly request euthanasia obviously cannot be justified by appeals to patient autonomy.

In reality, then, proponents of the slippery slope argument against legalizing euthanasia find important support for their position in what has actually been happening in the Netherlands, where it has not been possible to restrict euthanasia to the established guidelines for voluntary euthanasia even after its legalization. The evidence from Holland also raises questions about how honest physicians will be when it comes to reporting truthfully in accord with guidelines their practice of euthanasia. Of course some proponents of euthanasia argue that the Dutch slide down the slippery slope is not inevitable and that better safeguards could have prevented it. One wonders just what those effective safeguards could be.

It is also disturbing that the proponents of euthanasia in Holland have tended to ignore the illegal acts of euthanasia. Instead of calling for legal action against the physicians who violated the law, the attitude seems to be that the law is too restrictive and that the guidelines should be expanded to include the euthanasia of people who have not requested it and of children when parents and physicians think euthanasia is appropriate. This attitude tends to confirm the suspicion of many that legalizing voluntary euthanasia is only the first step down the slippery slope to widespread acceptance of nonvoluntary euthanasia.

What about Oregon? Is there any evidence of physicians not following reporting guidelines or sliding down the slippery slope toward nonvoluntary physician-assisted suicide? The short answer is that there is no such evidence thus far. However, we simply do not know what is really happening in Oregon because surveys to discover what is really going on, surveys such as those conducted in Holland for 1991, 1995, and 2005, simply have not been done. The Dutch deserve a lot of credit; they have made efforts to discover and publish the numerous failures of physicians to follow the legal guidelines. Oregonians have made no such effort, and supporters of legalizing physician-assisted suicide have shown no interest in pursuing how the laws they support are working in practice. The annual statistics published by Oregon merely summarize the reports submitted by physicians; they make no effort to conduct anonymous surveys that might uncover unreported or illegal incidents. Thus, everything looks as though protocol is being followed completely. As one critic wrote, in Oregon it is a case of "don't ask, don't tell."

We should note, however, that slippery slope arguments are never conclusive. A slippery slope or "wedge" argument can never prove absolutely that terrible consequences will follow if a certain line is crossed. A slippery slope argument does not enjoy logical necessity; the first steps are not premises leading necessarily to the next steps in the argument. The power of slippery slope arguments derives from experience and history; if we eat the first peanut, we may well eat a few more.

The slippery slope argument against euthanasia, however, has some plausibility because to this point in history no society has yet demonstrated just what set of guidelines and protections would be effective in preventing a slide from voluntary euthanasia of suffering, irreversibly ill, patients to euthanasia without the voluntary informed consent of the patient. The slippery slope argument can never prove that unwanted abuses will occur once we accept euthanasia, only that they might occur. But the argument remains a thought-provoking one because the practice of euthanasia in Holland, the one modern example we have where people have made efforts to find out what really happens in this situation, has shown how quickly legal acceptance of voluntary euthanasia easily leads to widespread tacit acceptance of illegal forms of euthanasia.

There is a final worrisome point: legalization of euthanasia and physician-assisted suicide can create financial conflicts of interest in the United States because of the lack of universal health care. Under our present payment system in some situations providers, hospitals, and physicians are losing money on dying patients, and thus they have a distinct financial incentive to end their care. Even if the experience with euthanasia and physician-assisted suicide did not slide down a slippery slope as in the Netherlands, the Dutch experience would not help us much because their payment system is so different from ours. The Dutch have universal health care, and physicians are on salary so they have no financial incentive to practice euthanasia. But American physicians and hospitals may be in financial arrangements with incentives for cutting expenses and thus may experience a financial conflict of interest as patients linger near death.

The Story of a Landmark Physician-Assisted Suicide

We turn next to a widely noted account of a physician-assisted suicide written by a physician and published in a major medical journal. It is a case that will reveal how complex the issue truly is and how good people may sometimes disagree on how physicians should act.

The Case of Diane

The Story

Diane, a middle-aged woman, presented with a rash and a chronic tired feeling. Her blood count was suspicious, and a bone marrow biopsy confirmed the worst: an acute form of leukemia. Without treatment she would die within a few months.

The treatment for this condition is not pleasant. It begins in the hospital with three weeks of induction chemotherapy that helps three out of four patients. If she is one of the three, she will receive additional chemotherapy with a two out of three chance it will benefit her. If it does, she will then undergo a two-month hospitalization for a bone marrow transplantation with a 50 percent chance it will be effective for her. The bottom line is that her chance of survival is zero with no treatment and about one in four (25 percent) with the difficult chemotherapy treatments and bone marrow transplantation.

Her husband and college-age son wanted her to start the treatments, as did her physician, Dr. Timothy Quill, but Diane refused. Dr. Quill was bothered by her decision because he knew her as a fighter, but he respected it.

Diane then made a disturbing request. She told Dr. Quill that she wanted to kill herself when she could no longer maintain control of herself and her dignity as she died. Dr. Quill, a former hospice physician, assured her that he could keep her comfortable, but Diane wanted no part of lingering in the relative comfort of heavy medication as she died.

A week later she requested barbiturates to help her sleep. Subsequent conversation with Dr. Quill revealed that she was having trouble sleeping, but it was also clear that she wanted to accumulate enough barbiturates to commit suicide. After assuring himself that she was not despondent and that she was truly making an informed decision, Dr. Quill prescribed the barbiturates, making sure that she knew how to use them for sleep and how many to take for suicide.

Over the course of three and a half months, bone pain, weakness, fatigue, and fevers began to dominate Diane's life. Time was rapidly running out. She told her friends that she would be leaving soon and said a tearful good-bye to Dr. Quill. Two days later, after her final good-byes to her husband and son, she asked to be alone for an hour. They found her on the couch covered by her favorite shawl.

Dr. Quill went to the house. He called the medical examiner, telling him the cause of death was "acute leukemia" to avoid any investigation a suicide might have triggered. He then wrote a moving account of the story for a respected and widely read medical journal, the *New England Journal of Medicine*, and many of the letters published in response to his article were favorable. His account helped stimulate the public debate on euthanasia and physician-assisted suicide in a thoughtful and sensitive way. For this we should be grateful, because intelligent and graceful discussion is the only way a society can resolve these issues.

Ethical Analysis

Situational awareness. We are aware of these facts in Diane's story.

1. Diane had terminal leukemia. With no treatment, she would die in a matter of months; with difficult treatment, she had one chance in four of surviving. She decided to decline treatment.

2. Dr. Quill, a physician with hospice experience, assured Diane that he knew "how to use pain medicines to keep patients comfortable and lessen suffering."

3. It was extraordinarily important to Diane to maintain control of herself and her own dignity during the time remaining to her. If she could not maintain this control, she wanted to kill herself.

4. When she requested barbiturates from Dr. Quill, he prescribed them and made sure she knew how to kill herself with them: "Knowing of her desire for independence and her decision to stay in control, I thought this request made perfect sense."

5. Diane committed suicide.

We are also aware of the following good and bad features in the story.

1. Diane's acute leukemia and the dim prospects of cure despite very difficult treatment were terrible realities for her, her family, and her physician.

2. Once she had declined treatment, her impending suffering and death were also significantly bad features. And for her, the inevitable loss of control at the end was a most upsetting aspect of what would be her final days.

3. The distress her physician, who had known her for eight years, would experience if he did not help her fulfill her last important wish was another bad feature in this case.

4. One good feature of the situation was that, unlike earlier times, the medications and knowledge to keep her comfortable to the very end were available.

5. Another good feature was that, judging from the written account, her physician was a caring and compassionate man. Convinced he was giving her "the best care possible," he was nonetheless honest enough to acknowledge the following: "I am not sure the law, society, or the medical profession would agree" with his assistance in her suicide.

Prudential Reasoning in the Story of Diane

Here we look at the story from the perspectives of the moral agents in this case, the patient and the physician. We ask how moral agents in such a situation might behave to achieve their personal good.

Patient's perspective. Once her leukemia had been diagnosed, Diane was faced with several difficult decisions. The first was whether or not to accept treatment. If she declined treatment, she could avoid the side effects and discomfort of chemotherapy and transplantation, but it meant certain death in a matter of months. If she underwent treatment, the chance of failure would be 75 percent, and she might well experience the burdens of treatment for nothing. Prudence suggests that this is one of those situations in which either decision is morally justified. A patient who decides to seek the chance of survival has good reasons for so acting, but so does a patient who decides to decline the burdensome treatment when history shows it fails most of the time. In an ethics of prudence, either decision of the patient in this situation can easily be justified from a moral point of view.

Once she had decided to decline treatment, Diane was faced with a second major decision: whether to endure her dying or, at some point, to kill herself. Neither of these decisions would lead to a good life in any meaningful sense of the term. Heavy medication is not good, and suicide ends life. Diane was in a tragic situation in which no option would bring what we call happiness and fulfillment in life. Her situation was analogous to Aristotle's soldier whose post is being overrun: he can stand firm and be killed, or he can desert and become a coward. In such a situation, the moral person can only choose the less worse. According to Aristotle, it is less worse for the soldier to fight courageously than to desert. Which choice is less worse for a person in Diane's tragic position—killing herself or accepting comfort care as she dies?

Her decision to kill herself is not easily justified in an ethics of prudence. The killing of a human being, even a human being dying of leukemia, is a momentous action. Whenever we deliberately kill, we need forceful reasons to justify it. The reasons that justify killing must be cogent reasons because destroying human life, even human life ravaged by final illness, is such a serious step that society has struggled to avoid it.

What reasons might justify suicide in a situation such as this? None are offered in the account of Diane's final months written by her physician. We do know that it was "extraordinarily important to her to maintain control of herself" and that she had a "desire for independence." These are important factors, but they are not pieces of moral reasoning. In ethics when the issue is damage to life, what someone desires or thinks important is not always the same as what is morally reasonable. The morally reasonable is determined by asking whether what we desire or think important is truly good for us or at least is the less worse option. And since our good is inextricably linked with others, we have to ask as well how what we do affects them and the community.

In this case, it is difficult to think of any reason to justify the suicide. The suicide would not save the lives of others, nor was it necessary to avoid severe uncontrollable pain. It might be argued that the thought of losing control caused her unbearable suffering and that this suffering could only be avoided by the suicide. There is some merit to this reasoning, and the account indicates Diane may well have felt this way, but such reasoning is questionable. In logical form the reasoning would look like this:

- Losing control as I die is bad (I view the loss of control as a terrible suffering).
- I am about to lose control.
- Therefore, I have a sufficient reason to kill myself. The bad features of killing myself are less important than the bad features of losing control as the disease advances and I need stronger medication for pain.

Most would agree that losing control is bad, but it is at least arguable that it is less worse than destroying a human life, even a human life that is almost over. The fear of losing control hardly seems a morally sufficient reason for killing a human being, even a dying human being. Losing control is terribly unfortunate, but not so unfortunate in these circumstances that it justifies killing in order to prevent it from happening.

The patient made a third major decision in this case: she decided to ask another human being, her physician, to help her kill herself. This adds another moral dimension to the case. Most people would find it an emotional burden to help someone kill herself, especially if the assistance were not really necessary. Although it is sometimes true that a person is unable to commit suicide without help, this was not the case here. At the time she killed herself, Diane could easily have done it without any help from her physician.

People find all sorts of ways to kill themselves without assistance in relatively painless ways. Everyone is familiar with the tragic newspaper accounts of people sitting in parked cars, with the windows up and motor running for warmth, who are found dead of accidental carbon monoxide poisoning. Apparently the passage from life to death is so painless they are not stimulated by discomfort to do the one simple thing that could save their lives—open the door and get out. The most recent physician-assisted suicides of Dr. Kevorkian remind us of how painless these deaths are; his "patients" killed themselves by putting a simple plastic mask over their faces and then breathing carbon monoxide from a canister.

For patients with as much mobility as Diane had, painless suicide is an action they can accomplish all by themselves without any assistance from anybody. Why, then, do so many still able-bodied patients seek assistance and complicity from their physicians? Some suspect it may well represent an inarticulate desire to have approval for the suicide. Physician assistance in suicide gives the act an approval in the eyes of some patients that it might not otherwise have. It reminds one of a case reported by the media in which a man insisted that he wanted his respirator withdrawn. The court approved his request but told him he would have to shut it off himself. He declined.

It may well be that some people want to commit suicide but do not want to do it themselves; they want their physician to do it with them. This not only places an awful burden on the physician but makes one wonder whether the unnecessary assistance of a physician in their suicide is at least partially motivated by the need to have an authority figure endorse the suicide and share the responsibility. If a person could easily commit suicide without physician assistance, but nonetheless seeks it, we have to wonder why. And we have to guard against the perception that killing and assisting in suicide by physicians are somehow more easily justified morally than killings and assistance in suicides by those who are not physicians.

Physician's perspective.   What is the moral response of a physician when a patient planning on suicide requests a prescription for barbiturates and for instructions on how to kill herself with them? Giving someone intent on killing herself a poison and teaching her how to use it in a lethal way makes the physician an accomplice in the killing that follows. He will need convincing moral reasons to justify his participation in the suicide.

In the original published account of this case, the physician did not provide any moral reasoning for his decision to help Diane kill herself. Although he acknowledged he had an uneasy feeling about the "spiritual, legal, professional, and personal" boundaries he was exploring, neither ethics nor morality was mentioned. Several of his remarks suggested moral reasoning, but they remained undeveloped.

For example, Dr. Quill's account speaks of his being an advocate of a patient's right to die with as much control and dignity as possible. The mention of a "right" suggests moral reasoning because some moralists argue that we have a moral obligation to respect another's rights. But the assertion of a right is not a substitute for moral reasoning. Before I can use a right in moral reasoning, I must show that the claimed right exists and contributes to the human good, something many deny about the "right to die." And if I can show that the right to die exists and is something morally good, I must still give reasons for extending the right to die to the "right to kill oneself," and then for extending it again to the "right to receive physician assistance" when the patient could do it herself. And if I can show all this, then I must also show that the exercise of that right to die, so understood, indicates, at this time and in these circumstances, that assisting in this suicide is morally reasonable behavior.

In other words, before a physician can use the "right to die" as a moral reason for helping a patient kill herself, he has to show (1) that the right to die is truly a right, (2) how the right to die can be expanded into a right to kill oneself, and (3) how the right to kill oneself justifies the physician's helping someone kill herself when no help is necessary. None of this appears in the analysis we have of Diane's suicide.

Another example of inchoate moral reasoning appears when Dr. Quill identifies several bad features that may develop if he does not help Diane kill herself. He feared the effects of a violent death on her family, the consequences if her suicide attempt was unsuccessful and left her damaged, and the possibility that a family member might try to help her and hence suffer legal and personal repercussions. Identifying the bad features that might happen if I choose not to act in a situation is an important first step in moral reasoning—but only that. Moral reasoning will also consider the bad features that will happen if I do choose to act in the situation. Helping someone kill is a notable bad feature. Good people do not kill or help others kill unless they can justify the action with reasons sufficiently strong to justify the destruction of human life.

The lack of an effort to develop moral reasoning that would justify helping someone kill herself may be the result of how the physician viewed his participation in the killing. He wrote: "Although I did not assist in her suicide directly, I helped indirectly to make it possible."

The distinction between direct and indirect roles in killing needs to be approached with care. Some ethicists do made a distinction between direct and indirect killing. They say, for example, that a pilot dropping a bomb on a military target in a city kills the soldiers directly but kills the civilians indirectly. Here direct and indirect killing depend on intention. The bombing pilot may intend to kill the enemy soldiers but not the civilians. Their deaths are foreseen but unintended side effects. It is clear, however, that this traditional use of direct and indirect killing is not what the physician is appealing to in this case.

Nonetheless, the physician believes his help was indirect. For the sake of argument, let us assume that this is so. This still leaves us with the major moral question: Was it moral for him to participate "indirectly" in the suicide? Describing a participation in a killing as indirect does not imply that the participant escapes responsibility for the killing.

To see this clearly, imagine the following. A neighbor tells you he wants to kill himself. He asks you to loan him your gun and show him how to use it. You loan him your gun, making sure he knows how to use it to kill himself. Some time later he shoots himself with your gun in just the way you instructed him. Obviously your "indirect" assistance does not absolve you of your responsibility for your role in the suicide. To see this it is important not to camouflage your role. You may call your role in the suicide indirect if you wish, but you still need to acknowledge that you played a significant role in the person's death, and we need to develop absolutely compelling reasons for playing significant roles in people's deaths.

The Legal Aftermath

This case occurred in New York, at that time one of the twenty-six states with laws making it a crime to help people kill themselves. The district attorney, however, decided not to prosecute Dr. Quill. He explained that "Diane" was never identified and that there was no evidence of a crime because there was no body to examine for possible evidence that would indicate a crime.

He was forced to change his mind and call for a grand jury investigation after a reporter identified Diane and located her body in a laboratory. Forensic investigation revealed the barbiturates in Diane's body, but the grand jury declined to indict Dr. Quill for assisting in the suicide. The disciplinary board of the New York State Health Department also investigated the incident and decided Dr. Quill was not guilty of misconduct since he did not "directly" participate in the suicide.

As we saw in the discussion of the battle in federal courts, Dr. Quill later joined with other physicians and dying patients in an unsuccessful effort to have the New York law prohibiting suicide assistance declared unconstitutional.

Ethical Reflections

Our desire for independence as we die is understandable, but it is a desire, not a reason. Maintaining control of ourselves is also important, very important for people such as Diane, but this importance does not automatically justify everything we can do to maintain control. Not every action designed to fulfill our desires or to achieve what is important to us can be morally justified. Whenever it is a question of damaging or destroying human life, something more is needed, and what are needed are reasons to justify the destruction.

In our culture there is a tendency to think we are authentically human only if we are in control. But that is not a realistic reaction to the human condition. At some time or other everyone is vulnerable and needs others. The desire to remain in control no matter what is not a reasonable desire because it is incompatible with the human condition. Only an almighty being could always be in control, and we are not almighty but vulnerable. We can, and should, control much in our lives, but it is unreasonable to think we can control everything. There are times when it is reasonable to place our lives in the hands of others, to let go, to acknowledge our humanity. In a cultural milieu that prizes control and autonomy, this can be difficult.

It is with great hesitation that we attempt to judge the dead, especially those who have died by their own hand. There is something almost disrespectful about it, and we should not do it unless we have a good reason. But we can learn from the dead. We learn from autopsy and the dissection of cadavers in medical school, and there is something almost disrespectful about this as well. So too, we can learn from published accounts of suicides. We can perform a postmortem moral examination, not to criticize the dead or embarrass their families but to work our way through the difficult moral issue of physician-assisted suicide. Unless we analyze the actions of people such as Diane and those associated with Dr. Kevorkian, our moral discourse about suicide will remain totally theoretical.

If we accept the idea that the taking of human life is such a serious personal and social event that it should be a last resort, then an ethics of prudence is hard pressed to justify this suicide and the physician's assistance in the suicide. This is not to say that suicide and assistance in suicide could never be morally justified but simply that this does not seem to be one of those cases. The main reasons why the moral arguments allowing suicide fail here are that Diane was not suffering uncontrollable pain and that her desire for control is not enough to justify killing a human being—herself. There is no question that she wanted to kill herself. But the ultimate moral issue when the destruction of human life is involved is not what one wants but whether what one wants is reasonable; that is, whether it contributes to the human good or at least is the less worse option.

This case is most difficult because we have every reason to believe that Diane and Dr. Quill were sensitive human beings doing what they thought was best. To disagree with what they thought is not in any way to imply a pejorative judgment about them as human beings. And we must acknowledge two things. First, their moral judgments may have been the right ones and the position presented here the wrong one. Second, their good intentions and personal beliefs are not sufficient to establish the morality of what was done—people with the best of intentions have often done what is not good.

CONCLUDING REFLECTIONS

Since we can expect the intense public debate about euthanasia and assisted suicide to continue, the following remarks may be helpful.

First, deliberately killing another human being and assisting in suicide are very serious actions. Our first reaction should be to avoid them and not allow them to happen except as a last resort. This is the thrust of our tradition in recent centuries.

Second, the burden of proof in the moral argument about euthanasia and physician-assisted suicide, therefore, rests on those proposing the moral rightness of these killings. They must establish the morality of euthanasia and physician-assisted suicide and show the wisdom of making these actions legal.

Third, opponents of euthanasia who argue that euthanasia is wrong because intentionally killing innocent people is always wrong are begging the question. They must show why it is immoral to kill suffering, hopelessly ill people who request it. It is not enough to state the absolute moral prohibition "do not deliberately kill innocent people" and ignore the very complicated circumstances surrounding euthanasia.

Fourth, since an individual good is not always a social good and therefore may not be morally justified, an exclusive focus on a patient-centered ethics in medicine is misleading. Any adequate ethics embraces both individual and social consequences of behavior. Physicians killing patients is not a private medical matter—people killing other people has always been a matter of great social and legal concern. Hence, no individual stories that seem to cry out for euthanasia or assisted suicide are ever, of themselves, sufficient arguments for allowing a social practice of euthanasia and assisted suicide. Since killing is involved, it is never a matter of purely private ethics; there is an important social dimension to it as well.

Fifth, the unfortunate publicity surrounding Dr. Jack Kevorkian's assisted suicides can all too easily blind opponents of euthanasia and physician-assisted suicide to the valid concerns of those proposing the legalization of these options. Dr. Kevorkian's behavior does not easily fit into what Aristotle would call good and noble behavior or virtuous activity. Most of the suicides Kevorkian has assisted would fall outside the carefully crafted guidelines of Oregon and Washington, and many proponents of physician-assisted suicide have no support for the way he enabled people to end their lives.

Sixth, the most prominent movement to eliminate the suffering of the dying, which reduces the need for physicians to kill them or help them kill themselves, is hospice care. The first modern hospice in America was opened in 1974; today there are more than four thousand programs caring for more than one million patients each year. Hospice studies show that most patients can be kept comfortable as they die, although some do require heavy sedation, usually only in the last few days of life. It is somewhat ironic that great improvements in hospice and palliative care in the last two decades in the United States have been matched by a growing movement to allow physicians to kill patients or help them kill themselves, lest they suffer from somatic pain or psychological distress as they die.

Seventh, in the last analysis, the ironic simultaneous growth of the hospice and euthanasia movements may well be partially generated by two different views of ethics. The action guides of modern ethics—the right to choose, the right to die, the right of privacy, the principle of autonomy, and the principle of beneficence—can all be used to justify euthanasia and physician-assisted suicide. An ethics of prudential reasoning aiming at living well, however, is hard pressed to find reasons for euthanasia and physician-assisted suicide now that pain management and palliative care can ease the suffering confronting some at the end of life. Even when the situation becomes truly tragic, and the only choice is between the less worse and the more worse, prudence directs one toward the less worse. And sedation is less worse than killing.

SUGGESTED READINGS

For the history of attitudes toward euthanasia and physician-assisted suicide, see Paul Carrick, 1985, *Medical Ethics in Antiquity*, Boston: D. Reidel Publishing. Two papers by Ludwig Edelstein are especially helpful in understanding the limited role of Hippocratic medicine and morality in the classical world. See Ludwig Edelstein, 1987, "The Hippocratic Oath: Text, Translation and Interpretation," and "The Professional Ethics of the Greek Physician," in *Ancient Medicine*, Owsei Temkin and C. Lilian Temkin, eds., Baltimore: Johns Hopkins University Press, pp. 3–63 and 319–48.

Aristotle's remarks on infanticide are in the *Politics* 1335b20–22, and his remarks on suicide are in the *Eudemian Ethics* 1230a1–4 (suicide to escape from trouble or pain shows a lack of courage) and in the *Nicomachean Ethics* 1138a6–14 (suicide that violates the civil law is an act of injustice against the city-state). A helpful collection on the various views of suicide in our cultural tradition is Baruch Brody, ed., 1989, *Suicide and Euthanasia: Historical and Contemporary Themes*, Dordrecht: Kluwer Academic Publishers.

Kant's stand against suicide is from his *Lectures on Ethics*, pp. 148–54. His question about whether Frederick the Great harbored an intention contrary to the moral law when he carried poison into battle lest he be captured is found in his *The Metaphysical Principles of Virtue in Ethical Philosophy*, James Ellington, trans., Indianapolis: Hackett, 1983, pp. 84–85. Here Kant also asks whether it is immoral for a person bitten by a mad dog to kill himself lest his incurable madness from the bite lead him to harm others.

"It's All Over, Debbie" appeared in *JAMA* 1988, *259*, 272. The particular author of this piece in the weekly column titled "A Piece of My Mind" was not identified. A year earlier, the same column had published an opposing view. See Carl Kjellstrand, "The Impossible Choice," *JAMA* 1987, *257*, 233. The article by twelve physicians, ten of whom thought it would be ethical for physicians to help patients kill themselves in certain situations, is Sidney Wanzer et al., "The Physician's Responsibility toward Hopelessly Ill Patients: A Second Look," *New England Journal of Medicine* 1989, *320*, 844–49. Derek Humphrey's book *Final Exit* was published in 1991 by the National Hemlock Society.

Among the many helpful articles on euthanasia and physician-assisted suicide are these: Dan Brock, "Voluntary Active Euthanasia," *Hastings Center Report* 1992, *22* (March–April), 10–22; Daniel Callahan, "When Self-Determination Runs Amok," *Hastings Center Report* 1992, *22* (March–April), 52–55; Willard Gaylin et al., "Doctors Must Not Kill," *JAMA* 1988, *259*, 2139–40; David Orentlicher, "Physician Participation in Assisted Suicide," *JAMA* 1989, *262*, 1844–45; Marcia Angell, "Euthanasia," *New England Journal of Medicine* 1988, *319*, 1348–50; Christine Cassel and Diane Meier, "Morals and Moralism in the Debate over Euthanasia and Assisted Suicide," *New England Journal of Medicine* 1990, *323*, 750–52; Timothy Quill, Christine Cassel, and Diane Meier, "Care of the Hopelessly Ill: Proposed Clinical Criteria for Physician-Assisted Suicide," *New England Journal of Medicine* 1992, *327*, 1380–84; Howard Brody, "Assisted Death—A Compassionate Response to a Medical Failure," *New England Journal of Medicine* 1992, *327*, 1384–88; Robert Miller, "Hospice Care as an Alternative to Euthanasia," *Law, Medicine & Health Care* 1992, *20*, 127–32; Susan Wolf, "Holding the Line on Euthanasia," *Hastings Center Report* 1989, *19* (January–February), supplement, pp. 13–15; Lisa Cahill, "Bioethical Decisions to End Life," *Theological Studies* 1991, *52*, 107–25; and John Paris, "Active Euthanasia," *Theological Studies* 1992, *53*, 113–26.

For a classic article reprinted in many anthologies see Yale Kamisar, "Some Non-Religious Views against Proposed 'Mercy-killing' Legislation," *Minnesota Law Review* 1958, *42*, 969–1042. On the difficulty of knowing just what motivates a person's desire for euthanasia or suicide, the view of psychiatrists is important. See Yeates Conwell and Eric Caine, "Rational Suicide and the Right to Die: Reality and Myth," *New England Journal of Medicine* 1991, *325*, 1100–02. For the impact of suicide assistance on physicians, see Steven Miles, "Physicians and Their Patients' Suicides," *JAMA* 1994, *271*, 1786–88. See also Thomas Preston, "Professional Norms and Physician Attitudes toward Euthanasia," *Journal of Law, Medicine & Ethics* 1994, *22*, 36–40.

Among the many books wherein euthanasia is discussed at some length are Germain Grisez and Joseph Boyle, 1979, *Life and Death with Liberty and Justice: A Contribution to the Euthanasia Debate*, Notre Dame: University of Notre Dame Press; James Rachels, 1986, *The End of Life: Euthanasia and Morality*, New York: Oxford University Press; Timothy Quill, 1993, *Death and Dignity: Making Choices and Taking Charge*, New York: Norton; and Margaret Battin, 1994, *The Least Worse Death: Essays in Bioethics on the End of Life*, New York: Oxford University Press, and its sequel, Battin, 2005, *Ending Life: Ethics and Way We Die*, New York: Oxford University Press. The New York State Task Force on Life and the Law has taken a strong stand against legalizing euthanasia and physician-assisted suicide. See its report titled *When Death Is Sought: Assisted Suicide and Euthanasia in the Medical Context*, 1994, Albany: Health Education Services.

The controversial Dutch experience with euthanasia is described and debated in Carlos Gomez, 1991, *Regulating Death: Euthanasia and the Case of the Netherlands*, New York: The Free Press; Maurice de Wachter, "Active Euthanasia in the Netherlands," *JAMA* 1989, *262*, 3216–19, and "Euthanasia in the Netherlands," *Hastings Center Report* 1992, *22* (March–April), 23–30; Alexander Capron, "Euthanasia in the Netherlands: American Observations," *Hastings Center Report* 1992, *22* (March–April), 30–33; Henk ten Have and Jos Welie, "Euthanasia: Normal Medical Practice?" *Hastings Center Report* 1992, *22* (March–April), 34–38; John Keown, "On Regulating Death," *Hastings Center Report* 1992, *22* (March–April), 39–43; Margaret Battin, "Voluntary Euthanasia and the Risks of Abuse: Can We Learn Anything from the Netherlands?" *Law, Medicine & Health Care* 1992, *20*, 133–43, and "Euthanasia: The Way We Do It, The Way They Do It," *Journal of Pain and Symptom Management* 1991, *6*, 298–305; Paul Van der Mass et al., "Euthanasia and Other Medical Decisions Concerning the End of Life," *Lancet* 1991, *338*, 669–74; Johannes van Delden et al., "The Remmelink Study: Two Years Later," *Hastings Center Report* 1993, *23* (November–December), 24–27; Gerrit Kimsma and Evert van Leeuwen, "Dutch Euthanasia: Background, Practice, and Present Justifications," *Cambridge Quarterly of Healthcare Ethics* 1993, *2*, 19–31.

For a follow-up of the Remmelink report see Paul van der Maas et al., "Euthanasia, Physician-Assisted Suicide, and Other Medical Decisions concerning the End of Life in the Netherlands 1990–1995," *New England Journal of Medicine* 1996, *335*, 1699–1705. For indications that the slide down a slippery slope continues to occur in the Netherlands, see J. K. M. Gevers, "Physician-Assisted Suicide and the Dutch Courts," *Cambridge Quarterly of Healthcare Ethics* 1996, *5*, 93–99. Gevers, a professor of law at the University of Amsterdam, recounts Dutch legal cases of euthanasia and physician-assisted suicide involving patients suffering from mental disease or from depression, thus showing how "as soon as PAS is allowed under strict conditions for a particular category of patients . . . other groups emerge and request for such assistance" [*sic*] (p. 98). An excellent introduction to the history of euthanasia in The Netherlands is John Griffiths et al., 1998, *Euthanasia and Law in the Netherlands*, Ann Arbor: University of Michigan Press. Griffiths, an American who teaches sociology and law at the University of Groningen, is sympathetic to the practice of euthanasia in the Netherlands. For recent developments see Agnes van der Heide et al., "End of Life Practices in the Netherlands under the Euthanasia Act," *New England Journal of Medicine* 2007, *356*, 1957–65; Timothy Quill, "Legal Regulation of Physician-Assisted Death—The Latest Report Cards," *New England Journal of Medicine* 2007, *356*, 1011–13; Susan Wolf, "Assessing Physician Compliance with the Rules for Euthanasia and Assisted Suicide," *Archives of Internal Medicine* 2005, *165*, 1677–79; Bregje Onwuteaka-Phillipsen et al., "Taking the Final Step: Changing the Law on Euthanasia and Physician-Assisted Suicide—Dutch Experience of Monitoring Euthanasia," *British Medical Journal* 2005, *331*, 691–93. For the Dutch debate on nonvoluntary euthanasia see Cess Hertogh et al., "Would We Rather Lose Our Life Than Lose Our Self? Lessons from the Dutch Debate on Euthanasia for Patients with Dementia," *American Journal of Bioethics* 2007, *7*, 48–56.

For the debate about euthanasia in Belgian Catholic hospitals see Chris Gastmans, "Caring for a Dignified End of Life in a Christian Health-Care Institution," *Ethical Perspectives* 2002, *9*, 134–45. This article contains the text of the 2002 Caritas Catholica recommendations, and this volume of *Ethical Perspectives* contains several important articles on euthanasia in the Netherlands and Belgium as well as the actual text of the euthanasia laws in both countries. See also Chris Gastmans et al., "Pluralism and Ethical Dialogue in Christian Healthcare Institutions: The View of Caritas Catholica Flanders," *Christian Bioethics* 2006, *12*, 265–80 and Chris Gastmans et al., "Prevalence and Content of Written Ethics Policies on Euthanasia in Catholic Healthcare Institutions in Belgium (Flanders)," *Health Policy* 2006, *76*, 169–78. For a critique of the Caritas position by defenders of the traditional Catholic position against euthanasia, see Daniel Salmasy, "Death, Dignity, and the Theory of Value," *Ethical Perspectives* 2002, *9*, 103–18; and Ana Iltis, "On the Impermissibility of Euthanasia in Catholic Healthcare Organizations," *Christian Bioethics* 2006, *12*, 281–90.

For an example of the sometimes heated debate about euthanasia see Daniel Callahan, "When Self-Determination Runs Amok," *Hastings Center Report* 1992, *22* (March–April), 52–55; and a response by John Lachs, "When Abstract Moralizing Runs Amok," *Journal of Clinical Ethics* 1994, *5*, 10–13; with a response by Daniel Callahan, "*Ad Hominem* Run Amok: A Response to John Lachs," *Journal of Clinical Ethics* 1994, *5*, 13–15. A 1993 survey in Washington State, where voters defeated a proposal allowing euthanasia and physician-assisted suicide known as Initiative 119 in 1991, revealed that physicians were sharply polarized on the issue. See Jonathan Cohen et al., "Attitudes toward Assisted Suicide and Euthanasia among Physicians in Washington State," *New England Journal of Medicine* 1994, *331*, 89–94. For a review of the referenda questions in Washington, California, and Oregon, see George Annas, "Death by Prescription," *New England Journal of Medicine* 1994, *331*, 1240–43.

For more recent material on the ethics of euthanasia and physician-assisted suicide see Linda Emanuel, ed., 1998, *Regulating How We Die: The Ethical, Medical, and Legal Issues surrounding Physician-Assisted Suicide*, Cambridge, MA: Harvard University Press; Robert Weir, ed., 1997, *Physician-Assisted Suicide*, Bloomington: Indiana University Press; John Keown, ed., 1997, *Euthanasia Examined: Ethical, Legal and Clinical Perspectives*, Cambridge, UK: Cambridge University Press; and David Thomasma, "An Analysis of Arguments for and against Euthanasia and Physician-Assisted Suicide," *Cambridge Quarterly of Healthcare Ethics* 1996, *5*, 62–76 (part 1) and 1998, *7*, 388–401 (part 2). This issue also contains a special section on euthanasia and public policy.

The growing public debate about euthanasia is hampered by controversies over terminology and the moral implications of the distinctions employed in the debate. See, for example, James Rachels, "Active and Passive Euthanasia," *New England Journal of Medicine* 1975, *292*, 78–80; Dan Brock, "Taking Human Life," *Ethics* 1985, *95*, 851–65; Bonnie Steinbock, 1980, *Killing and Allowing to Die*, Englewood Cliffs: Prentice Hall; Raymond Devettere, "The Imprecise Language of Euthanasia and Causing Death," *Journal of Clinical Ethics* 1990, *1*, 268–74, and "Reconceptualizing the Euthanasia Debate," *Law, Medicine & Health Care* 1989, *17*, 145–55; Howard Brody, "Causing, Intending, and Assisting Death," *Journal of Clinical Ethics* 1993, *4*, 112–17; Joseph Lombardi, "Killing and Letting Die: What Is the Moral Difference?" *New Scholasticism* 1980, *54*, 200–12; Gilbert Meilaender, "The Distinction between Killing and Allowing to Die," *Theological Studies* 1976, *37*, 467–70; Raanan Gillon, "Euthanasia, Withholding Life-Prolonging Treatment, and Moral Differences between Killing and Letting Die," *Journal of Medical Ethics* 1988, *14*, 115–17; and Lawrence Gostin, "Drawing a Line between Killing and Letting Die: The Law, and Law Reform, on Medically Assisted Dying," *Journal of Law, Medicine & Ethics* 1993, *21*, 94–101.

Debates over terminology have not abated. See, for example, Patrick Hopkins, "Why Does Removing Machines Count as 'Passive' Euthanasia?" *Hastings Center Report* 1997, *27* (May–June), 29–37; Thomas Cavanaugh, "Currently Accepted Practices That Are Known to Lead to Death, and PAS: Is There an Ethically Relevant Difference?" *Cambridge Quarterly of Healthcare Ethics* 1998, *7*, 375–81; and Timothy Quill et al., "Palliative Options of Last Resort: A Comparison of Voluntarily Stopping Eating and Drinking, Terminal Sedation, Physician-Assisted Suicide, and Voluntary Active Euthanasia," *JAMA* 1997, *278*, 2099–2104. In the last article the authors argue that there is no "principled ethical distinction [among] sedation, physician-assisted suicide, and euthanasia." A virtue-based ethic, however, considers intentions morally significant and thus makes an ethical distinction between actions intended to sedate or to remove unreasonable treatment and actions intended to kill. For a philosophically questionable attempt to show that the Supreme Court unintentionally embraced the constitutionality of euthanasia when it rejected a constitutional right to physician assistance in suicide, see David Orentlicher, "The

Supreme Court and Physician-Assisted Suicide: Rejecting Assisted Suicide but Embracing Euthanasia," *New England Journal of Medicine*, 1997, *337*, 1236–39.

For an example of a carefully crafted policy proposal that would allow voluntary euthanasia and physician-assisted suicide as a last resort when palliative and supportive treatments are inadequate, see Franklin Miller et al., "Regulating Physician-Assisted Death," *New England Journal of Medicine* 1994, *331*, 119–23. The choice of language in this article is not without interest. There is a growing tendency by those favoring legalization of euthanasia and physician-assisted suicide to speak of it as "physician-assisted death" and "death with dignity." Oregon, for example, now considers physician-assisted suicide not suicide but "physician-assisted death," and the laws allowing physician-assisted suicide in Oregon and Washington are called "Death with Dignity Acts." And the editorial introduction to several thoughtful articles in the *Hastings Center Report* for 2008 speaks of efforts "to legalize physician assistance in a patient's death." See Timothy Quill, "Physician-Assisted Death in the United States: Are the Existing 'Last Resorts' Enough?" *Hastings Center Report* 2008, *38* (September–October), 17–22. For a critique of the misleading language in the physician-assisted suicide controversy see Daniel Callahan, "Organized Obfuscation: Advocacy for Physician-Assisted Suicide," *Hastings Center Report* 2008, *38* (September–October), 30–32.

For the value of the slippery slope argument, an argument used by many opposed to euthanasia and physician-assisted suicide, see Douglas Walton, 1992, *Slippery Slope Arguments*, New York: Oxford University Press; Wilbren van der Berg, "The Slippery-Slope Argument," *Ethics* 1992, *102*, 42–65 (a condensed version appeared in the *Journal of Clinical Ethics* 1992, *3*, 256–68 with commentaries by Benjamin Freedman, Raymond Devettere, and David Ozar); Bernard Williams, 1985, "Which Slopes Are Slippery?" in *Moral Dilemmas in Modern Medicine*, Michael Lockwood, ed., Oxford: Oxford University Press, pp. 126–37; and Bruce Jennings, "Active Euthanasia and Forgoing Life-Sustaining Treatment: Can We Hold the Line?" *Journal of Pain and Symptom Management* 1991, *6*, 312–16.

Dr. Quill's article on the suicide of Diane and his role in it is "Death and Dignity: A Case of Individualized Decision Making," *New England Journal of Medicine* 1991, *324*, 691–94. For a sympathetic account of this suicide and a critical account of Dr. Kevorkian's assisted suicides, see Robert Weir, "The Morality of Physician-Assisted Suicide," *Law, Medicine & Health Care* 1992, *20*, 116–26. See also Timothy Quill, "Doctor, I Want to Die. Will You Help Me?" *JAMA* 1993, *270*, 870–73, and "The Ambiguity of Clinical Intentions," *New England Journal of Medicine* 1993, *329*, 1039–40.

Some advocates of euthanasia or physician-assisted suicide propose a psychiatric consult to be sure the patient is capable of giving voluntary, fully informed consent to be killed or to receive suicide assistance. This seems unreasonable for two reasons. First, it would make psychiatrists the gatekeepers of euthanasia and suicide assistance, and, second, if psychiatric consults are not required when very sick or dying patients request withdrawals of life support they should not be required for physician-assisted suicide. See Linda Ganzini et al., "Psychiatry and Assisted Suicide in the United States," *New England Journal of Medicine* 1997, *336*, 1720–22.

Sometimes people propose euthanasia and suicide assistance from a social justice perspective, arguing it is immoral to use expensive resources for dying patients when they want to end their lives. In other words, euthanasia will allow us to divert medical resources to more worthwhile endeavors. In fact, will euthanasia and suicide assistance save much money? Probably not. See Ezekiel Emanuel et al., "What Are the Potential Cost Savings from Legalized Physician-Assisted Suicide?" *New England Journal of Medicine* 1998, *339*, 167–72.

For the background and efficacy of hospice care, see Vincent Mor, David Greer, and Robert Kastenbaum, *The Hospice Experiment*, 1988, Baltimore: Johns Hopkins University Press; Robin Fainsinger et al., "Symptom Control during the Last Week of Life on a Palliative Care Unit," *Journal of Palliative Care* 1990, *6*, 5–11; and Robert Miller, "Hospice Care as an Alternative to Euthanasia," *Law, Medicine & Health Care* 1992, *20*, 127–32.

The Department of HHS's Agency for Health Care Policy and Research (AHCPR) has published an extensive (257-page) clinical guideline on pain management developed by an interdisciplinary panel of clinicians, patients, and others. The guideline includes a section on pain management for AIDS patients because the suffering associated with AIDS is similar to that of many cancers. The panel acknowledges that not all pain can always be eliminated but that available palliative care "can effectively relieve pain in most patients" (p. 2). See AHCPR, 1994, *Management of Cancer Pain*, Washington, DC: U.S. Government Printing Office.

Good palliative care at the end of life is receiving more and more emphasis. In 1997 the Robert Wood Johnson Foundation funded a project titled "Education for Physicians on End-of-Life Care (EPEC)" that developed a curriculum and presented nationwide conferences on end-of-life care for physicians, a subject that most had learned little about in medical school. Obviously, good end-of-life care will reduce tremendously the need for doctors to kill their patients or help patients kill themselves in order to prevent suffering. See Joanne Lynn, "Caring at the End of Our Lives," *New England Journal of Medicine* 1996, *335*, 201–2; Henry Foster, "The Supreme Court Speaks: Not Assisted Suicide but a Constitutional Right to Palliative Care," *New England Journal of Medicine* 1997, *337*, 1234–36; Diane Meier et al., "Improving Palliative Care," *Annals of Internal Medicine* 1997, *127*, 225–30. Linda Emanuel has suggested a thoughtful way to respond to patients' requests for suicide assistance by showing them that less drastic alternatives exist for achieving their goals of avoiding suffering and needlessly prolonged dying in "Facing Requests for Physician-Assisted Suicide: Toward a Practical and Principled Clinical Skill Set," *JAMA* 1998, *280*, 643–47. The 2008 AMA Council on Ethical and Judicial Affairs' report *Sedation to Unconsciousness in End-of-Life Care* (terminal sedation) is available at ama-assn.org/ama/pub/category/3840.

For the court battles leading to the 1997 Supreme Court decision that found no constitutional right to physician-assisted suicide, see especially Susan Behuniak and Arthur Svenson, 2003, *Physician-Assisted Suicide: The Anatomy of a Constitutional Law Issue*, New York: Rowman and Littlefield, which contains excerpts from many of the legal documents including *amici curiae* briefs in the various federal cases. See also Alexander Capron, "Death and the Court," *Hastings Center Report* 1997, *27* (September–October), 25–28; Cathleen Kaveny, "Assisted Suicide, the Supreme Court, and the Constitutive Function of the Law," *Hastings Center Report* 1997, *27* (September–October), 29–34; George Annas, "The Bell Tolls for a Right to Suicide," in Linda Emanuel, ed. *Regulating How We Die*, chapter 9. An earlier version of this chapter appeared under the same title in *New England Journal of Medicine* 1996, *335*, 683–87. Lawrence Gostin, "Deciding Life and Death in the Courtroom: From *Quinlan* to *Cruzan*, *Glucksberg*, and *Vacco*—A Brief History and Analysis of the Constitutional Protection of the 'Right to Die'," *JAMA* 1997, *278*, 1523–28, is a good summary of key court cases about actions (both treatment withdrawals and suicide) resulting in a patient's death. The Ninth Circuit case citation is *Compassion in Dying v. Washington*, 79 F.3d 790 (1996), and the Second Circuit citation is *Quill v. Vacco*, 80 F.3d 716 (1996). The Supreme Court reversals are *Washington v. Glucksberg*, 521 U.S. 702 (1997) and *Vacco v. Quill*, 521 U.S. 793 (1997). The Supreme Court decision ending the attorney general's efforts to render Oregon's law ineffective is *Gonzales v. Oregon*, 546 U.S. 243 (2006).

The report of the Oregon Health Division is Arthur Chin et al., "Legalized Physician-Assisted Suicide in Oregon—The First Year's Experience," *New England Journal of Medicine* 1999, *340*, 577–83. The report suggested that autonomy was a key factor in the decision of many who committed suicide. For a criticism of the report see Kathleen Foley and Herbert Hendin, "The Oregon Report: Don't Ask, Don't Tell," *Hastings Center Report*, 1999, *29* (May–June), 37–42. The official annual summaries of physician-assisted suicide in Oregon are available online at oregon.gov/DHS/ps/pas. See also John Safranek, "Autonomy and Assisted Suicide: The Execution of Freedom," 1998, *28* (July–August), 32–36; and Joan Woolfrey, "What Happens Now? Oregon and Physician-Assisted Suicide," *Hastings Center Report* 1998, *28*, *3* (May–June), 9–17. For a criticism of the language in the Oregon law, see Alexander Capron, "Legalizing Physician-Aided Death," *Cambridge Quarterly of Healthcare Ethics* 1996, *5*, 10–23; and Daniel Callahan, "Organized Obfuscation: Advocacy for Physician Assisted Suicide," *Hasting Center Report* 2008, *38* (September–October), 30–32. See also Margaret Battin et al., "Legal Physician-Assisted Dying in Oregon and the Netherlands: Evidence Concerning the Impact on Patients in 'Vulnerable' Groups," *Journal of Medical Ethics* 2007, *33*, 591–97; Timothy Quill and Margaret Battin, eds., 2004, *Physician-Assisted Dying: The Case for Palliative Care and Patient Choice*, Baltimore: Johns Hopkins University Press; Kathleen Foley and Herbert Hendin, eds., 2002, *The Case against Assisted Suicide: For the Right to End-of-Life Care*, Baltimore: Johns Hopkins University Press; and Mary Warnock, 2009, *Easeful Death: Is There a Case for Assisted Dying?* New York: Oxford University Press.

FOURTEEN

Medical Research

RESEARCH INVOLVING ANIMALS and human subjects is an important part of modern medicine. New techniques and technologies as well as new drugs are routinely tested on animals and humans before physicians use them in normal clinical practice. Since the tests can cause harm to both the animals and humans, they pose ethical concerns. We have to ask whether the actual or potential harms caused by the research are reasonable, that is, whether they are consistent with living well. Medical researchers undermine their own good when they do things that could cause suffering or damage life without sufficient reasons.

The primary ethical concern in medical research centers on what it does to the people who are the subjects of the testing. Of concern also is what the research does to human embryos and fetuses, and to animals. Embryos and fetuses are human life, and damaging human life without sufficient reason is contrary to human flourishing. Animals suffer and die, and causing them to suffer or to die needlessly also undermines living a good life.

A distinction is frequently made between therapeutic and nontherapeutic research. In therapeutic research the subjects are sick, and the hope is that the research will both benefit them as well as provide knowledge that can benefit others. In nontherapeutic research the subjects are not sick or, if they are sick, there is no real expectation of any benefit to them from the research. Nontherapeutic research is entirely for the benefit of people other than the subjects of the research.

The distinction between therapeutic and nontherapeutic research is not really helpful in ethical deliberation for several reasons. First, although the distinction is sometimes clear, it can be ambiguous. Many research protocols for drugs, for example, involve random clinical trials with sick people. Some patients receive the drug and others, a control group, receive placebos. For the patients actually receiving the drug, the research will be, or at least might be, therapeutic, but for those not receiving it, the research will be nontherapeutic. Thus, the same drug trial is both therapeutic and nontherapeutic. Of course, the reverse could also be true—the study could be counter-therapeutic by harming the patients receiving the trial drug, as sometimes happens.

Furthermore, even when the distinction is not ambiguous, it contributes little to ethical reasoning. The moral deliberations about the possible bad effects of the medical research and the reasons that justify risking them are the same whether the research is therapeutic or nontherapeutic. The balance between the expected benefits and burdens is what matters, not whether the research is therapeutic or not. In fact the distinction between therapeutic and nontherapeutic research can obscure good moral reasoning by suggesting that we can tolerate unreasonably high levels of harm and risks of harm as long as the intervention might help the patient. It can lead to the attitude that a dying patient has nothing to lose and can try anything. This is not good ethics—some medical research and unproven drugs are not good for dying patients.

Sometimes the words experimentation and experiment are used to describe medical research. Although literally correct, the word is not a happy choice. The idea of experimenting with human beings is not a comfortable one. It is too close to the notion of experiments in the natural sciences where the researchers manipulate nature to produce desired results. Medical research involving human subjects differs so greatly from scientific research in biology or physics that it seems best to avoid the term.

In this chapter we avoid both the distinction between therapeutic and nontherapeutic research and the word experimentation. We instead use the terms "medical research" to designate any medical or psychological testing on human subjects or animals; "human subject" to designate children and adults, as well as human embryos and fetuses; and "participants" to designate people who have given voluntary informed consent to participate in the research.

The current moral awareness about medical research and the various laws and regulations governing its practice developed in large measure as a reaction against earlier mistreatment of human beings in research projects. There is much to be learned from remembering how medical research became unethical when the desire to achieve scientific and medical progress overshadowed moral sensitivity to the well-being of the persons involved. A brief look at several well-known abuses in research is valuable for understanding current concerns in the ethics of medical research.

NOTORIOUS EXAMPLES OF QUESTIONABLE ETHICS IN RESEARCH

We now review a number of research studies with poorly thought-out ethical bases.

The Tuskegee Syphilis Study (1932–72)

When this study began in 1932, injection of various heavy metals, especially mercury and various arsenicals, was a standard treatment for syphilis. The treatment was controversial. There were some indications that the treatment helped patients with syphilis, but it also seemed to cause other problems and symptoms. Moreover, a Norwegian study dating from 1891 suggested that some people with syphilis had survived for decades with no treatment, sometimes without symptoms. This suggested that the disease was not always fatal and that populations without treatment might actually do better than those treated, and weakened, by the standard injections.

The U.S. Public Health Service wanted to find out just how lethal syphilis was if not treated. The Public Health Service could do this by studying the natural course of the disease over a long period of time in a rather large population. The study would compare the health and longevity of people infected with the disease with those not infected. The infected group, of course, would not be treated because treatments would interfere with the natural course of the disease.

The Public Health Service soon found a ready-made group for its syphilis study. In 1929 the Julius Rosenweld Foundation had funded an effort to eradicate syphilis in Macon County, Alabama, where about 40 percent of the men were infected. The foundation's laudable effort to eradicate the disease ended when its endowment shrank during the Great Depression a few years later. Subsequently, the U.S. Public Health Service decided to conduct its study of syphilis with the same population but, unlike the private foundation's efforts to cure, this was purely an information-gathering study. It selected about six hundred adult males for the research. About four hundred had syphilis, and the remaining two hundred served as a control group. The research was centered in Tuskegee, and hence the project became known as the Tuskegee Syphilis Study.

The infected men were not informed about the nature of the research and were merely told they suffered from "bad blood." They did not receive any treatment for their syphilis, although researchers sometimes told them that the procedure was a "treatment" when they wanted to perform spinal taps for analysis. During the study some men in the control group contracted the disease. They were transferred to the infected group but never told of their syphilis, thereby exposing their sexual partners to it.

The study continued long after the early 1940s, when it became known that penicillin was successful in treating syphilis. At this point there was no need to continue the study—the success of penicillin left the researchers with no reason for studying how syphilis develops in humans when it is not treated. But the research continued. Researchers were able to prevent the infected men from being drafted for military service in World War II lest military physicians discover their syphilis and treat it with penicillin. And the researchers provided local physicians with the names of those infected and asked them not to give these men antibiotics for any reason lest the medications undermine the study. Thus, bacterial infections unrelated to syphilis were not treated.

Finally, in the late 1960s Peter Buxton, a researcher working for the U.S. Public Health Service, complained about the morality of the ongoing research project, which was now under the auspices of the Centers for Disease Control (CDC) in Atlanta. After several years when the CDC made no move to stop the study, Buxton told his story to a reporter. In July 1972 the *New York Times* ran the story on its front page, and other newspapers soon picked it up. CDC officials tried to defend the study, but public outrage was strong. One cartoon in a newspaper showed a dead patient, covered by a sheet, and a nurse, holding a syringe of penicillin, asking the physician: "Now can we give him the penicillin?"

In February and March of 1973, Senator Edward Kennedy of Massachusetts chaired a highly visible congressional hearing on the research as public criticism grew. Many citizens were shocked that the Centers for Disease Control and the U.S. Public Health Service were involved in research involving deceit and the denial of treatment in order to obtain useless information about the natural development of syphilis without treatment. And many could not help but notice that all the subjects in the study were poor black men. The fact that many of the physicians in Macon County who had collected data in the later years of the study were also black did little to erase the idea that the decision not to offer treatment had racial overtones.

Once the terrible history had been exposed, survivors and families sought damages in federal court. In July 1973 they accepted an out-of-court settlement. The compensation, considering the personal damage and the risks to the men, was not much. Infected survivors received $37,500 and control group survivors received $16,000. Families of the men involved in the study who had died before 1973 also received compensation. If the deceased man had been infected, his family received $15,000; if he had not been infected, $5,000.

Although most people learning of the research in 1972 had no problem seeing how immoral it was, physicians who had known of the study for years apparently never saw how wrong it was. The research had never been a secret. Between 1936 and 1973 at least thirteen articles reported findings of the study in journals such as the *Archives of Internal Medicine* and the *Journal of Chronic Diseases*. The articles in the professional journals, unlike those in the press, expressed no moral discomfort about the poor men who were selected for the research and left without treatment long after the cure for the disease had been developed.

This bit of history shows how easily sensitivity to moral issues can diminish when groups with special interests are not sufficiently self-critical about the morality of what they do. It shows as well the need for public and professional scrutiny of medical research.

Experiments in Nazi Germany (1942–45)

During World War II prisoners and other detained people were forced into dangerous and painful medical experiments. Japanese physicians, for example, injected Chinese prisoners with syphilis, cholera, plague, and other diseases in order to observe how the illnesses progressed.

The most upsetting events, however, occurred in Europe under Nazi Germany. As is well known, about eight million people lost their lives in the death camps during the war, about six million of them Jews. At some of the camps, Buchenwald and Auschwitz for example, people were also used for crude medical experiments. Subjects were deliberately infected with diseases to test the efficacy of vaccines and treatments, placed in altitude chambers to gather data affecting air crews at high altitudes, exposed to cold so the revival of extremely chilled bodies could be studied, shot so treatment for gunshot wounds could be improved, given electric shocks to see how much electricity people could survive, exposed to radiation in experiments designed to sterilize them, and exposed to other gynecologic experimentation. Some subjects died from the experiments; others suffered terribly. Many of these people were later killed when they were no longer useful to the experiment.

Physicians designed and conducted these experiments. Perhaps the most widely known of them was Dr. Josef Mengele. He not only selected those to be killed as the trains arrived at the camp, and killed some himself, but also conducted extensive medical experiments. Of special interest to him were twins, and he experimented with many pairs of twins, sometimes killing them in order to dissect their bodies.

All of the medical experiments conducted in the camps were clearly immoral, not only according to standards widely accepted today but according to official German regulations governing novel treatments and medical research that had been in place since 1931. The German regulations governing medical research were very advanced for the time, and they required voluntary consent from the subjects of the research before it could begin. Physicians conducting research in the camps simply ignored the regulations—especially the requirement for voluntary consent.

After the Allied victory over Nazi Germany in 1945, trials of war criminals were held in the German city of Nuremberg, the site of huge Nazi rallies in the 1930s. The Nuremberg Military Tribunal indicted twenty German physicians and convicted fifteen of them on charges of performing medical experiments without the subjects' consent. Seven of these doctors were hanged; the other eight received long prison terms. Dr. Mengele, however, as did so many others, had escaped to South America before the trials. Despite efforts to capture him, he remained free. It is thought that he died in Brazil years later.

As the result of international outrage over the Nazi medical experiments, the judges at Nuremberg set forth certain basic principles for medical research. The first of these ten principles, known as the Nuremberg Code, says: "The voluntary consent of the human subject is absolutely essential." Other principles allow the subject to withdraw at any time, and they remind the physician that he must terminate the experiment if it is likely to injure or kill the subject and that he must avoid all unnecessary physical and mental suffering and injury.

The famous Nuremberg Code was published along with accounts of the trials by the U.S. Government Printing Office in 1949. One might assume that medical researchers in the United States would abide by the Nuremberg Code from that time onward. Unfortunately, they sometimes did not.

Hepatitis at the Willowbrook State School (1956–70)

The Willowbrook State School on Staten Island was an institution for children with severe developmental disabilities. When the research on hepatitis started in 1956, it had a population of about forty-five hundred and a staff of about one thousand. Because a large number of the children were not toilet trained, most of them became infected with hepatitis, usually a mild variety, within a year of admission. Wanting to study the disease and to develop an effective immunization to eradicate it, two researchers from the New York University School of Medicine, Saul Krugman and Joan Giles, conducted various trials. One of them consisted of inoculating newly admitted children with gamma globulin, then dividing them into two groups. Children in one group were then deliberately infected with hepatitis to learn how effective the inoculations were.

Researchers obtained the consent of parents before enrolling children in the study. However, the validity of this consent can be questioned. By 1964 Willowbrook was desperately overcrowded with about five thousand children in a facility designed for three thousand. Long waiting lists developed, but immediate placement was available if parents agreed to enroll their children in the hepatitis study. The inducement of immediate placement for children who were hard to manage at home undermined the validity of the parents' consent to the research.

After papers based on the study were published in respected medical journals, some people questioned the ethics of the research. Perhaps the most notable criticism was a letter by Dr. Stephen Goldby published in the prestigious British medical journal *Lancet* on April 10, 1971. In an editorial remark, the editors of the journal agreed with his criticisms of the research despite their earlier editorial support of the study. Goldby claimed the study was "quite unjustifiable" and that it was not right to experiment on children when it is of no benefit to them.

Goldby's criticisms were vigorously denied by the researchers at Willowbrook. They were only partially successful, however, in defending their research. A rather general consensus arose that adequate information had not been provided to the parents and that the consent in many cases was not truly voluntary because of the pressures on the parents to enroll their needy children, many of whom were difficult to care for at home, in the study in order to gain admission to the school. Moreover, some found it difficult to think the parents' consent could have considered the best interests of their child. Deliberately infecting a healthy child with hepatitis is hardly in the best interests of that child.

The research eventually ceased after the public outrage surfaced, but not everyone was convinced that the study had been immoral. When the *New England Journal of Medicine* published a report on the study in 1973, for example, the editor reminded readers that the journal does not publish unethical research, thus reassuring them of his opinion that the research had been morally acceptable. Nonetheless, many others were upset that a vulnerable population of retarded children in a state school could be deliberately infected with hepatitis, and the highly publicized incident served to raise consciousness about medical research in the early 1970s.

Cancer Research at the Jewish Chronic Disease Hospital (1963)

In 1963 Dr. Chester Southam, a physician at the Sloan-Kettering Institute for Cancer Research in New York, organized a study that was conducted at the Jewish Chronic Disease Hospital (JCDH) facility that involved injecting live cancer cells into twenty-two patients. Dr. Southam was doing research on the ability of the body's immune system to fight cancer. He knew that cancer patients were less able to fight cancer cells than healthy people, but he did not know why this was so. Was the weakened immune system caused by the cancer that was already in the body, or was it caused by the general debilitation experienced by people suffering from cancer?

He thought that the injection of cancer cells into debilitated patients would provide him with the answer. If they became less able to fight cancer after the injections, it would indicate that the cancer was the cause of the weakened immune system. If, on the other hand, they did not become less able to fight cancer after the injections, then general debilitation, and not cancer, was the reason cancer patients were less able to fight cancer. The research was funded in part by Sloan-Kettering, the U.S. Public Health Service, and the American Cancer Society.

The consent process in the study was terribly flawed. Some patients did not have decision-making capacity. Others had it, but they were not told they were being given injections of cancer cells. No written records of the consent process were kept.

An attorney on the JCDH's Board of Directors became concerned about the hospital's exposure to liability for injecting patients with cancer cells and the possible moral abuse of the patients. The research was then investigated, and Dr. Southam, along with the medical director at JCDH, who had approved of the study without submitting it to his hospital's research committee, were both placed on probation for a year. The Board of Regents of the State University of New York found the physicians guilty of fraud, deceit, and unprofessional conduct. The involvement of the U.S. Public Health Service in the obviously unethical study helped alert it and other government agencies to the need for ethical guidelines governing federally funded research.

Obedience Tests at Yale University (1960–63)

Behavioral research is also an issue for health care ethics, and in the 1960s and early 1970s attention was drawn to several ethically questionable studies in this field. A widely publicized case involved the studies on obedience conducted at Yale University by Stanley Milgram. Milgram was interested in learning about how human beings react to a person in authority, even when that person directs them to do things against their better judgment.

Subjects for the study were recruited by newspaper advertisements and were paid a nominal fee for their participation. Eventually, they numbered over a thousand. Researchers told the participants that the study was designed to determine how punishment might stimulate memory. They were then put at the controls of a device that generated electric shocks ranging from 15 volts ("Slight Shock") to 450 volts (a stage beyond "Danger—Severe Shock"). The person whose memory was being tested was strapped in a chair with electric wires from the device attached to his wrists. He was given lists of word pairs to memorize. Each time he failed to memorize the words, the person at the controls was ordered to apply an electric shock and to increase the voltage by 15 volts after each failure. The person at the controls had been given a sample of a 45-volt shock before the experiment started—it caused a mild jolt.

As the memory failures multiplied, the people receiving the shocks of increasing intensity began to manifest distress. They groaned at 75 volts, complained of pain at 120 volts, demanded to be released at 150 volts, and screamed in agony at 285 volts. By 300 volts they were speechless. Naturally the people applying the shocks began to hesitate as they saw the distress and questioned the researcher about continuing. The researcher assured them that the experiment must go on for the advancement of science, that the shocks were painful but not really dangerous, and that the researcher would accept full responsibility for whatever happened.

People giving the shocks expressed serious reservations. Some said they did not want to continue but they did give additional shocks after the researcher adamantly ordered them to continue. The test ended either when the person giving the electric shocks disobeyed the researcher and refused to continue or when the person failing to memorize the word pairs received the maximum shock—450 volts.

Researchers conducting the study were surprised by what happened. Even though nobody at the controls really wanted to give the full shock treatment, almost two out of three (62 percent) went all the way to 450 volts. In other words, most people obeyed the authority figures even though they were not threatened with any punishment for disobedience and even though they were convinced that they were inflicting pain on a screaming human being begging to be released from the experiment.

Of course, there were no shocks. The screaming "victims" were acting—they were not receiving any electrical charges. They were not being tested for memory or for anything else. It was the people giving the shocks who were being tested, and the results were upsetting. Researchers found that if people in authority give orders, many will follow them even though they feel what they are doing is wrong.

As the research became known, criticism grew. Critics pointed out that the subjects could not have given informed consent for the research project because they had been deceived about its true nature and that the researchers had not explained all the risks to them. Indeed, a number of subjects did become upset when they realized how weak they had been and how easily they had obeyed orders to harm others. They felt the experiment had truly harmed them, yet they had not been warned of any risks when they agreed to take part, and information about risks is crucial to informed consent.

REACTIONS TO THE QUESTIONABLE MEDICAL RESEARCH

By the 1960s a growing sense of discomfort about these and other studies led to several important initiatives that have raised the moral level of medical research. The major stages in that story are as follows.

The Work of Henry Beecher

A major turning point came in 1966 when Henry Beecher published an article in the *New England Journal of Medicine* titled "Ethics and Clinical Research." Beecher, a distinguished professor of research in anesthesia at Harvard Medical School, reported twenty-two research projects where he felt the researchers had failed to provide the subjects with adequate information or to obtain truly voluntary consent. Although the article did not identify the research projects (he did, however, identify the research for the editors of the *Journal*, and they verified that the facts were true), Beecher claimed they represented mainstream research in the past fifteen years.

In almost every study, the subjects selected were in situations where truly voluntary consent would be impossible or difficult to obtain. Many were military personnel, charity patients, newly born or retarded children (Willowbrook was one of Beecher's examples), very elderly, terminally ill, or alcoholics with advanced cirrhosis of the liver. One of Beecher's conclusions was that ethically questionable medical research was the rule and not the exception. He also believed that investigators failed to disclose risks fully or to seek true consent because they were under such intense pressure to achieve tenure on the faculties of medical schools and to advance their careers.

The research cited by Beecher was indeed mainstream. Published reports of the studies he identified had appeared in such journals as the *Journal of the American Medical Association*, the *New England Journal of Medicine*, *Circulation*, and the *Journal of Clinical Investigation*. Fourteen of the twenty-two protocols were in university medical schools and hospitals, including Harvard Medical

School, the University of Pennsylvania, Georgetown, Ohio State, New York University, Northwestern, Emory, and Duke. Three of the studies had been conducted at the National Institutes of Health (NIH). Funding for the research came from such sources as the Armed Forces Epidemiology Board, the NIH, the U.S. Public Health Service, the Atomic Energy Commission, and large drug companies including Parke-Davis and Merck. Beecher also reported that these twenty-two cases were not the only problems he found. He had identified another twenty-eight instances of ethically suspicious research but did not include them in the article for lack of space.

It is of interest to note, in passing, that Beecher did not believe that rules and regulations, although necessary, could solve the problem of unethical research. He argued that rules often do more harm than good and that they never curb the unscrupulous. Ethical abuses in medical research, he felt, will be eliminated only if researchers actually become good and decent people— that is, virtuous. His conviction that ethics is more a matter of being good, of being virtuous, rather than a matter of following rules and regulations (or principles or laws) echoes, of course, a fundamental theme of this book.

As we will see, however, government regulations did play a major role in elevating the moral level of medical research after Beecher's report. This history suggests that rules and regulations do play an important role in an ethics of virtue. Although following rules and regulations is not the essence of ethics, the rules and regulations can be very helpful in guiding people to a good life. And they are needed for medical researchers who have not developed a sufficient degree of character excellence to make good moral decisions. Aristotle, ever the realist, thought most people never develop adequate character excellence and thus he said that we need laws and regulations to force, if necessary, the achievement of the human good.

Beecher's work made an immediate impact. He enjoyed a reputation as a respected researcher himself and had previously published a book, titled *Experimentation in Man*, where he tried to increase awareness about the complex moral issues involved in research on human subjects. Once his 1966 article broke the ice by pointing out the widespread lack of ethical concern in many cases of medical research, other literature about questionable research soon followed. M. H. Pappworth's *Human Guinea Pigs: Experimentation on Man* appeared in 1967, Beecher's own *Research and the Individual* in 1970, and Jay Katz's *Experimentation with Human Beings* in 1972. Pappworth listed over five hundred papers where he found the research questionable from a moral point of view, and Katz presented a wide-ranging collection of materials from psychology and law as well as medicine that revealed the tension between protecting the humanity of the subject and advancing medical research to benefit humankind.

Early Federal Initiatives

Even before Beecher's article, some federal efforts to establish ethical guidelines for research had begun in the United States. In 1953, for example, an NIH policy called for peer review of research at the NIH to protect human subjects from undue risks. In 1966 the Surgeon General William Stewart issued a *Statement of Policy* on clinical investigations using human subjects. It required approval of research funded by the Public Health Service by a committee of the principal investigator's "institutional associates." The committee was to review three things: (1) the subject's rights and welfare, (2) the methods of obtaining informed consent, and (3) the risks and potential medical benefits.

After Beecher's revelations, the Department of Health, Education and Welfare ([HEW], the predecessor of the Department of Health and Human Services [HHS]) issued *The Institutional Guide to DHEW Policy on Protection of Human Subjects* (1971). This guide also emphasized both institutional review and informed consent in medical research. By this time the committees reviewing research proposals were being called "institutional review boards"; this phrase, sometimes shortened to IRB, remains popular today.

After the Tuskegee study became public in 1972, HEW appointed a panel to review that case as well as the then current policies for the protection of research subjects. In 1973 the panel recommended the immediate termination of the Tuskegee study and noted that sound policies for the protection of human subjects simply did not exist. That same year the American Psychological

Association adopted a code of research ethics titled Ethical Principles in the Conduct of Research with Human Participants. And from February to July 1973 the congressional committee chaired by Senator Kennedy continued to examine now well-known cases such as Willowbrook and Tuskegee and to hear testimony from Jay Katz and others on the lack of protection for human subjects in many research protocols, most of them funded by federal money.

The National Commission (1974–78)

The time was ripe for legislative action, and Congress responded by passing the National Research Act in July 1974. This act created the *National Commission for the Protection of Human Subjects of Biomedical and Behavioral Research* (henceforth, the National Commission). This commission existed until 1978 and was one of the most influential factors in the development of medical ethics during that decade.

When Congress set up the National Commission, it directed the members to "conduct a comprehensive investigation and study to identify *the basic ethical principles* which should underlie the conduct of biomedical and behavioral research involving human subjects" and to "develop guidelines which should be followed in such research to assure that it is conducted *in accordance with such principles*" (Sec. 202 [a][1][A], emphasis added). In effect, Congress directed the National Commission to develop not simply an ethics of medical and behavioral research but a particular kind of ethics, an ethics based on principles. Beecher's plea for an ethics of virtue was forgotten.

Yet it is doubtful that anything but federal guidelines would have been effective in the climate of that time. A virtue ethics, after all, takes a long time to develop in a moral agent. It assumes a period of moral education and requires a maturity that comes only with experience. Given the abuses and the pressing questions about new medical research, something was needed immediately. Regulations and rules were the answer, and it was assumed that principles were needed to justify the rules.

Prompted by Congress, the eleven members of the National Commission set out to identify the basic ethical principles of medical research and to develop effective mechanisms for their implementation. Their work lasted four years (1974–78) and resulted in two major reports. The first is known as *The Belmont Report: Ethical Principles and Guidelines for the Protection of Human Subjects of Research*, and the second is *Institutional Review Boards: Report and Recommendations*. It will be helpful to comment briefly on both of these reports.

The *Belmont Report* endorsed a model of ethics known as *applied normative ethics*, sometimes called *principlism* today. According to this model, ethics begins with a few basic principles. The commissioners defined a basic ethical principle as a "general judgment that serves as a basic justification for the many particular prescriptions for and evaluations of human actions." The report identified three such principles: respect for persons (treating people as autonomous), beneficence, and justice. These principles serve as the basis for developing more precise second-order norms or rules. The rules are then applied to individual cases to determine what actions are ethical.

Although the National Commission was concerned with medical research, the model of ethics whereby principles provide an "objectively or absolutely valid moral action-guide" was appealing to many people struggling to develop a coherent ethics for all medical practice in an age of rapidly developing new techniques and technologies. More recently, however, some ethicists are becoming uncomfortable with an ethics grounded on "objectively or absolutely valid" principles and their derived rules. Among the critics is a former member of the National Commission itself, Albert Jonsen, who stated: "As a Commissioner, I participated in the formulation of that (Belmont) Report. . . . Today I am skeptical of its status as a serious ethical analysis. I suspect that it is, in effect, a product of American moralism, prompted by the desire of Congressmen and of the public to see the chaotic world of biomedical research reduced to order by clear and unambiguous principles."

The model of applied normative ethics wherein principles and rules are applied to particular cases is not, of course, the model we are using in this text. Here the model is an ethics based not on principles but on the natural inclination of each moral agent to seek what is truly good for herself. Whatever contributes to this good, rightly understood, is considered ethical. Principles and rules remain important, but they do not determine in the last analysis how a moral agent behaves morally well. This is determined by prudence, and any principles or rules in an ethics of prudential reasoning are derivative guidelines, not foundational norms or absolutely valid action-guides.

The second report of the National Commission, *Institutional Review Boards*, was every bit as important as the *Belmont Report*. It recommended oversight of all proposed medical research by an institutional committee responsible for protecting human subjects. These IRBs are required by HHS in all institutions receiving federal money for research. The actual name of the board varies from facility to facility, but IRB is the generic title of these boards.

The primary purpose of the IRB is to balance protection of human subjects with the need for research on human subjects. Hence, a major responsibility of the IRB is to ensure that the subjects of research, or their appropriate proxies, receive adequate information and are able to give truly voluntary consent. Among the things a subject or proxy must know are these facts: the purpose of the study, that it involves research, the foreseeable risks or discomfort that may be experienced, benefits the subjects or others might receive, alternative treatments available, and, if the risk is more than minimal, whether or not compensation and medical care for injuries are available. Subjects must also be told that their participation is voluntary, that they may withdraw at any time, and that their refusal to participate or their decision to withdraw will not penalize them or detract from their proper medical care in any way.

The IRB is typically composed of physicians, nurses, social workers, chaplains, pharmacists, and administrators from the institution. It also includes several representatives from the community, people not affiliated with the institution. The federally mandated IRBs have been able to maintain a level of ethical integrity in medical research.

The major reason for the lasting impact of the National Commission is the fact that many of its recommendations became the basis for regulations promulgated by HEW, later HHS, and by the Food and Drug Administration (FDA). These agencies instituted an extensive set of regulations for research on human subjects in 1981 and have since added important amendments, most notably in 1991. The federal regulations are taken seriously because most hospitals that conduct research receive federal funding (chiefly research grants, Medicare, and Medicaid) and are therefore required to follow them.

The President's Commission (1980–83)

The *President's Commission for the Study of Ethical Problems in Medicine and Biomedical and Behavioral Research*, which met from 1980 to 1983, issued a number of reports pertaining to research on human subjects. The President's Commission supported the National Commission's insistence on informed consent, the IRBs, and the use of ethical principles (sometimes it called them values) as norms for making ethical judgments. The final report of the President's Commission acknowledged the National Commission had appealed to the now familiar ethical principles of autonomy, beneficence, and justice. It stated that these principles "are a basic part of the Western cultural and philosophical traditions" and cited both the National Commission's *Belmont Report* and an important text titled *Principles of Biomedical Ethics*, written by two leading ethicists, Tom Beauchamp and James Childress, as evidence that these principles have "special importance in evaluating the ethical implications of decisions, actions, and policies in medicine and biomedical and behavioral research."

The reactions to the morally questionable research of several decades ago led to many positive developments in the ethics of research involving human subjects. Thanks to increased moral awareness, the federal requirements of informed and voluntary consent, and oversight by IRBs, a significant level of moral responsibility has now been achieved in medical research.

Nonetheless, problem cases continued to be reported in the following years. Toward the end of 1993, for example, three cases of questionable moral procedures emerged. First, three prominent cancer researchers at the Montefiore Medical Center in New York admitted in statements to the U.S. Attorney that they had used an unapproved drug on sixteen patients with brain cancer in 1987. The FDA had approved the experimental drug for kidney cancer but not for brain cancer. When the project was investigated by the FDA, the NIH, and the FBI, the physicians involved, according to the *New York Times* (October 28, 1993), had lied in an effort to cover up the unapproved use of the drug.

It was also reported by the *New York Times* (October 5, 1993) that five of fifteen subjects in an NIH trial of a new drug (Fialuridine or FIAU) designed to combat hepatitis B died as a result of taking the drug. The consent form indicated that subjects had been told of six specific risks (fatigue, nausea, rashes, bone marrow suppression, seizures, and pains or numbness in the arms and legs) but not that the drug might be lethal. The consent form also said that "FIAU is a new medication, and its side effects have not been completely described." Although the researchers did not expect any deaths to result from the research, some ethicists felt that the IRB review of the research proposal was not adequate because the information given the subjects was vague, incomplete, and somewhat misleading, especially for sick patients looking for a cure after they had not benefited from the standard treatment for hepatitis B.

Finally, the *New York Times* reported on December 16, 1993, that one of the world's largest manufacturers of medical devices, C. R. Bard of New Jersey, agreed to plead guilty to many crimes, including the shipping of adulterated products for human experimentation. The company agreed to pay a fine of $61 million, the largest penalty to that date for health care fraud. The chairman of the company and five former executives also faced criminal charges.

What had happened? One of Bard's divisions manufactured catheters that are used in balloon angioplasty, a procedure designed to open blocked arteries. The procedure was first used in 1980 and is now performed frequently. In February 1988 Bard was aware that one of its catheter designs sometimes failed to deflate, but it concealed this information when it sought FDA approval for the product. Once the product had been approved, some of these catheters did fail to deflate, and a few people died as a result. Bard hastily redesigned the catheter and then sold the modified design without proper FDA approval. When the FDA finally caught up with the company, the FDA commissioner was quoted as saying that Bard was "using unsuspecting patients as guinea pigs and operating rooms as laboratories for unapproved products."

Stories such as these still appear all too frequently. They remind us of the ongoing vigilance needed to ensure the protection of human subjects in contemporary medical research and in the development of new medical techniques and technologies. And a series of disclosures in 1994 of earlier questionable government research involving radiation studies years ago also reminds us of how important moral oversight is in medical research.

Advisory Commiteee on Human Radiation Experiments (1994–96)

President Clinton formed the Advisory Committee on Human Radiation Experiments in January 1994 as the result of allegations that the United States had treated human subjects unethically in its radiation research in the thirty years prior to 1974, when HEW adopted research regulations and the National Commission for the Protection of Human Subjects began its work. The task of the Advisory Committee was to review the history of radiation experiments involving both medical research and nuclear weapons testing during the 1944–74 period as well as some current research programs and then to make recommendations to ensure that whatever abuses occurred in the past would not happen again.

The fourteen members of the committee and its staff did an extraordinary amount of work that included reviewing hundreds of thousands of government documents, some declassified at the committee's request; surveying or interviewing thousands of people including both researchers and research subjects; and offering a series of significant recommendations applicable to future research on human subjects.

To no one's surprise, the Committee found cases where medical researchers had ignored prevailing ethical standards. Singled out for harsh criticism were dangerous experiments conducted on patients without their knowledge or consent and of no possible benefit to them. Physicians, for example, had injected plutonium into unknowing patients at the Universities of Chicago and California at San Francisco and had injected uranium into dying patients at the University of Rochester and at Massachusetts General Hospital. Their goal was not to help their patients in any way but to observe the impact of radioactive substances on these patients.

After reviewing the radiation experiments of earlier years, the Committee looked at 125 research projects funded during fiscal years 1990–93 and found evidence suggesting that people enrolled in medical research were still not being adequately protected. The committee made a series of thoughtful recommendations to improve the work of the IRBs and to raise the moral level of both federally funded and non-federally funded research. Its *Final Report* published in 1996 is an important text for anyone interested in medical research.

What normative ethical framework did the members of the Advisory Committee rely on for making their numerous moral judgments? As did the National Commission in the 1970s and the President's Commission in the 1980s, it decided to forget theoretical foundations and simply set out some basic ethical principles. Whereas the earlier commissions had set forth three basic principles—autonomy, beneficence, and justice—the Advisory Committee proposed the following six principles:

- One ought not to treat people as mere means to the ends of others.
- One ought not to deceive others.
- One ought not to inflict harm or risk of harm.
- One ought to promote welfare and prevent harm (beneficence).
- One ought to treat people fairly and with equal respect (justice).
- One ought to respect the self-determination of others (autonomy).

The Advisory Committee's six ethical principles "state moral requirements; they are principles of obligation telling us what we ought to do." And where do these principles emanate from? What justifies the committee's claim that researchers ought to follow these six principles? There is no attempt at justification; the committee simply "settled on a list of immediately recognizable and widely accepted ethical principles that are not usually thought to require justification themselves." The committee held that these "basic ethical principles are general standards or rules that all morally serious individuals accept" and "are so basic that we ordinarily assume, with good reason, that they are applicable to the past as well as the present (and will be applicable in the future as well)."

However, the committee's claim that its six ethical principles or rules are "not usually thought to require justification" is puzzling. Philosophers advocating principle-based ethics have struggled for decades to provide a justification for their proposed action-guiding principles in utilitarian and deontological ethical theories or in some kind of universally valid common morality. Admittedly they have failed to develop any widely accepted justification for their principles, but they have not thereby concluded that the action-guiding principles do not require justification. Commissions and committees may not have the luxury of pursuing theoretical foundations for the principles they propose, but that does not mean that moral philosophers have concluded that principles do not require justification. Philosophy always looks for reasons, and if reasons cannot be given, it gives reasons why reasons cannot be given.

Moreover, not all morally serious people accept the committee's action-guiding principles and rules as basic. As we have seen, such a claim fails to recognize a long tradition of virtue-based ethics that does not consider moral principles and rules basic; in fact, virtue ethics considers principles, laws, and rules as premoral guides for those who are not yet ethical, that is, for those not yet able to manage their lives in a virtuous way. Finally, the committee's claim that its principles are "widely accepted" and applicable to the past and to the future is somewhat surprising in light of well-known cultural and historical differences of opinion concerning some of these principles.

National Bioethics Advisory Commission (1996–2001)

A presidential executive order established the National Bioethics Advisory Commission (NBAC) in October 1995 just as the Advisory Committee on Human Radiation Experiments was about to issue its final report with criticisms of recent federally funded research in the United States. The commission had two priority areas: the ethics of human subjects research and of the possible uses of genetic information. The presidential order establishing the commission also reinforced the principle-based ethics that had driven the National Commission in the 1970s by instructing NBAC to "identify broad principles to govern the ethical conduct of research."

After a slow start—its first meeting did not occur until almost a year after it had been created—the commission steadily gained momentum and was meeting regularly by the end of the 1990s. It received a big boost in 1997, as we saw in chapter 10, when President Clinton asked it to prepare a report on cloning within ninety days. Its June 1997 report was titled *Cloning Human Beings*. During its existence the NBAC issued a series of helpful reports that are available on online:

- *Research Involving Persons with Mental Disorders That May Affect Decisionmaking Capacity* (December 1998)
- *Research Involving Human Biological Materials: Ethical Issues and Policy Guidance* (August 1999)
- *Ethical Issues in Human Stem Cell Research* (September 1999)
- *Ethical and Policy Issues in International Research: Clinical Trials in Developing Countries* (April 2001)
- *Ethical and Policy Issues in Research Involving Human Participants* (August 2001)

The title of the NBAC's last report signals a shift in terminology. The *National Commission for the Protection of Human Subjects* (1974–78) and the subsequent literature of research spoke of the people enrolled in clinical trials as "human subjects." That phrase is now increasingly replaced by "human participants," an important shift emphasizing that the people in clinical trials are better viewed and better protected if they are not thought of as *subjects* of medical research but as *participants* and partners with the people conducting the trials.

President's Council on Bioethics (2001–09)

President George W. Bush established this Council in 2001, and in 2007 he extended its existence to September 2009 by executive order. However, in June 2009, the Obama administration directed the PCB to stop meeting, so it effectively ceased to exist at that time. It did not focus on research as much as did the NBAC, but several of its reports have some relevance to research:

- *Human Cloning and Human Dignity: An Ethical Inquiry* (July 2002)
- *Beyond Therapy: Biotechnology and the Pursuit of Happiness* (October 2003)
- *Monitoring Stem Cell Research* (January 2004)
- *The Changing Moral Focus of Newborn Screening* (December 2008)

The PCB also published an important white paper relevant to research titled *Alternative Sources of Human Pluripotent Stem Cells* in May 2005. We will look at this white paper in the next section of this chapter.

The task of moral awareness and oversight in research is made all the more difficult because some populations of human subjects present unique and complicated problems for ethical consideration. We now consider several such populations.

RESEARCH ON EMBRYOS

Discussion about doing research on human embryos actually goes back to the 1970s when people began to foresee the possibility of fertilizing ova in a Petri dish and then transferring them into a woman by the process of in vitro fertilization (IVF). When science began fertilizing ova in vitro, these ova became readily available for research, and thus, the ethical question of using them for research quickly arose. In August 1975 HEW issued a regulation requiring review by an ethics advisory board (EAB) before it would allow federal funding for research on in vitro embryos. HEW did not establish this EAB until September 1977. The next year, 1978, the world's first IVF baby was born in England.

In 1979 the EAB received its first proposal for federally funded research on in vitro embryos, and it responded with an analysis and recommendations. The Board recognized the intense debate over the moral status of the in vitro embryo: Is it deserving of protection as soon as it exists or only later in its development? The EAB concluded "that the human embryo is entitled to profound respect; but this respect does not necessarily encompass the full legal and moral rights attributed to persons." Hence, the EAB took the position that some research on human embryos would be ethically acceptable. However HEW did not adopt the EAB's recommendations and did not allow federal funding for research involving human embryos.

Then a rather strange situation transpired. The administration of Ronald Reagan, elected in 1980, declined to renew funding for the EAB, and thus, it ceased to exist. Yet the regulation requiring its approval for federally funded research on human embryos remained in force. In effect, then, there was a de facto moratorium on federally funded research on human embryos because federal funds could not be provided without EAB approval and there was no EAB to give approval after 1980. Only in 1993, when Congress omitted the regulation requiring approval from the nonexistent EAB in the National Institutes of Health Revitalization Act, did federally funded embryo research once again become a possibility. During this time, of course, much privately funded embryo research had continued.

After the 1993 NIH Revitalization Act gave NIH the authority to release federal funds for human embryo research, NIH set up the Human Embryo Research Panel to set guidelines for the federally funded embryo research. The Panel recommended that federal funds could be used for research in IVF clinics on human embryos that had been frozen but were no longer wanted and also for research on human embryos created *in vitro* precisely for research. The Panel based its recommendations on three factors: (1) the promise of significant benefit from the research, (2) human embryos deserve serious moral consideration but not the same consideration as infants because they lack sentience and suffer a natural high rate of loss, and (3) federal funding will provide federal regulatory and ethical oversight of the research, something that is now lacking in the private sector. President Clinton immediately rejected the use of federal funds to create embryos for research but accepted the recommendations for funding research on the "left over" or "spare" IVF embryos frozen in IVF clinics.

Before NIH released any funds for embryo research, however, a new Congress in 1996 stepped in to prevent any federally funded research that would create or destroy human embryos. Representative Jay Dickey of Arkansas authored an amendment to the annual NIH appropriations bill that prohibited NIH funds from being used to support research involving the creation of embryos in any way (fertilization, cloning, parthenogenesis, or any other way) or for research that would subject existing embryos to the risk of injury or death greater than the minimal risks that federal regulations allow for research on fetuses. The Dickey amendment, as it is called, was added to subsequent annual NIH appropriations bills. In effect it prevented federal funding for any research involving more than minimal risk to the embryo. Although it prevented federal funds from being used in research that destroyed embryos, it also pushed all embryonic research into the private sector where scientists could move forward without any federal oversight of their research on human embryos. The Dickey amendment thus actually undermined federal oversight of research involving human embryos.

Destructive Embryonic Stem Cell Research

In 1998 human embryo research took on a dramatic new urgency when scientists led by James Thomson at the University of Wisconsin, supported in large part by the biotechnology company Geron, published the first report showing that stem cells could be removed from human embryos and then multiplied indefinitely in cultured cell lines. The removal, of course, destroys the embryos. These embryonic stem cells have two very important properties. First, they are pluripotent; that is, they are not yet differentiated into specific cells (heart cells, liver cells, brain cells, etc.), but they will differentiate if placed with other differentiated cells (insert them in a liver and they will become liver cells). Second, they can be cultured to produce an almost unlimited supply of copies of themselves in cell lines.

Because of the significant therapeutic potential of the pluripotent human embryonic stem cells, some thought that Congress should now relax its ban on federal funds for embryonic stem cell research, but the renewal of the Dickey amendment each year continued to block federal funding. The problem, of course, is that retrieving the stem cells destroys the embryo, and this reawakened the intense abortion controversy that has played such a dominant role in the United States since the 1973 *Roe v. Wade* decision.

The ability of scientists to retrieve and cultivate embryonic stem cells with their immense therapeutic potential introduced a whole new chapter on embryo research and significantly raised the intensity of the debate about research on human embryos. In 1999 NBAC released its report on *Ethical Issues in Human Stem Cell Research*. It acknowledged "that although the human embryo and fetus deserve respect as forms of human life, the scientific and clinical benefits of stem cell research should not be foregone." It recommended federal funding for research on embryos left over after IVF fertility treatments but not for embryos created for research by fertilization or by cloning. It also recommended a comprehensive informed consent process that makes it clear to the donors of the embryos that the research will destroy the embryos. It further stipulated that researchers should disclose their source of funding and expected commercial benefits they might receive.

The Dickey amendment prevented NIH from following any of NBAC's recommendations. The NIH, trying to find a way around the Dickey amendment, suggested in 1999 that federal funds could be used for human embryonic research as long as the federally funded research was not involved in obtaining the stem cells from the embryos. In other words, research supported by private funds had to obtain the stem cells from embryos, but federally funded research could then work with cell lines developed by the private sources. Clinton left office before any such research took place, and the NIH under the new administration of George W. Bush showed no interest in pursuing this controversial interpretation of the Dickey amendment.

At the turn of the new century, then, the situation in the United States was that (1) privately funded stem cell research on human embryos was perfectly legal, but (2) federal funding for it was not possible if the creation or destruction of human embryos were involved (the Dickey amendment). This dual approach reflects two very vocal groups in the United States. One group believes that the failure to pursue human stem cell research is clearly immoral because of the tremendous good such research might well accomplish for suffering people. Another group believes human embryo research, including stem cell research, is clearly immoral whenever it involves the destruction of human embryos, an act that can never be right no matter what good may come from the research.

On August 9, 2001, President Bush stepped into the controversy. In a nationally televised speech he announced his decision to allow the limited use of federal funds for embryonic stem cell research provided the stem cell lines have been derived from embryos that were destroyed before the date of his speech. In other words he was allowing federal funding for embryonic stem cell research as long as the cell lines came from embryos already destroyed; he did not allow federal funding for research that would destroy existing embryos or that would create embryos for research. In the same speech President Bush announced that he would form "a President's Council to monitor stem cell research, to recommend appropriate guidelines and regulations, and to consider all of the medical and ethical ramifications of biomedical innovation." This Council is the President's Council on Bioethics (PCB), and it began meeting in January 2002.

In January 2004 the PCB published its report *Monitoring Stem Cell Research*. The report discusses both embryonic and nonembryonic or "adult" stem cells. As the title indicates, it focuses on *monitoring* stem cell research and does not recommend any guidelines and regulations beyond noting the guidelines President Bush set forth in his 2001 address; namely, federal funding for embryonic stem cell research will be available only for research with stem cell lines that existed before August 9, 2001. The report provides a useful summary of the scientific, ethical, and legal landscape in stem cell research through 2003. Much of chapters 3 and 4 remain relevant despite the passage of time. Chapter 3 provides an excellent overview of moral arguments for and against embryonic stem cell research, and chapter 4 is written to help the nonscientist understand the science of human stem cell research together with its therapeutic promise and the host of scientific and ethical problems that need to be solved before we will see clinical benefits from the research.

Nondestructive Embryonic Stem Cell Research

In May 2005 the PCB published a white paper titled *Alternative Sources of Human Pluripotent Stem Cells,* which enumerated four possible ways that embryonic stem cells might be obtained without destroying embryos:

- Extracting stem cells from very early IVF embryos (four to eight cells) that have spontaneously stopped developing. Sometimes stem cells that appear normal can be harvested from these "dead" embryos, and they might one day provide embryonic stem cells lines.
- Extracting stem cells from living embryos. We already know how to remove a cell from an early (eight cell) embryo and examine it for genetic mutations in a process known as preimplantation genetic diagnosis (PGD), a process that does not prevent the embryo from developing into a normal child. Perhaps science can find a way to extract stem cells from early embryos (eight to twenty-four cells) without harming them. This is sometimes called "embryo biopsy." One cell is removed and originates a cell line; the remaining seven cells develop into a normal fetus.
- Extracting cells from an artificially created embryo-like organism. There are several ways that this might be done. One scientist on the PCB, William Hurlbut, has suggested that a modified form of cloning called *altered nuclear transfer* (ANT) could be used to create an embryo-type entity that is not really a human embryo but would have human stem cells. In his version of ANT, the nucleus of a somatic cell is altered by deleting a gene known as Cdx2, an essential gene that directs the organization and development of an embryo. Then the altered nucleus that can no longer organize itself is put into an enucleated ovum that has also been altered to prevent expression of Cdx2. The result is a kind of clone, but the cells in the entity cannot become organized and develop. The cells of the entity begin dividing as in any embryo but soon become stuck in a disorganized state. Hence, Hurlbut and his supporters argue, the entity is not really an embryo, and its stem cells can be harvested for research. Hurlbut's proposal is often called ANT-Cdx2. A second version of ANT not mentioned in the White Paper is called ANT-Oocyte Assisted Reprogramming (ANT-OAR). Here the somatic nucleus and the ovum that will receive it are each altered by switching on the genes that make an entity pluripotent before the somatic nucleus is put into the ovum. The result is an entity that is pluripotent from the moment of fusion. Normally both SCNT and ANT cloning (and fertilization) first result in a single cell that is *totipotent*—it can become any human cell—and then that cell divides into two *pluripotent* cells, one with Cdx2 that can organize and develop all the cells forming the human body and one without Cdx2 that can develop the cells forming the placenta. The ANT-OAR technique forces the entity resulting from the fusion of a somatic nucleus with an enucleated ovum to skip the totipotent state from the very beginning and thus makes it not really an embryo. Hence, some argue that harvesting stem cells from an ANT-OAR clone is not destroying a human embryo. In addition to forms of ANT, the White Paper presents another way to produce an embryo-like organism—a process called *parthenogenesis*. Here an ovum is biochemically stimulated to begin developing as if it were an embryo. Once it develops fifty to one hundred cells, it may have stem cells that could be harvested. This would destroy the developing ovum, but it would not really be the destruction of a human embryo in the eyes of many people because the twenty-three–chromosome human ovum, even if stimulated to develop into a multicell embryo-like entity, is not the same as the forty-six–chromosome entity that we recognize as a human embryo.
- Reversing differentiated somatic cells back into pluripotent cells. Research in cloning (SCNT) has already shown that differentiated DNA in a somatic cell can be reversed back into a dedifferentiated or pluripotent state. In cloning, when the nucleus of a differentiated somatic cell is inserted into an enucleated ovum, its DNA begins to behave in pluripotent

undifferentiated ways somewhat like the nucleus of an embryo before it begins developing the differentiated cells that will compose the offspring. This suggests the possibility of finding a way to coax differentiated somatic cells back into the undifferentiated pluripotent state that would make them equivalent to embryonic stem cells. If this could be done, we would have a way to retrieve pluripotent stem cells without destroying human embryos.

As of 2005, none of these alternatives had been developed to the point where they were providing usable human stem cells, and not everyone agrees that all these methods are ethically acceptable. The PCB White Paper, for example, considers the second procedure, the embryo biopsy, unethical because it imposes unacceptable risks on living embryos destined to become children for the sole purpose of obtaining stem cells for research. And they also "at this time" have ethical concerns about the ANT procedure because some members of the PCB worry about the ethics of producing human-like entities that will be used as factories for human cells. Others are opposed to ANT because they view the product of the ANT procedure not as a biological artifact but rather as a human embryo with a severe disability.

In January 2007 the Bush White House (not the PCB) published a document titled *Advancing Stem Cell Science without Destroying Human Life* and then issued an updated version in April 2007. This document provides a summary of the Administration's efforts to support all forms of stem cell research that do not cause more destruction of human embryos. It reiterates the four potential nondestructive sources of pluripotent embryonic stem cells identified by the PCB report (from dead embryos, from biopsy, from embryo-like artifacts, and from dedifferentiated cells) and adds a fifth that scientists had just announced. In January 2007 scientists reported that amniotic fluid contains pluripotent stem cells that have been shed by the fetus, and they announced that they had been able to grow brain, bone, liver, and muscle cells from these amniotic stem cells. These stem cells can be easily retrieved without destroying an embryo or a fetus. The document also reported significant progress in reversing differentiated somatic cells so they can function as undifferentiated pluripotent stem cells.

Induced Pluripotent Stem Cells

In late 2007, two separate published studies announced a major breakthrough in obtaining pluripotent stem cells. Scientists had used genetic engineering to turn ordinary adult skin cells back into pluripotent stem cells biologically equivalent to embryonic stem cells. Scientists at Kyoto University in Japan and another group working independently at the University of Wisconsin used viruses to transfer several altered genes into skin cells, which then began switching off the genes that made them function as skin cells, and soon they became undifferentiated pluripotent cells equivalent to embryonic stem cells. Scientists called these new cells "induced pluripotent stem cells" (iPSCs or iPS cells).

James Thomson, the scientist at the University of Wisconsin who was the first to isolate and culture stem-cell lines from human embryos back in 1998, and who was involved in the latest breakthrough, said that the reprogrammed skin cells "meet the defining criteria we originally proposed for human ES cells, with the notable exception that the iPS cells are not derived from embryos." If this technique is successful, the intense controversy about obtaining pluripotent stem cells from embryos may fade away. In a published interview Thomson was quoted as saying as much: "The world has changed. . . . It is the beginning of the end of the controversy that has surrounded this field. Over time these cells will be used in more and more labs. And human embryo stem-cell research will be abandoned by more and more labs." The ethical debate over embryonic stem-cell research may never be resolved, but it may become irrelevant.

It is important to note that this research only establishes another way that pluripotent stem cells can be obtained; it does not show that the pluripotent cells are safe and successful ways to reverse diseases. The same is true for the pluripotent stem cells derived from human embryos— science has not yet established their safety and success. In fact, the FDA did not approve the first clinical trial using human embryonic stem cells until January 2009, when it allowed Geron to begin a phase 1 trial with ten people to see whether using embryonic stem cells to reverse spinal cord injuries is safe. Researchers must enroll the participants within two weeks of their injury and then monitor them for one year. Only if these participants are not harmed will Geron proceed to seek approval for additional and larger clinical trials to determine whether the human embryonic stem cells are actually therapeutic. From this we can see that no stem cell therapy will be a reality any time soon.

If the iPS cells (induced pluripotent stem cells) are truly equivalent to embryonic stem cells, they will probably become the pluripotent cells of choice for scientific research, and this for several reasons. First, since they can be derived without destroying embryos, there will be no restriction on federal funds available for the research. Second, pluripotent stem cells derived from a patient's own skin cells will no longer run the risk of triggering an immune response as do pluripotent stem cells derived from embryos and embryo-like biological artifacts. Third, it lessens the need for human cloning, which many oppose but that some have said is necessary so we can obtain pluripotent stem cells matching the patient's genome. Fourth, it lessens the need for human-animal cloning, which many oppose but that some have said is necessary so we can obtain human embryos for research. (Great Britain already allows scientists to put a nucleus from a human somatic cell into an animal ovum to produce an embryo whose nuclear DNA will be human.) However, even if human embryonic stem-cell research will become obsolete if somatic cells can be reprogrammed back into pluripotent cells equivalent to embryonic cells, other forms of embryo research will be pursued so the moral questions about creating and destroying human embryos for research will remain.

Ethical Reflections

A traditional virtue-based approach toward research on human embryos would begin by asking whether or not the research will likely contribute to or undermine human flourishing understood as people living a noble and virtuous life. And a key factor in answering this question is arriving at a reasonable determination regarding the moral status of the embryo. We need to decide, and it is truly a decision, what value to accord human embryos that are human beings. If we consider human embryos as human beings that are "one of us," then it would be hard to think research that harms or destroys them would be morally reasonable. If we do not consider human embryos as human beings that are one of us, then it would be possible to think research that harms or destroys them would be morally reasonable in some situations; for example, in a situation where the research is the only way to advance important and beneficial scientific work.

Is a human embryo one of us? As was pointed out in chapter 6, human embryos are living human entities whose cell genomes are clearly human. This makes them human beings; that is, living beings with human DNA. But they are human beings in a unique state: immediately after fertilization they are microscopic beings of only one cell, and for the first few days of their existence after that they are multiple-cell beings that are not yet organized or differentiated, and whose future development to infancy is not very likely because most human embryos fail to implant; and some of those that do implant are lost during pregnancy because of spontaneous miscarriages. Moreover human embryos are human beings that can divide after several days into two distinct human beings that become identical twins, a possibility that does not favor thinking of early embryos as "one of us."

Analysis in virtue ethics tends to avoid extreme views, and in discussions about the moral status of an embryo there are two extreme views. One holds that even a one-cell human embryo is a person or equivalent to a person, or is a human individual with rights, including the right to life. People viewing human embryos this way generally conclude that it is immoral to destroy them intentionally even if the goal is to advance important and beneficial science. The other extreme view holds that an embryo is little more than a ball of undifferentiated cells. People viewing human embryos this way inevitably conclude that they can be created and used for research in view of the cures that might be achieved; in fact, they think it might be immoral not to use them for such important research.

There are more moderate positions. For example, NBAC said in its report *Ethical Issues in Human Stem Cell Research* (1999) that: "In our judgment, the derivation of stem cells from embryos remaining following fertility treatments is justifiable only if no less morally problematic alternatives are available for advancing the research." NBAC's view avoids the extremes by acknowledging that research harming human embryos is "morally problematic" yet can be justified as the lesser of evils if morally better alternatives are not available. Thus, NBAC recognizes that human embryos have moral value yet not a moral value equivalent to what we accord to "one of us." An analysis in virtue ethics would tend to explore, as did NBAC, a middle position whereby embryos are valued as human beings but not as what were described in chapter 6 as human beings-in-the-world, which would make them one of us.

A second factor that needs to be considered in determining whether research on human embryos contributes to or undermines human flourishing is considering whether scientists should produce these embryos in the laboratory, perhaps by fertilization in vitro with commercial ova and sperm or by cloning (putting the nucleus of a somatic cell into an enucleated ovum). It is one thing to argue, as some do, that embryo research is moral because it will use unwanted leftover embryos from IVF clinics that are going to die anyway, and it is quite another thing to advocate creating human embryos with the intention of destroying them for research. Intentions do count in ethics. Moreover, producing them by cloning, which has some medical advantages because a person in need of stem-cell treatment could thereby have stem cells with his own nuclear genome, introduces a whole new moral debate about human cloning, which many people find morally suspect even if it is restricted to embryos for research and not allowed for producing a child.

A third factor that needs to be considered in determining whether research on human embryos contributes to or undermines human flourishing is securing proper informed consent for the embryos that come from IVF clinics. Even before human stem cells were isolated and cultured in 1998, the NIH Human Embryo Research Panel (1994) concluded that the consent process must give donors specific information about the nature and purpose of the research as well as anything else reasonable persons might want to know before making a decision to release their embryos for scientific research. NBAC's 1999 Report on stem-cell research recognized the need for informed consent but did not go into details. The NIH Guidelines for Embyonic Stem Cell Research, which were published in the August 25, 2000, *Federal Register* but never became effective, were a little more explicit. They called for telling the patients who agreed to donate their excess embryos for research such information as the following: the cells or cell lines derived from your embryos may be around for many years; the embryo research may have commercial benefit, but you the donors will not receive any financial benefit from it; and the derivation of stem cells will destroy your embryos.

In 2005 the National Academy of Sciences and its Institute of Medicine, aware that the prohibition against using federal funds in most human embryonic stem-cell research meant that there was no federal oversight over much of human embryonic stem-cell research, published its *Guidelines for Embryonic Stem Cell Research*. It amended the *Guidelines* in 2007. Among other things, the *Guidelines* recommend that informed consent for donation to scientific research should be given at the time the embryos are released for research and not simply when the couple gave consent for the IVF procedures and that people should not be paid for donating their embryos or for donating sperm or eggs to make embryos for science. They also recommend informing people that their cell lines might exist for years, that they might be mixed with nonhuman cells in animal models, that the research with the cells might have commercial value for others but not for the donor of the embryos, that the embryos will be destroyed when the cells are taken, and that there could be risks of donating the embryos, e.g., if the couple changed their mind and wanted to use them for pregnancy at a later date, only to discover that they had been used for research.

And the NAS guidelines added an additional interesting recommendation: If the couple used gametes from other people to create the embryo, then the person whose sperm or ova was used must give consent before the embryo can be donated for research. In effect this means most embryos created in fertility treatments using commercial sperm or ova cannot be donated to research because sperm and egg donors (sellers) tend to remain anonymous. Fortunately there is growing concern about truly informed consent when it comes to people giving consent for researchers to use their embryos for research because, as a review of consent forms for the cell lines that are eligible for federal funding under the Bush guidelines reveals, there are some serious problems with the informed consent process.

A fourth factor that needs to be considered in determining whether research on human embryos contributes to or undermines human flourishing is recognition of the importance of prudent legislation and regulation. Political leaders need to consider what might make sense in a society where many people are ardently opposed to human embryonic research, some of them because of sincerely held religious beliefs. One reasonable solution might be what actually happened: political leaders might legally allow the research on embryos to take place but not support it with federal funds. In that way, people opposed to such research are not forced to see their tax dollars funding it. Some critics find this approach incoherent. If, they argue, you deny federal funds for destructive embryonic research because it is wrong but then you support it by allowing it to proceed with private funds, your position is contradictory. This criticism fails to recognize what Aristotle called political prudence. It may not be unreasonable, given the deeply held views of a considerable portion of citizens and despite a political dimension that is in play, for a person in a leadership position to accept the legality of human embryonic research but not support it financially with tax dollars.

A fifth factor that needs to be considered in determining whether research on human embryos contributes to or undermines human flourishing is the possibility of obtaining pluripotent cells functionally equivalent to embryonic stem cells without destroying embryos. If embryo-equivalent pluripotent cells can be obtained without destroying human embryos, and there are now indications this might be possible, then arguments favoring the destruction of human embryos to harvest their stem cells will cease to be reasonable.

RESEARCH ON FETUSES

The 1974 public law authorizing the National Commission contained two important items that affect research on the fetus: it directed the commission to produce a report on fetal research within four months after it began work, and it imposed a moratorium on federally funded fetal research while that report was being prepared. There were several reasons why Congress wanted immediate action on questions of fetal research. In January 1973, the *Roe v. Wade* decision had struck down all state laws protecting fetuses in the first two trimesters, and many feared that this would become an open invitation for unscrupulous research on human fetuses. The great fear was that the demands of fetal research would actually encourage the abortion of healthy fetuses for the wrong reasons and would not show respect for fetal human life.

At the same time, some upsetting reports of research on live fetuses both before and after abortions resulted in public demonstrations at NIH headquarters, although NIH had not been involved in the research. Then, in Boston, a grand jury indicted four physicians for allegedly violating an 1814 statute forbidding "grave-robbing," a law originally designed to prevent stealing from cemeteries. The physicians were conducting research to learn whether antibiotics given to a pregnant woman would also affect the fetus. Several women planning an abortion at Boston City Hospital agreed to take the antibiotics, and the physicians retrieved their fetuses after their abortions for examination. The district attorney claimed that the women had given consent for the medications, but not for the postmortem examinations of the fetuses. Hence, he accused the physicians of "grave-robbing." Although the charges were eventually dropped, the case made a significant impact on medical researchers.

More than a dozen state legislatures, no longer able to prevent abortions in the first two trimesters after *Roe v. Wade*, reacted by passing laws designed to prevent the use of aborted, or about to be aborted, fetuses in medical research. Some national guidelines were obviously needed, and this explains why the Congress pressed the National Commission for an early report on fetal research.

The National Commission produced its report in record time. Its *Research on the Fetus* appeared in April 1975, and its recommendations became the basis for federal regulations promulgated the following July. These regulations, with some changes and additional amendments over the years, are the regulations governing fetal research today.

Federal Regulations on Fetal Research

Some of the important highlights as found in Title 45, Code of Federal Regulations, Part 46 (45 CFR 46) are the following:

1. The fetus is a human subject deserving of care and respect. A fetus begins at implantation and continues for the duration of the pregnancy. Once expelled or extracted, the living human subject is still considered a fetus unless it is mature enough to survive outside the uterus, in which case it is no longer a fetus but an infant (46.203).

2. The federal regulations are not concerned with research on dead fetuses, or on fetal parts taken from them. Regulations for research on dead fetuses or on fetal materials (cells, tissue, etc.) are determined by state or local laws (46.210). Many states do have laws governing research on dead fetuses.

3. No research can be carried out on fetuses—even fetuses destined for legal abortions—unless first tried on animals (46.206).

4. No research can be carried out on pregnant women—even on women planning legal abortions—until experiments have also been conducted on women who are not pregnant (46.206). This is to ensure that the research on the woman will not put her fetus at risk.

5. Strict limitations govern research on fetuses during pregnancy, regardless of whether the woman desires a healthy birth or an abortion. The regulations allow research on a fetus in only two cases: if its purpose is the health needs of the fetus or if its purpose is important biomedical knowledge that cannot otherwise be obtained, and the risk to the fetus is "minimal" (46.208). Both parents must give consent for the research, although the man's consent is not necessary under certain specified conditions.

The definition of "minimal risk" to a fetus for research undertaken not for its health needs but for general scientific knowledge is difficult to determine. Some have suggested that "minimal risk" should be a variable notion tied to the age of the fetus. Thus, researchers should be very careful about harming a thirty-eight-week fetus but need not be so careful about harming a six-week fetus. In other words, the protection of immature fetuses in research need not be as great as the protection of mature fetuses. Hence, "minimal risk" for a mature fetus would not be the same as "minimal risk" for an early fetus.

Many object to this approach, claiming that the same level of protection should apply to fetuses of any age. Their position seems reasonable. It certainly is reasonable if the woman is hoping to give birth, but it also seems reasonable if she is planning on an abortion. Fetuses are defined as human subjects, and it is at least arguable that subjecting human subjects destined for destruction to risky research does not enhance but undermines the moral character of the researcher. Some, of course, will argue the other way and claim that it makes no sense to protect fetuses destined for abortion from research risks.

6. The regulations for research on fetuses after the pregnancy is ended are more complicated (46.209). The regulations envision three situations.

- *The fetus is living but not viable.* Research is permitted only if (1) the purpose is obtaining important biomedical knowledge not otherwise available, (2) the interventions will not cause cardiopulmonary arrest, and (3) the vital functions of the fetus will not be artificially maintained.
- *The fetus is viable.* The regulations are not concerned with research on a viable fetus. A viable fetus outside the uterus is an infant, and it is thus subject to the regulations governing research on children.
- *The fetus may be viable.* When it is not known whether or not the fetus is viable, research is not permitted unless (1) the purpose is to enhance the chances of its survival to viability or (2) the purpose is to obtain important biomedical knowledge not otherwise available and the research presents no risk to the fetus.

7. The regulations also direct the secretary of HEW to establish one or more ethics advisory boards to deal with the ethical, legal, social, and medical issues of fetal research (46.204). The EAB would be made up of people not employed by HEW and would include ethicists as well as representatives of the professions and of the general public. With the approval of the EAB, the secretary may waive or modify the regulations. The EAB would also offer advice on the ethical issues of fetal research and, if requested, on HEW's general policies, guidelines, and procedures. Finally, the EAB would approve all research on IVF. As we have already noted, the EAB never received funding after 1980, and thus it ceased to exist shortly after it began its work.

The government's discouragement of fetal research intensified in 1988. The assistant secretary of HHS, Dr. Robert Windom, imposed a moratorium on funding for any fetal research involving the transplantation of fetal tissue derived from elective abortions. Windom then appointed a panel—the Human Fetal Tissue Transplantation Research Panel or HFTTR—to study the issue. As we saw in chapter 11, the panel recommended that the research on fetal tissue transplantation be funded, provided certain ethical restrictions were observed. The NIH accepted the HFTTR panel's recommendations, but HHS continued the moratorium against funding fetal transplantation research.

When President Clinton took office in 1993, the moratorium on fetal tissue research was lifted, and in January 1994, the National Institute of Neurological Disorders and Stroke provided the first federal funding for fetal tissue research. It awarded $4.5 million to three institutions for research in transplanting fetal tissue from elective abortions to patients with Parkinson's disease.

Ethical Reflections

Research on fetuses is morally sensitive for many reasons. First, a fetus is human life, and whenever there is a question of real or possible damage to human life, moral deliberation and judgment are required. Damaging human life is not moral unless we have reasons that will justify the harm we cause or could cause. Moral reasoning about fetal research is an effort to strike a delicate balance between the risks imposed on the fetus and the benefits expected from the study.

Second, research requires informed consent. When the human subject is still a minor (under eighteen), the parents would normally be the ones to give consent for the research. In consenting to research affecting their children, parents are expected to protect their children from undue risks and harms. When the human subject is still a fetus, the pregnant woman would normally be the one to give consent for the research. In consenting to research affecting her fetus, she is expected to protect it from undue risks and harm. Although she certainly is motivated to protect the fetus if she intends to give birth, she has no reason to protect it if she intends to abort it. This creates a serious problem about the legitimacy of her giving consent for research on her fetus. The main purpose of informed consent in medical research is to protect the human subject, in this case the fetus. This purpose is lost if the woman giving the consent has already decided to destroy the fetus in an abortion. This is why some ethicists insist that a woman who has decided to abort a fetus is not the proper person to give consent for research on it, at least while it is alive.

Third, fetal research is often associated with abortion, and abortion is a highly controversial issue. Some researchers see great advantages for fetal research in legal abortion because once a woman has decided to abort her fetus, there is an opportunity to do research on drugs or diagnostic interventions that would be too dangerous for the fetus if the mother were intending to give birth. Other people take a different view. They fear that the use of fetuses for medical research will encourage more abortions because the promise of making a contribution to medical science will overshadow the moral issues involved in the abortion itself. Some people fear that desperate women may even become pregnant for the purpose of selling their aborted fetuses for research.

Fourth, the risks of fetal research are difficult to establish. We simply do not know as much about risks to the fetus as we do about risks to adults or children. For example, many fetuses (some say more than 15 percent) are spontaneously aborted after the pregnancy has begun. If these fetuses were the subjects of research, it would be difficult to know whether the research or some other factor were the cause of the miscarriage. The difficulty in assessing risks to fetuses makes moral judgments about fetal research difficult.

Fifth, the father's role in giving consent for the research is a sensitive issue. Some say that the father should assume some responsibility for the pregnancy he caused, and this implies that he should share in making decisions about medical interventions on the fetus. Others see the man's participation in decisions about the fetus as an intrusion into the control a woman should have over what happens inside her body. The issue remains a troubling one.

For these reasons research on fetuses is a very complicated moral subject. Given the sensitive nature of fetal research and the undeniable medical benefits that can accrue from it, what might be a reasonable ethical approach to the issue?

The recommendations of the National Commission and the subsequent federal regulations based on them that we outlined above are a good starting point. The Commission insisted that the fetus is a human subject from the time of implantation and thus deserves protection, as does any human subject of medical research. Unlike the *Roe v. Wade* decision, which offers no protection for a fetus before viability, the federal regulations governing fetal research do protect fetuses even before viability, and this is a positive first step.

In any moral evaluation of research on fetuses there are at least three major ethical concerns. First, we want to protect all human life and fetal human subjects from harm, yet acknowledge the benefits of research on fetal human subjects. Second, we want to acknowledge the importance of fully informed appropriate consent and insist on a proper place for it in fetal research. If a woman has decided to destroy her fetus, the issue of informed consent becomes complicated because she no longer has an interest in protecting it from risky interventions. Hence, some argue that the person intending to abort a fetus is not the proper person to give consent for research on it. Third, we want to separate fetal research from abortions that are not morally reasonable, otherwise researchers run the risk of being complicit in immoral actions. Certainly, people disagree on what reasons justify an abortion, but many people admit that some abortions are morally suspect. If we can adequately respond to these concerns with intelligent guidelines and, in addition, if we can avoid causing suffering in a fetus that has developed awareness, there are reasons for saying some fetal research is morally reasonable to acquire beneficial knowledge not otherwise available.

RESEARCH ON MINORS

In 1983 the HHS issued specific regulations governing research on children. The regulations (45 C.F.R. 46, Subpart D) allow four kinds of research on children:

- Research with no more than minimal risk is permitted.
- Research with more than minimal risk is permitted if it is intended to benefit the child.
- Research with a "minor increase" over minimal risk is permitted if it is likely to yield "generalizable knowledge" about the child's condition; that is, knowledge of benefit to others.
- Research not meeting these three conditions but which a panel of experts determines will present a reasonable opportunity to understand, prevent, or alleviate serious problems affecting the health and welfare of children, and which will be conducted in accord with sound ethical principles and the assent of the children, is also permitted.

Unfortunately, these categories are open to a rather wide range of different interpretations by the local IRBs reviewing the research proposals. The regulations governing research on adults (45 C.F.R. 46 Subpart A) do define "minimal risk" as a risk not greater than what a person encounters in routine physical or psychological tests, but no definition is given of a "minor increase" over minimal risk.

A major controversy has existed for years over the issue of informed consent for research on children. Parents or guardians normally give informed consent for medical interventions on children, unless the child is an emancipated minor or covered by one of the "minor treatment statutes" discussed in chapter 5. Informed consent given on behalf of people without decision-making capacity, however, normally follows the best interests standard; that is, parents should only consent to what is in the best interests of the child. Some research, of course, will be of no benefit to the child; in fact, it might even pose some risk or actually cause harm. This has created a controversy among ethicists.

Some ethicists have argued that no parent or guardian can give consent for any intervention that is not for the benefit of the child. One well-known health care ethicist, Paul Ramsey, held just such a position. Ramsey argued from the moral principle known as "respect for persons." According to this principle unless a person consents, we cannot use him for any experiments not directly beneficial to him, even if there is no risk involved. Since young children cannot give valid informed consent, no research involving them is morally justified.

Others disagree. Richard McCormick, for example, has argued that we can presume children would, if they could, consent to research posing no more than slight risk, even if it is of no benefit to them. Although McCormick's position appears reasonable, his reasoning in defense of it may not be the best. It is open to the same criticisms directed against the Massachusetts Supreme Judicial Court and its use of substituted judgment in cases involving children; namely, we have no reason for saying that we know what never-competent children would want if they were competent.

We can, however, morally justify limited research on children another way. In our discussion of permanently unconscious patients whose wishes are not known, we have acknowledged that the two usual standards of proxy decision making—substituted judgment and best interests—do not apply. We appealed to a third standard—reasonable treatment—to decide whether to continue treatment or medical nutrition. We could appeal to the same standard here for research on children not able to give consent. The reasonable treatment standard, for example, would allow parents to consent to something like drawing blood from a five-year-old child for research, even if the research would be of no conceivable benefit to the child. This reasonableness standard is consistent with the federal regulations allowing research of no benefit to the child, provided it creates no more than minimal risk for the child.

The federal regulations governing research on children also introduce an important consideration relevant to informed consent. They acknowledge that children usually cannot give informed consent but that something called "assent" is often possible. Under the regulations, the local IRB determines whether or not the child incapable of giving informed consent can nonetheless give or withhold assent to the research. In making the determination, the IRB considers the age, maturity, and psychological state of the child. In effect, the child's assent to the research means that she agrees to the procedures even though she is not yet capable of giving a truly informed and voluntary consent.

RESEARCH IN DEVELOPING COUNTRIES

Researchers from developed countries often sponsor medical research in undeveloped or developing countries. This international research introduces a number of unique ethical issues, especially when the research is conducted on people in poor countries facing severe public health problems. Among the ethical concerns are worries about truly informed and voluntary consent and about the exploitation of vulnerable and poorly educated people unlikely to receive any benefit from the research. The ethical questions are many. When, if ever, would it be ethical to use a placebo group in a random clinical trial when a known treatment already exists? When, if ever, would it be ethical to conduct research in other countries that would not be considered ethical in the United States? When, if ever, would it be ethical to conduct research in countries so poor that it is unlikely many people will ever receive the treatment that might be proven effective by the research? Finally, when, if ever, would it be ethical for Americans to conduct research abroad in violation of federal regulations?

Before looking at this controversial research we need to recognize the widespread scientific consensus that the best way to conduct drug research is by a double-blind random clinical trial with a control group that receives a placebo instead of the drug under investigation. We also need to know that there is a general moral consensus that clinical trials involving placebos should not normally be done when an effective treatment for the problem being studied already exists. This is so because the people in a placebo group will receive nothing during the trial—neither the known effective treatment nor the possibly effective treatment under study—and will thus be harmed by being denied a known treatment. There is an additional moral consensus that researchers should not conduct research in a foreign country that would not be allowed in their own country. There is also a moral consensus that research done in another country should somehow benefit the people of that country and not simply benefit the people of the country sponsoring the research.

Two Cases of Controversial HIV/AIDS Research in Developing Countries

Among the many ways people can become infected with HIV are two that involve natural and morally acceptable forms of human behavior: perinatal or vertical transmission, whereby mothers unfortunately infect their babies during pregnancy, birth, and nursing; and heterosexual marital transmission, whereby one spouse unfortunately infects the other. Ethically questionable research on both these forms of transmission has been conducted in developing countries, as the following case studies show. The first research project focused on a search to find less expensive ways to prevent perinatal HIV transmission, and the second focused on determining the relation of possible risk factors such as the viral load in the infected partner and the presence of a sexually transmitted disease in the uninfected partner to HIV transmission in conjugal couples.

Seeking Inexpensive Antiretroviral Treatment to Prevent Perinatal HIV Transmission

Each day about sixteen hundred HIV-positive mothers transmit HIV to their infants as they give birth or nurse their infants. Any research designed to reverse this tragic statistic confronts an explosive mix of ingredients: most of the human subjects will be poor and people of color living in developing countries, all the human subjects will be pregnant women and babies, there is an effective preventative treatment that prevents perinatal HIV transmission but is too expensive for widespread use in developing countries, and any people who develop the targeted disease—AIDS—seldom receive proper treatment as they die in great pain and discomfort.

In the 1990s a major controversy erupted over some AIDS research in several African countries and in Thailand. The studies focused on finding less expensive treatments to prevent the transmission of HIV from mothers to their infants during birth and nursing. By 1994 research had established that zidovudine (AZT) could reduce the vertical transmission of HIV from mothers to infants by as much as two-thirds. The landmark study is known as AIDS Clinical Trials Group study number 076 (ACTG 076). Unfortunately the antiretroviral treatment proven effective by ACTG 076 has two major drawbacks for developing countries. First, it is expensive—it costs almost $1000 a person, an exorbitant amount in countries where the annual income of most people is many times less than that and the per-capita expenditure on health care might be only a few dollars a year. Second, it is complicated—women must be seen early in pregnancy, take the AZT orally five times a day for at least twelve weeks, receive AZT by an IV line during delivery, forgo nursing, and give their babies oral AZT four times a day for six weeks after delivery. In countries of great poverty and minimal obstetrical care, then, the hope that many HIV-positive pregnant women will receive the 076 AZT protocol to protect their babies is not realistic. Understandably, researchers wanted to find a less expensive and a less complicated way to reduce vertical transmission of HIV to babies.

In September 1997 the *New England Journal of Medicine* published an article with the provocative title "Unethical Trials of Interventions to Reduce Perinatal Transmission of the Human Immunodeficiency Virus in Developing Countries." The language is strong—the authors claimed that fifteen of the sixteen ongoing studies on perinatal transmission of HIV in the developing world were unethical. What was happening here?

The Story

Recognizing the need for a simpler and more economical intervention than the ACTG 076 regimen to prevent the transmission of HIV from mothers to their babies, the World Health Organization (WHO) Global Program on AIDS convened a meeting in Geneva shortly after the 076 protocol was found successful in 1994. Twenty-eight researchers and other interested parties (but no ethicists) from eight developed and six developing countries quickly reached a consensus to begin drug trials designed to find less expensive and simpler ways to reduce the vertical transmission of the HIV infection.

Soon sixteen trials outside the United States were evaluating several simpler interventions of antiretroviral drugs, most notably whether a shorter course of AZT (perhaps as short as two or three weeks) would be as effective, or almost as effective, as the long and complicated 076 protocol. Ten of these sixteen trials were funded by the U.S. Government through agencies such as the Centers for Disease Control (CDC) and the NIH. Nine of the ten federally funded trials enrolled people in a placebo group and thus deprived them of a known effective treatment (the 076 AZT protocol). The major moral question, which will become clearer as we analyze the story, was: Is it ethical for researchers to conduct these studies and for the CDC and NIH to support them even though federal regulations would not allow these trials in the United States?

Ethical Analysis

Situational awareness.   We are aware of these facts in the AZT story.

1. The HIV infection is being transmitted to more than a half million babies a year through the placenta, body fluids at birth, and breast-feeding.

2. The proven 076 AZT protocol can reduce this number by more than half, but it is not a realistic option in poor countries because the regimen is expensive, complicated, and rules out breast-feeding.

3. Many researchers believed a shorter protocol of a few weeks might also be effective and wanted to use standard clinical trials with a randomized placebo group to find out. The World Health Organization's Global Program on AIDS supported this approach.

4. The CDC and the NIH funded many of the studies in foreign countries and thus supported clinical trials with the placebo group.

5. These clinical trials with a placebo group could not have been done in the United States because they would violate federal regulations. Moreover, a widespread consensus would consider them unethical because people randomized to the placebo would be deprived of an already known effective treatment during the trials.

We are also aware of these good and bad features in the story.

1. Transmission of the HIV infection from mothers to their babies is a terrible problem calling for an intense effort to reverse it.

2. It is unfortunate but true that the ACTG 076 regimen is too expensive and too complicated to save children in many countries where it is needed most.

3. The primary intention of the international researchers is good—they want to stop the spread of HIV and AIDS to babies in poor countries as quickly as possible.

4. Trials with a placebo group will knowingly let hundreds of babies enrolled in the program die, because researchers will withhold all antiretroviral drugs from them and their mothers to preserve the scientific value of the clinical trial.

Prudential Reasoning in the Perinatal AIDS Research Story

Here we look at the story from the perspectives of the researchers who followed the approach suggested by the WHO group, of the directors of the NIH and the CDC, and of the critics who claimed the placebo-based research was unethical.

Researchers' perspective. From the scientific point of view, the researchers' desire to use clinical trials with a placebo group is the best way to proceed. Double-blind clinical trials with a randomized placebo arm are the gold standard of drug research because they best show whether or not the drug regimen will be safe and effective in the particular population. The researchers could have conducted *equivalency* studies wherein both groups would receive AZT, one group the long 076 dose and the other the short experimental dose. Scientifically, however, an equivalency study is not as valuable as a clinical trial with a placebo group because we are not showing whether the group receiving the medication will do better than those not receiving it. There is no question, then, that from a scientific and probably from an epidemiological perspective the best way to proceed is by clinical trials with a placebo group.

Researchers also argued that trials with a placebo group, although not allowed in the United States because they would subject that group to unnecessary risk, are morally acceptable in undeveloped countries because those populations do not currently have any effective treatment available to prevent the mother-infant transmission of HIV, and hence, their risk is not increased by being in a placebo group. In other words, babies in a placebo group in the United States would be subjected to unnecessary risk because the 076 protocol is available in this country, but babies in a placebo group living in undeveloped poor countries would not be subjected to *unnecessary* risk because the 076 AZT regimen is simply not available in their country.

Finally researchers argued that they are not exploiting people who were put at risk in their research but will probably not benefit from it because their job is research and not resource allocation. All they can do is to supply local health authorities with good scientific data. If those authorities do not allocate the resources to provide effective treatments for their populations, then they are the ones deserving of ethical criticism, not the researchers who are providing data with the hope that political leaders will use it wisely to help their people.

NIH and CDC perspective. Once criticism of the federally funded trials surfaced, the directors of the NIH and the CDC, Drs. Harold Varmus and David Satcher, respectively, defended the ethics of these random clinical trials with a placebo group. They based their moral reasoning on the 1979 *Belmont Report* and its principle-based approach, that is, the principles of autonomy, beneficence, and justice. They pointed out that the *principle of autonomy* was correctly applied because the people gave voluntary informed consent to become subjects in the study. The *principle of justice* was also correctly applied because the goal was not to exploit people in the developing countries but to develop something they could use. Finally, the *principle of beneficence* was correctly applied because the benefits of a successful study for many babies outweighed the risks incurred by the relatively few in the placebo group who would not receive any treatment. This last point is the heart of the NIH and CDC ethical reasoning and is captured in the following text: "[A] placebo-controlled trial may be the only way to obtain an answer that is ultimately useful to people in similar circumstances. If we enroll subjects in a study that exposes them to unknown risks and is designed in a way that is unlikely to provide results that are useful to the subjects *or others* in the population, we have failed the test of beneficence" (emphasis added).

In other words, the directors of NIH and CDC claim that the principle of beneficence allows them to deprive babies in the placebo group of any treatment that might prevent them from being infected with HIV as long as the research might save the lives of many other babies when the trial is over. This argument reflects the moral theory known as *act–utilitarianism*—whatever actions are most useful for bringing the greatest good (beneficence) for the greatest number are ethical, regardless of the damage a few might suffer in the effort to achieve the greatest good. Most ethicists, including most utilitarians (who are *rule*-utilitarians and not *act*-utilitarians), consider act-utilitarianism and its tendency to neglect the few for the many to be morally defective. It is not enough for researchers to show that their actions are designed to benefit many people; they also need to show that their behavior is ethical when one group in the clinical trial will be left without any treatment to prevent a lethal infection so that others can benefit at a later date.

Critics' perspectives. Among the moral reasons critics advanced against these trials are the following. First, it is unethical for researchers to use a placebo group once an effective treatment is known because it is treating the human subjects in the placebo group merely as a means so others can benefit. Second, it is unethical to conduct trials in foreign countries that would not be allowed in the researchers' country. Third, it is unethical to conduct trials in foreign countries unless researchers are assured that successful results of the trials will actually benefit the populations of those countries, something unlikely to happen in many developing countries given their histories of failing to provide basic health care or even such basic needs as potable water, sanitation, penicillin, oral rehydration fluids, and so forth. Fourth, it is unethical to expose babies to serious harm (e.g., AIDS) by putting them in a placebo group when equivalency studies without a placebo group could provide much of what researchers want to know. Finally, it is unethical to conduct trials that conflict with the *Declaration of Helsinki* published by WHO and with the *International Ethical Guidelines for Biomedical Research on Human Subjects* published by the Council for International Organizations of Medical Sciences (CIOMS)

Risk Factors in Heterosexual HIV Transmission

In March 2000 the *New England Journal of Medicine* published another disturbing study on HIV research in Africa. It was so disturbing that Marcia Angell, the editor of the *Journal* at that time, wrote an editorial questioning the ethics of the trial but, acknowledging that the two ethicists she asked to review the study disagreed about its moral status, decided to publish the study. What was going on with this HIV research that gave rise to moral concerns?

The Story

Researchers wanted to learn more about risk factors affecting the heterosexual transmission of HIV. Specifically they focused on two questions: Does having a sexually transmitted disease (STD) increase the risk of becoming infected, and do higher viral loads increase the risk of transmitting the infection? They also decided to observe whether the male's being uncircumcised increased the risk of female-to-male HIV transmission. The study recruited people from rural villages in the Rakai district of Uganda.

To answer the first question researchers identified thousands of HIV-negative people, including pregnant women, in conjugal relationships who had asymptomatic STDs (e.g., syphilis, gonorrhea, bacterial vaginosis, chlamydia) and divided them into two groups. Researchers treated one group with antibiotics and left the other group without treatment. Both groups received identical education on preventing HIV infection and received free condoms. The people recruited for the study were not paid, although each family did receive a free bar of soap.

Researchers planned to evaluate both groups five times at ten-month intervals to see whether the rate of HIV infection varied depending on whether or not the STDs were being treated with antibiotics. The study was stopped after the third evaluation because, rather unexpectedly, the data showed no significant difference between the groups. In other words, the study showed that having an STD does not increase the risk of contracting AIDS from an HIV-positive partner. This part of the study was published in the *Lancet*.

To answer the second question—whether higher viral loads increase the risk of heterosexual HIV transmission—researchers tested thousands of people and identified 415 couples with one HIV-positive partner. All persons were encouraged to ask for their HIV status, received instruction on the prevention of HIV infection and condom use, and were provided with free condoms. The HIV-positive people were encouraged but not obliged to inform their spouses or partners of their status, and the researchers assumed no responsibility for informing HIV-negative people in the study about the status of their HIV-positive partner.

Researchers checked the couples five times at ten-month intervals and discovered that ninety (22 percent) of the original HIV-negative partners had become HIV positive by the end of the study. Not surprisingly, higher viral loads increased the risk of transmission. The research also uncovered two other pieces of information: No HIV-negative circumcised male became infected during the study, and no partner of an HIV-positive person with a low viral load (a serum HIV-1 RNA viral load of less than 1,500 copies per milliliter) became infected during the study. This suggested that sexual contact with an HIV-positive partner is less risky if he or she has a low viral load or if he has been circumcised.

Ethical Analysis

Situational awareness.   We are aware of these facts in the Uganda trial.

1. Heterosexual HIV transmission is widespread in many regions of Africa, and it is thought that numerous risk factors exist (e.g., existing STDs, nonuse of condoms).

2. Researchers believed that a better understanding of the role that STDs and high viral loads play in the spread of HIV is important because it could "facilitate efforts to prevent transmission of the virus."

3. The trial was approved by NIH, by the IRBs at Columbia University and Johns Hopkins University, and by the AIDS Research Subcommittee of the Uganda National Council for Science and Technology.

4. The trial could not have been conducted in the United States because it would violate federal regulations designed to protect human subjects in clinical trails. Researchers could not enroll asymptomatic people with STDs in their clinical trials and then leave them untreated for years, nor could they enroll couples with one HIV-positive partner in their clinical and then watch to see if the other partner became HIV positive.

We are also aware of some good and bad features—values and disvalues—in the story.

1. Heterosexual transmission of HIV is a major problem, and we might be able to reduce it if we learn more about the role STDs and viral loads play.

2. A primary intention of the scientists is good—they want to learn more about risk factors for heterosexual transmission of HIV.

3. Researchers knowingly declined to treat more than 6,000 people enrolled in the study who tested positive for syphilis and other STDs while the trial was conducted. This allowed researchers to compare their rate of HIV infection with the rate of those who received standard STD treatments.

4. Researchers also knowingly declined to treat more than 400 HIV-positive people in relationships with HIV-negative partners. This put the infected people at greater risk for developing AIDS, and it put their partners at risk for HIV infection.

5. Researchers did offer treatment for STDs to all participants after the study had been completed.

Prudential Reasoning in the HIV Transmission Research Stories

Here we look at the story from the perspectives of the researchers and their critics.

Researchers' perspective.   Supporters of the research believe that that aspect of the clinical trial that sought scientific evidence about the relation of STDs and viral loads on HIV heterosexual transmission was morally justified. They argue that it was approved by the IRBs at Columbia

University and at Johns Hopkins University as well as by the NIH Office for Protection from Research Risk and the Uganda National Council for Science and Technology.

Regarding the STD phase of the trial, they argued that it was not unethical to withhold treatment for the STDs in the control group (those not receiving treatment in the trial) because all participants in the study could have obtained the results of their tests for STDs if they had asked for them. Furthermore, members of the control group could always go to the government clinics, which the researchers had stocked with free penicillin, if they wished. Moreover, the researchers also treated the control group for their STDs when the trial was over so everyone ultimately received treatment thanks to the research trial. Researchers also pointed out that the HIV situation in Africa has reached epidemic proportions, and this situation allows research methods that would not be considered appropriate in other parts of the world.

With regard to the the viral load phase of the trial, researchers argued that it would breach confidentiality and set up a risk of stigma and discrimination if they informed people that their asymptomatic partners were HIV positive and that disclosure of HIV status would also have undermined the national program of confidential HIV testing in Uganda. Furthermore, they pointed out that survey staff provided people with information about HIV transmission and encouraged abstinence and safe sex practices. Hence, all people enrolled in the study received benefits that they would not have received if the study had not been done. They also argued that the untreated HIV-positive people in the clinical trials did not receive less than standard care because HIV-positive Ugandans in rural villages are generally not diagnosed, and, if they are diagnosed as HIV-positive, they seldom receive antiretroviral drugs. Hence the trial provided no less than the standard of care for the population it was studying.

Critics' perspectives. Critics of the research argued that research should not have been done in Uganda because federal regulations would not have allowed it in the United States, thus making it inconsistent with both the Declaration of Helsinki and the CIOMS guidelines. Moreover, a 2001 NBAC report recommends that clinical trials conducted by U.S. researchers in developing countries should meet the ethical standards required for trials in the United States. Critics also pointed out that it is difficult to see how people in rural sections of Uganda would be sufficiently literate and educated to understand the trial and give fully informed consent for their participation.

Critics further argued that diagnosing STDs in research participants and then leaving the disease untreated for months is morally questionable even though the people could have gone to government clinics for treatment. Critics also contended that it was unethical to design a study that enrolled asymptomatic people, discovered that some were HIV positive, measured their viral loads, and then let them go untreated for up to thirty months while watching to see if they infected their partners. Moreover, critics argued that it was ethically questionable for researchers not to insist that the HIV-positive spouses inform their partners of their diagnosis.

Ethical Reflections

From the perspective of virtue ethics, the statements and principles of the 2008 Declaration of Helsinki and the 2002 CIOMS guidelines provide helpful starting points, but not final conclusions, for international research in developing countries. Virtue ethics will always subject principles and guidelines to constant reevaluation in light of circumstances to be sure these principles and guidelines preserve their fundamental purpose—setting up situations conducive to human flourishing. Researchers do not flourish by exploiting human beings, and people living in developing countries, who are often living less than robust flourishing lives, sometimes could benefit from research that would not be possible in the researchers' own country. The great challenge is to find a promising course of action that improves the lot of people in the developing world without exploiting the few for the sake of the many.

A starting point for our ethical reflection begins with some pertinent quotations from some key statements from the 2008 Helsinki Declaration.

- It is the duty of the physician to promote and safeguard the health of patients, including those who are involved in medical research. (3)

- In medical research involving human subjects, the well-being of the individual research subject must take precedence over all other interests. (6)
- It is the duty of physicians who participate in medical research to protect the life (and) health . . . of research subjects. (11)
- At the conclusion of the study, patients entered into the study are entitled to be informed about the outcome of the study and to share any benefits that might result from it. (33)

The latest (2002) CIOMS *International Ethical Guidelines for Biomedical Research Involving Human Subjects* includes the following guidelines.

Guideline 3. An external sponsoring organization and individual investigators should submit the research protocol for ethical and scientific review in the country of the sponsoring organization, and the ethical standards applied should be no less stringent than they would be for research carried out in that country.

Guideline 10. Before undertaking research in a population or community with limited resources, the sponsor and the investigator must make every effort to ensure that . . . any intervention or product developed, or knowledge generated, will be made reasonably available for the benefit of that population or community.

Both the HIV perinatal transmission trials and the HIV heterosexual transmission trial raise many of the ethical issues that arise in almost any international research not allowed in the researchers' home country. A virtue-based prudential approach to the problem would acknowledge the possibility of relevant extenuating circumstances that might find such research reasonable. However, it is hard to see that the perinatal HIV trials with placebo groups were reasonable given that researchers could learn much of what they needed to know from comparative studies (one group receiving the proven treatment and the other the short course) without leaving a group without any treatment whatsoever.

It is also hard to see that the heterosexual HIV transmission trials looking at risk factors such as STDs or viral loads were reasonable; in fact, it could be argued that they were morally unreasonable because the information uncovered could do more harm than good. For example, trying to discover whether the presence of an STD makes it more likely that a person will become infected with HIV meant that investigators, some of them physicians, would discover that participants in their trials have a treatable STD and then leave some of them untreated, putting them and that partners at risk. Moreover, once researchers discovered that STDs do not make infection more likely, then it became easier for researchers focusing on preventing AIDS to overlook the plight of those at risk from STDs. And trying to correlate heterosexual HIV infection rates with the viral load of the infected party meant that investigators would discover that participants in their trials are HIV positive and then leave them untreated, putting them and their partners at risk of developing AIDS, very often a fatal disease in Uganda. Moreover, once HIV-positive people learn from the trials that low viral loads indicate little or no risk of infecting someone, then it becomes easier for them to ignore safe sex practices.

OTHER SPECIAL POPULATIONS IN RESEARCH

We note in passing that other populations pose particular problems for medical research. Most of the ethical problems arise because these populations do not have sufficient capacity to give informed consent or, if they do have decision-making capacity, are in a position where the voluntary aspect of their consent may be easily undermined. Prisoners, for example, are in a vulnerable position and could easily be exploited. Special regulations exist to protect them.

The mentally ill, the handicapped, and the disabled are also vulnerable, and special care must be taken so they will not be exploited. Care must also be taken that the elderly are not coerced or unduly influenced to participate in research protocols.

Military personnel represent another vulnerable population. During Operation Desert Storm in 1991, unapproved drugs were used on soldiers without their informed consent. Because the drugs had not been fully tested and approved by the FDA, their use was not medical but experimental. The FDA did issue an interim regulation allowing the military to use the unapproved drugs. A serviceman challenged the FDA ruling in federal court but lost. The court said that the FDA could issue an interim regulation allowing the use of unapproved drugs without informed consent if those administering the drugs believed obtaining informed consent from the recipients was not feasible. This decision (*Doe v. Sullivan*, 938 F. 2d 1370 [1991]) is notable in that it runs counter to the careful protection of human subjects found in most government regulations and court decisions. Its impact is undoubtedly limited by the special circumstances of military personnel's preparing for combat and by the reasonable belief that the drug would benefit most of the military people going into combat in the Persian Gulf area.

ANIMALS AND MEDICAL RESEARCH

The last special population we want to mention is composed of research subjects who are not human—animals. Many therapies are first tested on animals before they are tested on human subjects, and this research on animals has contributed to important developments in human health care. Experiments on dogs helped to isolate insulin in 1921, and this led to the development of insulin therapy that has been so beneficial for many people suffering from diabetes. Research on animal primates was a key factor in the 1953 development of polio vaccines. So many other examples of beneficial research using animals could be given that it is impossible to deny the value for humans of biomedical research using animals.

Until recently many people were unaware that the use of animals in medical research involved any moral issues. In most cultural traditions, people simply assumed that they could use animals for their own purposes. They hunted them down and killed them, sometimes for food, sometimes for clothing, sometimes for decoration, sometimes for sport. They used them for work, for transportation, and for amusement. They domesticated some of them and made others into personal pets.

The roots of this attitude run deep. The book of Genesis 1:28 depicts God giving humans dominion over all other living things—the fish in the sea, the birds of the air, and the animals of the earth—implying that people can use these creatures, although care for the well-being of domesticated animals is mandated in at least two places in Deuteronomy. Jewish and Christian theology emphasized the disparity between humans and animals by insisting that God created only humans in his "image and likeness," and that this gives humans a dignity not shared by animals.

Nor is there much respect for animals in Greek thought. The early Pythagoreans did respect animals because they thought that an animal might embody a reincarnated human soul, but Socrates and Plato rejected this idea. They taught that once the human soul leaves the body at death, it never returns to another body. The Pythagorean reason for respecting animal life was thus lost when its doctrine of reincarnation was superseded by the Platonic and later Christian teachings of an immaterial human soul living after death in a disembodied state.

René Descartes, known as the "father of modern philosophy," is a more modern example of one who did not accord any moral standing to animals. He compared them to machines. If someone designed a clever machine, he said, that looked like a human being, we would not be fooled for long that it really was a human being. In particular, we would notice two things. First, even though the machine may have been programmed to make the sounds of words, it would be incapable of participating in a meaningful conversation. Second, even though the machine may have been programmed to act in many different ways, it would be unable to learn how to act in all sorts of circumstances as humans can, thanks to their ability to reason. On the other hand, if someone designed a clever machine that looked and acted like a monkey, we would never be able to tell the difference between the machine and the monkey. The implication of Descartes' argument is obvious: if animals are like machines and may one day be indistinguishable from them, they have no important moral standing.

It is not surprising, then, that ethical concerns for animals are largely absent from the major works of moral theology and moral philosophy in our cultural traditions. Ethics has traditionally centered on how we treat ourselves and other human beings and not on how we treat animals or the environment. In the past few decades, however, concern for our treatment of animals and for our relationship with the environment has been growing as more and more people become aware of the ethical issues in these areas of life.

Of the three main modern approaches to ethics—natural rights, the Kantian moral law, and utilitarianism—two (natural rights and utilitarianism) offer some support for the ethical treatment of animals. Moral theories based on rights can be expanded to include an ethics about animals by simply extending the notion of natural rights to animals. Once we claim animals have rights, especially the right to live naturally, we have given animals a moral standing that we must respect. The attribution of rights to animals reminds us that they are not there simply for our purposes.

The second major moral theory, utilitarianism, can also be extended to provide a moral standing for animals. The fundamental moral principle of utilitarianism is the "greatest happiness principle"—the action or the rule that brings the greatest happiness or pleasure to the greatest number is what is morally required. Now, since higher animals obviously experience pleasure and pain, they can easily be counted among the "greatest number" who will be affected by our actions. The utilitarian obligation to increase pleasure and reduce pain can easily be extended to include the pleasure and pain of animals. One of the founders of utilitarianism, Jeremy Bentham, took issue with Descartes on this very point. Descartes had thought that animals are like machines because they cannot speak or reason. Bentham countered: "The question is not Can they *reason*? nor Can they *talk*? but Can they *suffer*?"

Unfortunately, the third major moral theory, that of Kant, offers little to support the moral standing of animals. His ethics centered exclusively on respect for humanity. One version of his fundamental moral principle was: Act in such a way that you treat humanity, whether in your own person or in the person of another, always at the same time as an end and never simply as a means. Since he derived all moral laws from this fundamental moral principle, his moral laws pertain only to humanity, not to animals. Kant did suggest that mistreatment of animals is wrong, but it is wrong not because it is bad for the animals or because animals have moral worth but because the mistreatment undermines the humanity of those tormenting the animals.

Fortunately, a biblically based theological approach to animals (and the environment) has been gaining ground in recent years. It is driven by the biblical idea of creation and stewardship: the planet and all living entities are creatures of God, and this implies that we should take care of them. There has also been a renewed interest in the goodness of creation in biblical texts found in the writings of medieval Christian theologians, most notably Augustine, Chrysostom, and Aquinas. The general idea is that we need to think of the stewardship of God's creation and not simply of usefulness when it comes to animals and the environment.

Today, considerable debate swirls around the ethics of our relationships with animals. As we have noted, this is a new moral concern since the older religious, theological, and philosophical ethics of our tradition did not give priority to moral questions about the welfare of animals. And, as we might expect, the debate about the morality of behavior toward animals embraces a wide range of positions. At one extreme are those who argue against almost all use of animals for human purposes. They say it is immoral to use animals for medical research, to hunt, to use animals for work or transportation, to breed animals for food, to eat animals, to confine them as pets, or other uses. At the other extreme are those who maintain a more traditional position. They say almost any use of animals is morally acceptable as long as it contributes to human well-being. They have no problem using animals for medical research, plowing fields with them, trapping them for fur, raising them for food, confining them in cages, or hunting them for sport.

The debate over the ethics of how we should relate to animals will undoubtedly continue for some time. It is a whole new area for moral philosophy and moral theology, and it will take time to develop. In the meantime, by following the ethics of prudence and the human good that we have been developing in this book, several helpful points can be made about the use of animals in medical research.

First, deliberately doing anything that causes suffering or damage to life does not contribute to our good unless we have cogent reasons to offset the bad things resulting from our actions. This ethics of right reason demands good reasons for research that will hurt or kill animals.

Second, this ethics encourages us to cherish, and not damage, all life—human life as well as the life of all living things, including animals and the environment. Yet it acknowledges the morality of employing living beings (including human beings) as the subjects of medical research even though no benefit, and some pain or damage, may ensue in their lives, provided certain moral safeguards are in place to prevent exploitation and provided beneficial advances in medicine are anticipated.

Third, biomedical research on animals is important, and sometimes crucial, for understanding and treating some human diseases. Research using computer models, plants, and live cultures can only go so far. Often the research must involve animals (and humans) before the therapeutic intervention or drug can be accepted as normal medical practice. Hence, there are good reasons for some animal research. The moral debate in this ethics of the good, then, centers on what reasons are strong enough to justify the suffering, damage, and death of animals used in research.

Fourth, undoubtedly, some animal research today is morally questionable. Better efforts are needed to reduce unnecessary pain and suffering. One thing we need is more explicit federal regulations, analogous to those developed in the past few decades for research on human subjects, to guide research on animals. These regulations would not require that animals be treated the same as human subjects in research, but they would protect animal subjects from morally unreasonable treatment by requiring convincing reasons for any harmful experimentation.

Another way to prevent immoral animal research is by requiring approval by the local animal welfare board similar to an IRB operating under appropriate guidelines. By way of example, we can look at the review process used at Stanford University Medical Center to prevent the abuse, inappropriate use, or neglect of animals in research.

All the animal research at Stanford must be approved by the university's Panel on Laboratory Animal Care. Among recent members of the panel were a hospital chaplain and several veterinarians from the community with no other relationship to the university. Before beginning research involving animals, the investigator must give reasons why the animals have to be used and explain all the procedures that will involve them. He must also show how any pain or distress greater than that caused by a routine injection will be minimized and list the anesthetics and pain-killing drugs that will be used. If surgery is involved, the preoperative, surgical, and postoperative interventions must be outlined in detail.

Perhaps the best way to prevent immoral animal research is to increase the effort aimed at reminding researchers of two things. First, the traditional ethics of our culture, both religious and philosophical, failed to a considerable degree to acknowledge our moral relationship with animals. This failure has left us with a sort of moral vacuum where animals are concerned, so our traditional attitudes of dominion over them are not morally well founded and cannot be trusted.

Second, an ethics based on the human good recognizes that our good is not achieved by causing unnecessary suffering and death in this world. This recognition serves as the basis for the humane treatment of all animals, including laboratory animals. The day may come when none of us will kill and eat animals or use them in research, but that day is not now realistic. Our immediate moral concerns, then, center on providing humane care for the animals we use, with good reasons, for nourishment and research.

SUGGESTED READINGS

The Tuskegee study is treated at length in James Jones, 1981, *Bad Blood: The Tuskegee Syphilis Experiment*, New York: The Free Press. See also articles by Arthur Caplan, Harold Edgar, Patricia King, and James Jones in a special section entitled "Twenty Years After: The Legacy of the Tuskegee Syphilis Study," *Hastings Center Report* 1992, *22* (November–December), 29–40; William Curran, "The Tuskegee Syphilis Study," *New England Journal of Medicine* 1973, *289*, 730–32; and Allan Brandt, "Racism and Research: The Case of the Tuskegee Syphilis Study," *Hastings Center Report* 1978, *8* (December), 21–29.

Among the many treatments of the Nazi medical experiments are George Annas and Michael Grodin, eds., 1992, *The Nazi Doctors and the Nuremberg Code: Human Rights in Human Experimentation*, New York: Oxford University Press; Robert Jay Lifton, 1986, *The Nazi Doctors: Medical Killing and the*

Psychology of Genocide, New York: Basic Books, chapters 15 and 17; Jay Katz, 1972, *Experimentation with Human Beings*, New York: Russell Sage Foundation, chapter 1; and Leo Alexander, "Medical Science under Dictatorship," *New England Journal of Medicine* 1949, *249*, 39–47. Alexander was a psychiatrist who served as a consultant to the American Chief of Counsel for War Crimes at the Nuremberg trials. The Nuremberg Code is frequently reprinted in books on medical research. For a copy of the Code and an excellent article on its significance, see Evelyne Shuster, "Fifty Years Later: The Significance of the Nuremberg Code," *New England Journal of Medicine* 1997, *337*, 1436–40. The first principle ("The voluntary consent of the human subject is absolutely essential") is not always easy to arrange in practice. Some years ago, physicians in St. Paul, Minnesota, were testing a hand pump that both compressed and then decompressed the chest of a person in cardiac arrest outside the hospital. Emergency medical technicians and paramedics were using the pump in some sections of the city in an effort to determine whether it was more effective than the standard CPR used in other sections. Of course, a person in cardiac arrest cannot give informed consent for the experimental pump, so the FDA (which approves medical devices) stopped the trial. Unfortunately, it is very difficult to see how one could ever obtain informed consent for trials involving resuscitation equipment designed for use by emergency medical personnel in cases of unexpected cardiopulmonary arrest outside a medical setting. Prudential reasoning suggests, therefore, that there may be cases (cardiac arrest, for example) where the informed consent of the subject for some unapproved equipment is not absolutely essential. See Keith Lurie et al., "Evaluation of Active Compression-Decompression CPR in Victims of Out-of-Hospital Cardiac Arrest," *JAMA* 1994, *271*, 1405–11; Carin Olson, "The Letter or the Spirit: Consent for Research in CPR," *JAMA* 1994, *271*, 1445–47; and Robert Truog et al., "Is Informed Consent Always Necessary for Randomized, Controlled Trials?" *New England Journal of Medicine* 1999, *340*, 804–7.

Paul Ramsey's criticism of Willowbrook is found in 1970, *The Patient as Person*, New Haven: Yale University Press, pp. 47–56. The editorial defense of Willowbrook as "not unethical" is by Franz Ingelfinger, "Ethics of Experiments on Children," *New England Journal of Medicine* 1973, *288*, 791–92. An excellent summary of the cancer research at the Jewish Chronic Disease Hospital can be found in Katz, *Experimentation*, chapter 1.

Accounts of the obedience studies can be found in Stanley Milgram, 1974, *Obedience to Authority: An Experimental View*, New York: Harper & Row; Sissela Bok, 1979, *Lying: Moral Choice in Public and Private Life*, New York: Random House, pp. 193–95; and Ruth Faden and Tom Beauchamp, 1986, *A History and Theory of Informed Consent*, New York: Oxford University Press, pp. 174–77. Milgram defended the ethics of his research—see, for example, his "Subject Reaction: The Neglected Factor in the Ethics of Experimentation," *Hastings Center Report* 1977, *7* (October), 19–23. Here he argues that misinformation has a place in behavioral research if it is unavoidable and that almost no subjects in his experiments were harmed since questionnaires returned after the tests showed over 98 percent of the people were "glad" or "very glad" they had participated in the experiment.

Among the articles and books sparking the public reaction to the questionable morality prevailing in medical research were Henry Beecher, "Ethics and Clinical Research," *New England Journal of Medicine* 1966, *274*, 1354–60; M. H. Pappworth, 1967, *Human Guinea Pigs: Experimentation on Man*, Boston: Beacon Press; Henry Beecher, 1970, *Research and the Individual*, Boston: Little, Brown and Co.; and Jay Katz, *Experimentation*. See also David Rothman, "Ethics and Human Experimentation: Henry Beecher Revisited," *New England Journal of Medicine* 1987, *317*, 1195–99; Jay Katz, "Reflections on Unethical Experiments and the Beginnings of Bioethics in the United States," *Kennedy Institute of Ethics Journal* 1994, *4*, 85–92; and Jay Katz, "'Ethics and Clinical Research' Revisited: A Tribute to Henry K. Beecher," *Hastings Center Report* 1993, *23* (September–October), 31–39.

The influential textbook that helped establish the ethical model of principles in medical ethics was Beauchamp and Childress, *Principles of Biomedical Ethics*, 1979 (1st ed.), 1982 (2nd ed.), 1989 (3rd ed.), 1994 (4th ed.), 2001 (5th ed.), and 2009 (6th ed). Chapter 2 of the sixth edition titled "Moral Character" introduces an expanded and helpful introduction to virtue ethics. However, the core of the book, chapters 4 through 8, continues to rely on the authors' traditional principle-based and rule-based approach to decision making. Albert Jonsen's criticism of the principlism found in the National Commission's *Belmont Report* (he was a member of the Commission) can be found in his "American Moralism and the Origin of Bioethics in the United States," *Journal of Medicine and Philosophy* 1991, *16*, 115–29; the quotation is from p. 125.

For federal regulations governing research see Title 45 of the Code of Federal Regulations, Part 46 (45 CFR 46) published in 1991. In 1998 a number of ethicists reviewed the regulations and made some important recommendations for change. See Jonathan Moreno et al., "Updating Protections for Human Subjects Involved in Research," *JAMA* 1998, *280*, 1951–58. The President's Commission reports on research are *Protecting Human Subjects* (1981), *Whistleblowing in Biomedical Research* (1981), *Compensating for Research Injuries* (1982), and *Implementing Human Research Regulations* (1983). They were originally published by the U.S. Government Printing Office and are now available in a six-volume set from William S. Hein & Company (1997). The quotations showing the central role played by the three principles in the commission's work are from the final report, *Summing Up* (1983), p. 67.

For the report and recommendations of the committee that studied the radiation research, see Advisory Committee on Human Radiation Experiments, 1996, *The Human Radiation Experiments: Final Report of the President's Advisory Committee,* New York: Oxford University Press. See also Ruth Faden et al., "Research Ethics and the Medical Profession: Report of the Advisory Committee on Human Radiation Experiments," *JAMA* 1996, *276*, 403–9, and the articles and commentaries in the special issue of the *Kennedy Institute of Ethics Journal* 1996, *6*, 215–322, especially the lead article by Ruth Faden, the chair of the Committee.

A good overview of the stem-cell controversy is Ronald Green, 2001, *The Human Embryo Research Debates: Bioethics in the Vortex of Controversy,* New York: Oxford University Press. For background on ANT see William Hurlbut et al., "Seeking Consensus: A Clarification and Defense of Altered Nuclear Transfer," *Hastings Center Report* 2006, *36* (September–October), 42–50, reprinted in *National Catholic Bioethics Quarterly* 2007, *7*, 339–52. Hurlbut first presented his proposal for ANT to the PCB on December 4, 2004. It is available at bioethics.gov under transcripts for that day and reprinted as "Altered Nuclear Transfer as a Morally Acceptable Means for the Procurement of Human Embryonic Stem Cells," *National Catholic Bioethics Quarterly* 2005, *5*, 145–51.

For the promising work on obtaining pluripotent stem cells without embryo destruction see Junying Yu et al., "Induced Pluripotent Stem Cell Lines Derived from Human Somatic Cells," *Science* 2007, *318*, 1917–20; and Kazutoshi Takahashi et al., "Induction of Pluripotent Stem Cells from Adult Human Fibroblasts by Defined Factors," *Cell* 2007, *131*, 861–72. See also Young Chung et al., "Human Embryonic Stem Cell Lines Generated without Embryo Destruction," *Cell Stem Cell* 2008, *2*, 113–17; In-Hyun Park et al., "Reprogramming of Human Somatic Cells to Pluripotency with Defined Factors," *Nature* 2008, *451*, 141–46; Douglas Higgs, "A New Dawn for Stem-Cell Therapy," *New England Journal of Medicine* 2008, *358*, 964–66; and Nicanor Austriaco, "Primate Cloning and Nuclear Reprogramming (iPS) Technology: The End of the Stem Cell Wars," *National Catholic Bioethics Quarterly* 2008, *8*, 131–35. James Thomson's remarks about the end of embryonic stem cell controversy can be found in Colin Nickerson, "Breakthrough on Stem Cells," *Boston Globe*, November 21, 2007, available at boston.com. Also see Gina Kolata, "Scientists Bypass Need for Embryo to Get Stem Cells" and "Man Who Helped Start Stem Cell War May End It," *New York Times*, November 21 and 22, 2007, available at nytimes.com. See also Martin Fackler, "Risk Taking Is in His Genes," *New York Times*, December 11, 2007, available at nytimes.com. The last story is about Shinya Yamanaka, who led the team at Osaka University and who is quoted as saying "I thought, we can't keep destroying embryos for our research. There must be another way."

For problems with informed consent documents that were used in obtaining the embryos that gave rise to the stem-cell lines that are eligible for federal funding under the Bush administration's guidelines, see Robert Streiffer, "Informed Consent and Federal Funding for Stem Cell Research," *Hastings Center Report* 2008, *38* (May–June), 40–47.

Among the many articles on embryonic and fetal research are Leon Kass, 1985, *Toward a More Natural Science,* New York: The Free Press, especially chapter 4, titled "The Meaning of Life—in the Laboratory"; Richard McCormick, 1985, *How Brave a New World?* Washington, DC: Georgetown University Press, especially chapter 5, titled "Public Policy and Fetal Research"; Henry Greely et al., "The Ethical Use of Human Fetal Tissue in Medicine," *New England Journal of Medicine* 1989, *320*, 1093–96; John Fletcher and Joseph Schulman, "Fetal Research: The State of the Art, the State of the Question," *Hastings Center Report* 1985, *15* (April), 6–12; and John Fletcher and Kenneth Ryan, "Federal Regulations for Fetal Research: A Case for Reform," *Law, Medicine & Health Care* 1987, *15*, 126–38. The conclusions and recommendations of the National Commission relevant to fetal research can be found in the *Hastings Center Report* 1975, *5* (June), 41–46. This issue of the report also contains a valuable collection of abridged papers that were submitted to the commission during its deliberations. Also important is Steinbock, *Life before Birth,* chapters 5 and 6. See also George Annas et al., "The Politics of Human Embryo Research—Avoiding Ethical Gridlock," *New England Journal of Medicine* 1996, *334*, 1329–32.

For Paul Ramsey's criticism of all research on minors, see "The Enforcement of Morals: Nontherapeutic Research on Children," *Hastings Center Report* 1976, *6* (August), 21–30. McCormick's defense of limited research on children can be found in *How Brave a New World?* chapters 4, 6, and 7. The crucial point in his argument is: "I believe my own analysis is precisely at root and in substance a best-interests test: The fetus/child would choose nontherapeutic experimentation of minimal risk because it is compatible with and not opposed to his best interests" (p. 113). This is more of an assertion than a reason. We can never say that we know a human being who never had decision-making capacity would choose to participate in medical research. In fact, some people do decline to participate in medical research even when the risk is minimal or absent.

The landmark article that claimed that the clinical trials to discover a less expensive way to reduce the vertical transmission of the HIV infection to babies were unethical is Peter Lurie and Sidney Wolf, "Unethical Trials of Interventions to Reduce Perinatal Transmission of the Human Immunodeficiency Virus in Developing Countries," *New England Journal of Medicine* 1997, *337*, 853–56. See also Marcia Angell, "The Ethics of Clinical Research in the Third World," *New England Journal of Medicine* 1997, *337*, 847–49; Praphan Phanuphak, "Ethical Issues in Studies in Thailand of the Vertical Transmission of HIV," *New England Journal of Medicine* 1998, *338*, 834–35; Eliot Marshall, "Controversial Trial Offers Hopeful Results: HIV Transmission from Mother to Child," *Science* 1998, *279*, 1299; Leonard Glantz et al., "Research in Developing Countries: Taking 'Benefit' Seriously," and Carol Levine, "Placebos and HIV: Lessons Learned," both in the *Hastings Center Report* 1998, *28* (November–December), 38–42 and 43–48. An account of the one trial that refused to use a placebo group is reported in Marc Lallemant, "AZT Trial in Thailand," *Science* 1995, *270*, 899–900. For an excellent analysis of the ethical debate, concluding that the trials were unethical, see Peter Clark, "The Ethics of Placebo-Controlled Clinical Trials for Perinatal Transmission of HIV in Developing Countries," *Journal of Clinical Ethics* 1998, *9*, 156–66. For articles claiming the trials with placebos were ethical see Harold Varmus and David Satcher, "Ethical Complexities of Conducting Research in Developing Countries," *New England Journal of Medicine* 1998, *337*, 1003–5; Robert Levine, "The 'Best Proven Therapeutic Method' Standard in Clinical Trials in Technologically Developing Countries," *IRB* 1998, *20* (January–February), 5–9, reprinted in the *Journal of Clinical Ethics* 1998, *9*, 167–72; Merlin Robb et al., "Studies in Thailand of the Vertical Transmission of HIV," *New England Journal of Medicine* 1998, *338*, 843–44; Robert Crouch and John Arras, "AZT Trials and Tribulations," and Christine Grady, "Science in the Service of Healing," both in *Hastings Center Report* 1998, *28* (November–December), 26–34 and 34–38. Crouch and Arras's support is a "qualified support."

For the Uganda HIV trial see Maria Wawer et al., "Control of Sexually Transmitted Diseases for AIDS Prevention in Uganda: A Randomized Community Trial," *Lancet* 1999, *353*, 525–35; Thomas Quinn et al., "Viral Load and Heterosexual Transmission of Human Immunodeficiency Virus Type 1," *New England Journal of Medicine* 2000, *342*, 921–29. For a defense of the trial see correspondence from Ronald Gray et al. in *New England Journal of Medicine* 2000, *343*, 361.

For a critique of the Uganda heterosexual HIV trial see Marcia Angell, "Investigators' Responsibilities for Human Subjects in Developing Countries," *New England Journal of Medicine* 2000, *342*, 967–69. The 2001 NBAC report is *Ethical and Policy Issues in International Research: Clinical Trials in Developing Countries*, and it is available at bioethics.georgetown.edu/nbac. For a balanced and nuanced approach to research in developing countries see David Winkler et al., "The Standard of Care Debate: Can Research in Developing Countries Be Both Ethical and Responsive to Those Countries' Health Needs?" *American Journal of Public Health* 2004, *94*, 923–28, and the policy statement from a 2001 conference on the ethical aspects of research in developing countries titled "Fair Benefits for Research in Developing Countries" in *Science* 2002, *298*, 2133–34. See also Ruth Macklin, 2004, *Double Standards in Medical Research in Developing Countries*, New York: Cambridge University Press; and Ezekiel Emanuel et al., "What Makes Clinical Research in Developing Countries Ethical? Benchmarks of Ethical Research," *Journal of Infectious Diseases* 2004, *189*, 930–37.

The latest Council for International Organizations of Medical Sciences (CIOMS) *International Ethical Guidelines for Biomedical Research on Human Subjects* was published in 2002 and is available at cioms.ch. The World Medical Association *Declaration of Helsinki* was first adopted in 1964; the latest revision, approved in October 2008, is available at wma.net. See also the National Bioethics Advisory Commission (NBAC) 2001 report titled *Ethical and Policy Issues in International Research: Clinical Trials in Developing Countries*, available at bioethics.georgetown.edu/nbac, and "Ethical Aspects of Clinical Research in Developing Countries," a 2003 opinion of the European Group on Ethics in Science and

New Technologies (EGE), available at ec.europa.eu/european group ethics; and an article by participants in a 2001 conference on ethical aspects of research in developing countries titled "Moral Standards for Research in Developing Countries: From 'Reasonable Availability' to 'Fair Benefits,'" *Hastings Center Report* 2004, *34* (May–June), 17–27.

Descartes's remarks on animals can be found in part five of his *Discourse on Method*, first published in 1637. In an early work, Kant's lack of moral concern for animals emerged clearly: "But so far as animals are concerned, we have no direct duties. Animals are not self-conscious and are there merely as a means to an end. That end is man." Kant, *Lectures on Ethics*, p. 239. (These lectures were recorded by Kant's students at the University of Königsberg during 1775–80 and first published in 1924.) Jeremy Bentham's remark on the ethical importance of animal suffering is from chapter 17 of his *An Introduction to the Principles of Morals and Legislation*, first printed in 1780.

For critical comments on the NBAC report "Research Involving Persons with Mental Disorders That May Affect Decisionmaking Capacity" (1998), see Robert Michels, "Are Research Ethics Bad for Our Mental Health?" *New England Journal of Medicine* 1999, *340*, 1427–30. For a defense of the NBAC recommendations see Alexander Capron, "Ethical and Human-Rights Issues in Research on Mental Disorders That May Affect Decision-Making Capacity," *New England Journal of Medicine* 1999, *340*, 1430–34.

A leading proponent of animal rights in our country is Tom Regan. He advanced his theory in *The Case for Animal Rights*, 1983, Berkeley: University of California Press, and several articles including "The Moral Standing of Animals in Medical Research," *Law, Medicine & Health Care* 1992, *20*, 7–16. A leading proponent of the utilitarian approach to the moral treatment of animals is Peter Singer. See his *Animal Liberation*, 1977, New York: Random House. See also Tom Regan and Peter Singer, eds., 1976, *Animal Rights and Human Obligation*, Englewood Cliffs: Prentice Hall; Barbara Orians, 1993, *In the Name of Science: Issues in Responsible Animal Experimentation*, New York: Oxford University Press; H. J. McCloskey, "The Moral Case for Experimentation on Animals," *Monist* 1987, *70*, 64–70; Arthur Caplan, "Beastly Conduct: Ethical Issues in Animal Experimentation," *Annals of the New York Academy of Sciences* 1983, *406*, 159–69; Christina Hoff, "Immoral and Moral Uses of Animals," *New England Journal of Medicine* 1980, *302*, 115–18; Charles McCarthy, "Improved Standards for Laboratory Animals," *Kennedy Institute of Ethics Journal* 1993, *3*, 293–302; and Gary Varner, "The Prospects for Consensus and Convergence in the Animal Rights Debate," *Hastings Center Report* 1994, *24* (January–February), 24–28. Information about the procedures for protecting research at Stanford University Medical Center was taken from James Thomas et al., "Animal Research at Stanford University," *New England Journal of Medicine* 1988, *318*, 1630–32.

An excellent resource for considering the ethical issues in animal studies is Barbara Orlans et al., 1998, *The Human Use of Animals: Case Studies in Ethical Choice*, New York: Oxford University Press, especially the introductory chapter titled "Moral Issues about Animals." See also the special section of nine articles "On Animal Experimentation: Seeking Common Ground" in the *Cambridge Quarterly of Healthcare Ethics* 1999, *8*, 9–87; and David Thomasma and Erich Loewy, "A Dialogue on Species-Specific Rights: Humans and Animals in Bioethics," *Cambridge Quarterly of Healthcare Ethics* 1997, *6*, 435–44, with a commentary by Peter Whitehouse on pp. 445–48. An overview of published international policies on research involving both animals and human subjects (mostly the latter) can be found in Baruch Brody, 1998, *The Ethics of Biomedical Research: An International Perspective*, New York: Oxford University Press.

The recent literature on research ethics is vast, and some good starting points for further reading are these: James Childress, Eric Meslin, and Harold Shapiro, eds., 2005, *Belmont Revisited: Ethical Principles for Research with Human Subjects*, Washington, DC: Georgetown University Press; Timothy Murphy, 2004, *Case Studies in Biomedical Research Ethics*, Cambridge: MIT Press; William LaFleur, Gernot Bohme, and Susumu Shimazono, 2008, *Dark Medicine: Rationalizing Unethical Medical Research*, Bloomington: Indiana University Press; and Ezekiel Emanuel et al., eds., 2008, *The Oxford Textbook of Clinical Research Ethics*, New York: Oxford University Press.

FIFTEEN

Transplantation

Surgeons have been inserting organs and tissues, as well as artificial devices, into patients for several decades. These surgeries often raise profound ethical questions. In this chapter we consider the ethical issues generated by the transplantation of organs and by the implantation of artificial hearts.

Although successful transplantation of a kidney from one dog to another was reported at the beginning of the twentieth century, transplanting a human kidney did not become a realistic possibility until 1947, when surgeons at Boston's Peter Bent Brigham Hospital attached a kidney taken from a cadaver to the arm of an unconscious patient. The external kidney produced urine until it was rejected by the patient's immune system several days later. By that time the woman's kidneys had regained adequate functioning, and she eventually recovered. The rather crude procedure convinced many that human kidney transplantations could succeed.

In 1953 Dr. David Hume performed a somewhat successful kidney transplantation, also at the Peter Bent Brigham Hospital. The patient was able to leave the hospital and survived for almost six months. In 1954, again at the same hospital, Dr. Joseph Murray transplanted a kidney from one identical twin to another. This transplantation is now considered the first successful kidney transplant—Richard Herrick lived eight years after receiving his brother Ronald's kidney. Using a kidney from an identical twin avoided the usual problems of rejection triggered by the recipient's immune system. Improved immunosuppressive drugs were soon developed, and in 1962 the transplantation of a kidney from a donor unrelated to the patient was successful.

Dr. Christiaan Barnard performed the first heart transplantation in South Africa on December 3, 1967. The patient was Louis Washkansky, a fifty-five-year-old man with diabetes, coronary artery disease, and congestive heart failure. The heart came from a twenty-five-year-old woman fatally injured when she was struck by a car less than a mile from the hospital. After her pulse had ceased for several minutes, she was placed on a heart-lung machine to nourish her heart, while Washkansky was prepared for surgery in a nearby operating room. After surgeons implanted her heart in Washkansky's chest, they restarted it with electric shocks. The patient recovered from the surgery and made good progress for almost two weeks. Then his condition rapidly deteriorated. He was in pain, lost control of his bodily functions, and required both feeding tube and a respirator. His transplanted heart went into fibrillation, and after some discussion, physicians decided not to put him back on a heart-lung machine. He died less than three weeks after the transplant, on December 22, 1967.

On December 6, 1967, three days after Washkansky received his transplant in South Africa, Dr. Adrian Kantrowitz performed the first successful heart transplantation in the United States at Maimonides Hospital in Brooklyn. The heart came from an anencephalic infant. Earlier, in June 1966, Dr. Kantrowitz had tried to transplant a heart from another anencephalic infant, but the implanted heart did not restart. This time the donor baby was chilled by immersion in ice water while still alive, and the heart was removed immediately after it stopped beating. Although the recipient lived only six and a half hours, the operation was considered successful, and it is now acknowledged as the first heart transplant in the United States.

In the next few years scores of heart transplants were attempted, but most patients died in the first few months after the surgery. Liver transplants also began in 1967, but success in the early years was very limited.

A major problem affecting organ transplantation in the early years was the rejection of the new organ by the body's immune system. A giant step in overcoming this rejection came with the development of the immunosuppressive drug cyclosporine. This drug was approved by the Food and Drug Administration (FDA) in 1983. Despite some toxic reactions caused by the drug, it noticeably reduced the rejection problem and significantly increased survival rates. More recently, other promising immunosuppressive drugs have been introduced.

Transplanted organs include the pancreas, heart, lung, kidney, liver, and intestine. Corneas, heart valves, skin, bone, bone marrow, partial livers, blood vessels, tendons, and ligaments are also transplanted. In December 1989 a leading transplant surgeon, Dr. Thomas Starzi, implanted a heart, a liver, and a kidney into a young woman; she died four months later of hepatitis. That same month, physicians began transplanting liver lobes from living parents to their children at the University of Chicago Medical Center. In November 2005 surgeons in Amiens, France, transplanted a partial face (lips, chin, and nose) from a cadaver to Isabelle Dinoire in the world's first facial transplantation. In some cases, organs and tissues from animals have been transplanted into humans.

Efforts have also been made to implant mechanical devices as substitutes for organs, most notably, artificial hearts. In 1969 Dr. Denton Cooley implanted the first totally artificial heart in Haskell Karp at the Texas Heart Institute in Houston. Haskell died in a matter of days. His wife sued Dr. Cooley, claiming that the innovative nature of the implantation, which offered no real hope of good health for her husband, was never explained to her or to her husband. The case was dismissed, but questions about appropriate informed consent for what was really a radical medical experiment lingered.

In 1982 Dr. William DeVries implanted a permanent artificial heart into Barney Clark at the University of Utah Medical Center in Salt Lake City. It was a cumbersome device, requiring a bedside air compressor weighing over three hundred pounds to drive the internal pump known as the Jarvik-7. Numerous complications developed, and Barney Clark needed several additional surgeries. His condition deteriorated, and four months later, after many of his vital organs failed, the pump was shut off and he died.

In this chapter we consider the ethical issues surrounding the use of transplanted organs and artificial hearts in the following order:

1. Transplantation of organs from dead human donors
2. Transplantation of organs from living human donors
3. Transplantation of organs from animals
4. Implantation of artificial hearts

TRANSPLANTATION OF ORGANS FROM DEAD HUMAN DONORS

In our culture most people readily accept the transplantation of organs retrieved from a donor after death. Indeed, many think, with good reason, that donating organs after death is morally admirable. At least part of the reason why so many in our culture are morally comfortable with retrieving organs from cadavers is the long history of using cadavers in our medical schools and of performing autopsies to learn about diseases and the causes of death. These practices have made many comfortable with using dead bodies to help the living.

This cultural comfort is reflected in the Uniform Anatomical Gift Act (UAGA), first approved in 1968 by the National Conference of Commissioners on Uniform State Laws and the American Bar Association and now adopted, in some form, by all fifty states and the District of Columbia. This UAGA allows people of sound mind who are at least eighteen years of age to donate all or any part of their bodies for various uses after they die, including transplantation. People can designate the gift in a will or in a document signed in the presence of two witnesses. In some states, people can express their desires to donate their organs on their drivers' licenses.

The UAGA also allows family members, or the person's guardian at the time of death, to donate organs of the deceased, provided the person had not indicated his opposition to organ retrieval while he was alive. Those empowered to make these decisions fall into a list whereby those higher on the list, if they are available, take precedence over those listed at a lower level. The UAGA list of family members who can donate the organs of a deceased person sets the following order of priority: the spouse, an adult child, either parent, an adult sibling, legal guardian at the time of death, any other person authorized or obliged to dispose of the body.

The UAGA allows a person low on the list to donate the organs of the deceased person provided no one at the same level or a higher level on the list objects. Thus, a sister could donate her brother's organs as long as neither his wife nor any of his children nor one of his parents objected.

The UAGA also allows potential recipients to refuse the donation of a cadaver for organs. Thus, if the organs are not usable, the transplant team can refuse the donation.

According to the UAGA, the donated organs cannot be removed until the donor's attending physician or, if there is no attending physician, another physician has determined that the person is dead. The physician determining death may not participate in removing organs or in transplanting them to the recipient. The UAGA also protects physicians acting in good faith from both civil and criminal litigation. This means, for example, that transplant surgeons with good reasons for believing a patient wanted his organs donated could not be prosecuted or sued if it were later discovered that the patient had revoked his consent to donation.

Although one might expect that the clear wishes of persons to donate their organs after death would always be respected, this is not the case. In reality, if family members object to the organ retrieval, the transplant team will almost always decline to retrieve the organs despite certain knowledge and clear documentation that the deceased person wanted the organs donated. The reluctance of transplant teams to retrieve donated organs against the wishes of the family is motivated in large part by their desire not to upset the family at a time of loss and grief. The team also wants to avoid possible negative publicity about organ transplantation. Moreover, the body of a deceased person belongs, in a sense, to the family, and delaying its release in order to harvest organs against family wishes would place members of a transplant team in an uncomfortable position.

The UAGA and the various state laws derived from it have facilitated and encouraged the donation of cadaverous organs. Most ethicists believe the UAGA is, in general, morally sound, and many ethicists encourage the donation of organs after death. In an ethics of virtue it is clearly an expression of the virtue of love, defined by Aristotle as doing something for another for the sake of the other and not for any personal gain.

Despite the general agreement about the morality of cadaverous transplantations as long as appropriate consent is obtained from the donor or from the family, these transplantations have spawned two major ethical questions. The first centers on determining the moment of death; the second centers on the allocation of scarce organs. These questions need to be discussed in some detail.

Death and Organ Retrieval

Transplantation requires organs that are well nourished by oxygenated blood. This means the team must remove them as soon as possible after death. Determining the moment of death thus becomes a crucial issue. Taking the heart out of a person not yet dead is not an act of organ retrieval but an act of killing someone to get his organs. This is why people speak so often of the "dead donor rule."

The two criteria now used to determine when a person is dead were explained in chapter 6. The first, and traditional, criterion of death is the irreversible cessation of the cardiopulmonary functions. When this occurs, the person is dead. Unfortunately, relying on this criterion of death undermines the possibility of retrieving the organs in most cases. Cardiopulmonary functions often weaken over a period of time before they finally stop, and the organs are often damaged while the person is dying. Moreover, the surgeon cannot retrieve organs after the cardiopulmonary arrest until he is sure that the cessation is irreversible. This determination takes time, and the delay usually causes so much additional damage to the organs that they are unusable. This is why, as we noted in chapter 6, physicians have developed protocols whereby surgeons can begin harvesting organs from an organ donor a few minutes (usually five) after the heart stops even though we cannot say for sure that the arrest is absolutely irreversible and even though the transplanted heart might be restarted in the recipient's body. The procedure is called donation after cardiac death (DCD) and usually works this way. The organ donor is on life support that is going to be withdrawn. If the cardiac arrest occurs within thirty minutes after withdrawal, the physician declares death after five minutes, and then the organ retrieval team moves in to harvest the organs.

The second criterion of death is the irreversible cessation of all brain functions, including those of the brain stem. Ordinarily, the cessation of all brain functions in a person leads almost immediately to the irreversible cessation of cardiopulmonary functions as well, but life-support equipment or a heart-lung machine can sometimes support the cardiopulmonary functions after the brain functions have ceased. When this occurs, it presents an ideal opportunity for organ retrieval. The brain-dead patient on life support is truly dead, but the organs are being nourished as if she were alive. In fact, almost all transplantable organs obtained after death are from people determined to be dead by the whole brain death criterion. It is not surprising, then, that one of the factors driving the discussion and eventual acceptance of the whole brain death criterion in the 1960s was the need for fresh organs in the emerging field of transplantation.

Although the two criteria of human death are relatively clear and widely accepted, the need for fresh organs has generated several concerns relevant to organ retrieval and the criteria of death.

Concerns Related to Attempting Resuscitation

The cardiopulmonary criterion of death is normally the way death is determined, but organs from people determined dead by this criterion are rarely usable. If CPR is attempted, it will delay for many minutes organ retrieval from a donor whose cardiopulmonary arrest is, in fact, irreversible even though the irreversibility is not yet clear to those attempting resuscitation. Two worthy causes collide in these cases. The team performing CPR is working diligently to save the donor's life while the donor wants his organs retrieved if he dies. The longer CPR is attempted, the less chance there is of retrieving viable organs, and the CPR team knows this. Their moral problem centers on how to integrate the patient's desire to donate his organs with their efforts to resuscitate him if possible.

Another ethical problem can arise when resuscitation will not be attempted, perhaps because the person is subject to a DNR order. Here there may be a temptation to retrieve the organs almost immediately after the heart stops. In the first few minutes after a cardiopulmonary arrest, however, it is not known for sure whether the cessation of cardiopulmonary functions is irreversible. There is always the chance, in the first few minutes, that the cardiac arrest could be reversed if CPR were attempted. Hence, it cannot be said that these patients have clearly suffered the irreversible cessation of cardiopulmonary functions. Of course, when CPR will not be attempted, the arrest will not in fact be reversed, but this is not the same as saying the arrest is irreversible. Under the present criterion, only when we are certain that the cessation of all the cardiopulmonary functions is irreversible can we say the person is dead, and this certainty is not present in the first few minutes after the arrest of a person because CPR, if attempted, might just reverse the arrest.

It can be argued that moral concern about this is groundless. Cardiopulmonary arrests seldom reverse themselves, so a decision not to attempt CPR after an arrest means that the arrest will be permanent. Still, the accepted cardiopulmonary criterion of death states that the arrest must be *irreversible* and not simply an arrest where reversal might occur if CPR is attempted. If we do not want to chance harvesting organs from the still living, we cannot begin until we know that the cessation of the cardiopulmonary functions is truly *irreversible*, and this takes time. Even after ten minutes, some arrests are reversible, although there may well be some irreversible neurological damage.

Hence, the new DCD protocols that we discussed in chapter 6 that allow for organ retrieval from donors a few minutes after their heart stops are morally problematic because we cannot say for sure that the cardiopulmonary arrest is irreversible in such a short time. These donors are called non-heart-beating donors (NHBDs) or asystolic cadaveric donors. Once they or their proxy consents to life-support withdrawal, the attending physician waits several minutes (usually between two and five depending on the hospital protocol) and then declares the person dead, allowing the organ transplant team to begin harvesting the organs. As we discussed in chapter 6, this organ retrieval procedure seems to ignore the standard cardiopulmonary criterion for determining death, yet there are some good reasons for pursuing donation after cardiac death.

Concerns Related to Consent

Transplant teams normally do not attempt retrieval of organs from a donor without the permission of the family. Now, if the death of a person not on a life-support system was unexpected, by the time permission is obtained from a family member, the organs are often too damaged for use. The process of obtaining consent from family members is time consuming, especially if the deceased person had not indicated she wanted to donate organs. Physicians have to explain what donation entails to a family who are grieving a death. They have just been told a loved one is dead, and now they must decide immediately whether or not to give consent for the retrieval of her organs. If they delay more than a short time, the organs will be too damaged for use.

In an attempt to save organs while permission for transplantation is being sought, some physicians have injected ice-cold saline solutions into the bodies of potential donors as soon as they have died. Cooling the organs reduces their need for blood and oxygen and gives the physicians time to seek permission or consent for organ retrieval from the family. If the family grants permission or consent, the organs can be used. If the family does not consent to organ retrieval, no real harm was done to the potential donor because the person was already dead when the cooling solution was injected. Nonetheless, there are legitimate ethical concerns over treating a dead body this way without any consent by the person or by the family.

Concerns about Living, Breathing Bodies

Organ retrieval from people declared dead by the whole-brain criterion of death can create a certain level of moral discomfort for some people. After the determination of brain death is made, the life-support equipment will be continued to preserve the organs until the transplant team and the recipients are ready for the procedure. When all is ready, the organ retrieval will begin, sometimes without stopping the life support. For some, this appears to be taking organs from a living person, and it is morally upsetting. In fact, however, if the brain death criterion is accepted, and if the clinical verification has been accurate, there are no moral problems associated with retrieving a kidney, for example, from a donor while life-support equipment continues to sustain his respiratory and circulatory functions. Despite appearances, it is simply another case of cadaverous organ donation.

Concerns about the Brain-Death Definition Itself

Other legitimate moral problems, however, do surround the use of the brain-death criterion in organ transplantation. For example, the brain-death criterion of death requires that "all functions of the entire brain" have irreversibly ceased, but the meaning of "all functions of the entire brain" has never been clearly defined. Sometimes small pockets of dying brain cells remain functioning and small amounts of electrical activity persist in people who are determined to be dead according to the current clinical criteria for brain death. And it has been reported that organ retrieval has triggered hemodynamic responses in the blood circulation of brain-dead patients. Since these hemodynamic responses are thought to originate in the brain, their detection raises questions about the clarity of the phrase "all functions of the entire brain."

The need for organs has prompted some people to suggest that the brain-death criterion should be made less demanding. They propose requiring only the irreversible cessation of higher brain functions, what some call neocortical death. If brain death were understood as neocortical death, it would permit retrieval of organs from people in a persistent vegetative state and permanent coma; that is, from some permanently unconscious patients sustained only by feeding tubes. At the present time, however, the permanently unconscious are not considered brain dead, and reasons for not adopting this criterion of death were noted in chapter 6.

Concerns Related to Brain Death in Children

Some controversy exists about the ability to determine brain death in children, especially very young children and neonates. The President's Commission report titled *Defining Death* (1982) noted that the brains of infants and young children have more resistance to damage than older brains and that they may recover substantive functions after longer periods of unresponsiveness. The commission therefore urged physicians to be cautious about applying the standard clinical criteria of brain death to children under five years of age.

A special group called the Task Force on Brain Death in Childhood (1985–86) recommended various clinical criteria for determining brain death in three categories of young children: those over one year of age, those between two months and one year, and those between seven days and two months. These carefully crafted criteria are helpful, although they do not apply to infants under seven days of age. Several medical centers have also developed clinical criteria for diagnosing brain death in young children. Still, the difficulty of diagnosing brain death in children, especially infants, remains, and it has inhibited the use of the brain death standard for infants whose parents have consented to organ donation.

Concerns Related to Anencephaly

Some see anencephalic infants as a promising source of organ donations. These infants usually do not live long, and often their organs are healthy. Some suggest we should consider infants with anencephaly "brain dead" even though they never had a living brain that could have died. Several years ago physicians in Germany considered two anencephalic infants brain dead, placed them on ventilators, and harvested their kidneys within an hour of birth.

One of these infants was a twin whose anencephaly had been diagnosed at sixteen weeks of gestation. In what was an obvious inconsistency in moral reasoning, the parents declined an elective abortion because it was "morally unacceptable," yet they consented to the lethal action of removing the living infant's kidneys. In effect, they thought it was immoral for physicians to destroy the fetus before birth but not immoral for physicians to destroy the infant by taking the kidneys an hour after birth. Apparently, it never dawned on them that if the baby was "brain dead" after birth and could therefore be destroyed (by the act of retrieving its organs), then it was also "brain dead" before birth and could therefore be aborted without moral objection.

Of course the anencephalic infant was not brain dead at all, and the kidneys should not have been taken from the living infant. The legal authorities in Germany have since put a stop to the retrieval of organs from anencephalic infants, and rightly so. As much as we need organs for transplantation, it is hard to see how taking them from dying infants who are not dead by currently accepted criteria will help us flourish as noble and decent human beings. Today, the debate about retrieving organs from anencephalic infants has abated somewhat because the numbers of such cases are decreasing. Many cases are discovered by prenatal diagnosis, and abortion often follows, thus reducing the number of infants born with anencephaly.

The need for infant organs moved physicians at Loma Linda Hospital in California to try a different approach. They put infants suffering from anencephaly on life support, and then withdrew the infant from the ventilator at periodic intervals to determine whether or not the infant could breathe without ventilation. If the infant breathed spontaneously, he was put back on the ventilator; if not, he was declared dead and the organs were retrieved. The lack of spontaneous respiration was taken as a clinical sign that the child had recently died while on the life support.

What criterion of death was being used in this protocol? Strictly speaking, neither of those currently in use. Mere cessation of spontaneous respiration does not fulfill the cardiopulmonary criterion of death—this criterion requires irreversible cessation of respiratory functions. And cessation of spontaneous respiration does not fulfill the brain death criterion of death—this criterion requires extensive neurological testing and is not satisfied by observing that a ventilator-dependent infant cannot breathe without the ventilator. After moral objections were raised about treating anencephalic infants in this way, the hospital abandoned the practice.

The need for infant organs has led others to suggest still another approach. Admitting that we cannot say anencephalic infants are dead according to either of the two current criteria (brain death or irreversible cessation of cardiopulmonary functions), they advocate changing the criteria or, if the criteria are not changed, making a special case for anencephalic infants so their organs can be retrieved before they die. As you may well imagine, many ethical objections have been raised against these strategies. It is simply not a good idea, many argue, to change the criteria of death in order to harvest more organs from living infants, even those suffering from anencephaly.

In summary, a number of issues surrounding the determination of death are still associated with organ retrieval. The chronic shortage of organs for transplantation is one reason why these ethical issues linger. The shortage puts pressure on physicians to make every donated organ count, and this means retrieving organs as soon as possible after death.

The unfortunate organ shortage also creates the second major ethical question emerging from donation after death—allocation of the organs we do retrieve. We will now consider some of the vexing ethical problems associated with the distribution of organs.

Allocation of Scarce Cadaverous Organs

Organ transplantation is an example of a major social and ethical dilemma in health care—the distribution of scarce resources. Organ transplants save lives, but at the present time, we cannot supply organs to everyone who needs them. How, then, do we select the lucky ones, knowing that many of those not selected will die? It is a hard choice, captured well in the question: "Who shall live when not all can live?"

In 1984 Congress responded to the chaotic and unfair distribution of organs in the United States by passing the National Organ Transplant Act, which calls for a single national network for allocating organs. The Reagan administration was at first reluctant to support government involvement in allocation. However, the publicity surrounding the cases of Jamie Fiske and Jesse Sepulveda, covered later in this chapter, helped the government overcome its hesitations, and by 1986 a single national network—the Organ Procurement and Transplantation Network (OPTN)—was in place. A nonprofit group called United Network for Organ Sharing (UNOS) began managing OPTN under a federal contract that gives the Department of Health and Human Services (HHS) ultimate control over organ distribution in the United States.

By December 2008 OPTN had more than 100,000 Americans on its waiting list, up from about 60,000 in 1998 and 16,000 in 1988. Only about 28,000 people would receive an organ in 2008, and many on the waiting list will die still waiting for organs.

UNOS divides the country into eleven geographic regions. Organs, except for perfectly matched donor kidneys, are first offered to patients within the area where they were donated. If the organ is not needed there, UNOS offers it to patients in other parts of the country. There was a good reason for this geographical allocation system—organs do not last long once they are removed from the body. The ideal preservation time for hearts and lungs is about four hours; for pancreases and livers it is about ten hours. Kidneys, however, can be preserved for many more hours. Fortunately, newer preservation techniques are extending these times.

Unfortunately, the geographical distribution system has created a serious ethical problem of fairness because the lines are shorter in some areas of the country than in others. Hence, organs are sometimes going to less needy recipients in the area where they were retrieved, whereas more needy patients in an adjoining area have been waiting, perhaps in vain, for an organ to be retrieved in their area.

In February 1998 the secretary of HHS, Donna Shalala, announced new federal regulations that would dismantle the geographical hierarchy and make organs available to the most needy person anywhere in the country. The proposed regulations caused such a controversy that Congress delayed its implementation until late in 1999. Essentially, the pending HHS regulation directed UNOS to abandon the geographical system and set up a nationwide allocation system with a standardized set of criteria to determine ranking on the list. UNOS, however, objected to such a plan, claiming that it would not work as well as the existing geographical system.

Certainly it would not work as well for some small transplant centers. Under the existing system some small transplant centers could continue to operate only because they had first access to organs donated in the area. They would lose this privilege if the organs were distributed nationally because organs harvested in their area would go to sicker people outside their area. As a result some of the smaller medical centers probably would not receive enough organs to keep their transplant centers open. This would hurt them financially because organ transplantation is one of the areas where medical centers earn a profit or surplus and receive extensive favorable publicity.

The battle over changing the system took a new turn when states began passing laws prohibiting organs that had been retrieved within the state from going to other states. By early 1999 five states had such laws, and others were considering them. This forced HHS to revise its proposed regulations. When the revised final rule appeared in March 2000, several states, including New Jersey and Wisconsin, sued for relief in federal court, but the suit was dismissed in November 2000. The current HHS regulation retains a general geographical distribution system but directs OPTN to distribute organs beyond geographical areas and to consider the urgency of needs for organs outside region where they were harvested.

The battle over a local or a national allocation system, however, is only the tip of the complicated allocation and scarcity problem for several reasons. First, it is not easy to design an ethical system of distributing organs that will be fair to everyone and capture major ethical values such as the urgency of need and the likelihood of significant benefit for the recipient. Second, the scarcity of organs available for allocation in the United States is exacerbated by the cultural preference for self-determination and autonomy. Americans thus far have tended to feel that organs should not be taken from cadavers unless there is a process of explicit consent: either the donor gives consent while living and the family does not object after death, or, if the donor did not give consent, the family gives consent after death. The assumption is that people would not want organs taken after death so we have to ask for permission. There is some value in this approach, but it has also resulted in a tremendous scarcity of organs, and hence needless deaths, in the United States.

Many other countries have taken a different approach. In general, they assume that a person would want her organs used to save lives, and so the organs will generally be harvested if they are usable unless the person has formally registered her opposition to organ donation. Spain, for example, passed its presumed consent law in 1979, and now Spain has the highest rate of organ donation in the world. Belgium also increased organ donation by its presumed consent law of 1986, and other countries (e.g., Austria, France, Norway, and Italy) have followed suit. In Austria the rate of organ donation increased 400 percent after its presumed consent law was introduced. Countries with presumed consent laws harvest more organs and save more lives than countries such as the United States, Canada, and Great Britain that still require asking people and families to give consent for harvesting organs after death.

Ethicists in the United States are divided on instituting a policy of presumed consent to increase the supply of organs and save lives. Utilitarians tend to favor such a policy, but rights-based ethicists tend to oppose it, arguing that we cannot assume people would give consent for their organs to be taken after death. Virtue ethics might well readily support presumed consent. Surveys show that many more Americans are willing to donate their organs than actually so indicate on their driver's license renewal forms or elsewhere, and this provides some reason for presuming consent in many cases. Moreover, tailoring public policies so they will support the social good is a major goal in virtue ethics, and saving many lives with organs that would otherwise be wasted provides yet another reason for presuming consent provided those opposed had ample opportunity to opt out and provided the immediate family does not object.

Given the shortage of organs, selecting people for transplants in a fair way is a difficult challenge. Roughly speaking, it is a two-stage affair. In the first stage, the selection determines who will be placed on the waiting list for an organ. In the second stage, the selection determines who on the waiting list will receive the next available organ. Selecting organ recipients is so difficult that extensive controversy still exists over the criteria used for the selection.

The Case of Jamie Fiske

The Story

Jamie was born in 1983 with biliary atresia, an incurable malfunction of the liver. Her only hope of survival past infancy was a liver transplant. The family's insurance plan, Blue Cross and Blue Shield of Massachusetts, did not pay for liver transplants at that time because it did not consider liver transplants a "generally accepted" surgical procedure. Few had been performed, and no Massachusetts hospital had a liver transplantation program set up in 1983.

Charles Fiske, Jamie's father, immediately complained to Tom McGee, Speaker of the Massachusetts House, and to a local TV station, that Blue Cross and Blue Shield refused to pay for his daughter's transplant. Within twenty-four hours Blue Cross and Blue Shield agreed to make a special exception and pay for the surgery. The governor of Massachusetts also pledged Medicaid funding for the surgery. The guaranteed funding enabled the parents to place Jamie's name on a waiting list in Minnesota, and she was transferred there to await a liver.

Six weeks went by and nothing happened. The parents contacted the AMA for help. They also contacted the American Academy of Pediatrics, looking for the addresses of pediatric surgeons. They planned to write them all, hoping one of them would encounter a brain-dead child whose liver could be retrieved. It so happened that the academy was having its national convention in New York at that time, and Charles Fiske asked to address the group. He received an equivocal response. The pediatricians were sympathetic, but they reminded him that other babies were on the list awaiting organs.

Jamie's parents turned once again to political figures and to the mass media. They contacted their senator and their representative in Washington, as well as the speaker of the U.S. House of Representatives, who came from their state. They appealed to the local TV stations and to ABC, NBC, and CBS as well. Their plight received national coverage.

Less than a week later, a baby boy in Utah was killed in an accident. His parents had heard of Jamie Fiske on TV and decided to donate their child's organs to her. The liver was successfully transplanted into Jamie, and her life was saved.

Ethical Analysis

Situational awareness.   We are aware of these facts in the Fiske story.

1. Jamie would not survive without a liver transplant. Although some liver transplants fail, some do succeed and save lives.

2. The family insurance did not cover liver transplants, and the family did not have the money to pay for it.

3. Funding was obtained, but then a donor had to be found. Weeks on a waiting list produced nothing, and her condition worsened. Her parents resorted to political pressure and to media attention in a desperate effort to save her life.

We are also aware of these good and bad features in this case.

1. Clearly, Jamie's life is good and her death would be bad, and a terrible thing for her parents.

2. The media campaign accomplished some good. It raised national awareness about insurance coverage for liver transplantations and about the donation of cadaverous infant organs. It also influenced the parents of a deceased baby to donate his liver, and the liver saved a life.

3. The media campaigns and political pressure to obtain funding and organ donations for a needy child also gave rise to several bad features. Among them are the following.

- Extensive and emotional publicity about the plight of one child diverts resources from other needy children, and this is bad for them.

- The publicity about expensive interventions can lead to an excessive emphasis on these interventions to the neglect of routine and less expensive medical care for needy children, and this is bad for them.
- Publicity undermines the basic equality of opportunity that should characterize the allocation of scarce resources. Obtaining organs by publicity is a discriminatory process—it favors families with political connections and with the ability to present the case well to reporters and TV audiences.
- The publicity given to some patients heightens the anxiety and frustration of the parents of other children, who realize their children may be bypassed in favor of the case before the public eye.

Prudential Reasoning in the Fiske Story

Parents' perspective. It would be difficult to say that Jamie's parents acted in a morally inappropriate way. Their primary responsibility was to Jamie, and they worked hard to save her life. Their use of media publicity and political pressure is hard to fault. Their actions were actions of love, and there is a priority in the virtue of love whereby we will go to greater lengths for family than for others, for friends than for strangers. Modern ethical theories, those reflecting Kant and utilitarianism in particular, tend to overlook this order of love in their emphasis on treating everyone with equal respect and impartiality. In an ethics of virtue and right reason, however, the order of love or charity is more easily acknowledged. Given the predicament Jamie's parents faced in 1983 when the social system of organ distribution was not yet organized as it is today, their extraordinary efforts to save their daughter were not only reasonable but laudable.

Providers' perspective. From a clinical perspective, it is also hard to fault the transplant team in Minnesota. Their primary clinical responsibility is doing good for their patient. However, there are limitations to clinical beneficence. Most ethicists agree, for example, that it would be unethical for a transplant surgeon to buy organs from living patients on the black market in order to benefit his patient. The black market in commercial organs harvested from the living is not a morally good distribution system. Neither is an organ distribution process based on media publicity. Hence, from a social perspective, physicians cooperating with organ distribution by media campaigns are participating in an unethical distribution program. Clinical beneficence in organ transplantation becomes morally unreasonable whenever the organ procurement or distribution systems are morally unreasonable by reason of the disproportionate damage they do to the human good. What is truly beneficial for one patient can be unethical, as it is when it involves unreasonable (that is, morally unjustified) damage to others.

Social perspective. It was a wonderful event for Jamie and her family when the publicity resulted in the life-saving organ, but was the social system that allowed and abetted this kind of allocation process fair? It seems not. Other babies were on the waiting list, but their parents did not use political and media pressure to find an organ for them. As happy as everyone is for Jamie and her family, there is something morally disturbing about the babies of bright, articulate, well-educated, and determined parents receiving organs, while the babies of parents without these qualities fail to receive them. And it is disturbing to think that parents must use political influence and national media coverage to help their sick children.

The moral problems involved in this case, then, are not personal but medical and social. The parents acted reasonably and pursued what was truly good in their lives. The physicians acted in a responsible way, but by agreeing to transplant organs designated for their patients in a process lacking in fairness, their behavior raises moral concerns. If the allocation of organs by media appeals and talk shows is not a fair way to distribute organs, then there are good reasons for saying transplant surgeons should refuse to participate in this kind of allocation. And there are good reasons for saying that politicians and responsible people in the print and electronic media should refuse to assist parents in finding organs this way.

The Case of Jesse Sepulveda

The Story

Jesse was born on May 25, 1986, at Huntington Memorial Hospital in Pasadena with hypoplastic left-heart syndrome, a congenital defect that is usually fatal. Physicians immediately referred the parents to Loma Linda University Medical Center, which by then had transplanted five infant hearts in the first six months of its new program. The parents, seventeen-year-old Deana Binckley and twenty-six-year-old Jesse Sepulveda, Sr., were interviewed at Loma Linda. Their request to have Jesse placed on the waiting list for a heart was sent to the twenty-member hospital committee that reviews the transplant requests. The committee, by a unanimous vote, declined to accept Jesse as a candidate. The committee did not give Deana and Jesse a reason, but physicians at Huntington told them that it was because they were young and not married.

When Father Michael Carcerano, the priest who baptized baby Jesse, heard of the rejection, he contacted Susan McMillan, the California spokesperson for the National Right to Life Committee. She began a media campaign. In the face of the publicity, much of it critical of the hospital, Loma Linda agreed to accept Jesse as a candidate for a transplant, provided his parents would give custody of the baby to the paternal grandparents. In an effort to save their child, the parents agreed. Loma Linda then accepted Jesse as a candidate for a heart.

The hospital denied that it had originally refused to list Jesse as a candidate for a transplant because his parents were not married and said that its decision had been based on concern about what kind of postoperative care Jesse would receive at home. It declined to reveal why it doubted that Jesse's parents could provide the necessary care, but press reports indicated that Deana may have had a substance abuse problem.

Meanwhile, a baby named Frank Clemenshaw died in Michigan. The parents at first refused to donate his organs, but after hearing of Jesse's plight on television news programs and realizing that he had been born on the same day as their son, they decided to donate his heart to Jesse. Physicians in Michigan notified Loma Linda that a heart was available for Jesse, but the hospital did not immediately notify Jesse's parents or grandparents.

The next day, still unaware that a heart had been found, Jesse's parents, Susan McMillan of the Right to Life Committee, and Rev. Carcerano appeared on the Phil Donahue Show in New York. They made a moving plea for a heart for Jesse. During the live program, the phone rang and a spokesperson from the hospital in Michigan told the nationwide audience that it had a heart for Jesse. There was great rejoicing on the set and in the audience as people cheered, cried, and applauded. After a few emotional moments, Phil Donahue excused the parents so they could fly back to California for the operation. Mr. Donahue assured the audience that the hospital's call had not been prearranged, but later accounts told a different story. The woman making the call claimed the producers of the Donahue program had learned of the donation and then pressed her to call during the show to announce it on national television.

Jesse received Frank's heart and became the fourth baby in the world to receive a successful heart transplant. Seven years later, this heart began to fail. In June 1993 Jesse became the second child in the world to receive a second heart transplant. Unfortunately, drugs could not prevent his immune system from rejecting the second heart, and physicians at Loma Linda declined to try a third transplant. Jesse died in July 1993.

Ethical Reflection

Jesse's story is sufficiently similar to Jamie's story that we need not repeat the facts in a situational analysis nor provide an ethical analysis of the behavior of the various moral agents who played a major role in the case. When a baby needs an organ to live, it is difficult to fault parents when they use the media or a national TV talk show to appeal for that organ. And it is difficult to fault the child's physicians for implanting an organ produced by the publicity, although the participation of physicians in an allocation system based on publicity remains morally questionable. The main point of telling Jesse's story is to illustrate how such an allocation process, although good for one baby, is not a morally good allocation system.

Although we can acknowledge the good intentions of the priest and the spokesperson for the National Right to Life Committee whose efforts enabled Jesse to receive his first heart, we cannot overlook the other side to the story. Their efforts found a heart for Jesse, but they also skewered the allocation process.

When the heart was given to Jesse, it meant the baby designated to receive the next heart was bypassed. His name was Robert Cardin. Robert was in a hospital in Kentucky and first in line to receive the next available heart. When Frank's heart became available, however, Robert did not receive it. National media attention on Jesse's plight so influenced the allocation process that the heart went to him and not to Robert, the baby first in line. This delay created an unnecessary risk for Robert.

When Robert's physician realized how his patient had lost his chance for a heart, he contacted the news media to gain publicity for his side of the story. Soon Baby Robert's plight became national news, and another heart was donated for him. This still meant, of course, that the baby next in line was left waiting. The danger is that hearts will be distributed on the basis of publicity, rather than by medical need, and within a social system of allocation based on triage.

The stories of Jamie and Jesse reveal the two sides of ethics. The publicity efforts of the Fiskes and of Ms. McMillan saved the lives of these two babies, and that is undeniably good for those individuals. But there are good reasons for saying that their efforts undermined an ethical allocation system, and this is bad for other unknown babies and their parents. To put it another way, there is no moral justification for distributing scarce organs in this country on the basis of publicity.

Of course it can be argued that Jamie's liver and Jesse's heart would not have been donated but for the publicity and that the publicity actually produced organs that otherwise would not have been donated. The publicity, then, did not deprive anyone on the established waiting list of an organ because it actually produced an additional organ. This argument has some merit, but it is not sufficiently strong to overcome the other negative social aspects of retrieving and allocating organs by media publicity focused on desperate families. More reasonable, and hence more ethical, ways of allocating organs are available.

The stories of Jamie and Jesse are not simply about the ethically questionable role of media attention in the organ allocation process; they also raise questions about what we might call designated donation. The parents of the deceased babies in these stories actually designated Jamie and Jesse as recipients of their children's organs. The idea of people or their proxies designating recipients of the donated organs presents another moral issue. Given the shortage of organs, is it ever morally justified to override the national waiting list by designating the recipient, or a class of recipients, for organs? The morality of the donor designating the recipient of his organs is complex because there are plausible reasons both for and against such a practice. The following reasons favor designated donation:

- Since people can donate their bodies to a designated medical school for research, there should be no moral objection to donating an organ to a designated person.
- Since living people can donate a kidney to a designated recipient, usually a sibling, there should be no moral objection to designated donation after death.
- Since there is a unique bond within families, there should be no moral objection if one member wishes to designate another member as the recipient of his organ after death.
- Since some people would not donate unless they could identify a recipient, it is better to allow designated donation than to lose the organ.

The main reason against designated donation is based on social justice. Organ transplantation is not just a personal matter—it is also a social process involving hospitals and surgical teams, and sometimes public funding. Transplantation, therefore, falls within the realm of social justice, and social justice is undermined when institutions and practitioners participate in a program that favors people for reasons unrelated to medical need and benefit. Allocating organs on the basis of personal designations is not an allocation process that meets the requirements of a fair and equitable distribution of organs. Designating a particular person means that others higher up on the list may wait longer for their chance. It could also result in a valuable organ being wasted because the designated recipient may not be a person with a high probability of benefiting from it.

There are, however, situations where it can be reasonably argued that designated donation is morally acceptable. One example is donation within families. The special love and support that exist, or should exist, within families are an important consideration that could be allowed to override the impartial demands of equality and fairness that characterize social justice. As we pointed out earlier, the modern theories of utilitarianism and Kantian deontology have difficulty recognizing this kind of partiality in ethics.

In an ethics of virtue, however, there is room for a complementary balance between the virtues of justice and love. The virtue of justice is primary in our relationships with strangers and in our responsibility to the community, but the virtue of love is primary in our relationships with our family and close friends. Love, by its very nature, allows us to act in a preferential way toward those whom we love. The virtue of love means, in an important sense, that some people in our lives count more than others; love is not a virtue whereby we treat everyone impartially. In an ethics that embraces personal love as a virtue, there are reasons for saying designated donations within loving relationships are morally acceptable.

TRANSPLANTATION OF ORGANS FROM LIVING HUMAN DONORS

Moral questions about donation from living donors center on two fundamental issues: how can we justify the harm done to the donor, and how can we ensure that the donor's consent is truly voluntary? Recently, a third issue has begun to emerge—the purchase of a kidney from a living person. The first issue was paramount when transplanting organs from living donors began, but now it has receded as most people have become morally comfortable in justifying the harm done to the donor by the surgery and the loss of a healthy organ. The implications of the second issue were not fully appreciated at first, but now the voluntary aspect of informed consent is receiving most of the attention.

The Risks and Harm Affecting the Donor

The most common form of donation from the living involves kidneys. Retrieving a kidney from a live donor requires major surgery and leaves the person less able to cope with kidney disease should it ever occur in her life. From a medical point of view, the donor is harmed, not helped, by the surgery. In some traditional moral approaches, this raises a serious moral problem. One of the ancient principles of medical ethics is *"primum, non nocere"* (that is, "first, do no harm"). The principle is captured today in the principle of nonmaleficence, often listed as a major action-guide along with the principles of autonomy, beneficence, and justice. The principle of nonmaleficence (meaning "do not harm") would seem to oblige us not to remove somebody's kidney when the removal harms her without producing any medical benefit for her.

A similar problem arose in Catholic moral theology in the 1950s as live donations became a reality. Theologians had earlier worked out a principle to justify surgery—the principle of totality. This principle allows the mutilation or destruction of part of the body in order to save the whole body. Ordinarily, the theologians taught, it would be wrong for a person to mutilate his body by surgery or to destroy a part of it. However, if the mutilation or destruction could contribute to the benefit of the body as a whole, then it could be morally justified by the principle of totality. For example, if a person has a cancerous kidney, the mutilation of the body necessary to remove the kidney can be morally justified because it contributes to the total health of the body.

In an ethics of principles, the principle of totality worked well for surgeries that contributed to the overall total health of the body. Moreover, the principle also conveniently ruled out surgeries that the Catholic Church opposed—sterilizations, the surgeries designed to prevent pregnancy. Theologians argued that vasectomies and tubal ligations are not justified by the principle of totality because they are not performed to benefit the whole body but to prevent conception.

When surgery to retrieve a kidney from a live donor became a reality, the theologians who had been justifying surgery by the principle of totality were perplexed. Obviously, their principle of totality ruled it out. The surgery taking a healthy kidney out of one person to give it to another in no way contributes to the totality of the donor's health. On the contrary, the donor's health is actually undermined by the risks of the unnecessary surgery and by the life-long deprivation of the healthy kidney.

Some theologians, faithful to their principle of totality, drew the obvious conclusion and considered organ retrieval from a living donor immoral. Others were not so sure. They thought, almost intuitively, that donating an organ to a person in need was a kind of Christian thing to do. Since Christianity had always taught that it was an act of great love to lay down one's life for another, they wondered why it would not also be an act of love to donate a life-saving kidney to another person.

Today, when it comes to organ donation from the living, medical ethicists who rely on a principle-based approach ignore their principle of nonmaleficence, and the theologians have all but forgotten their principle of totality. Most of them acknowledge that the living person who freely donates a kidney is acting in a morally admirable way. Fortunately, moral discernment triumphed over the moral principles of nonmaleficence and totality.

Surgery to retrieve organs for transplantation from the living is not, however, without legitimate moral concerns. Before retrieving the first kidney from a living identical twin in 1954, physicians at the Peter Bent Brigham Hospital sought court approval. Only when the judge ruled that the donor child would be more harmed by the loss of his twin brother than by the loss of his kidney did the surgeons proceed to remove the healthy kidney. The hospital's seeking court approval suggests concern about the legal liability for the medically unjustified harm its surgeons were about to do to the healthy twin by removing his kidney.

And there is still reason for this worry. Some kidney donors have died as the result of complications from the surgery, and others have been negatively affected by the surgery and by subsequent medical problems exacerbated by the loss of a kidney. The time may come that live donations will no longer be needed. As better immunosuppressive drugs come on line, and as more people arrange to donate their organs after death, it may no longer be necessary to harvest kidneys or parts of livers from the living. Until that happens, and it probably will not happen for a long time, most agree that organ donation from the living is morally acceptable, even admirable and virtuous.

However, the second serious moral question about live donation—the question of truly voluntary informed consent—remains. Unlike the questions about the harm and mutilation to the body, questions now resolved for ethicists and theologians, the question of informed consent for the retrieval of organs from living donors is now looming larger than ever.

Questions about Voluntary Consent

Consider, first, an adult whose family member needs a kidney, and the match is perfect or almost perfect. The adult will have to give informed consent for the surgery to remove her kidney. The question is, can the consent be truly voluntary in such circumstances? Consider the predicament the woman is in. If she refuses the surgery, think of the guilt she will experience when her sister needing the kidney dies, and think of the way other family members may treat (or mistreat) her after she refuses to donate. It is quite possible that the intense pressures, both real and perceived, on the potential donor destroy the possibility of truly voluntary consent. And surgery on an adult with decision-making capacity without her voluntary consent is immoral (and illegal).

Consider, second, a child whose kidney is the best match for a sibling. For surgery on children, the parents must give consent. And when parents are deciding to give consent for surgery on their children, they normally rely, as we saw in chapter 5, on what is known as the best interests standard. In other words, the parents decide on the basis of what is in the best interests of the child. Now, in a very important sense, surgery to take a perfectly healthy kidney from a child is simply not in that donor child's best interests.

Some will argue that it is. Following the reasoning of the Massachusetts court in the first live kidney donation, they will claim that losing the sibling would be more harmful to the child than losing the kidney. But this is no more than a gratuitous claim; it is not, with all due respect to the court, a judgment based on evidence. We simply do not know that the child would agree with this opinion. Undoubtedly, some children may grow up delighted that their parents decided to use their kidney to save a sibling before they were old enough to make the decision. But others, especially if the surgery has harmed them or shortened their life, may resent what happened. Also, as happens in some families, hostile relations can develop between a child and parent or between sibling and sibling. In such situations, the donor may grow old very unhappy that his parents authorized the surgery or that a particular sibling received his kidney.

The pressing moral problem about obtaining truly voluntary consent from a living donor, both consent by the adult donor and consent by parents on behalf of a child, remains troublesome. At the very least, great care must be taken to ensure truly voluntary consent.

An example of serious attention to the ethical problems of donation from living donors occurred before the first partial liver transplant from a mother to a child. In November 1989 the first partial transplantation of a liver was made at the University of Chicago when a mother donated for her child. One of the most encouraging aspects of this transplantation of liver lobes was the thorough discussion of the ethical issues related to the experimental surgery before it took place. People were sensitive to the risks for the donor as well as the benefits for the donor and for the recipient and to the need for a consent that was truly voluntary. At the very least this intense ethical scrutiny will diminish the fears that consent to donate an organ while the donor is still living may not be truly voluntary.

Buying Organs Harvested from the Living

Stories about selling organs harvested from living people have persisted for years. In its issue of March 13, 1989, *Time* magazine reported that a poor Turkish peasant sold a kidney in London for about $4,500 to raise money for an operation for his daughter. In September 2008 station KABC in Los Angeles broadcast the story of a man who traveled to Pakistan to receive a kidney sold by a poor woman. He said that he paid the Aadvil Hospital in Lahore about $30,000 for the transplant and that he was told the kidney seller received about $4,500. The TV station provided him with a video camera so he could film his trip for them, and KABC put the video on the Internet. It is not clear when the trip was made. Pakistan made organ sales illegal in September 2007, and published reports have indicated that the number of kidney transplants at the Aadvil Hospital, most of them using kidneys bought from poor people, has dropped significantly from its annual rate of five hundred a year. Abdul Sheikh, the CEO of the hospital, was quoted in the press in May 2008 as saying: "The government has turned a $1 billion medical tourism business into a $1 million one." His hospital's website now states that a recipient must make arrangements for his own donor, yet also includes the comment: "You may contact us by email for necessary guidance on the donor."

The World Health Organization and the laws of most countries make organ sales illegal. Nonetheless, reports indicate that the practice continues in a kind of black market, and a few countries, the Philippines for example, have declined to make selling organs illegal. In the United States the 1984 Organ Procurement and Transplantation Act prohibits the sale of organs for transplantation.

What might an ethics of right reason conclude about people selling their organs? From the perspective of the person selling his organ, the action can be considered reasonable, and even laudable, if it is a last resort to prevent starvation. When survival is at stake, some behaviors not normally ethical can be considered morally reasonable. For example, stealing is normally immoral, but a long, and reasonable, ethical tradition condones stealing to prevent a greater harm—starving to death. In the same way, it could also be argued that a person should not sell his kidney—unless the act were necessary to prevent an even greater threat to his life or the life of a loved one.

Of course, a person should not have to sell a kidney to save his life or the life of his child, but life does not always unfold as we would like. It would be a strange ethics indeed that would allow a person to give up his place on a crowded life raft voluntarily so another could live but would condemn a person for giving up a kidney to provide life-saving medical care for his family.

From the perspective of the people in the commercial system who would be buying and selling kidneys bought from living people, organ sales are not so easy to justify as reasonable and virtuous. In fact, many reasons have been advanced against allowing the practice. Some say that the system exploits poor people, since only needy people would agree to sell a kidney, and many sellers receive little or no follow-up care after their surgery. Some say the practice would result in lower quality kidneys, since the sellers would probably already be in less than optimum health. Some say the practice would undermine an allocation system based on medical criteria, since the purchased kidneys would go to the well insured and the rich. Some say the practice would undermine the sense of altruism motivating organ donation today, since a market in organs could destroy the powerful feeling of "giving a gift of life" that motivates some donors.

All these arguments have some merit, but so do the responses to them advanced by those defending the sale of organs in a carefully regulated environment. They argue that exploitation can be prevented, that measures of quality control to ensure retrieval only of healthy organs are possible, that equitable allocation systems are possible, and that buying kidneys would provide a greater supply of healthy kidneys than the current system of donation from the dead.

There are, however, two stronger arguments against allowing a system whereby living people could sell their organs. First, there is a legitimate concern about truly voluntary informed consent. We can assume that people willing to sell a kidney are under great pressure, and this coercive pressure all too easily subverts the requirement for truly voluntary consent. Moreover, there are grave concerns about whether the poor people selling a kidney actually receive and understand the information they need for fully *informed* consent. Second, it is difficult to see how a social system that allowed living people to sell kidneys would be compatible with an ethics of the human good. This ethics seeks a good life, and thus cherishes life. Commercial systems that damage life—and removing a healthy kidney from a living person is damaging to him—introduce bad features that an ethics of the good will seek to avoid, not encourage.

Thus, an ethics of the good would likely not condone commercial systems of slavery or prostitution, even if some people think their autonomy should permit them to choose slavery or prostitution, because these forms of commercial practices are not compatible with a good and noble life. In the same way, it can be well argued that a commercial system of buying organs from willing people is inconsistent with living a good life. Slavery, prostitution, and paying people for organs are arguably not beneficial practices for societies because whatever benefit they might achieve is outweighed by the bad features inherent in the systemic commercialization of slavery, of prostitution, and of organ harvesting from poverty-stricken people who benefit little from the medically risky procedure.

Would the offer of money for organs given up after death meet with the same moral objections? Here the issue of the voluntary consent, so very important before surgical interventions on the living, is significantly reduced. A person can more easily agree to donate an organ freely after death than during life because he knows that the removal after death brings no harm to him. And the money paid for the organ is not a coercive inducement since it does him no good. The bad features of commercialization involving the living are also reduced because the organ retrieval is no longer from one of us, and the retrieval does not result in a person suffering from the surgical retrieval and facing the rest of his life without a kidney. There may be ways to increase the supply of organs by reasonable financial inducements that do not undermine the common good. Some, for example, have proposed a system whereby funeral costs would be subsidized if organs were harvested from the deceased.

TRANSPLANTATION OF ORGANS FROM ANIMALS

In November 1963 Dr. Keith Reemtsma transplanted chimpanzee kidneys into a forty-three-year-old poor African-American man in New Orleans Charity Hospital. Jefferson Davis was dying and thought his only chance was a transplant from an animal. According to a transcript of a conversation with his doctors after the surgery, he said: "Well, I ain't had no choice." He lived about two months and died in January 1964. That same month, at the University of Mississippi Medical Center, Dr. James Hardy transplanted a chimpanzee heart into sixty-eight-year-old Boyd Rush, another poor dying man. Mr. Rush, who was deaf and mute, was unconscious when he was admitted to the hospital, and his stepsister gave consent for a "suitable heart transplant" if necessary. He lived less than two hours.

Although ethical sensitivity about what was, in effect, medical research was not as high in 1963–64 as it is now, these transplantations are suspect under moral restraints known by all at the time. It is difficult, for example, to see how these experiments could be justified under the Nuremberg Code of 1947. Of course, these men were dying, and when people are dying, some think almost any medical intervention intended to save their lives is justified. That thinking, however, is not morally sound. In fact, it is morally dangerous because it can easily cause unreasonable suffering for the dying patient.

The cases of Jefferson Davis and Boyd Rush, and those of a few other patients who received animal organs years ago, did not generate extensive public debate about the procedure. However, that debate exploded in 1984 when Dr. Leonard Bailey and his team transplanted a baboon heart into a newborn baby girl at Loma Linda University Medical Center in California. The plight of Baby Fae fascinated the nation for weeks, a fascination fueled in no small way by a two-part series in *People* magazine that ran in December 1984. A review of this case will help us sharpen our prudential reasoning about animal transplants or, as they are sometimes called, xenografts.

The Case of Baby Fae

The Story

On October 14, 1984, in southern California, a baby girl suffering from hypoplastic left-heart syndrome, a fatal condition, was delivered three weeks prematurely. She was transferred to Loma Linda University Medical Center, and the world soon knew her as Baby Fae.

Physicians and families faced with a baby suffering from this heart problem had few options at the time. They could do nothing, they could seek a human heart for transplantation, or they could try an experimental surgery developed by Dr. William Norwood of Philadelphia (sometimes known as the Norwood procedure). Physicians at Loma Linda decided on a fourth option: the transplantation of a baboon heart. For this, they needed the consent of the parents.

Baby Fae's parents, who were not married but had lived together for about four years, had separated a few months before her birth. Her mother had not completed high school and was on welfare when the baby was born. Her father did not know he had a daughter until she was several days old. Both parents were upset about the baby's condition and wanted to do everything possible to save her life.

In a long conference that began about midnight and ended seven hours later, the mother, grandmother, and a male friend of the mother who was staying at the mother's home spent hours with Dr. Leonard Bailey discussing what could be done. As a result of this discussion, the mother signed an informed consent form allowing transplantation from an animal. Later, the father also gave consent, although he had not been involved in the extensive deliberations with the others.

Since transplantation from an animal to a human is an unorthodox procedure, it would have been a challenge to compose an appropriate informed consent form. The actual form signed by the parents, however, has never been made public despite the interest many have in reviewing it. Ultimately, the adequacy of the information on the form may not be that important; more important than the record of informed consent is the actual process that took place. The form may well be inadequate, but, as we pointed out in chapter 4, it is the reality of the consent process, and not the piece of paper, that is crucial.

After receiving IRB approval, Dr. Bailey transplanted the heart of a freshly killed baboon. Baby Fae died twenty days later. Her type O blood proved incompatible with the type AB blood of the baboon, and blood clots led to kidney failure. Autopsy also revealed some mild rejection by her immune system despite the immunosuppressive drugs.

Ethical Analysis

Situational awareness.   We are aware of these facts in the Baby Fae story.

1. Baby Fae was expected to die from heart failure in a matter of weeks.

2. Although there was a chance a human heart could be found and transplanted, no serious effort was made to pursue this option. There was also a chance that the Norwood procedure could save her, but no effort was made to pursue this option.

3. Dr. Bailey believed that it was medically feasible and morally acceptable to use animal organs in human beings. He had performed more than 150 transplantations in animals in the course of his research. In an interview ten days after the transplantation, he praised Dr. James Hardy, the physician who had transplanted a chimpanzee heart into Boyd Rush twenty years earlier, as his "champion." He said Hardy is "an idol of mine because he followed through and did what he should have done . . . he took a gamble to try to save a human life." Dr. Bailey also believed that the rare operation may have benefited Baby Fae and that it was not simply a medical experiment on a dying infant.

4. Baby Fae's parents were unmarried and separated when she was born. This fact is important because parental difficulties can undermine the process whereby parents work together as a team to decide with the physician what is in the best interests of their child.

5. Although both transplantation of a human heart and the Norwood procedure had been previously used with limited success, transplantation of an animal heart to a baby had never been attempted, and animal studies had not, and still have not, established its feasibility.

6. Baby Fae's parents were poor and had no health insurance. The hospital provided the baboon transplant at no charge. There is no evidence that it would have provided a human transplant for free or that the Norwood procedure would have been done for free.

We are also aware of these good and bad features in the case.

1. Baby Fae's death, as any human death, would be unfortunate and be a great loss for her parents.

2. Transplanting a baboon heart and providing the necessary preoperative and postoperative treatments would cause significant pain and suffering to Baby Fae. Her body would be placed on a heart-lung machine and her blood temperature lowered to sixty-eight degrees before the surgery. After the surgery, interventions would be necessary to support the transplant and prevent its rejection.

3. If the transplantation succeeded, Baby Fae could live longer than she would have lived with her own heart, and life is always a good. But we really do not know how much longer she might have lived if her body did not reject the baboon heart. Dr. Bailey said that she could someday celebrate her twenty-first birthday, but there is no compelling reason to believe a baboon heart could support an adult human body that long.

4. If the transplantation occurred and failed, physicians could still gain valuable information that would help future babies. There are not enough human hearts for infants, and it could save lives if a way were found to use animal hearts.

5. A baboon, a healthy animal with a high level of neurological development, was killed to retrieve his heart. Although this would not bother some people, the loss of life (including animal and environmental life) is always a bad feature in the ethics of the good, and concern for the loss is part of any complete moral deliberation.

Prudential Reasoning in the Baby Fae Story

The major moral agents in this case were the parents, the physician proposing the use of a baboon heart, and the members of the IRB that approved the experiment.

Parents' perspective. Unfortunately, personal difficulties prevented the parents from acting as a team in this case, but both parents did agree to the transplantation. Parents normally achieve their good by doing what they think is in the best interests of their child. However, parents can only work with the realistic options given them. As we noted earlier, hospitals routinely require insurance or a large down payment before attempting a heart transplant; Baby Fae's parents had neither. The Norwood procedure is also costly, and it would require transportation to and lodging in Philadelphia. Hence, the parents had only two realistic options if they were not offered a free human transplant or a Norwood procedure: no corrective interventions or a baboon transplant.

Faced with doing nothing to save the life of a child or doing something, no matter how unusual or unorthodox, many parents will think it reasonable to do something. But "doing something" is not always the reasonable response. Sometimes, as we saw in chapter 11, interventions are so burdensome and the possibility of significant success so slim that doing something to a very sick child is not morally justified.

Today, more than twenty-five years after the Baby Fae case, it would still seem unreasonable to subject an infant to a transplantation of an organ from an animal. Not enough promising research on transplantation from one species to another has been done with animals for us to begin the research on human beings, especially human beings who cannot give consent to the experiments. Parents have to be very careful about giving consent for research on their children. And when they do consent to research on their children, the risks should be minimal. The understandable urge to save the life of an infant can never blind parents to the concern for the baby's best interests. Faced with the impending death of their baby, they cannot agree to everything and anything; they can only agree to what is reasonable. And if the intervention on babies is experimental, they have to be very careful lest the legitimate goals of research pursued by physicians blind them to the child's best interest.

It is also worth noting that Baby Fae's father, although he signed the consent form, was not involved in the seven-hour conference that comprised the major part of the consent process. Signing a consent form is not enough. A parent has to be fully informed, and the very first effort to transplant an animal heart into a baby would obviously require a considerable amount of time for the father to grasp adequately the required information about the risks, side effects, alternatives, prognosis, and so forth.

Physician's perspective. Dr. Bailey of Loma Linda was out of town when Baby Fae was admitted to the hospital. When he returned several days later, he contacted the parents and suggested the baboon transplant. During the all-night session with Baby Fae's mother, he provided a film and showed slides explaining his research. He also gave reasons why he believed a baboon heart might work. In the interview after the surgery, he acknowledged that "We were not searching for a human heart. We were out to enter the whole new area of transplanting tissue-matched baboon hearts into newborns who are supported with antisuppressive drugs."

Physicians engaged in medical research always live and work under a potential conflict of interest. As physicians, they want to give the best medical care and comfort to a particular patient; as researchers, they want to test interventions. The two aims often collide. When they do, the situation becomes very delicate. If the patient has decision-making capacity and adequate knowledge about the burdens and risks of the experimental intervention, he may voluntarily give consent to the unusual intervention, and there may be no moral problem. But when the patient cannot consent, physicians must proceed much more carefully. The goal of good patient care must remain primary, and not the goal, no matter how laudable, of medical research.

As we saw in chapter 14, experiments on children can sometimes be morally justified. A physician can argue that it is morally good to subject an infant to the trauma of any transplant surgery only if there are good reasons to think the expected benefits significantly outweigh the anticipated burdens.

IRB members' perspectives.   Members of IRBs are also moral agents in this case—they approved the surgery. In March 1985 the National Institutes of Health sent a team to review the Baby Fae case at Loma Linda. The team found some problems with the consent document, reporting that it did not include the possibility of a human heart transplant, and that it seemed to overstate the chance of a good outcome for the baby. In general, the committee was critical of the IRB's oversight of the informed consent process in the case.

Public information showing how the IRB members were satisfied that Baby Fae was adequately protected in this case is not available. We do not know what reasons IRB members used to justify killing an animal and implanting its heart into Baby Fae. We do know, however, that the IRBs exist for the protection of human subjects (in this case, for the protection of Baby Fae). The physicians may want to try something, and the parents may agree to have it done, but the IRB members have to protect vulnerable human subjects who cannot give informed consent for unorthodox medical interventions. Maybe some members of the IRB tried to stop the transplantation, but the IRB did give its approval for the baboon transplant. We are left wondering how it could have justified the procedure, but the board has made no effort to explain its position.

Ethical Reflection

Since the Baby Fae case, animal heart transplants have not been used in humans. Dr. Leonard Bailey has turned his attention to using human hearts to help babies born with hypoplastic left-heart syndrome and has achieved notable success. Nonetheless, in a reflective article on organ transplantation published in 1990, Dr. Bailey opined that Baby Fae would still be alive if the baboon's blood type had been a better match with hers. In the same article he was critical of what he called the "reactive bioethical rhetoric" generated by the Baby Fae case: "Much of what was said and written did not reflect well on the fledgling profession of biomedical ethics. It was all too quick, too ill-informed, too self-assured. Furthermore, some of it hurt my feelings. I have often compared the ethical rhetoric of those days to the phenomenon of 'pack journalism,' and have considered it 'semi-ethics'—close, but not quite the real thing. What was missing was *wisdom* and a sense of perspective."

Little is gained by remarks of this kind. Many of the ethical responses to the transplantation of the baboon heart into Baby Fae were written by prominent ethicists and well argued. If physicians disagree with the ethical criticisms of their medical research on human beings, we would all be the richer if they would engage the ethicists in moral reasoning and not dismiss their work as reactive rhetoric. This is especially so since some ethicists are convinced that what was "all too quick, too ill-informed, too self-assured," and missing "wisdom and a sense of perspective" was not the ethical reaction to the Baby Fae case but the transplantation itself, especially since no sustained history of xenografts between animal species existed and no serious effort was made to find a human heart for the child.

Surgeons continue seeking ways to transplant animal organs into human beings, as Dr. Thomas Starzl did when he transplanted a baboon's liver into a thirty-five-year-old man dying of hepatitis B in 1992. The ethics of doing so, however, is not yet clear. Perhaps these xenografts are truly beneficial, or perhaps they represent an unreasonable and overly zealous effort to rebuild failing human bodies and thus are a diversion of time, talent, and resources from other efforts that would help many more people live better. Yet one thing is clear: there is no moral justification at this time for experimenting with xenografts on children. Fully informed dying adults may freely choose to become subjects of xenografts, and one may applaud their willingness to take a chance, knowing something might be learned that will help others even if they do not benefit. But children cannot make that choice, and we have no moral reason for forcing it upon them.

Implantation of Artificial Hearts

The effort to develop artificial hearts is driven by the fact that only several thousand human hearts are available for transplantation each year while tens of thousands more patients could benefit from a transplant. The first artificial heart was implanted in 1969 at St. Luke's Hospital in Houston by Dr. Denton Cooley. The device kept forty-seven-year-old Haskell Karp alive until a human heart was found and transplanted three days later. Karp died within a day.

The operation received widespread publicity and started several controversies. Critics accused Dr. Cooley of using an artificial heart prematurely since the procedure had not succeeded in animals; of being motivated more by publicity than by the welfare of the patient; and of not obtaining a truly informed consent. Mrs. Karp sued him, claiming that neither she nor her husband realized the implant was experimental and being done for the first time. Dr. Michael DeBakey, the head of artificial heart research at Baylor University, where Dr. Cooley was also on the faculty, was also critical of the attempt. A local medical society censured Dr. Cooley for his enthusiasm in seeking publicity after the surgery, but it declined to take disciplinary action against him. Dr. Cooley soon resigned from Baylor but continued to practice.

Haskell Karp's artificial heart was designed to be temporary; Barney Clark's was not. Dr. William DeVries implanted the first permanent artificial heart, known as the Jarvik-7, into Barney Clark at the University of Utah Medical Center in 1982. Clark lived but suffered numerous complications including respiratory failure, renal failure, rampant fevers, aspiration pneumonia, and sepsis until he died of multiple organ failure 112 days after the artificial heart transplant.

After Barney Clark died, Dr. DeVries moved his practice to the Humana Hospital in Louisville. Humana Hospital was part of a large chain of for-profit hospitals that owned stock in Symbion, the manufacturer of the patented Jarvik-7. Humana promised Dr. DeVries funding for 100 artificial heart implants. The corporation hoped that DeVries's presence would generate favorable publicity that would attract patients needing artificial hearts to the hospital.

Dr. DeVries implanted the Jarvik-7 as a permanent implant in three other patients, William Schroeder, Murray Haydon, and Jack Burcham. Schroeder lived 620 days but suffered four strokes and chronic infections that caused significant mental and physical deterioration. Haydon also lived more than a year but spent much of it in the ICU supported by a respirator. Burcham, the last patient to receive the Jarvik-7 artificial heart, died ten days after his April 1985 implantation. Only one other person received a permanent artificial heart at this time. Dr. Bjarne Semb of Sweden implanted one in Leif Stenberg; he died of a massive stroke several months later.

The initial burst of enthusiasm over the use of permanent artificial hearts soon waned after these five cases. In 1988 several articles, including one by DeVries himself, acknowledged a major problem with the permanent artificial heart—inevitably it became a site for infection and a source of clots that caused strokes.

In May 1988 Claude L'Enfant, director of the National Heart, Lung and Blood Institute (NHLBI), announced that the institute would no longer support research on artificial hearts. The ban lasted only two months. Proponents of federal funding for the artificial heart program convinced lawmakers to reverse it. Senators Orin Hatch and Edward Kennedy—the latter was chair of the committee that approves NIH's budget—led a successful effort to continue federal funding for the artificial heart program. However, problems with the Jarvik-7 heart led to an FDA moratorium on its use in 1991, but efforts to develop a permanent artificial heart continued. The challenges are great. The machine, for example, has to beat about 100,000 times a day without causing damage to the delicate blood cells flowing through the pump.

In July 2001 surgeons implanted the first fully self-contained artificial heart—the AbioCor—into fifty-eight-year-old Robert Tools in Louisville, Kentucky. The AbioCor had an internal battery that could be recharged without breaking the skin. The internal batteries last about thirty minutes, which allows the recipient to take a bath or shower, whereas an external battery pack lasts about four hours. When the patient is not using batteries, the power comes from an electrical outlet.

Robert Tools lived about five months before he had a fatal stroke. Abiomed, the manufacturer of the AbioCor, soon began a phase I trial of the AbioCor artificial heart. By 2004 nine research participants had received it. They lived an average of five months, although one patient lived for seventeen months and was actually able to leave the hospital. In September 2006 the FDA allowed limited use of the AbioCor under a Humanitarian Device Exemption (HDE) approval for patients who have no other treatment options and are expected to die within thirty days. In June 2009 a seventy-six-year-old man in New Jersey received the first AbioCor outside of a clinical trial.

Artificial hearts are often used on a temporary basis while the patient is awaiting a human transplant. One such device is the SynCardia Systems device known as the CardioWest, a modern version of the Jarvik-7 artificial heart. The CardioWest unit was originally designed as a permanent replacement but is currently used only as a bridge to a human heart transplant. As of 2008 it is the only FDA-approved temporary artificial heart for use in those awaiting a human heart transplant. It requires an external power supply, but the company has developed a portable unit that allows people to return home while awaiting a human heart. European countries have fully approved the portable power supply for use, but the FDA has limited it to investigational use in the United States. Over 750 people have received the CardioWest, and some have used it for more than year before receiving a human heart. Seventy-nine percent of those with the CardioWest had subsequent successful human heart transplants, and the five-year survival rate of these people is about 64 percent. Unlike the AbioCor, the CardioWest is being implanted in patients outside the United States.

In addition to artificial hearts, pumps known as ventricular assist devices (VADs) are increasingly being used. The VADs help a failing heart to function rather than replace it and seem to generate fewer infections. In 1991 the FDA approved the use of VADs as a temporary measure for people awaiting a heart transplant. As technology improved, patients using these devices were able to have a fairly normal life while awaiting their transplant, and they were in much better health when they received it. By early in the twenty-first century VADs were being used as permanent therapies for people with end-stage cardiac disease who were not candidates for a human heart transplant, much as dialysis is used for people with end-stage renal disease.

And just what are some of the ethical concerns about the use of artificial hearts? There are several. First, some are concerned about just how voluntary a patient's informed consent can be when he is threatened with fatal heart failure and no human heart is available. In such circumstances patients may actually think that they have no choice but to accept an artificial heart, and if they do so think, then their consent is clearly not voluntary.

Second, the early permanent artificial hearts brought little in the way of benefits to those receiving them and introduced significant physical and psychological burdens into their lives. It is doubtful that the recipients were fully informed about just how difficult it would be to live with an artificial heart. After watching what happened to them, few physicians or patients are seeking permanent artificial hearts to replace failing hearts at the present time. This may change if better products are developed.

Third, the temporary artificial hearts and temporary VADs present us with an ambiguous situation: they save individual lives but do not, in the long run, save any lives. To understand this apparently contradictory claim, it is necessary to remember that there are not enough human hearts for those needing them. Many people needing a human heart, then, will die while waiting for one. Putting an artificial heart into any one of these people on the waiting list may keep her alive until a human heart is available for her. The human transplant will then save her life, but this means that that heart will not be available to save the life of another person who would have received it had not the first person been kept alive by the artificial heart.

The net result, then, is that the temporary artificial hearts such as the CardioWest do not increase the number of lives saved by the human heart transplant programs. In effect, the temporary artificial heart affects the allocation of human hearts, but it does not affect the number of lives saved because it does not increase the number of human hearts available for transplantation.

True, if an artificial heart will keep your loved one alive until a human heart is found, it is an attractive option. The dark side of this option, however, is that someone else would have received that heart had your loved one not been kept alive with an artificial heart. The artificial heart saves one life only at the expense of losing another. It is not easy to defend this practice. Not only does it skewer the waiting list for human transplants (those with artificial hearts usually jump over others on the list), but it presents a clear example of spending additional money for life-saving treatments that do not save any additional lives. If there were enough donated human hearts, of course, then the temporary use of the artificial heart would no longer be subject to this objection. There is, unfortunately, no reason to think an abundance of donated hearts will happen in the near future. Given the fact that temporary artificial hearts cannot increase the net number of lives saved in the foreseeable future, it is hard to escape the conclusion that most of the interest in the temporary artificial hearts is driven by the glamour and prestige of keeping people alive and by the desire for commercial profits.

There is a growing consensus that permanent VADs are now a morally reasonable option and that a permanent artificial heart such as the AbioCor may soon be morally reasonable as a last resort. At the present time, however, we have learned that temporary use of artificial hearts such as the CardoWest or ventricular assist devices that enable people to survive while awaiting a human heart neither increases the number of lives saved nor preserves equitable access to the scarce human hearts that are available, and it does expend additional financial resources without saving additional lives.

Suggested Readings

Information about the Organ Procurement and Transplantation Network (OPTN), which sets policies for organ allocation and collects nationwide data, can be found at optn.org, and information about the United Network for Organ Sharing (UNOS), the nonprofit organization that carries out the policies of the OPTN, can be found at unos.org. A good introduction online to various ethical issues in organ transplantation is the September 2005 issue of the AMA *Journal of Ethics* at virtualmentor.ama-assn.org/2005/09. Stories of the world's first heart transplant and first artificial heart can be found in Gregory Pence, 2004, *Classic Cases in Medical Ethics*, 4th ed., chapter 12. For the early history of transplantation, see Renée Fox and Judith Swazey, 1978, *The Courage to Fail: A Social View of Organ Transplants and Dialysis*, 2nd ed., Chicago: University of Chicago Press. In a more recent work titled *Spare Parts: Organ Replacement in American Society*, 1992, New York: Oxford University Press, these authors review and express concern about some of the troubling aspects of transplantation. These concerns are summarized in their article "Leaving the Field," *Hastings Center Report* 1991, *22* (September–October), 9–15.

For an excellent collection of articles on a range of issues more broad than the title would indicate, see Howard Kaufman, ed., 1989, *Pediatric Brain Death and Organ/Tissue Retrieval: Medical, Ethical and Legal Aspects*, New York: Plenum Medical Books. A special section on organ ethics, including an extensive bibliography, appeared in the *Cambridge Quarterly of Healthcare Ethics* 1992, *1*, 305–60. To alleviate the shortage of organs available for transplantation, two solutions have been proposed. The first would require people to make a decision about donation when they renew licenses or pay taxes, and the second would presume consent for donation unless the person or family objected. The AMA Code of Medical Ethics (2.155) supports the legalization of mandated choice but states that presumed consent raises serious ethical concerns. See the AMA Council on Ethical and Judicial Affairs Report titled "Strategies for Organ Procurement: Mandated Choice and Presumed Consent," *JAMA* 1994, *272*, 809–12. As noted in the chapter, many countries have legalized presumed consent and thereby increased their organ donation rates. See Sheldon Zink et al., "Presumed versus Expressed Consent in the US and Internationally," at virtualmentor.ama-assn.org, September 2005. The *Kennedy Institute of Ethics Journal* devoted its March 2003 and September 2004 issues to the organ procurement problem in the United States, yet none of the articles advocated the presumed consent approach. See also the PCB staff discussion paper by Sam Crowe, "Increasing the Supply of Human Organs: Three Policy Proposals," at bioethics.gov/background (February 2007), which also ignores presumed consent as a policy option. However, see also the PCB staff background paper "Organ Transplantation: Ethical Dilemmas and Policy Choices" at bioethics.gov/background (January 2003), which does include presumed consent as one of its five possible procurement proposals. See also Aaron Spital and Charles Erin, "Conscription of Cadaveric Organs for Transplantation: Let's at Least Talk about It," *American Journal of Kidney Diseases* 2002, *39*, 611–15; and Aaron Spital, "Conscription of Cadaveric Organs for Transplantation: Neglected Again," *Kennedy Institute of Ethics Journal* 2003, *13*, 169–74.

Fourteen articles on donation after cardiac death (DCD), whereby physicians take organs a few minutes after life-sustaining treatment is withdrawn from living patients (and thereby raising the question of whether the cessation of cardiopulmonary functions has become truly irreversible), can be found in a special issue of the *Kennedy Institute of Ethics Journal* 1993, *3*, 103–278. An appendix to this issue contains the policy adopted by the University of Pittsburgh Medical Center in May 1992, whereby the cardiopulmonary criterion of death is considered to be met two minutes after the heart stops, goes into fibrillation, or manifests electromechanical dissociation (disharmony involving the natural electrical pacemakers in the heart). For a description of the first organ procurement when cardiopulmonary death was assumed only two minutes after the heart stopped, see Michael DeVita et al., "Procuring Organs from a Non-Heart-Beating Cadaver: A Case Report," *Kennedy Institute of Ethics Journal* 1993, *3*, 371–85. See also Roger Herdman et al., "The Institute of Medicine's Report on Non-Heart-Beating Organ Transplantation," *Kennedy Institute of Ethics Journal* 1998, *8*, 83–90; and the Institute of Medicine (IOM) publication *Non-Heart-Beating Organ Transplantation: Practice and Protocols*, 2007, Washington, DC: National Academies Press. A national conference on DCD was held in 2005; for its report see J. Bernat et al., "Report of a National Conference on Donation after Cardiac Death," *American Journal of Transplantation* 2006, *6*, 281–91. For an excellent summary of DCD see the New York State Task Force on Life & the Law 2007 report titled *Donation after Cardiac Death: Analysis and Recommendations*, available online at health.state.ny.us/task_force.

Also helpful is W. Land and J. B. Dossetor, eds., 1991, *Organ Replacement Therapy: Ethics, Justice and Commerce*, Berlin: Springer-Verlag. For a well-argued position advocating retrieval of vital organs from imminently dying but not yet dead patients, see Franklin Miller and Robert Truog, "Rethinking the Ethics of Vital Organ Donations," *Hastings Center Report* 2008, *38* (November–December), 38–46; and Truog and Miller, "The Dead Donor Rule and Organ Transplantation," *New England Journal of Medicine* 2008, *359*, 674–75. Miller and Truog argue that people declared dead by the neurological criterion are not truly dead, yet we take their organs, and that, as withdrawing life support is part of a morally acceptable causal sequence that leads to death, so might we accept the ethics of organ retrieval with consent as yet another step in the causal sequence leading to death that is already under way when the life support is withdrawn. See also James Bernat, "The Boundaries of Organ Donation after Circulatory Death," *New England Journal of Medicine* 2008, *359*, 669–71; and Robert Veatch, "Donating Hearts after Cardiac Death—Reversing the Irreversible," *New England Journal of Medicine* 2008, *359*, 672–73.

The report that physicians in Germany had removed kidneys from two anencephalic infants who had been placed on ventilators for this purpose appeared in Wolfgang Holzgreve et al., "Kidney Transplantation from Anencephalic Donors," *New England Journal of Medicine* 1987, *316*, 1069–70. Shana Alexander's landmark article creating public awareness about the committees selecting patients for dialysis appeared in *Life*, November 9, 1962, pp. 102–25. The Jamie Fiske story is taken from Charles Fiske's testimony at the 1983 House Subcommittee hearings on H.R. 4080, a proposed bill on organ transplants, pp. 212–18. Jesse Sepulveda's story is taken from the *New York Times* of June 15, 1986, p. 1, and July 18, 1993, p. 36. Accounts of designated organ donation include Eike-Henner Kluge, "Designated Organ Donation: Private Choices in Social Context," *Hastings Center Report* 1989, 19 (September–October), 10–16; and Wayne Arnason, "Directed Donation: The Relevance of Race," *Hastings Center Report* 1991, 21 (November–December), 13–19. It is interesting to note that the Uniform Anatomical Gift Act (UAGA) does allow designated donation: "The gift may be made to a specific donee or without specifying a donee" (Section 4 [c]).

Dr. Thomas Starzl, one of the best known transplant surgeons in the country, has noted the growing difficulties in retrieving organs from living donors in a short piece titled "Will Live Organ Donations No Longer Be Justified?" *Hastings Center Report* 1985, *15* (April), 5. The ethical considerations of partial liver transplantation are well described by Peter Singer et al. in "Ethics of Liver Transplantation with Living Donors," *New England Journal of Medicine* 1989, *321*, 620–22. For the sale of organs by living people, see Lori Andrews, "My Body, My Property," *Hastings Center Report* 1986, *16* (October), 28–38; George Annas, "Life, Liberty, and the Pursuit of Organ Sales," *Hastings Center Report* 1986, *16* (February), 22–23; Norman Fost, 1989, "Reconsidering the Ban on Financial Incentives," in *Pediatric Brain Death and Organ/Tissue Retrieval*, Howard Kaufman, ed., London: Plenum Medical Book Company, pp. 309–15; and Ellen Paul, "Natural Rights and Property Rights," *Harvard Journal of Law and Public Policy* 1990, *13*, 10–16.

The story of Baby Fae is taken from Leonard Bailey et al., "Baboon-to-Human Cardiac Xenotransplantation in a Neonate," *JAMA* 1985, *254*, 3321–29; Eleanor Hoover, "Baby Fae: A Child Loved and Lost,"

People, December 3, 1984, pp. 49–63; Dennis Breo, "Interview with Baby Fae's Surgeon: Therapeutic Intent Was Topmost," *American Medical News*, November 16, 1984, p. 1; and "Is 'Baby Fae' Transplant Worth It? Experts Mixed," *American Medical News*, November 9, 1984, p. 1. See also Pence, *Classic Cases*, chapter 12; a series of seven brief commentaries on the case in *Hastings Center Report* 1985, *15* (February), 8–13 and 15–17; and Robert Veatch, "The Ethics of Xenografts," *Transplantation Proceedings* 1986, *18*, suppl. 2, pp. 93–97. Concern about the moral misuse of animals in transplantation research and therapy is voiced by James Nelson, "Transplantation through a Glass Darkly," *Hastings Center Report* 1992, 22 (September–October), 6–8. The early work of Dr. Bailey with human hearts after the Baby Fae case is described in Leonard Bailey et al., "Cardiac Allotransplantation in Newborns as Therapy for Hypoplastic Left Heart Syndrome," *New England Journal of Medicine* 1986, *315*, 949–51. Dr. Bailey's criticism of what he called "reactive bioethical rhetoric" in the wake of the Baby Fae case can be found in Leonard Bailey, "Organ Transplantation: A Paradigm of Medical Progress," *Hastings Center Report* 1990, 20 (January–February), 24–28. An excellent overview of the ethical issues in the Baby Fae case is the 1985 Scope Note by Judith Mistichelli titled "Baby Fae: Ethical Issues Surrounding Cross-Species Organ Transplantation," available online at bioethics.georgetown.edu/publications.

Information about the renal center at Aadil Hospital in Lahore, Pakistan, can be accessed at aadilhospital.com/renal. The video of an anonymous American who purchased a kidney at the Aadil Hospital was accessed in November 2008 at abclocal.com. The quotation about the decline in kidney transplants by Aadil's CEO is from the *Sydney Morning Herald* of May 12, 2008, available at smh.com.au/news. A good overview of the commercial organ business is the review article by Yosuke Shimazono, "The State of the International Organ Trade: A Provisional Picture Based on Integration of Available Information," *Bulletin of the World Health Organization* 2007, *85*, 955–62, available online at who.int/bulletin. According to the article, "transplant tourism" continues to thrive and expand, and the motivating force behind everyone's decision to sell one of his or her kidneys is poverty, and studies show that the few thousand dollars the seller receives provides little or no lasting economic benefit. Most countries have made selling organs illegal, and the WHO has taken a strong stand against it because it exploits the poor and undermines their health. See also the excellent book by Mark Cherry, 2005, *Kidney for Sale by Owner: Human Organs, Transplantation, and the Market*, Washington, DC: Georgetown University Press.

For assessments of the artificial heart, see Margery Shaw, ed., 1984, *After Barney Clark: Rejections on the Utah Artificial Heart Program*, Austin: University of Texas Press; Pence, *Classic Cases*, chapter 11; Judith P. Swazey, Judith C. Watkins, and Renée Fox, "Assessing the Artificial Heart: The Clinical Moratorium Revisited," *International Journal of Technology Assessment in Health Care* 1986, 2, 387–410; Michael Strauss, "The Political History of the Artificial Heart," *New England Journal of Medicine* 1984, *310*, 332–36; William DeVries, "The Permanent Artificial Heart: Four Case Reports," *JAMA* 1988, *259*, 849–59; William DeVries, "The Physician, the Media, and the 'Spectacular Case.'" *JAMA* 1988, *259*, 886–90; William Pierce, "Permanent Heart Substitution: Better Solutions Lie Ahead," *JAMA* 1988, *259*, 891; Albert Jonsen, "The Artificial Heart's Threat to Others," *Hastings Center Report* 1986, *16* (February), 9–12; and Gideon Gil, "The Artificial Heart Juggernaut," *Hastings Center Report* 1989, *19* (March–April), 24–31.

A prominent critic of the artificial heart programs is George Annas. See his "Consent to the Artificial Heart: The Lion and the Crocodiles," *Hastings Center Report* 1983, *13* (April), 20–22, "The Phoenix Heart: What We Have to Lose," *Hastings Center Report* 1985, *15* (June), 15–16; "No Cheers for Temporary Artificial Hearts," *Hastings Center Report* 1985, *15* (October), 27–28; and Annas, 1993, "Death and the Magic Machine: Consent to the Artificial Heart," in *Standard of Care*, New York: Oxford University Press, chapter 15, pp. 198–210.

For a study of the CardioWest artificial heart see Jack Copeland et al., "Cardiac Replacement with a Total Artificial Heart as a Bridge to Transplantation," *New England Journal of Medicine* 2004, *351*, 859–67. See also Kenneth Baughman and John Jarcho, "Bridge to Life—Cardiac Mechanical Support," *New England Journal of Medicine* 2007, *357*, 846–49; Sandeep Jauhar, "The Artificial Heart," *New England Journal of Medicine* 2004, *350*, 542–44; and Dale Renlund, "Building a Bridge to Heart Transplantation," *New England Journal of Medicine* 2004, *351*, 849–51.

For the need to make the allocation system more equitable, see Paul Hauptman and Kevin O'Connor, "Procurement and Allocation of Solid Organs for Transplantation," and Robert Steinbrook, "Allocating Livers—Devising a Fair System," both in *New England Journal of Medicine* 1997, *336*, 422–31 and 436–38. See also P. E. Ubel and Arthur Caplan, "Geographic Favoritism in Liver Transplantation—Unfortunate or Unfair?" *New England Journal of Medicine* 1998, *339*, 1322–25. A readable book on transplantation is Arthur Caplan, 1998, *Am I My Brother's Keeper?* Bloomington: Indiana University Press. For some social distribution problems, see Caleb Alexander and Ashwini Sehgal, "Barriers to Cadaveric Renal Transplantation among Blacks, Women, and the Poor," *JAMA* 1998, *280*, 1148–52. A difficult moral problem in organ distribution is giving people with serious disabilities scarce organs. In 1996 Sandra Jensen, a thirty-five-year-old victim of Down syndrome, received a heart-lung transplant and lived almost another two years. See Angela Whitehead, "Rejecting Organs: The Organ Allocation Process and the Americans with Disabilities Act," *American Journal of Law & Medicine* 1998, *24*, 481–97.

SIXTEEN

Medical Genetics

THE MODERN STORY OF GENETICS began in 1865 with an obscure scientific paper published in German by an Austrian monk. It was a slow beginning because few realized the significance of Gregor Mendel's painstaking observations in the monastery garden. Mendel had carefully formulated precise laws for predicting the various ways certain traits—tall and short, for example—are inherited in successive generations of his pure-bred and crossbred pea plants. The patterns of inheritance he stumbled on showed that each plant receives two sets of instructions for each trait, one set from each parent plant, but only one set shows itself in the offspring.

In 1892 a German scientist named August Friedrich Weismann theorized that some sort of physical substances or particles in the chromosomes must contain the instructions for these inherited traits. By 1910 scientists were calling these instructional substances "genes." The root of the word is from Greek words such as *genesis* (beginning, source, or birth) and *genos* (race, kin, clan, family). Genes account for the family traits present in an organism from its beginning.

In 1952 James Watson and Francis Crick made the momentous discovery that the acid that forms the 46 chromosomes inside the nucleus of each human cell, an acid known as deoxyribonucleic acid, or DNA, is structured like a spiral staircase with each "step" composed of a pair of interlocking chemical bases. It was soon realized that each human cell contained about three billion of these chemical pairs. Fortunately there are only four kinds of chemical bases forming the DNA, and they are identified by the first letter of their chemical names as *A*, *G*, *C*, and *T*. Because of their chemical structure, an *A* base can only lock with a *T* base and a *G* base can only lock with a *C* base.

Once this was understood scientists could begin to "read" the DNA; that is, they could identify the sequence of bases along one side of the DNA in the cells. The result would be a long series of letters such as *AGT CCA TGT TGA CC. . . .* Except for a few random mutations, the sequence of letters in all the cells of one individual is identical and also unique to that person. A massive effort to read all the base pairs in a human cell—the Human Genome Project (HGP)—began in 1990.

Fewer than 2 percent of these base pairs in the cells compose the instructions for proteins; hence, most of the base pairs in the genome are idle. Most cells have two copies of each instruction, but the cells of sperm and ova have only one copy. Generally only one set of instructions manifests itself in the host body, but either set can be passed on to offspring, depending on which copy happens to be in the sperm or ova. The sequences of base pairs composing the instructions for traits and functions are the genes we talk about today.

After Watson and Crick's discovery of the DNA structure, the field known as genetics or molecular biology exploded. Medical genetics soon became one of the hottest fields in medicine. The implications of genetics for health care, as we will see, are tremendous. More and more decisions about health care will become decisions about genes as we learn how to test and screen for the genetic basis of inherited and acquired disease and then develop gene therapies to prevent, ameliorate, or cure gene-based diseases and abnormalities.

We need some idea of molecular biology and its terminology if we are to understand the rest of the chapter. What follows is a very rough outline to help readers unfamiliar with the field of genetics.

The basic unit of our bodies is the *cell*. There are two kinds of cells—*germ* cells and *somatic* cells. Germ cells are the reproductive cells, spermatozoa in males and ova in females. All other cells in a human body are somatic cells (the Greek word for body is *soma*).

All our cells have, except for some random mutations, the same sequence of base pairs no matter where they are working in the body. The cells in our brain are the same as the cells in our blood, or in our kidneys, pancreas, lungs, bladder, and other parts of the body. The only difference is this: the cells functioning as brain cells are not using the same base pairs as the cells functioning as blood cells or as cells anywhere else.

After fertilization the first few cell divisions produce cells that are undifferentiated; that is, they have the potential to generate any kind of somatic cell and even germ cells. Cells at this early stage are therefore called *totipotential*. Later cells become more restricted; that is, they can no longer become any kind of cell. These cells are called *plutipotential*. Finally all cells become differentiated; that is they will function in a set way—as a brain cell or a blood cell, for example—for the rest of their existence. However, some recent reports suggest it may be possible to reprogram differentiated cells so they can function in new ways in the body.

Roughly speaking, the structure of our cells is as follows. Inside the outer shell is the cytoplasm surrounding a nucleus. Most of the DNA is in the nucleus but a few pieces are in the cytoplasm. Under a microscope the DNA in the nucleus looks a little like forty-six pieces of thread (the forty-six chromosomes) arranged in twenty-three pairs. If all the DNA threads in one cell were put end to end, they would be about six feet long.

About 95 percent of the bases (the *A*s, *G*s, *T*s, and *C*s) forming the DNA apparently do nothing. Some people call them "junk" DNA. The remaining base sequences are instructions for producing *amino acids*. Amino acids compose *proteins*. Proteins make up the major part of our tissues and organs. Whatever stretch of base pairs combines to provide the instructions for one particular protein is called a *gene*. No one yet knows exactly how many genes are in a human cell, although the number suggested by the HGP seems to be about 25,000, which is not many more than we find in the cells of worms, flies, and plants.

Unfortunately the sequences of base pairs for a particular gene are usually scattered at different places on the chromosome and are mixed with the stretches of junk sequences or with sequences that are coding for other genes. Sometimes sequences coding for a particular gene are located on different chromosomes. This makes decoding the genetic identity of a human cell very difficult.

A few more key concepts and terms will complete this brief introduction to the challenging field of genetics.

- Recombinant DNA (rDNA). When segments of DNA are cut from one source and inserted into a new strand of DNA the result is recombinant DNA or rDNA for short. It simply means DNA has been severed and then recombined with other DNA. This is often called *genetic engineering*.

- RNA. Cells transfer relevant DNA instructions in the nucleus onto molecules known as ribonucleic acid (RNA) in the cytoplasm. The RNA then directs the making of the protein. The process from DNA to RNA deletes the noncoding bases in the DNA, leaving the RNA an edited version of the DNA. RNA is thus like an abridged copy of the DNA. It contains only the sequences actually coding for genes. It is possible to make a DNA copy (cDNA) of the RNA and thus produce DNA that contains only the bases coding for genes.

- Allele. Normal cells have two versions of each gene in the nucleus, one inherited from the father and one from the mother. Each copy is called an allele. Usually one allele dominates the other.

- Genetic code. The chemical bases of the DNA with instructions for proteins and designated by the letters *A*, *G*, *C*, and *T* comprise the genetic code. The letters are combined into the three-letter "words" called *codons*. The sequences actually coding for genes are called *exons* and the noncoding sequences are called *introns*.

- Genotype. This is the total genetic code of an individual—the totality of genetic instructions carried in each of his cells. Many genetic instructions are inherited, but others are the result of sporadic mutations during cell division and of the interaction of genes with each other and with the environment. Hence, our genotype is not fully determined at fertilization; it evolves over the course of life.

- Phenotype. This is the actual physical manifestation of the hidden genetic code—the totality of physical characteristics appearing as the result of the genotype. Not every hidden genetic characteristic will appear in the phenotype. It is very important to distinguish genotype and phenotype. (The "pheno" in phenotype comes from the Greek word *phenomenon* meaning "that which shows itself"; a phenomenon is the appearance of something.) The phenotype is whatever genetic program actually shows up as a physical characteristic in the organism. An individual's phenotype is the physical appearance of his genetic traits. Some traits in a person's genotype will never appear in the phenotype, although they may appear in the phenotype of that person's children.

- Mutations. The genetic code in a cell can become scrambled in many different ways. Some mutations occur spontaneously, and some are caused by external agents. The simplest mutation occurs when a single codon is "misspelled." A *GAG* base sequence might appear as *GTG*, while the rest of the long chain is perfect. A simple misspelling can cause major problems. For example a child inheriting the *GTG* codon on a particular gene instead of *GAG* from both his parents will have sickle-cell anemia. More complicated mutations also occur. One codon might be deleted or added to a strand, thus altering the entire code from that point forward. Whole strands of DNA can appear in duplication or be deleted or break off and attach somewhere else. Some mutations cause no problems and may confer an advantage for the organism, but others cause problems. Some cause no problems in the host body but may cause problems in offspring. Some cause problems in the host but not in the offspring. And some cause problems both in the host and in the offspring.

- Genome. All the sequences coding for genes in a cell compose the genome. However, descriptions of the HGP often use "genome" to mean all the DNA in a cell even though only about 5 percent of it codes for genes.

- Carrier. In ordinary language, a carrier would be anyone carrying a particular genetic code. In genetics, however, carrier refers to abnormal genetic mutations appearing in the genotype but not in the phenotype. A carrier has the mutation, but it does not, and may not ever, manifest itself as the disease. Thus, a cystic fibrosis carrier has a cystic fibrosis mutation on one of its alleles, but the person will never develop the disease, and a young person with the mutation for Huntington's disease is considered a carrier only until the symptoms manifest themselves in middle age. People with a genetic disease also obviously carry the abnormal mutation, but they are not normally referred to as carriers.

- Genetic diseases. These are diseases wholly or partially caused by inherited or acquired genetic mutations. Some genetic diseases are caused by mutations in a single gene, others by mutations in several genes, others by chromosomal disorders, others by the interaction of genes with agents in the genes' environment, and still others by combinations of the above. Some inherited genetic diseases are apparent before or at birth, others are not apparent until months, years, or even decades into life. About 5 percent of humans are born with genetic diseases. Some are relatively mild; others are virulent.

- Gene therapy. Interventions on the genetic level designed to correct or to override disease-causing genetic mutations are referred to as gene therapy. No proven gene therapy or treatment yet exists and may not for some time because the biotechnical complications are greater than first imagined. Genetic interventions on people are not yet genetic therapies for patients but genetic research on human subjects. Some research subjects have experienced therapeutic improvement, but we should not confuse research on human subjects with the treatment of patients. Unfortunately, the clinical trials involving genetic interventions are often misleadingly called "gene therapy" or "gene therapy trials" or "genetic therapy research" when they are actually clinical experiments on human beings.

With these notions in mind we can now turn to several areas of ethical concern in genetics: (1) genetic testing, (2) genetic screening, (3) genetic research on humans, (4) genetic enhancement, and (5) the HGP.

GENETIC TESTING

Genetic testing is now available for more than fifteen hundred conditions, and it generates special ethical concern for several reasons. First, genetic tests expand greatly the power of medical tests. Most medical tests are diagnostic; they are designed to identify the problem after symptoms have appeared. Genetic tests can certainly do that, but they can also predict future diseases or the propensity for diseases long before any symptoms appear, and they can identify healthy people who are carriers of disease-prone genes that will or may affect only their offspring. The vast predictive power of genetic tests sets them apart from traditional medical tests, which are devoted mostly to the diagnosis of symptom-causing problems.

Second, genetic testing threatens our privacy. Testing can produce a tremendous amount of very personal information about an individual from an easily obtained source, usually blood. Only a few undamaged cells are needed for a genetic test, and soon it will be possible to retrieve the information of our entire genome from the nucleus of one cell. This information can easily be stored on a microchip or in a computerized data base, making it all too easy for people such as our employers, government agencies, and insurance companies to gain access to a great deal of genetic private information and use it to discriminate against us. Fortunately, the 2008 Genetic Information Nondiscrimination Act (GINA), mentioned at the end of the chapter, makes it illegal for health insurance companies and employers to discriminate on the basis of genetic information.

Third, the genetic testing of one individual often threatens the privacy of other individuals as well. If a person tests positive for an inherited disease or predisposition to a disease, then that test also reveals that one or both of the person's parents, depending on the disease, are carriers of the defective gene, and other members of the family, including relatives and children, are at risk of developing the disease or of having a predisposition toward it or of being carriers of the disease-causing gene. An inherited genetic defect is seldom a purely private matter; it is almost always a family matter as well. This raises the moral problem of communication: When might it be good for a person to inform family members of a genetic flaw that might also affect them? And conversely, when might it be good for a family member to have access to a relative's medical record to learn something of his own genetic risks?

Finally, the public grasp of genetic testing is fraught with misunderstanding. Many believe genes are the holy grail—the key to the great mysteries of human life, the determining factors in human behavior, and even the explanation of art, morality, religion, and culture. Some say we are nothing but our genes. Moreover, in the minds of many, molecular biology will enable us to predict and control the future, something modern science has dreamed of for a long time. Ironically this view of genetics, often thought to be based on science, really does not have a scientific basis. Molecular biology reveals that genes alone do not determine the structure and function of an organism. What do determine the structure and function of organisms are the genetic instructions in the cells plus the unpredictable interaction of genes with each other and with their environment as well as nongenetic factors such as choice and accident.

With some idea of the higher stakes in genetic testing, we can next consider two of the more sensitive areas in more detail.

Testing Children

Diagnostic testing of children to discover a genetic cause of symptoms is normally not morally problematic. However, pressures are mounting for *prognostic* testing of children without symptoms to detect their status as carriers or as subjects of a genetic disease that will or may develop later in life. Biotechnology companies, at considerable expense, are developing commercial tests, and they will want to market their products. Some pediatricians and parents may be tempted to see them as advantageous. After all, parents have an understandable curiosity about what will happen to their children.

The major ethical question here centers on determining whether the genetic testing of children will be a net benefit for them. As children they cannot consent to a test that may produce harmful repercussions, so our reasoning is guided by seeking their best interests. If the tests are for conditions that can be corrected easily during childhood, then finding reasons for testing the child is not difficult.

If, however, the tests are to determine carrier status or to uncover genetic liabilities that will not appear until adulthood, then finding good reasons for testing is much more difficult and often impossible because the test is of no benefit to the child at this stage of his life. Knowing carrier status becomes relevant only when the person is thinking of reproduction; knowing about adult-onset conditions becomes relevant only when the person is an adult. If parents suspect their child has carrier status or adult-onset genetic liabilities, it would be far more reasonable for them to wait until the child is old enough to give his own informed consent for the tests.

Parents and physicians need to be aware that positive results of a genetic test can impact negatively on how the child will be treated by others: his parents, family, friends, school authorities, future employers and insurers, and others, a risk they have no reason to impose unless a timely benefit for the child is likely.

Moreover, the child may not really want to know about his genetic condition when he is an adult. Studies show that some people at risk for late-onset genetic disease prefer not to be tested; that is, they prefer not to know. A test for Huntington's disease has been available for several years, for example, yet most adults at risk for the disease have thus far decided not to be tested.

Prudential reasoning suggests that genetic testing in the absence of any threat to the child in childhood should be postponed until the child has enough maturity to make the decision for herself. Some parents have an intense desire to know about their child's genotype, but their desire for this information is not the crucial factor in moral reasoning. Rather, the crucial factor is the awareness that they will live virtuously by seeking what is best for their children, and, in the absence of any possible benefit to a child in childhood, genetic testing for possible future problems is seldom a benefit for a child.

Testing Adults for Genetic Predispositions

Genetic tests showing a high degree of likelihood for some forms of Alzheimer disease, colon cancer, ovarian cancer, and breast cancer now exist. Testing for these genetic predispositions brings us into uncharted waters as it were, and we are just beginning to grasp the possible benefits and burdens of knowing about a genetic predisposition for a terrible disease long before any symptoms emerge.

Consider cancer. The disease itself is apparently not inherited, but all cancer cells contain genetic mutations. We now know that most of the mutations predisposing cells to malignancy are acquired during the person's lifetime, but some can come from a person's parents. In other words, the cancer is not an inherited disease, but some genes predisposing a person to cancer can be inherited. This explains why some cancers—breast, ovarian, and colon cancers, for example—sometimes run in families.

To get an idea of the medical and ethical complexity of decisions to test for a genetic predisposition to a disease, we can discuss one example—testing women from families with high rates of breast cancer for a genetic predisposition to the disease. By the mid 1990s researchers discovered that between 5 percent and 10 percent of the 180,000 new cases of breast cancer discovered every year are related to inherited defective mutations (over two hundred have been identified) on one of two genes. These genes are now known as BRCA1 and BRCA2 (BReast CAncer gene 1 and BReast CAncer gene 2). A primary function of these genes is to repair the minute abnormal mutations that inevitably occur in the DNA of cells. If the BRCA genes are flawed, the repair action does not occur properly, and the minute mutations can multiply and cause malignancy.

Inheriting a defective BRCA gene does not mean a woman will inevitably develop breast cancer; it means only that she is much more susceptible to developing breast and ovarian cancers than women without any such defective mutations. The BRCA genes can be inherited from either parent. They predispose males as well as females to breast cancer, although the risk of breast cancer developing in males is much less than in females. Some ethnic groups are at high risk for the BRCA genes—estimates indicate as many as 2 percent of American Jewish women of Ashkenazi descent may have one of the mutated genes.

The impact of inheriting a BRCA gene is considerable for a woman. Whereas the general population of women has approximately a 10 percent chance of developing breast cancer over a normal life span, a woman with mutations on either of the two BRCA genes has a much higher chance of breast cancer—some say it is as high as 85 percent—and of developing it in a more virulent form and at an earlier age than women without the BRCA genes.

Most women—those whose relatives have suffered breast or ovarian cancers no higher than the overall average, for example—are at very low risk of having the BRCA genes, and testing would seldom be a reasonable consideration. Women in families with incidence of these diseases higher than normal, however, are at higher risk of these cancers, especially if some of their relatives developed the disease at an early age. For these women, testing is a consideration.

Now that testing for the BRCA genes is possible, the people involved—primarily the physician, the woman at risk, and a genetic counselor—are faced with some serious ethical issues. Deciding what to do is difficult because testing for a genetic predisposition is a new reality in human history, and we lack the advantages of experience. Moreover, evaluating genetic tests for a predisposition involves probabilities and statistics, and figuring these out can be challenging. We have enough intelligence to know, however, that genetic testing for a predisposition toward cancer and other serious diseases has great potential for good as well as for harm.

What follows is a hypothetical case to show how prudential reason could help a woman and her physician make a good decision about being tested for genes predisposing her to breast cancer. It is an example of how we can engage in ethical decision making about any genetic testing designed to identify a predisposition to serious disease, including other cancers and Alzheimer disease. The decision to test or not test is not simply a medical decision. It is also an ethical decision, because it can so profoundly affect the quality of life.

A Case of Concern about Cancer

The Story

Imagine a twenty-five-year-old woman worried about breast cancer because several of her relatives have suffered from breast or ovarian cancer at relatively young ages. She has heard about the genetic test for breast cancer and is wondering about being tested. Is the test likely to do more good than harm? Since she is not sick, this is more of an ethical question than a medical question. A reasonable answer will require considerable background knowledge and prudent deliberation. Let's walk through one of the many ways prudential reasoning, faced with a decision on testing for a genetic predisposition, could unfold.

Ethical Analysis

Situational awareness. We are aware, at this time, of the following factors relevant to this woman's decision making.

1. Mutations on the BRCA genes give rise to only about 10 percent of all breast cancers. However, these defective genes are not distributed evenly throughout the population. The rate

runs higher than 10 percent in some population clusters and lower in others, something to be expected with an inherited characteristic. Can she estimate whether she is in a group with higher or lower risks of the BRCA genes? To a great extent she can, because the inherited BRCA genes are *dominant* genes; that is, the genetic predisposition occurs in 50 percent of offspring when either parent has the gene. Dominant genes run high in families. This means she is probably at a risk higher than 10 percent, because more than the average number of early breast or ovarian cancers have occurred in her extended family.

2. The test will not be conclusive. Testing positive for a defective BRCA gene does not mean she will inevitably develop breast cancer. Unlike some inherited genes—the genes for Huntington's disease or Tay-Sachs, for example—the BRCA mutations do not always cause the disease. The mutated BRCA genes only show a predisposition for breast cancer; that is, a risk higher than normal. Conversely, testing negative for a BRCA gene does not mean that she will not get breast cancer; it only means she will probably not be among the 10 percent of women who get breast cancer associated with inherited BRCA genes. A negative test for the BRCA mutations leaves her with the same approximate risk for breast cancer as the general population. The negative genetic test simply removes the risk for less than 10 percent of breast cancers—those involving the known inherited genetic predisposition. Moreover, a negative test could give her a false sense of security. There are hundreds of possible mutations of bases on the BRCA genes indicating a predisposition for cancer, and no test checks them all. And even if her particular test does cover a mutant base, it could still be misread and result in a false negative.

3. Professional uncertainty exists about the merits of testing for mutations on the BRCA genes. The National Advisory Council for Human Genome Research (NACHGR) has taken the position that genetic testing for the BRCA genes should not be done, except in medical research projects, because it could be harmful to patients. The National Breast Cancer Coalition generally agreed with this and wanted the FDA to ban commercial testing. On the other hand, the American Society of Clinical Oncology has advocated clinical testing for selected patients—patients thought to be at a risk greater than 10 percent of having the mutations.

4. A potential conflict of interest exists in reporting research on many genetic tests. Some articles published in medical journals reporting research results and making recommendations for testing are authored or co-authored by researchers who are affiliated with biotechnology companies. These companies are obviously interested in having doctors use their tests. For example a 1997 article in the *Journal of the American Medical Association* criticized NACHGR's position and advocated tests for women with family histories with as few as one or two cases of early-onset breast or ovarian cancer. The lead author and several other authors of the article, however, also disclosed they had affiliations with a company called Myriad Genetics, one of several biotechnology companies involved in bringing BRCA tests to market. Obviously commercial biotechnology companies want doctors to order their tests so they can recoup their research costs and make a profit.

5. The woman's doctor, aware of her family history, has suggested testing for mutations on her BRCA genes. She says the test is noninvasive, and a positive result will enable the woman to take precautions. What precautions? She could change her diet and lifestyle in a more healthy anticancer direction, and she could have more frequent breast exams and mammograms. And her physician mentions yet another surprising precaution—some women testing positive for ominous mutations on their BRCA genes have chosen to have double mastectomies to reduce their risk of breast cancer. The physician recommends that the woman see a genetic counselor.

Prudential Reasoning about Testing for the BRCA Genes

Patient's perspective. The woman is worrying, with some reason, about breast cancer and wondering whether to have the genetic test to determine if she has inherited the genetic predisposition for breast cancer. How might she make an intelligent decision? She could begin by learning as much as she could about genetics and genetic testing for a predisposition to the breast and ovarian cancers triggered by inherited mutations on the BRCA genes. Then she would consider the situational factors we just mentioned, and finally, she would evaluate the likely good and bad features of her being tested or not being tested. She would want to make sure she has enough information about the advantages and disadvantages of being tested, including the possible psychological risks if she tests positive, so that her decision will be a truly *informed* decision.

If she tests negative, one benefit is the relief she will feel when she realizes she probably does not have a dangerous mutation on these genes. However, her relief at testing positive is a restricted relief—she will only learn that she is probably not at increased risk for 10 percent of breast cancers; her risk for the other 90 percent of breast cancers not associated with inherited mutations remains the same as that of the general population.

If she tests positive, a possible benefit is the program of risk reduction—lifestyle changes and more frequent checkups—she can pursue. However, the impact of lifestyle changes and diet on the breast cancers caused by the inherited genetic mutations is unknown at this time. And it is also unknown at this time whether increasing watchfulness for the beginning of the disease will actually reduce the chances of illness and death; in fact, earlier and more frequent mammograms may actually increase the risk of cancer. In other words, it might not do any real good to know she has a deleterious mutation on a BRCA gene, although it will be upsetting. And remember, the mental anguish might be for nothing, because breast cancer does not always occur in women with the BRCA genes.

Hence, despite some indication of elevated risk in her family, she may well decide a test for mutations on the BRCA genes indicating a predisposition to 10 percent of breast cancers is not a reasonable choice at this time. She can set up a healthy anticancer diet and lifestyle and have more frequent checkups without the test, and she realizes, short of a double mastectomy which she has no interest in pursuing, there is not much else at the present time she could do if she were to learn that she had a deleterious BRCA gene.

Physician's perspective.   The physician is recommending a test. He knows, given his patient's family history, that she has a heightened risk of having mutations on one or both of her BRCA genes, and he wants to clarify her status. This is understandable—physicians do value the added clarity provided by diagnostic tests.

The physician cannot help but think of his interests also. If, knowing the family history, he does not recommend the test and she does have a defective BRCA gene and also develops breast cancer, he could find himself in a very awkward position if she then accuses him of being negligent for not recommending the test. If he recommends the test when she asks about it, he avoids this risk. Moreover, he may be involved in research about the BRCA genes and would like to include data from this case in his work.

What might a morally prudent physician do in a situation such as this? No ethical physician will proceed with any genetic testing in the absence of symptoms without obtaining the patient's informed consent. Obtaining truly informed consent means someone, normally either the physician or a genetic counselor, will have to do a tremendous amount of education before ordering a genetic test because most people do not know much about genetics and will be bewildered by the statistical array of probabilities involved in evaluating results of testing for genetic mutations predisposing them to disease.

And once a person understands the basic concepts of genetics and grasps something of the probabilities involved, the physician still needs to explain the psychological and social risks as well as the possible benefits of the genetic tests, the likelihood of false positives and negatives, and the medical interventions and psychological counseling that are available if the test is positive.

Genetic counselor's perspective.   Since the early 1970s genetic counseling has received professional standing in health care. Most genetic counselors have completed a master's program in human genetics or genetic counseling. In 1993 the newly formed American Board of Genetic Counseling began certifying genetic counselors.

From the beginning genetic counselors have emphasized the value of a neutral stance in counseling sessions with patients. Great emphasis is placed on avoiding any tinge of eugenics—the attempt to enhance good genes and eliminate bad genes in the population—and on respecting the autonomy of the patient or client. To this end the counselor is encouraged to be nondirective and nonjudgmental, that is, to avoid letting her opinions influence the client.

Hence, the genetic counselor was totally nondirective. She laid out the information and the probabilities and said she would support whatever decision the woman made. The counselor gave facts and statistics but not advice. She was nondirective in no small part because that attitude accords with her understanding of patient autonomy and a patient-centered ethic of care.

Ethical Reflection

This hypothetical case shows how difficult a decision about testing for a genetic predisposition can be. It also reveals how the perspectives of a physician and a genetic counselor can differ in important ways from that of the patient. The counselor did not make any recommendations but simply gave the facts and supported the woman's decision. Her nondirective stance invites comment. Although it is most important for patients to make the ultimate decision about being tested, it is at least arguable that a nondirective approach is not the most reasonable tack for a counselor to take. Genetic information is often overwhelming, and most of us have some trouble grasping the statistical probabilities, especially when several sets of probabilities have to be juggled at the same time.

Nondirective counseling certainly respects patient autonomy, but patient autonomy can too easily be exaggerated. As far back as the early 1980s the President's Commission, while still advocating autonomy, recommended a shared model of decision making, a model steering the middle course between extremes of physician paternalism and patient autonomy. In this model, as we saw in chapter 4, the provider, in this case the genetic counselor, shares her thoughts and feelings in a truly human dialogue. A counselor's experience and knowledge, no less than that of a physician, can be a tremendous source of advice without, of course, usurping the prerogative of the patient to make the final decision. Nondirective counseling may not be the best way for genetic counselors to counsel, and some people are suggesting a change in attitude. Some honest human dialogue and sharing may achieve more good in the counseling setting. Recently some have begun questioning the nondirective role of genetic counselors.

Perhaps the key question a person needs to ask before undergoing a genetic test for a predisposition to a disease is what she is going to do with the information if the test is positive. One possible response to a test for BRCA mutations is a double mastectomy, but if the woman is not ready to pursue that option, there is little else she can do after the test that she could not be doing now—healthy diet, exercise, no smoking, frequent checkups, and so on. The possible benefits of a prophylactic double mastectomy for women with mutations on a BRCA gene are not yet established. A significant study published in 1999 did show that prophylactic mastectomies in 639 women with family histories of breast cancer resulted in fewer deaths from breast cancer than expected (two instead of the expected twenty—a figure that is not all good news because it also shows that 621 of these women had unnecessary mastectomies), but no study has yet assessed the benefit of mastectomies for women with BRCA mutations. Hence, unless the woman is planning on a double mastectomy if the test is positive, it is difficult to see how having the test could make her life better. Often, when genes are involved, it is better not to know what the future might hold.

Finally, this breast cancer case reminds us how fear can distort decision making. There is widespread fear about breast cancer among women and among the men who care about them. Everyone is aware of how in the 1990s the American Cancer Society, in an effort to encourage mammograms and research, emphasized that "one in nine" women would develop breast cancer. The one in nine figure is approximately true but misleading. First, it is based on a life span projection of eighty-five years for all nine women. Second, most breast cancers develop late in life and are not the cause of death. Although figures show that about one in nine women living to eighty-five will develop breast cancer, only one in twenty-seven will die of it. Cardiovascular disease is six times more lethal than breast cancer for women, yet most women fear it much less. One study showed that the following could be expected to happen in a group of one thousand females over a period of eighty-five years: thirty-three will be dead of breast cancer, but two hundred and three will be dead of cardiovascular disease. The lesson here is this: Good decision making is undermined when the foresight into what might happen is distorted by exaggerated and hence unreasonable fears.

Genetic Screening

A distinction can be made between genetic testing and genetic screening, although genetic screening always includes some kind of genetic test. The distinction is this: the word "testing" refers to a search for genetic mutations in an individual and perhaps in his close relatives, whereas the word "screening" refers to a search for genetic mutations in populations. Both advantageous and deleterious mutations collect in population groups because people have historically tended to reproduce in their own geographical areas with people of similar genetic backgrounds. Hence, inherited diseases run at higher rates in some populations, as people inevitably pass on the mutant genes to some of their children who in turn become sick or carriers. Thus, for example, the frequency of cystic fibrosis is higher in whites than in most other ethnic and demographic groups.

Examples of other well-known genetic diseases with higher than normal occurrence in certain populations, in addition to cystic fibrosis, include these conditions:

- Tay-Sachs disease, a lethal disease characterized by physical and mental retardation, convulsions, and death within a few years of birth, occurring among Jewish people with genetic roots in eastern Europe
- Sickle-cell anemia, occurring among people of African descent
- Thalassemia, a disease characterized by chronic anemia, retarded growth, low energy, and ultimately early death if untreated, occurring in people living in a belt stretching from the Mediterranean through the Middle East to Southeast Asia

Next we will look at a well-known *medically* successful screening program that reduced drastically a disease called beta-thalassemia that can help us see how ethical issues are so often present in genetic screening.

Screening for Beta-Thalassemia Carriers on Sardinia

Beta-thalassemia occurs frequently in the Mediterranean region. It presents in the first year of life with severe anemia, failure to thrive, and enlargement of the baby's spleen and liver. Without treatment it usually causes death within about six years. Treatment can extend the patient's life for several decades, but the treatment is difficult. It includes transfusions and drugs infused via a pump over ten to twelve hours every day. A bone marrow transplant can actually cure the disease, but the right matching marrow from a sibling often does not exist, and the transplant would be very expensive in any case.

There is good news and bad news about the mutations on the thalassemia gene. The good news is that the deleterious mutations causing the problem are usually small—often only a single base in the DNA chain is added, deleted, or changed. This raises hopes that some kind of genetic therapy may someday correct the mutant base or override the faulty gene.

The bad news is that many different mutations in the thalassemia gene can cause the disease, and the most common mutations in one population are almost never the most common in other populations. The eight to ten most frequent mutations accounting for most of the disease in the Mediterranean basin, for example, are not the same as the eight to ten mutations accounting for most of the disease in Southeast Asia. Hence, as in cystic fibrosis, the genetic story is complex, and the most any test can do is to target the more common mutations in each population. A negative test never means the person is not carrying a mutation for cystic fibrosis or thalassemia. No test checks all possible mutations.

In the 1970s a major effort was launched to screen people for carrier status on the large island of Sardinia off the western coast of Italy. Preliminary analysis indicated that about one person in eight was a carrier, and about 1 child in 250 actually inherited the disease. A public education effort through television, radio, newspapers, magazines, posters, and other media was mounted. Community-based lectures and workshops as well as pamphlets and booklets were also used. Doctors, nurses, and midwives were briefed and asked to spread the word. Secondary schools showed educational programs with videos. Thanks to these efforts, the population was well educated about how carriers transmit the disease to their children, and people were encouraged to undergo testing before having babies. The last point is important—the people were encouraged to undergo screening; they were not coerced. The screening was voluntary.

In the early years most of the people screened were couples with a pregnancy. In recent years, however, more and more couples without a pregnancy as well as single people have been requesting the genetic tests as the screening gains momentum. Prescreening carrier counseling is provided; it includes information about the disease and its inheritance patterns, and also about reproductive options such as adoption, contraception, and artificial insemination. The possibility of fetal testing at about ten weeks into a pregnancy is also explained.

And what is the result of this intensive screening program? The rate of children born with beta-thalassemia on Sardinia fell from 1 in 250 in 1975 to 1 in 4,000 by 1995. A significant reduction also occurred on Cyprus, where a similar program was in place. In the Greek part of the island, babies born with thalassemia, expected to average about seventy a year, have been averaging only two a year since 1984.

All the factors causing the reduced numbers of affected babies are not fully known. Perhaps some carriers are avoiding marriage with other carriers, and some married carrier couples may be avoiding pregnancy. However, the major factor accounting for the reduction in the number of babies with beta-thalassemia is known: it is abortion. One center on Sardinia screened 4,973 known carrier couples as of 1997 and detected 1,282 fetuses with beta-thalassemia, a number confirming the expected disease ratio of one in four. Almost all (99 percent) of the women with fetuses carrying the two genes for thalassemia chose abortion. With a 75 percent chance that a child will not have thalassemia, many carrier couples are apparently starting their pregnancies and then using prenatal diagnosis and abortion to end 25 percent of the pregnancies in order to prevent the birth of a child with beta-thalassemia.

Ethical Reflections

Obviously this raises ethical questions. Abortion, the destruction of a human fetus, is ordinarily not compatible with an ethic whose norm is living a good and noble human life. As we saw in chapter 11, however, prudential reasoning does suggest that destroying fetuses may be the less worse option in some tragic situations where all possible choices result in bad outcomes. We gave some admittedly easy examples of morally reasonable abortions—ectopic pregnancy, fetal destruction in pregnancies of an exceptionally high number of fetuses, and serious lethal diseases that will allow a child no more than a few years of life with intense suffering.

Is beta-thalassemia a serious enough disease to make the abortion of the fetus at about eleven weeks morally reasonable? Virtuous people may well disagree about this. Prudential reasoning weighing the good and the bad involved in the destruction of these fetuses is difficult. Beta-thalassemia appears in varying degrees of severity. It can be so mild that it does not require transfusions, and the child will live a relatively normal life. And even the more frequent cases—called thalassemia major—requiring drugs and transfusions appear in a wide range of severity. Sometimes, but rarely, prenatal diagnosis predicts a mild case, sometimes it predicts a severe case, but often it cannot predict the severity with any accuracy. This uncertainty makes moral reasoning about the abortion of fetuses with beta-thalassemia difficult for morally sensitive people.

Moreover, relying on abortion as a form of birth control to prevent the birth of babies with this genetic disease is morally troublesome in a virtue-based ethics. The prudential reasoning that might support abortion after the unexpected discovery of a severe problem during pregnancy is not quite the same as prudential reasoning for relying on abortion to control genetic diseases in high-risk populations. Other options for avoiding beta-thalassemia in children could be considered.

Perhaps widespread carrier testing and public health information may encourage some beta-thalassemia carriers to avoid having children with another known carrier. This may at first sound unrealistic, but some people do avoid reproducing with people for health reasons. For example, a person knowing that a possible mate is infected with HIV, or is an alcoholic in a family of alcoholics, or is the child of a parent with Huntington's disease, may decide not to have children with him or her.

Providing IVF with preimplantation genetic diagnosis may be another alternative when both parents are carriers, although this will be expensive. Discarding a preimplantation embryo with serious deleterious mutations does not compromise the human good to the same extent as a second trimester abortion. In any case, some way of preventing the reproduction of fetuses with thalassemia may be less worse in a virtue-based ethic than planning to abort them if they appear. At the very least, prudence suggests looking at alternatives to parents' ignoring carrier status because they plan to abort any fetus with the genetic flaw discovered in prenatal testing. Admittedly the ethical reasoning in this kind of situation is difficult.

The different reactions of two major religious groups show the difficulty in determining a good course of action in prenatal screening for the disease. On Sardinia the Roman Catholic Church, the dominant religious tradition, has steadfastly opposed prenatal testing for beta-thalassemia, fearing it will increase abortions. On the Greek part of Cyprus, the Greek Orthodox Church, the dominant religious tradition there, has encouraged prenatal testing when both parents are carriers, knowing that almost all fetuses testing positive for the disease will be destroyed.

Screening of populations for genetic mutations will expand rapidly in the near future as more tests become available and more people want the information about themselves and their fetuses. Widespread screening raises many ethical issues that will take time and effort to resolve. For example, the Greek Cypriot government now requires carrier testing for thalassemia before granting a marriage license. Unfortunately, the published accounts of the medical success of the programs on Sardinia and Cyprus fail to grapple with the moral implications of the abortion solution.

GENETIC RESEARCH ON HUMANS

Gene *therapy* for human beings is the new dream of medicine, but it is only that—a dream. All we have now are genetic *research* trials using human participants. Significant gene therapies do not yet exist, although many people seem to think they do. Given the role genetic mutations play in so many diseases, however, the dream is for genetic therapies to correct or override the deleterious mutations. Undoubtedly that hope will be realized to some extent in the future. At the present time (2009), however, we need to acknowledge, contrary to media hype and public opinion, that genetic clinical research trials on hundreds of human subjects have not yet produced an approved gene therapy that doctors can use for their patients.

Genetic diseases fall roughly into four classes: single-gene diseases, multigene diseases, multifactorial diseases, and acquired diseases.

Single-gene inherited diseases are the least complicated because all the known mutations causing the disease are located on one identifiable gene in the cells. These diseases are inherited in the patterns Gregor Mendel first observed in his pea plants. Hence, they are usually called Mendelian diseases. The single-gene disease is dominant when the flaw on one copy (allele) of the particular gene is enough to cause the disease. The disease is recessive when the flaw has to occur on both copies of the gene to cause the disease.

Most of the mutations for these diseases occur on one of the autosomal chromosomes, the twenty-two pairs of nonsex chromosomes in the nucleus of human cells, and generally follow the Mendelian inheritance patterns. However, there are two important exceptions. One is when the mutations occur on a sex chromosome known as the X chromosome. Because the female has two X chromosomes and the male one X and one Y, a male child can inherit an X-linked genetic flaw only from his mother. This is so because a child inherits only one sex-linked chromosome from each parent and, since boys have one X and one Y, their X chromosomes had to come from their mothers, because the Y chromosomes could only have come from their fathers. Daughters, of course, can inherit X-linked genetic flaws from either or both parents. An example of an X-linked genetic disease is Duchenne muscular dystrophy, a lethal disease usually causing death by the early twenties.

A second exception occurs when the mutations are on the mitochondrial DNA in the cytoplasm outside the nucleus. These mutations are also passed on to children only by mothers. This is because the mitochondria in spermatozoa are located in the tail, and the tail is lost when the spermatozoon penetrates the ovum in fertilization. Hence, only the mother's mitochondrial genes are inherited.

Multigene inherited diseases are inherited diseases caused by mutations on two or more genes. Often they are known as chromosomal disorders. This is because so many genes are involved that the chromosome itself is notably deformed. Among the better known chromosomal or multigene disorders is Down syndrome, where chromosome 21 appears not as a pair but as a triplet. Hence the disease is often called trisomy 21. Most trisomies affect autosomal chromosomes, but a few affect the sex chromosomes—instead of XX (female) or XY (male), the person might be XXY or XXX or XYY. Not all multigene disorders involve an abnormal number of chromosomes. People with Wolf-Hirschhorn syndrome, for example, have the right number of chromosomes, but the genes that should form one arm of chromosome 4 are missing. Numerous other multigenetic deletions, additions, and translocations can also occur.

Multifactorial genetic diseases are diseases caused both by inherited genetic mutations on one or more genes and by interaction of the genes with environmental factors. Examples of multifactorial disease are the neural tube defects known as anencephaly and spina bifida (see chapter 12). Although the causes of these conditions are not fully understood, recent research indicates that neural tube defects appear when two events occur: a defective gene in the fetus fails to produce a crucial enzyme *and* the woman's diet is low in either folic acid or vitamin B_{12}.

Both the defective gene and the low dietary intake are necessary; neither one alone will cause the spina bifida or anencephaly. Hence, extra folic acid taken before and during pregnancy can prevent many neural tube defects from occurring even though the defective gene is present in the fetus. This is why neural tube defects are now considered multifactorial genetic diseases—both the gene and an environmental factor (diet) together cause the disease.

Acquired genetic diseases are diseases caused by spontaneous mutations occurring in a person's genes during his lifetime. A few sporadic mutations of the base pairs inevitably occur when the cells divide and multiply. Most of them are harmless, but sometimes the mutations on genes do play a role in disease. Mutations also occur in a person's lifetime as the result of environmental influences such as radiation, smoking, diet, and so forth. Many cancers and autoimmune diseases are examples of genetic diseases where acquired sporadic and environmental mutations rather than inherited mutations are the major causal factors.

Sometimes a particular disease can occur either through inheritance or through acquisition in the patient's lifetime. Retinoblastoma, cancer of the retina that affects children, is one example. Retinoblastoma arises from deleterious mutations on both copies (alleles) of the relevant gene. Rarely does a child inherit two mutated genes. Usually *hereditary* retinoblastoma occurs when the child inherits the mutation on one allele and then something triggers the mutation on the other allele. The rarer *spontaneous* retinoblastoma occurs when both mutations are acquired during the child's life. In other words, in the language of geneticists, you need "two hits," one on each copy of the gene, to develop this retinal cancer. Most affected people inherit one hit and then acquire the second hit during their life; this is the multifactorial version of the disease. A few people, however, acquire both hits during their lives; this is the acquired version of the same genetic disease. And a very few people inherit both mutations; this is the inherited version of the disease.

Breast cancer, as we saw, can be a multifactorial or an acquired disease. About 10 percent of breast cancers are multifactorial: the person has one of the BRCA genes (the first hit), but a second "hit" during life is required if the cancer is actually to appear. The other 90 percent of breast cancers are apparently acquired during life without an inherited causal factor.

By looking at these four broad categories, we can see that genes underlie most diseases, not simply those arising from inherited genes but those arising from genetic mutations that take place during the life of the cells. And the genetic factors in disease can be extremely complex, involving different mutations, many genes, and various interactions of genes with their environment. It is easy to see that trying to develop gene therapies to prevent or correct deleterious genetic mutations underlying genetic diseases is an awesome task.

How Gene Therapy Will Work

Gene therapy means, in general, any technique to repair, replace, or override malfunctioning genes in a patient's cells. In theory there are many ways to do this. Deleterious mutant genes could be removed from the DNA strings and replaced with properly functioning genes, or they could be simply repaired by correcting their errant codons. In fact, however, almost all current research in gene therapy forgoes direct intervention on mutant genes and simply adds normal genes to the patient's cells. If all goes well the additional normal genes will produce enough proteins to offset the failure of the dysfunctional genes.

How do scientists do this? How do they add genes to the patient's cells so they will code for the needed normal proteins? Usually they achieve this by using delivery vehicles they call *vectors*. They package the DNA in vectors, the vectors invade the cells, and once inside the cell, the DNA carried by the vector merges with the DNA in the nucleus of the cell, changing its genetic sequence or code.

The delivery of additional normal genes to cells by vectors is theoretically possible in several ways. The most desirable way would be to insert the vectors with the needed normal genes into the bloodstream so they could be delivered to the cellular sites in the body where their functioning is needed. Once perfected this could make delivery of normal genes a simple process using intravenous lines.

A second way of adding normal genes to a patient's cells is to deliver them directly to the cells at the diseased site in the body. Thus, normal genes, usually carried by a vector, could be inserted into a malignant tumor or sprayed into the lungs of a patient with cystic fibrosis. Once on site, the normal genes could provide the missing proteins to prevent the cancerous cells from multiplying wildly or the lung secretions associated with CF from arising. Some modest success has come from these efforts.

By far the most promising way of delivering additional genes to a patient's genome consists of removing cells from the patient, adding normal genes to those cells in the laboratory by vectors, and then placing the cells with the normal genes back into the patient. This is the technique being used in most clinical trials.

Although several different vectors have the capability of introducing DNA into cells, the ones used most frequently are viruses. Viruses are tiny strands of DNA or RNA that can, as we all know from the common cold, infect cells and cause mischief. It is their ability to get inside cells that makes them so important for medical geneticists. Scientists take a virus, alter its DNA so it will not cause problems in a human cell, and then add the desired normal human gene to it. Then they allow the altered viruses to invade human cells, something viruses love to do. The altered DNA in the virus is sometimes called recombinant DNA. This simply means strands of DNA have been cut and then recombined in a new way.

Especially helpful are a class of RNA viruses called retroviruses. These are very "clever" viruses. Once inside the host cell their RNA produces DNA that penetrates the nucleus and integrates itself with the cell's DNA. Then, when the infected cell's DNA divides into daughter cells, the virus-altered DNA is carried into the next generation of cells, and they in turn pass it on to their daughter cells. Soon, if all goes well, there are enough normal functioning genes in the genotype to make a difference in the phenotype; that is, we begin to see the disease caused by the defective gene or genes abate as the amount of normal proteins increases in the body.

Public Concerns

When scientists began cutting and recombining DNA in 1973, people became nervous about what they called "playing God." In response NIH set up an oversight committee known as the Recombinant DNA Advisory Committee (RAC) to review the safety of federally funded recombinant DNA research.

Public concern about the genetic engineering, however, continued to rise. American molecular biologists embraced a moratorium on research beginning in July 1974 that lasted almost a year. Controversy flared anew in 1976 when Cambridge, Massachusetts, home of Harvard University and the Massachusetts Institute of Technology, imposed its ban on genetic engineering. Then, in 1980 the general secretaries of three major religious organizations—the National Council of Churches, the Synagogue Council of America, and the United States Catholic Conference—wrote a letter to the newly formed President's Commission expressing their concerns about the religious, moral, and ethical questions arising from making new forms of DNA. The organizations asked for more government oversight and broad public consideration. The President's Commission did study the issue and in 1983 issued its report titled *Splicing Life*. Among other recommendations, it called for revising RAC so it could better consider the social and ethical implications of genetic alterations.

In response, RAC then set up the Working Group on Human Gene Therapy in 1984. The following year this group published a key document titled *Points to Consider in the Design and Submission of Human Somatic–Cell Gene Therapy Protocols*. The points are guidelines for those submitting proposals involving research on human subjects to RAC. The *Points to Consider* document, revised in the *Federal Register* of April 27, 1995, remains a key check on genetic research.

Genetic Research on Human Subjects

The Working Group soon evolved into the Human Gene Therapy Subcommittee. In 1990 this Subcommittee received its first proposal for genetic research on human beings. The proposed research subjects were two children suffering from a rare immunodeficiency disease known as ADA deficiency that is caused by a malfunctioning gene in the bone marrow. Researchers drew some of the children's blood, used a retrovirus to introduce normal copies of the ADA gene into its T cells, and then infused the blood back into the children in stages. As the cells with the normal ADA gene increased in the children, their immune systems improved. Researchers claimed success, and the public applauded.

Despite the glowing reports and extensive publicity, however, the first gene trial was at best only partially successful. One of the two girls, Ashanti DeSilva, did improve significantly, and about 50 percent of her blood cells carried the healthy new genes after three years. The other girl, however, did not experience great improvement—only 1 percent of her blood cells showed evidence of the healthy gene. Moreover, the clinical trial was somewhat compromised because the researchers continued giving synthetic ADA—the standard treatment for ADA—to the girls while they were also receiving the experimental genetic treatment. Since the genetic intervention was added to the ongoing treatments, we have no way of knowing how much of Ashanti's improvement was the result of the experimental genetic interventions and how much was the result of the traditional treatment.

By the end of 1998 the subcommittee had approved about 250 additional gene trials on human subjects, most of them using retroviruses as vectors to transport normal genes into human cells. Note that these protocols are medical research, not clinical therapies. Unlike genetic testing and screening, true gene therapy has not yet begun. It is, however, almost certain to create in the future a major revolution in health care. Already professional groups are gearing up to inform and encourage providers of health care. The National Coalition for Health Professional Education in Genetics was formed in 1996 and includes over a hundred professional organizations, including the AMA and the ANA, governmental and nongovernmental agencies, and managed care organizations. In 1998 the AMA sponsored a special meeting titled "Genetic Medicine for the Practicing Physician." The curricula in schools of medicine and nursing are changing rapidly to accommodate the genetic revolution and help practicing physicians, nurses, and other providers keep abreast of developments.

Recently an important shift has occurred in genetic research. In the 1980s the early genetic research focused on inherited diseases or propensities for disease caused by mutations on a single gene. This was understandable: working with mutations on one gene is a lot easier than looking at many genes, let alone the interaction of these genes with each other and with the environment.

This explains why single-gene inherited diseases such as ADA deficiency, thalassemia, cystic fibrosis, Tay-Sachs disease, and retinoblastoma received a lot of attention.

By the 1990s, however, there was a distinct shift in genetic research away from inherited diseases caused by single-gene mutations toward the multigene mutations found in more common diseases such as cancer, AIDS, diabetes, Alzheimer, and heart diseases. There are at least two reasons for this. First, there was a growing realization that genetic mutations play a major role in these acquired common diseases.

Second, although federal funds support some genetic research, a great deal of private capital is also at work. Genetic research is very expensive, and biotechnology companies, no less than drug companies, are looking at potential markets for their tests and therapies so they can offset the costs of development and realize a profit for their investors. Clearly, the market for genetic therapies to cure or prevent cancer, heart disease, and AIDS is much larger than the market for therapies to correct the inherited diseases such as ADA, cystic fibrosis, or thalassemia. These diseases affect fewer people and, as prenatal screening grows, will affect even fewer people in the future as couples opt for abortion. Hence, curing the symptoms of inherited diseases has a much less promising future than curing the acquired diseases. Numbers tell the story. As of mid-1998 the NIH had registered 244 gene therapy research protocols, mostly for cancer (150) and AIDS (23). Only thirty-three are for inherited genetic diseases.

The situation is commercially reasonable but medically ironic. The easiest genetic therapies to develop would be for the inherited single-gene diseases, but market forces slant the research toward the more complicated multigene environmentally triggered diseases such as cancer and heart disease.

Genetic research on human subjects raises a number of ethical questions. One set of ethical questions arises from the commercial promise of a successful genetic therapy. Once patented and licensed, such a therapy could make a lot of money. For some researchers the exciting science is the motivation, for others the potential for significant income is the motivation, and for still others both the science and the money together provide the motivation. The huge commercial potential of future genetic therapies can all too easily tempt researchers to ignore federal regulations, IRB requirements, fully informed consent, and, most importantly, the harms to human subjects that genetic research can cause. The push to develop genetic therapy and get it to market introduces a conflict of interest that, if not managed in an ethical way, can cause tremendous harm, even death, for those who volunteer for the clinical trials. An account of the first death caused by genetic research that raised numerous ethical and regulatory questions is a story that illustrates this conflict of interest in a tragic way.

The Case of Jesse Gelsinger

The Story

When Jesse was growing up in New Jersey he was diagnosed at the Children's Hospital of Philadelphia with ornithine transcarbamylase (OTC) deficiency, a rare genetic disorder affecting about one of every eighty thousand babies. An OTC deficiency means a person lacks an enzyme in liver cells that converts the nitrogen generated when the body absorbs protein into urea that can be excreted by the kidneys. Unless this conversion occurs, the nitrogen builds up in the blood as excessive ammonia, and this causes neurological damage and liver problems. Most babies with OTC deficiency die not long after birth.

The genetic mutation that causes this problem is located on the X chromosome. Women have two X chromosomes, so a defective gene on one of them makes them carriers but with few or no symptoms because the normal gene usually functions well. Men, however, have only one X chromosome, so if they happen to receive the defective X chromosome from their mothers (a 50 percent chance), they inherit the life-threatening OTC deficiency disease.

Jesse's mother, however, was not a carrier. Doctors therefore attributed his OTC deficiency to spontaneous mutations in some of his liver cells while other liver cells remained normal. Hence his OTC deficiency was mild. His disease was manageable as long as he stayed on a low-protein diet and took his medications.

In September 1998 when Jesse was seventeen and living in Arizona with his father Paul and his stepmother, a physician monitoring his disease at a metabolic clinic informed him and his father that researchers at the University of Pennsylvania were working on a clinical trial that the physician described as "gene therapy" to see whether they could find a cure for OTC deficiency. During his April 1999 visit to the metabolic clinic the subject of the clinical trial and gene therapy came up again. Both Jesse and Paul were interested, and, since the family was already planning a trip to New Jersey in June, they agreed to visit the Institute for Human Gene Therapy (IHGT) at the University of Pennsylvania to see whether Jesse would be a candidate for the gene therapy clinical trial that was already under way.

The design of the clinical trial, titled "Recombinant Adenovirus Gene Transfer in Adults with Partial Ornithine Transcarbamylase Deficiency" was relatively simple. Researchers were engineering an adenovirus (which gives us colds by working its way into our cells) so it would not replicate once it invaded the liver cells. Then they inserted good genes with the OTC capability into the altered virus and infused the altered virus carrying the good genes into the liver. Researchers hoped that the healthy genes in the liver would soon produce enough OTC to overcome the deficiency and prevent ammonia from building up in the body. At this point researchers were conducting only a phase I trial: that is, a trial to see how high a load of the OTC gene bearing viruses they could safely infuse into people's livers without causing adverse reactions.

For the phase I trial researchers were looking to recruit eighteen adults who either had some OTC deficiency or who were carriers. Originally researchers had hoped to try the experiment on babies suffering from the OTC deficiency, but a well-known ethicist at the university, Arthur Caplan, had raised objections to this plan. Caplan argued that the parents of children dying from OTC deficiency would be so devastated that many would agree to enroll their child in a clinical trial out of desperation, and thus their informed consent would not be truly voluntary. Moreover, the proposed trial was a phase I study where the goal was not to evaluate a therapeutic benefit but to see whether the intervention had unacceptable side effects, a distinction that desperate parents might not well understand.

Researchers planned to divide the eighteen participants into groups of three, with two women and one man in each group. Their plan was to give the three people in the first group a low dose of the altered virus and then monitor them for safety for at least three weeks. If all went well, they would give the second group of three subjects a higher dose of the altered virus and monitor them for three weeks, then infuse the third group, and so forth until all six groups have been tested. The women would receive the virus first, and only if the dose did not cause adverse reactions in them would the researchers give it to the man in the group, who would be more seriously affected by the OTC deficiency. Researchers were now nearing the end of the phase I clinical study; Jesse would be the third member of the sixth group, the last person to receive the altered virus.

In June 1999, Jesse and his father met with Dr. Raper at the University of Pennsylvania. Since Jesse turned eighteen that June he would be old enough to give voluntary informed consent for the clinical trial. Dr. Raper, a surgeon involved with the gene transfer trial, explained the procedure to Jesse and his father. He would insert a catheter into the artery leading to Jesse's liver and a second one into a vein leading from his liver. He would put the modified adenovirus with the healthy genes into the artery leading to the liver. Hopefully the virus with the genes would invade liver cells and thus deliver the good genes. A check of the blood in the vein leaving the liver would indicate how much of the gene-bearing virus remained in the liver. By measuring the viral input and output, researchers could determine whether the liver was absorbing the virus with the good genes embedded in it. A week later they would do a needle biopsy of the liver to confirm the results of the attempted gene transfer.

Dr. Raper told Jesse that there were risks involved. He would probably develop some flu-like symptoms after the infusion of the virus, and there was some small chance of hepatitis, which could be treated. There was also a remote possibility that he might die from the liver biopsy (Dr. Raper told him that the risk of death from a liver biopsy is about one in ten thousand). Dr. Raper also made it clear that the clinical trial, even if it worked as they hoped, would not reverse Jesse's OTC deficiency because his immune system would reject the virus with the healthy genes in a matter of weeks. On the other hand, if the gene transfer proved successful, then it would be a big step forward toward developing a genetic therapy for babies with the OTC deficiency as well as for dozens of other genetic diseases affecting the liver. Both Paul and Jesse agreed to participate if tests showed that Jesse would be a good candidate for the clinical trial.

A month later Dr. Mark Batshaw, another one of the physicians conducting the study, wrote both Paul and Jesse in Arizona about the clinical trial and then spoke with them by phone. According to Paul Gelsinger, Dr. Batshaw said that the treatment had worked temporarily in mice, even preventing death when mice were injected with lethal doses of ammonia. He also said that there were about twenty-five other liver disorders affecting a half-million people in the United States and twelve million worldwide that could be treated with the same technique if it worked and that a recent human participant in the study had experienced a 50 percent increase in her ability to excrete ammonia. In other words, the research was showing signs of therapeutic value that potentially could benefit millions of people. This clinched the matter for Jesse and his father; they considered this promising news and became excited about participating in the "genetic therapy" research at the IHGT.

The chief investigator in the study was Dr. James Wilson, the head of the IHGT at the University of Pennsylvania. He had become interested in developing genetic therapies for liver diseases after reading about a well-known patient named Stormy Jones whose liver cells had a genetic mutation that prevented the liver from removing LDL cholesterol from the blood. This genetic defect allows high levels of the dangerous LDL cholesterol (the "bad" cholesterol) to develop in the body, and most patients suffering from it die prematurely from heart attacks. Mr. Jones was in imminent danger of dying from very high LDL cholesterol levels when he received a heart and liver transplant. The transplanted liver began removing LDL from his bloodstream, and the healthy transplanted heart gave him a new lease on life. Wilson began to think it would be better for patients if a way could be found to insert normal cells into their liver rather than transplanting a new liver.

In experiments on human participants that began in 1992, Wilson and other researchers surgically removed part of the person's liver, cultured cells from it in the laboratory, used retroviruses to convey healthy genes into the DNA of these liver cells, and then infused the modified cells back into the liver through a catheter in the artery leading to the liver. Eighteen months after performing the procedure on a twenty-eight-year-old research subject, Wilson reported in 1994 that the genetic intervention was safe and had successfully lowered the person's LDL level.

Wilson realized, however, that removing cells from a patient, modifying them *in vitro*, and then putting them back into the patient would have limited application in genetic therapy. A more promising procedure would be the development of what he called "injectable genes." Using these, doctors would be able to transfer healthy genes directly into the body's liver cells, perhaps by viruses. If the technique worked, this would be an in vivo genetic therapy. In animal experiments, Wilson was actually able to lower the cholesterol level of rabbits by injecting healthy genes into their bloodstream.

Wilson soon began working on another genetic disease of liver cells, the OTC deficiency. He thought he could overcome this deficiency by using modified viruses to carry healthy cells with the OTC enzyme directly into the liver so there would be no need to remove part of the liver and add the genes in the laboratory. Scientists and biotech companies were watching his work with great interest. If it proved successful, many people could be cured of diseases caused by deleterious mutations on the genes in liver cells, and biotech companies could profit handsomely thanks to patent protection for the engineered viruses that could reverse the diseases.

Jesse flew to Philadelphia on September 10, 1999. Dr. Raper inserted the catheters on the following Monday, and a large dose of the modified virus with the healthy genes flowed into Jesse's liver. As expected, Jesse suffered flu-like symptoms that evening. Soon, however, things got worse. He spiked a high fever and rapidly deteriorated. Before long he was in a coma, on a ventilator, and receiving dialysis. Then he needed an ECMO machine. By Thursday he was so bloated that his father hardly recognized him. On Friday morning it was obvious that he had suffered massive brain damage and that his organs were shutting down. After the family gathered and a chaplain said a prayer, a doctor withdrew the life support and Jesse was pronounced dead at 2:30 p.m.

An autopsy failed to identify the cause of the problem that led to his death. Obviously the infusion of the altered viruses caused a reaction that killed him, but doctors could not determine how this happened. Paul Gelsinger, shocked over the loss of his son, nonetheless supported the doctors and felt that they had done the best they could.

The doctors at the Institute promised to conduct a complete investigation and to inform Paul of everything they discovered. About two months after Jesse's funeral Dr. James Wilson, the head of the Institute and the sponsor and chief investigator of the OTC deficiency study, flew to Arizona and met with Paul Gelsinger. He explained that Jesse's death had been totally unexpected and still remained unexplained. He spoke of how important the work of his IHGT was, and he sought Paul's continued support. He asked Paul to come to a three-day meeting of the RAC in December that would be reviewing the clinical trial. Paul agreed and flew to Philadelphia where he visited Wilson's IHGT and then drove to Bethesda the next day for the RAC meetings.

As the RAC meeting progressed, however, Paul began to see another side of the clinical trial that had taken the life of his son. He heard FDA officials say that Jesse should not have been infused with the virus because his ammonia level was too high at that time. Originally candidates with blood ammonia levels of more than 50 micromoles per liter (mol/L) were not considered eligible to participate; later researchers raised that level to 70 mol/L. When Jesse arrived in Philadelphia for the clinical procedure his blood ammonia level was 114 mol/L, and NIH officials said that he should have been rejected. However, researchers had lowered the level to 91 mol/L with medication before they infused the virus.

Paul also learned that researchers had failed to report to the FDA in a timely manner or to inform him and his son that some earlier participants had experienced significant side effects from the viral infusions. He also learned that the informed consent form that Jesse had signed differed from the one the FDA had approved and in fact omitted the important information that two monkeys had died in animal studies after being given high doses of the virus.

Paul now began to think that Jesse had signed the informed consent form without having been well informed about possible side effects and risks. He also heard that the viral infusions had not provided any clinically significant therapeutic impact on earlier participants, something that raised questions in his mind about Dr. Batshaw's remarks that one woman had achieved a 50 percent gain in ammonia excretion. Based on that remark both he and Jesse had thought the research was showing some sign of therapeutic advantage. Paul was also upset to learn that researchers had not provided NIH, which had funded the study, or the FDA, which had monitored it, or the IRB at the university that oversaw it with other information in a timely manner as was required by federal regulations.

In remarks to reporters outside the RAC meeting, Dr. Wilson objected to the FDA criticisms. He insisted that no data from either animal or human studies could have foretold that Jesse would die, that the FDA had eventually been told of the two participants who experienced the side effects before Jesse was infused yet did not stop the study, and that the ammonia level in Jesse's liver had been functioning within the protocol parameters when he was enrolled in the study three months before his infusion. Wilson, however, did not respond to criticisms about the informed consent form, and he declined to take questions.

On February 14, 2000, the IHGT responded formally to FDA criticisms and pointed out, among other things, that every patient did give informed consent for the clinical trial, that the two monkeys who had died were in a genetic experiment for a different problem—colorectal cancer—and that there was no evidence that the high ammonia level in Jesse was a cause of his death. However, these remarks still left important questions unanswered. Simply because there is a record of informed consent does not mean that the person actually had all the information he needed to give informed consent. And the issue about the two monkeys is not that they received a different gene for a different problem but that they received a similar viral vector to transport genes into their bodies. And although it is true that there is no evidence that Jesse's high ammonia level caused his death, the point of the FDA criticism was that the approved protocol did not allow researchers to infuse the virus into participants with such high ammonia levels, and researchers are expected to abide by the approved protocols.

After months of publicly supporting the doctors at the university and their research despite the loss of his son, Paul Gelsinger now became their critic and soon sought legal redress. Before looking at what happened next, we consider the case from an ethical point of view.

Ethical Analysis

Situational awareness.   We are aware of the following facts in the Gelsinger story.

1. When Jesse was seventeen, he and his father heard of some important gene therapy research at the University of Pennsylvania for people suffering from OTC deficiency, a genetic condition that takes the life of so many afflicted children. He and his father were interested in participating in the gene therapy research because they believed it might save the lives of babies and might even lead to some future curative therapy that would help Jesse eat a normal diet and not rely on medications to control his condition. When he turned eighteen, Jesse visited the Institute for Human Gene Therapy at the university and consented to becoming a participant in the phase I trial. According to his father, part of his reason for participating was to do something that would allow development of a genetic therapy to help prevent future babies from being ravaged by the deadly disease.

2. Unlike most children with OTC deficiency, Jesse's disease was controlled with medications and a low-protein diet. However, the teenager found taking his medications was a hassle. He did not always take them on schedule or stay on his diet, and hence he suffered occasional relapses. Dealing with his disease sometimes left him frustrated and angry. At one point, he actually jumped out of his father's vehicle in a fit of anger while it was still moving, and his arm ended up under a wheel. It is possible that Jesse hoped for a long shot—that enough progress could be made so a genetic therapy might actually benefit him by allowing him to go off his medications and enjoy a normal diet.

3. Dr. James Wilson, chief of Molecular Medicine and Genetics at the University of Pennsylvania and head of its Institute for Human Gene Therapy, was a leading researcher in the field of genetic research on liver diseases. Wilson thought it might be possible to transfer healthy liver genes into patients.

4. Jesse was the eighteenth and last participant in the phase 1 OTC deficiency clinical trial, and he would receive the highest dose of the viral vector with the healthy genes.

5. NIH funded the clinical trial, and the FDA approved it. The FDA provided oversight and required progress reports, especially about adverse reactions if they occurred. There was some hesitation when the trial was first proposed because infusing large amounts (trillions) of viruses into people is risky business. Viruses will trigger, and may overload, the immune system even though these viruses have been engineered not to replicate. Actually some earlier participants in the OTC trial did experience adverse effects serious enough to require FDA notification, but the doctors never informed the Gelsingers of this.

6. Researchers at the University of Pennsylvania were also doing animal studies that used adenoviruses to transfer genes. Two monkeys in one experiment had died and a third became ill, but the physicians did not inform the Gelsingers of these deaths.

7. Inserting genes into a person's body is a major challenge. Genes are mostly in the nucleus of our cells, and there is much we do not yet know about the DNA molecule that harbors them. Viruses have the capability of getting into the DNA of our cells (an adenovirus is what causes the common cold), so they are promising vehicles for transferring genes. The trick, of course, is to render the virus harmless and then use it to transport healthy genes into the DNA of the cells.

8. Genetic research is more challenging than drug research because we have to study not only the impact of the agent (the altered genes) on the body but also the impact of the vehicle we

use to transfer the altered genes into the body. The vehicle, or vector as it is called, is often a virus, and putting massive doses of viruses into a person's body even without any altered genes can trigger or even overwhelm the body's immune system.

9. The Bayh-Dole Act of 1980 allows universities to patent their discoveries and then assign patent rights to biotech companies in order to develop these discoveries into commercial products. Universities like the Bayh-Dole Act because it permits them to collect license fees and royalties from the biotech products their researchers develop. Academic researchers like the Act because it allows them an opportunity to profit from their research by investing in biotech companies that could support their research and then market what might be commercially viable. Both the University and Dr. Wilson had invested in a company known as Genovo, a biotechnology company that Wilson and others had founded. Penn's equity share in Genovo was 5 percent, and Wilson's share was 30 percent.

We are also aware of numerous good and bad features in the case.

1. Clinical trials with human participants are essential for medical progress, and they have done a tremendous amount of good. Medical research cannot progress very far without them, especially when it comes to drugs, medical devices, and genetic alterations.

2. People who volunteer for clinical trials do so for a number of reasons. Some are dying and will try anything with a meager possibility of cure, some volunteer for money (some trials pay the participants) or free health care, some do it in the hope they will receive therapeutic benefit, and some do it with a sense of altruism because they want to help researchers find a cure for diseases that afflict or kill others. Jesse was not dying, and he did not volunteer for the money. His father has indicated that he had a desire to help find a cure for the lethal disease that afflicts babies and also a hope that researchers might find something that could benefit him. These motivations are morally sound in a virtue-based ethics that focuses on flourishing and helping others to flourish.

3. Medical researchers inevitably find themselves enmeshed in numerous conflicts of interest. A major interest of ethical research is, or should be, protecting human participants from harm, but numerous other interests can conflict with this. First, good medical researchers have an intense interest in accomplishing successful breakthroughs, and this can clash with their responsibility to protect human participants in research from harm. Second, researchers often have an interest in winning recognition for their work and in seeing it published and accepted, and this can clash with protecting human participants. Third medical researchers, especially if they are trained physicians, often have an interest in finding something that will help many future patients, and this interest can clash with protecting the small number of human participants in their clinical trials. Fourth, in the past thirty years since the 1980 Bayh-Dole Act many researchers and their nonprofit academic institutions have developed an intense interest in profiting financially when they develop something with considerable commercial value. Obviously the desire to bring a treatment to market rapidly can clash with the responsibility to protect carefully the people enrolled in the clinical trials.

4. Researchers had a moral responsibility to provide adequate and honest information to the Gelsingers when they recruited Jesse Gelsinger for their clinical trial. They also had a responsibility to provide timely information about adverse events to the university IRB, to the NIH, and to the FDA. Further, they had a responsibility to adhere strictly to the approved protocols for the clinical research. Published reports indicate numerous lapses of their responsibilities in these areas. This is bad for the participants in the research, and it is bad for clinical trials in general because people will not volunteer if they think doctors are acting irresponsibly.

Prudential Reasoning in the Gelsinger Story

Participant's perspective.   Is it morally reasonable for a teenage person in Jesse's position to agree to enter a clinical trial such as this? Based on the information he was given and the guidance of his father, it is hard to fault his decision to enter the trial. He expected flu-like symptoms that would pass. The informed consent form also noted that the altered virus could be toxic to his liver, but he had been reassured that this toxicity could be treated. His biggest worry seemed to be the liver biopsy with its very slight risk of death.

The problem, of course, is that he and his father did not receive important information about the adverse effects of the virus transfer in monkeys or in previous participants in the trial, nor did they receive any concrete information about the entangled financial arrangements involving Dr. Wilson, the IHGT, and the University of Pennsylvania. It should be noted that at the end of the eleven-page informed consent form there was a statement indicating that both Dr. Wilson and the University of Pennsylvania had "financial interest in a successful outcome." The problem, of course, is that Jesse and his father had no idea what that interest was or that it potentially involved millions of dollars.

Parent's perspective. Jesse's father Paul provided a great deal of guidance and support for his son. It is hard to fault his role based on the information he was given. He subsequently pursued legal action against the researchers, which also is morally reasonable in a case such as this one because the researchers did not disclose important information and great harm was done: the clinical trial caused the death of a relatively healthy teenager who had no need of genetic therapy to control his genetic disease. Paul Gelsinger has continued to speak and write about the tragedy, and this has served to call attention to the need to improve patient protection in clinical trials.

Researchers' perspective. There are good moral reasons for doing research with human participants designed to develop genetic therapies correcting mutations in human liver cells. Someday genetic research might lead to a significant revolution in medicine that will help many human beings. It is not morally reasonable, however, for researchers not to follow meticulously the approved protocols; not to inform prospective participants of adverse reactions in previous subjects, or of animal deaths in viral transfers; not to inform prospective participants of financial arrangements relevant to clinical research; and not to provide timely information required by the protocols and by regulations to the NIH, the FDA, and the local IRB that oversee the clinical trial.

University's perspective. Officials at the University of Pennsylvania were aware of some of the conflicts of interest between Wilson's work as a university faculty member and his significant financial stake in Genovo, a company he had helped found to market the products of his research. In 1994 the university's Conflicts of Interest Standing Committee (CISC) had looked into the conflicts of interest that would exist between Wilson's research and the potential for great financial gain for him and his company that that research could generate. The CISC made an effort to reduce the potential negative impact of this conflict by imposing some restrictions on Wilson: he could not sit on Genovo's scientific board; he could not be paid for his work as a consultant for Genovo; and he could not do clinical studies funded by Genovo. Yet the university allowed Dr. Wilson to own 30 percent of Genovo stock, and it accepted an equity share in Genovo for itself. The university also agreed that the IHGT could accept $4 million a year for five years from Genovo for genetic research, and in return it allowed Genovo to seek licenses and patents and to earn profit on future developments by the IHGT or its researchers. They also agreed to accept $25,000 a year from Genovo toward the salary of Arthur Caplan, the well-known bioethicist at the university. Professor Caplan was professor of bioethics in the Department of Molecular and Cellular Engineering, which Dr. Wilson chaired at that time.

The Aftermath

In December 1999 the NIH and the FDA held hearings in Bethesda regarding the clinical trial, and Paul Gelsinger attended. After investigating the circumstances surrounding Jesse Gelsinger's death, the NIH reminded all researchers with similar genetic experiments that federal regulations required them to report adverse events that occur in the trials. Up to that point, 39 adverse events had been reported; after the NIH reminder, the number of adverse events reported suddenly jumped to 691! Clearly scientists were routinely disregarding the NIH reporting regulations.

On January 21, 2000, the FDA shut down all clinical genetic trials at the University of Pennsylvania because of numerous regulatory violations.

In August 2000 Targeted Genetics Corporation, a biotech company, acquired Genovo. Published reports indicate that Wilson's equity interest in Genovo brought him $13.5 million in Targeted Genetics stock and that the university's equity interest in the company was worth $1.4 million at the time of the sale.

In September 2000, one year after Jesse died, his family brought a wrongful death/fraud/intentional misrepresentation lawsuit against the university, the Children's National Medical Center in Washington (CNMC) , the Children's Hospital of Philadelphia, Drs. Wilson, Raper, Batshaw, and Kelley (the dean of the medical school), Genovo, and the bioethicist Arthur Caplan. The suit alleged, among other things, that the informed consent process had been seriously flawed because the defendants had failed to inform Jesse and his family of the risks to him suggested by the illness and death of the research monkeys and had failed to disclose the adverse effects the virus had caused in some earlier human participants. It also alleged that the defendants had failed to disclose adequately the conflict of interest that existed on the part of Dr. Wilson and the university that resulted from their financial interests in seeing Genovo succeed by bringing the viral vector to market as rapidly as possible. The implication of the lawsuit was that the researchers and the university had cut corners in the clinical trial in their haste to develop what would be a blockbuster biotechnology product.

The defendants in the lawsuit decided not to defend their actions in court. About a month after the lawsuit was filed, they quickly agreed to settle the case out of court and paid the Gelsinger family an undisclosed amount of money, estimated in a newspaper article posted on the web page of the Gelsingers' law firm (sskrplaw.com) to be about $10 million, to drop the lawsuit. Both the FDA and the Justice Department, however, continued their investigations.

In February 2002 the FDA formally notified Dr. Wilson that he had failed to address adequately numerous issues that the FDA had raised about the clinical trial; among them were the following serious issues:

- The study was not stopped as required by the approved protocol after some participants developed grade 3 or higher toxicities.
- Researchers injected the virus into subjects who did not meet the criteria required by the approved protocol.
- Researchers injected the virus into a male as the second person in a group of three despite written agreement that the sequence in each group of three would be two female subjects followed by one male (males with the disease are more at risk than female carriers).
- Researchers failed to perform prestudy ammonia tests three days and one day before the viral infusion on all participants as required by the protocol.
- Researchers failed to submit accurate and timely reports to the IRB. In the annual report to the IRB in August 1997, Dr. Wilson stated that the first person in the study developed mild anemia probably because so much blood had been drawn, and that the next two participants did not develop anemia after the amount of blood drawn had been reduced. In fact, however, those two participants actually did develop grade 1 anemias, but this fact was not reported. In the annual IRB report of August 1998, after the first ten participants had received the virus, Dr. Wilson stated that "there have been no significant treatment-related or procedure-related toxicities" when in fact a significant adverse event had occurred on June 25, 1998. Also, the 1998 annual report did not present a table of adverse events according to the protocol; this information was not submitted until the 1999 annual report. In the annual report of August 1999 Dr. Wilson stated: "No serious adverse effects have occurred as a result of this study." The FDA alleged this statement is false because the record shows there were some serious adverse effects, namely, grade 3 toxicities in six participants.
- The protocol stated that researchers will halt the study if a single participant develops a grade 3 or higher toxicity; yet they did not halt the study despite instances of grade 3 toxicities in dose cohorts 4, 5, and 6.

- Researchers failed to obtain proper informed consent in accord with federal regulations. The FDA requested that Dr. Wilson inform participants not to donate blood or gametes, and he confirmed in writing that he had added that information to the consent form when in fact this information was not in the informed consent form.
- Researchers also failed to inform potential participants that higher doses of the virus were associated with disseminated intravascular coagulation (DIC)—a life-threatening generalized bleeding that is hard to stop—in monkeys and might cause a similar problem for humans. Three monkeys received viral vectors in late 1998; one received the same virus vector as the humans, and the other two a different vector, but all three developed DIC. Yet the consent form was never changed to reflect this important fact, and Jessie did in fact develop DIC after he received the virus. Researchers also failed to inform the later participants in the trial that, in addition to "flu-like symptoms," they were likely to experience significant periods of chills, nausea, and vomiting. Moreover, the protocol said that they would be given only Tylenol for discomfort when in fact researchers had to use other pain medications to reduce the discomfort participants were experiencing.

In April 2002 Wilson relinquished his post as director of the IHGT. In September 2002 *Dateline NBC* did a program on Jesse's death and the family's search for answers. In February 2003 *BBC Two* devoted a program to the tragic story.

In February 2005 the U.S. Department of Justice announced a civil settlement in the case that the Department of Justice had brought against the institutions and the researchers involved in the OTC trial. The Department of Justice had accused the researchers (Wilson, Raper, and Batshaw) and their institutions (the University of Pennsylvania and the Children's National Medical Center [CNMC]) of violating the civil False Claims Act between July 1998 and September 1999 when the study was halted by their having (1) submitted false statements and claims on the grant applications, progress reports, and annual reports submitted to the NIH; (2) submitted false statements and claims to the FDA, which was monitoring the research; (3) submitted false statements to the IRBs that reviewed the research over a period of several years; and (4) submitted false statements and claims that prevented the human research participants from giving properly informed consent.

In the settlement with the Department of Justice, the University of Pennsylvania agreed to pay a fine of $517,496, and the CNMC agreed to pay a fine of $514,622. The Department of Justice settlement did not require Dr. Wilson and the other physicians to pay fines, but it did impose restrictions on their work. Dr. Wilson, as the sponsor of the FDA-regulated clinical trial paid for by NIH, had to agree not to participate in research involving human subjects until he completed training in protecting human subjects. He also had to accept severe restrictions on his research with human participants until February 2010. Dr. Wilson also agreed in the settlement to lecture and write an article on the lessons learned from the OTC study and to include statements from the Gelsinger family in the article. Two other physicians involved in the research, Drs. Mark Batshaw and Steven Raper, were also required to complete training in protecting human subjects, and both had restrictions placed on their clinical research for three years. As is customary in this kind of settlement, the accused parties (the two institutions and the three physicians) did not admit the allegations and contended that their behavior was at all times lawful and appropriate.

In January 2008 Dr. Wilson, now the editor-in-chief of the journal *Human Gene Therapy*, wrote an editorial on adverse events in gene transfer trials in which he encouraged genetic therapy organizations to put in place more effective ways for human participants in clinical trials to have "a full and unbiased understanding of the risks and benefits of their participation." The editorial mentioned the adverse events in the severe combined immune deficiency (SCID) and arthritis trials discussed in the next section, but it did not mention the adverse events and the death of Jesse Gelsinger in his OTC trial at the University of Pennsylvania. As of late 2008, an extensive search has failed to locate the article on lessons learned from the Gelsinger tragedy that Dr. Wilson agreed to write in the 2005 settlement with the Justice Department.

In the same issue of *Human Gene Therapy*, two authors recommended the appointment of advocates to help people considering participation in genetic experiments understand the risks of genetic research and to advise them whether participation in a study is truly in their best interest. Yet more than a participant-advocate was needed in the Gelsinger case. The subject needed to be informed about numerous major problems in his clinical trial, namely, the failure of researchers to provide information about the recent monkey deaths, the failure of researchers to inform him (and the IRBs, the FDA, and the NIH) of the earlier adverse events experienced by people enrolled in the study, the failure of researchers to abide by and eventually to stop the study in accord with the approved protocol, and the failure of researchers to mention the extent of the financial gain that Wilson and the University of Pennsylvania stood to receive if they could market the viral transfer procedure.

Ethical Reflection

The story of Jesse Gelsinger ranks with other landmark bioethics cases such as Quinlan, Conroy, Cruzan, and Baby Doe. Investigations into Jesse's death by the NIH, the FDA, the Justice Department, and attorneys representing the Gelsinger family uncovered numerous instances of actions and omissions on the part of researchers that appear less than admirable from a virtue ethics perspective and that are contrary to federal regulations guiding research on human participants.

We cannot flourish as human beings, that is, we cannot develop moral integrity by being less than fully honest with other human beings in matters that affect their health and well-being and by failing to manage well conflicts of interest where the well-being of research participants collides with the potential for huge profits and the desire for scientific acclaim. Jesse's death was the first time somebody in a clinical trial involving gene transfer died, and thus it serves as a wake-up call for everyone involved in genetic research.

The Gelsinger story also raises our consciousness about a whole new set of ethical issues that arise in the entanglement of campus-based research funded by the NIH with tax dollars with the commercial biotech industry funded with venture capital and seeking a profit for its shareholders sooner rather than later. The desire to make serious money all too easily conflicts with the moral responsibility to protect human subjects and to treat fellow human beings with honesty and decency. There is clearly a conflict when both the nonprofit universities and the researchers who work for them have an interest in the potential financial gain that could be generated from the federally funded research.

There is no way to root out conflicts of interest in medical research. Researchers, especially if they are physicians, generally have an interest in helping mankind by curing disease. But they also often have personal interests (they want public acclaim and awards), professional interests (they want to expand scientific knowledge, discover something new, and advance their careers), and financial interests (they want to make money). If we cannot root out conflicts of interests what can we do?

One suggestion for this dilemma is disclosure. Some insist that researchers should disclose their conflicts of interest to potential participants in their studies. As Theodore Friedman, who served as chair of the NIH RAC, wrote in the journal *Science* after the Gelsinger tragedy, "The single most important mechanism for ensuring patient protection from inherent risks of clinical experiments, unrealistic expectations, and potential conflicts of interest of the investigator is accurate and full disclosure of potential risks and benefits and a well-executed informed consent process."

This is a step in the right direction, but it is not enough because informing potential human participants does not adequately protect them from being harmed by the inherent risks or financial conflicts of interest. We need more than disclosure; we need protection for vulnerable human participants entering the world of clinical research. In addition to their disclosing conflicts of interest, we can insist on better oversight by IRBs, the NIH, and the FDA and better procedures to protect vulnerable human participants who do not really understand how the research culture is driven by money as well as by the desire to achieve breakthroughs in science and medicine.

Some have suggested that people considering enrollment in clinical experiments involving genetics be provided a knowledgeable advocate who will help them understand the genetic science, including the relevant studies on animals, and the financial background of the research so they can give fully informed consent before becoming human subjects in the genetic experiments. This is an idea worth exploring because the implications of scientific genetics are difficult to grasp, and serious money is often involved in the ties among researchers, universities, hospitals, and the biotechnology industry. In the Gelsinger case, according to published reports, Dr. Wilson's IHGT at the University was receiving 20 percent of its $25 million annual budget from Genovo, and Dr. Wilson himself held a 30 percent equity interest in Genovo (the maximum allowed by the university).

Most important, we can work to ensure that another interest receives serious attention in the way we educate future researchers—the ethical interest whereby researchers realize that the most important thing in their life is not discovering a cure or making a lot of money but flourishing as decent human beings; that ethics trumps personal, professional, and financial success; and that character integrity cannot be achieved unless we treat other people with respect and decency.

In addition, more accurate language in genetic research will help. The phrases "genetic therapy" and "gene therapy" are ubiquitous in both the professional and popular literature, but they are terribly misleading. At this point (2009) no genetic *therapies* exist, and we should not speak or write as if they do. All we have is genetic *research* and genetic *experimentation*. Calling an institute the *Institute for Human Gene Therapy*, for example, when the Institute's primary function is not providing any therapy for anyone but conducting experiments on human beings, is misleading. A more accurate title would be something like the *Institute for Human Gene Research*. Human beings enrolled in clinical research involving gene transfers can easily misunderstand what is going on if they are told they are participating in genetic therapy trials rather than in genetic research. As was stressed in chapter 3, inappropriate language often distorts understanding and moral reasoning.

Finally, we can also rethink the ethics of conducting research on children. Federal regulations governing federal funding for research on children (45 CFR 46.406) that brings more than a minor increase over the minimal risk may be conducted only if it is anticipated that the trial will benefit them. Normally we do not anticipate that children will receive a benefit in phase 1 clinical trials. Moreover, Arthur Caplan's advice to researchers at the University of Pennsylvania when they wanted to conduct their genetic research on babies carries some weight. Caplan said that research would be unethical because parents, distraught over hearing about the lethal disease affecting their child, would not be able to give truly voluntary consent on behalf of their children. He advised enrolling only people capable of giving consent. Caplan's advice captures an important insight: we cannot morally permit desperate parents to volunteer their babies for risky research.

However, federal regulations (45 CFR 46.407) allow the secretary of the Department of Health and Human Services to make an exception for research on children not otherwise approvable if it "presents an opportunity to understand, prevent, or alleviate a serious problem affecting the health or welfare of children" and if it "will be conducted in accord with sound ethical principles" that include the permission from parents or guardians. Hence, federal funding could, by way of exception, support research on children that brings more than a minor increase over minimal risk.

The federal regulations governing federal funding for research on children focuses on minimal or almost minimal risk, and Caplan's objection to enrolling children in the OTC genetic trial focused on parental voluntary informed consent. But maybe the focus in cases like this should be on whether the research has a reasonable balance of possible benefits for others compared with what is at stake for the children dying of OTC deficiency. If we focus on this, we might view the OTC research in a different light. We might see it as more appropriate for the babies than for people like Jesse. This is so because adults who have survived the disease are at risk for much greater harms than the babies who are dying from it. The research exposed the few adult males in the study to great harm—their lives were at risk from the experiment and not the potentially lethal disease. On the other hand, the lives of the babies with the OTC deficiency were already at risk from the lethal disease, and they would almost certainly soon die from it. They are already in grave medical condition, and if the experiment caused their death, it would be bad but less harmful than if it caused the death of somebody not at risk of imminently dying from OTC deficiency.

There is something of an analogy here with people who may be dying of cancer and who want to try a risky experimental treatment. These patients have a lot less to lose than a person who is not dying, so it is reasonable for them to take greater risks than a person who is not dying. So too, dying babies with OTC deficiency have a lot less to lose than adults such as Jesse who are surviving with mild forms of OTC deficiency. Even if he were fully and properly informed of the research, which he was not, it still might have been more reasonable not to admit him to the study because he had so much to lose. The more reasonable approach here might have been to allow parents to consent for their dying babies, as Dr. Wilson had wanted to do in the first place.

This does not mean we can use babies or children as guinea pigs for medical research. What is does mean is that, in some cases, a reasonable prudential argument can be made that, just as dying adults might think it is reasonable to enroll in a risky clinical trial hoping against hope that it may help them and, if it does not, that researchers might learn something that will help others, parents in extraordinary situations might think it reasonable to enroll their dying children in risky research that would not be reasonable if the children were expected to survive.

A final remark is in order. One can argue that it would be morally admirable for researchers to offer families of those harmed or killed in a poorly conducted clinical trial at least an apology for their various failures, especially after the litigation was settled. The FDA, the NIH, the Department of Justice, a settled civil lawsuit, and widespread ethical commentary found numerous lapses with the way the university, Wilson, Roper, and Batshaw conducted the Gelsinger clinical trial, yet no one is on record as apologizing for the misdeeds and omissions. The lack of an apology continues to bother Paul Gelsinger years after the tragic death of his son in a trial with numerous regulatory and ethical lapses.

Jesse Gelsinger was the first person to die in a genetic research trial but tragically not the last. In 2005 several of the eleven children enrolled in a clinical genetic trial in France developed leukemia-like disease, and one of the children died. The children had a form of SCID, an inherited genetic disease that leaves patients without a functioning immune system. White blood cells lack an enzyme needed to maintain the immune system, and without the enzyme they cannot fight off infections of any sort. Currently there really is no good treatment for the problem. Researchers led by Dr. Alain Fisher of the Necker Hospital in Paris were experimenting with a retrovirus to introduce genes with the enzyme into blood stem cells to see if they could provide a functioning immune system.

For a while the procedure seemed to work. In April 2000 Dr. Fisher reported in the journal *Science* that two babies in his study had normal immune systems ten months after receiving the gene transfers. On April 28, 2000, Gina Kolata reported in the *New York Times*: "For the first time, gene therapy has unequivocally succeeded scientists say." Eventually eight of eleven children receiving the gene transfer showed marked improvement. The gene transfer looked like a success. In 2002, however, a serious problem appeared: one of the children developed T-cell leukemia. Soon a second child developed the same problem. In January 2003 the FDA temporarily halted all twenty-seven SCID trials in the United States that were similar to the trial in France. Eventually four of the eight children who initially had benefited from the gene transfer developed T-cell leukemia. Then, early in 2005, tragedy struck: one of the children in France died from the leukemia. In effect, the genetic transfer did indeed reverse the SCID—but at the cost of a very high risk of leukemia and death in a few years. The hype about a successful genetic therapy had been premature; the experiment provided a functioning immune system but brought with it an unacceptable risk of cancer and death. In late 2007 it was reported that a child in a somewhat similar trial at the UCL Institute for Child Health in London also developed T-cell leukemia.

In July 2007 there was yet another death associated with genetic research on human beings. A thirty-six-year-old woman named Jolee Mohr, who was enrolled in a clinical trial by Targeted Genetics (the company that bought Dr. Wilson's Genovo), died after receiving an injection of adeno-associated viruses carrying genes into her arthritic knee in a phase 1–2 (safety plus the possibility of improvement) trial. Her rheumatologist, Dr. Robert Trapp, injected the adeno-associated virus into her knee on Monday, July 2. The next day her temperature was 101. She continued to get worse, and on Saturday, July 7, she went to the ER with a temperature of 104.1. She was sent home under the care of her primary care physician. Aware of the virus injection, he called the rheumatologist and told him of the adverse reaction. Dr. Trapp assured him that the virus was safe. Jolee's condition continued to worsen, and on Friday, July 12, she was admitted to the local hospital.

On July 19 she was transferred to the University of Chicago Hospital where doctors, learning of the gene transfer, notified the FDA of the adverse reaction. Targeted Genetics also notified the FDA the next day, and the arthritis study was halted. After life support was withdrawn from Jolee on July 24, she died in twenty minutes, leaving behind her husband and five-year-old daughter.

The FDA immediately halted the trial and other similar research studies, but then it lifted the ban in December 2007, a move that seems to indicate it believed that the genetic transfer was not the cause of Jolee's death. On the other hand, the NIH RAC reviewed the case and said it could not rule out that the genetic transfer via the viral vector was a factor in her death because of lack of data. Hence, in this case we are left not knowing whether or not her death was related to the gene transfer.

Even if Jolee's death were unrelated to the gene transfer, this clinical trial raises important ethical issues. First, the move to treat arthritis, which is not a lethal disease, by experiments using gene transfer with large doses of viruses is morally controversial. It raises ethical concerns because risking a person's well-being or life in connection with a nonlethal disease is seldom a prudent or reasonable thing to do. Moreover Jolee's husband said, according to published reports, that she was only mildly affected by her arthritis and was living a relatively normal life. In fact she had spent the weekend before she received the injection of the virus boating with her family.

Second, it should also be noted that she had been recruited for the study by Dr. Robert Trapp, her rheumatologist. Patients tend to place great trust in what their physicians suggest, and this could have biased her consideration of the risks. She also signed the consent agreement immediately after he told her of the clinical study. It would have been more prudent for Dr. Trapp to insist that she take the document home, read it carefully, and then think about it and discuss it with her husband. The document, by the way, did speak of "unknown side effects" and "in rare circumstances, death," but the language was buried in the middle of the fifteen pages.

A third ethical issue in this case is that her rheumatologist did not provide an important piece of relevant information: Targeted Genetics was paying him for every patient he recruited for the study. At least there was no mention of this in the informed consent document. It seems reasonable that many people would want to know whether the doctor recruiting them for a clinical experiment is being paid for having them sign up; otherwise, they may think their doctor is recommending their involvement solely for their best interests. Many researchers, however, continue to think that it is not ethically relevant to explain what their financial interest is in recruiting research subjects or in obtaining results quickly from trials that will bring them or their companies financial profit.

A fourth ethical issue is the IRB review in this case. Targeted Genetics did not use an IRB at a hospital or university; it submitted the protocol to a private commercial IRB under contract with the company. The IRB was approved by the FDA, but the problem is that these for-profit IRBs risk losing business if they are too demanding about studies that biotech companies want to pursue. Hence, there is yet another conflict of interest here; the IRB has a financial interest in approving studies for the biotech companies as well as a regulatory interest in protecting human subjects, and the danger is that the former interest might overshadow the latter.

Germ-line Genetic Research

One particularly thorny issue centers on future therapy affecting what are called *germ-line* cells, the cells of sperm and ova forming the next generation. Alterations of DNA in our somatic cells normally affect only our bodies and not those of our children, although some somatic cell alterations do appear in children. Alterations of DNA in germ cells, on the other hand, pass almost totally into the bodies of children and will modify genetic sequences in a whole line of future generations.

Altering only somatic cells is both an advantage and a disadvantage. It is an advantage because it confines any unintended and unwanted consequences of the genetic alterations to the actual patient. If something does not turn out well, and this often happens in medical research on human subjects, then the problem will affect only the patient and not future generations.

Yet it is also a disadvantage because successful gene therapy in somatic cells only helps the patient and does not correct the mutation children will receive from parents through the germ cells that form the fertilized ovum. It would be nice to correct the genetic error in subsequent generations as well as in the actual patient. It would be nice, in other words, to develop effective gene therapy for germ cells so that deleterious inherited genetic mutations can be stopped once and for all. Germ-line gene therapy, unlike somatic gene therapy, would alter the DNA of future generations. This is what makes it so promising—and so dangerous. Germ-line therapy could prevent disease in future generations, but it could also introduce unwanted alterations in the gene pool that could haunt us forever. The stakes are so high no germ-line research has yet been approved, although some want to try it.

Germ-line genetic alterations could occur in either ova and spermatozoa before fertilization or in early embryos. Alterations to cells in early embryos are germ-line alterations because the cells are not yet differentiated; that is, not yet functioning as specific cells such as brain cells, or kidney cells, or blood cells, or sex cells, and so forth. Any alterations made in the undifferentiated cells of an early embryo will thus appear in all that cell's daughter cells, and some of the altered daughter cells will eventually function as germ cells—spermatozoa or ova. This is how a change in the genome of the embryo affects its future germ cells.

An intense debate about germ-line therapy is now gathering momentum. The 1982 President's Commission report *Splicing Life* took a dim view of germ-line alterations but was not overly concerned because at the time germ-line genetic engineering seemed a long way off. This is no longer true. Germ-line alterations are now technically possible; debate about the moral and social issues is intensifying. In 1997 most European countries took a strong stand against germ-line therapy by signing the Convention on Human Rights and Biomedicine, which states: "An intervention seeking to modify the human genome may only be undertaken . . . if its aim is not to introduce a modification in the genome of any descendants" (Article 13).

The attitude toward germ-line therapy in the United States slants in the opposite direction. Many ethicists encourage caution but advocate moving forward, believing the potential benefits will outweigh the possible harms. Typical arguments favoring germ-line research and therapy include the following reasons:

- The desire to avoid producing children with inherited genetic flaws
- The desire to correct a genetic defect in a preimplantation embryo
- The desire for cost-effective ways to reduce inherited genetic diseases in the population
- The desire of researchers to explore all modes of treatment
- The desire of clinicians to offer patients the most effective treatments

Typical arguments against advancing germ-line research and therapy include the following reasons:

- The desire to avoid causing unintentional problems in the DNA of future generations
- The claim that discarding a genetically defective embryo is better than altering its genome with the attendant risk of causing deleterious mutations in future generations
- The social injustice of germ-line alterations—they are so expensive only the rich could afford them
- The limited impact of germ-line therapy on the population—only a small percentage of IVF embryos will benefit
- The claim that germ-line interventions will amount to eugenics in the pejorative sense—the effort to cleanse the race of "bad" genes, however they might be defined
- The claim that germ-line alterations would be used to breed various classes of human beings well suited to provide various desired services (if this sounds far-fetched, recall how some groups once castrated young boys so they could sing soprano in choruses and choirs)
- The claim that children have the right to receive from their parents DNA that has not been subject to tampering
- The claim that germ-line research for therapy will inevitably slide down a slippery slope toward germ-line research for *enhancement*; that is, for genetic alterations to achieve desired characteristics such as tall build, thin body, blue eyes, blond hair, and so forth in children

This last argument, the slippery slope argument claiming germ-line interventions will inevitably move from therapy to enhancement, is suggestive. After all, the need for germ-line therapy is really quite limited compared to many other more common problems affecting human beings. It is seldom needed for germ cells because people have so many of them, and deleterious mutations affecting all of them are rare. Normally, then, it would make more sense to discard defective ova or spermatozoa than to attempt correcting their genetic structure.

Moreover, germ-line therapy is not available for most embryos because only ova fertilized in a laboratory are candidates, and relatively few women attempt reproduction with IVF. And when women do attempt reproduction with IVF, they normally produce some normal embryos along with the abnormal ones. Prudential reasoning suggests the less worse behavior would be to discard the defective embryos and implant only those without deleterious mutations, thereby avoiding any upset with the germ-line. True, this solution will not work with mitochondrial mutations because all the embryos will probably have the flawed gene. However, mitochondrial diseases are rare, making it difficult to say that curing them is what is driving the push for germ-line therapy.

Given the limited opportunity for germ-line therapy, then, one does wonder why there is considerable interest in pursuing it. One answer may be the large role the market plays in American health care. The need for germ-line therapy is limited, but a vast potential market exists for germ-line enhancements. Unlike germ-line therapy to make abnormal genes normal, germ-line enhancement tries to make normal genes better in some way. It promises to make your children taller, stronger, brighter, more handsome, and more beautiful. Since a lot of parents find this prospect so appealing, commercial interests see a large potential market for germ-line enhancement as well as somatic enhancement. Given this interest in genetic enhancement we need to consider it, however briefly.

GENETIC ENHANCEMENT

Genetic enhancement is the alteration of the human genome not to cure or prevent genetic diseases but to augment some desirable features in the appearance and functioning of the body. The desired improvement could be physical, mental, or behavioral; and it could be for oneself (somatic enhancement) or for one's children (germ-line enhancement).

Genetic enhancement lies in the future but, given the accelerating pace of genetic progress, perhaps not that far into the future. In 1979 engineers from a firm known as Genentech took the RNA from pituitary gland cells, made a DNA copy of it, located in the copy the gene that programs the hormone for growth in the body, and then put that gene into bacteria. As the bacteria multiplied rapidly, so did the gene programming the growth hormone. Genentech had thus found a way to "manufacture" great quantities of the human growth hormone (HGH) in bacteria using recombinant DNA techniques. When given to children, HGH increases growth and height, something many parents would consider desirable.

In the 1990s a gene was found in mice that codes a protein for appetite control and resultant weight loss, now called the obese gene (*ob* gene). A similar gene probably exists in the human genome. If a gene coding for appetite control were ever successfully developed, it would find a vast market among those interested in weight control.

The potential for genetic enhancement is not confined to the physical realm—intellectual and behavioral characteristics can also be genetically enhanced. *Behavior genetics* is a growing field studying the role of genes in human behavior. Efforts to enhance the genetic codes for desirable behavior and cancel those for undesirable behavior are not far off. Few doubt that normal personality traits such as extroversion and introversion, shyness, aggression, risk taking, sociability, and other qualities also have some basis in the genes and hence could possibly be altered genetically.

Ethical Reflections

The ethical arguments for and against genetic enhancement are too complex to discuss thoroughly here. There are two pitfalls plaguing the discussion: reliance on misleading distinctions and predictions of dehumanization and social unrest.

Two misleading distinctions. The first misleading distinction is the distinction between gene therapy and gene enhancement. Usually people make the distinction with the idea of supporting the former but not the latter. They find genetic alterations to prevent or cure disease morally acceptable but not alterations to enhance normal height, weight, intelligence, personality, and so on.

However, the distinction between genetic therapy and genetic enhancement is confusing and misleading in so many instances that it is not helpful in ethical deliberation. Think, for example, of two boys who will be five feet tall as adults. One has a growth hormone (GH) deficiency, one does not. Giving the two short boys the GH to add eight inches to their heights would be, according to the therapy-enhancement distinction, therapy for the boy with the GH deficiency (and thus morally acceptable) but enhancement for the normally short boy (and thus morally questionable). Prudential reasoning would not, as we saw in chapter 3, draw moral conclusions from such misleading distinctions. Rather, it would ask whether adding the growth hormone would, all things considered, be a net benefit for each boy. It would find some genetic therapy good and some bad, and some genetic enhancement good and some bad. Genetic enhancement for the naturally short boy might well be a reasonable option in our society.

The second misleading distinction in the debate about enhancement is the attempt by supporters of enhancement to draw a line between the human body and the human soul (or mind, rationality, free will, spirit, true self, inner self, or whatever is thought to provide our uniquely human dignity). The distinction between the body and the soul, or between the body and whatever else one claims is the source of human dignity, is made to reassure critics of genetic enhancement that genetic enhancement will only affect the body and not really alter whatever nonbiological reality provides our human dignity. In other words, advocates of genetic enhancement claim enhancement will affect only the body and not the true "self," and hence is not a threat to the humanity of the species.

Underlying this distinction are variations of the familiar dualities in Western philosophy: body/soul (Socrates, Plato, and Augustine); mind/body (Descartes); body/immaterial self (Locke); and body/noumenal self (Kant). But this tradition of locating human dignity and freedom in a metaphysical and metabiological reality such as soul, mind, or self somehow embedded within a human body is becoming more and more difficult to sustain given what we learn from evolutionary biology and cognitive science as well as from reflection on our experience.

It may be more helpful, as suggested in chapter 6, to think of ourselves as uniquely human not because we have a nonbiological mind or soul somehow united to our bodies but because our bodies (and brains) normally have the capacities to feel, to think, to reason, to choose, to love, to form communities, and to seek justice, truth, beauty, and goodness, and so on. We thereby transcend the merely physical cells, DNA molecules, genes, base pairs, atoms, and subatomic particles constituting our bodies, and in that possibility for transcendence lies our dignity.

Fears of dehumanization and social unrest. The second pitfall we need to note is the fears that critics of enhancement often raise as arguments against any effort to develop genetic enhancement of behavior. One fear is that any admission that a genetic alteration can change our behavior will undermine such cherished spiritual and humanistic values as human freedom, human equality, the sacredness of human life, and responsibility for one's actions. Another fear is that attributing behavior to people's genes will reinforce prejudicial attitudes in a society already haunted by racial discrimination, fear of crime, and homophobia. The fear is that acknowledging the genetic basis of behavior will make it easier to claim some races have better genes for intelligence or that some races have genes for crime and laziness or that some people can be categorized as genetically abnormal because they have the genes for homosexuality, and so forth.

Yet denying the role of genes in behavior and the possibility of behavioral genetic enhancement for fear of undermining our dignity or equality or reinforcing discrimination is shortsighted. We already know physical alterations (diet and exercise, for example) and drugs can enhance our thinking and behavior. Genetic enhancement is a more profound, and admittedly more unsettling, acknowledgment of this reality, but one that could do great good if not misused.

We are our bodies, and the stretches of DNA comprising our genotype represent the codes for significant aspects of our bodies and of behaviors including thinking, choosing, loving, and hating. Acknowledging the influence of genes on our intelligence and behavior, and acknowledging that these genes, as all genes, are distributed in populations with some variation is simply acknowledging what is the case. Our genes are not the only things that account for our intelligence and behavior, but they are part of the story. Prudential reasoning will consider carefully when efforts to enhance our intelligence and behavior as well as our bodies will likely contribute to the good life for ourselves and our communities and when they will likely undermine it.

HUMAN GENOME PROJECT

Before we conclude this long chapter on the emerging field of genetic medicine, we need to say a word about the HGP. By the 1980s a general consensus emerged for a complete decoding of human DNA—all three billion of its base pairs. Backed by reports of the National Academy of Sciences and the Office of Technology Assessment, Congress approved funding for the project known as the Human Genome Project. Work also began in several other countries, and in 1988 the Human Genome Organization (HUGO) was formed to coordinate international efforts.

The same year, the NIH created the Office of Genome Research. It became the National Center for Human Genome Research in 1989 and is now known as the National Human Genome Research Institute (NHGRI), one of the institutes comprising the NIH. The first director of the HGP was James Watson, the well-known scientist who discovered the DNA double helix with Francis Crick in 1953. By 1990 federally funded work began in earnest at NIH and at the Department of Energy as well as at other laboratories throughout the world to identify the exact sequence of all the bases—identified by the letters *A*, *C*, *G*, or *T*—in the DNA of a human cell by the year 2005. Crick resigned in 1992 after a public dispute with the NIH director over patenting strings of DNA (Crick was opposed), and Francis Collins assumed the position and managed the project to its completion.

The project had two main tasks, mapping and sequencing. The task of mapping involves making various maps, each with increasing magnification, of the genome. The rougher maps are *genetic* maps. They spot patterns of bases on DNA that serve as genetic markers giving a rough idea of where certain genes are located. Before the genes for Huntington's disease and cystic fibrosis were discovered, for example, scientists had discovered markers indicating that these genes were present somewhere in a particular stretch of the DNA. A more precise map is a *physical* map that shows the location of coding and noncoding stretches of DNA.

The second main task was sequencing or identifying in order all the chemical bases in human DNA. Sequencing one person's genome provides more than 99.9 percent of the basic genetic code of anyone's genome. Whereas this is a most exciting thought, the morally loaded questions center on what this information means and on what we are going to do with it.

By the mid-1990s some people, eager for genetic information that is potentially worth millions of dollars in revenue to drug and biotechnology companies, became impatient with the federally funded HGP programs and their target completion date of 2005. They wanted to focus on faster but less accurate sequencing, a kind of first version that could be improved later, or on sequencing only the bases constituting the genes, estimated to be about 5 percent of the total number of bases.

One privately funded company named Celera Genomics, working with new, faster sequencing machines, predicted that sequencing the entire DNA could be accomplished several years earlier than the government's 2005 goal and at a fraction of the original cost estimates. Another company, Human Genome Sciences, began working not with the DNA in the nucleus but with DNA copied from RNA in the cytoplasm (cDNA). This is a quicker way to sequence genes because DNA copied from RNA contains only the DNA coding for genes. Hence, cDNA is only one-twentieth of the original DNA, and yet it contains all the functioning sequences of interest to medical geneticists with patients in mind and to investors with profits in mind. Dedicated molecular biologists, on the other hand, want to know the sequence of all the DNA bases and not just those coding for proteins—the genes. By June 2000 scientists had developed a rough draft of the human genome, and by April 2003 they had completed mapping and sequencing the human genome. Surprisingly they found that the human genome has only about twenty-five to thirty thousand genes, far fewer than what was originally thought.

Obviously the information unleashed by the HGP will have staggering implications for our understanding of life and of ourselves as human beings. The international HUGO has set up an Ethical, Legal, and Social Issues Committee to make recommendations about the use of genetic material and of information contained in the DNA. James Watson, the director of the original program, was sensitive to the humanistic implications of the HGP from the outset and set aside 3 percent of the funding for an important program called Ethical, Legal, and Social Implications (ELSI). The formation of the ELSI program was a prudent move. Advances in genetics give rise to great apprehension among many people. Fears of eugenics, of "playing God," of discrimination in insurance and employment, of racial discrimination, and of creating Frankenstein monsters hover over the new discoveries.

The ELSI initiative has developed programs and awarded grants to help people identify and understand the ethical, legal, and social implications of the genome project and to propose policy options to enhance the benefits and reduce the burdens. In recent years it has focused on four areas: (1) privacy issues arising from genetic information in people's records, (2) diagnostic and treatment issues as medical genetics becomes an ever larger part of clinical care, (3) protection of human subjects in genetic research, and (4) education of health care professionals and of the public about genetics and the implications of genetic information and interventions in their lives. In 1995 the NHGRI took another step forward and established an Office of Ethics at the Institute to provide ethics education, consultation, and research on-site.

A big step in protecting people from the misuse of their genetic information occurred in May 2008 when President George W. Bush signed the Genetic Information Nondiscrimination Act (GINA), which makes it illegal for employers (as of November 2009) and health insurers (as of May 2010) to discriminate against people on the basis of their genetic information. By genetic information the Act means test results from the individual or relatives up to and including fourth-degree relationships or the appearance of a genetic disease or disorder in family members. Specifically the Act prohibits health insurers (but not insurers for life, disability, or long-term care) from requesting or requiring a person (unless he or she is a member of the military) to undergo a genetic test, and from using genetic information to determine enrollment in the insurance plan or the premiums. It also prohibits employers from using genetic information to make decisions about hiring, firing, and other terms of employment. If the federal law is well enforced, it will be a major step in protecting human beings from many forms of genetic discrimination.

Ethical Reflections

Making ethics an integral part of the human genome project from the beginning is a welcome move. All too often in the past new medical techniques and technologies were developed in research and moved into the clinic with little thought about their ethical impact. Only when problems arose did people begin to ask about the ethics of using and withdrawing ventilators and feeding tubes, or performing CPR every time a cardiac arrest occurs, or doing research on unsuspecting patients or children, or trying to "do everything" to salvage extremely defective infants, or manipulating sperm, ova, and embryos in artificial reproductive technologies and medically assisted fertility and surrogate mother arrangements, and so forth. It is far better to think through ethical issues before new developments are widespread. Prudential reasoning is very much foresight—looking ahead to figure out how best to live well.

Protecting people from discrimination arising from genomic information is also an important good. Both health insurers and employers have a significant financial interest in using genetic information to treat those afflicted with known problematic genetic mutations differently from other people, and this could cause serious harms to those people. GINA may be able to prevent this new kind of discrimination.

This chapter is unusually long because of the complexity of medical genetics and the need to offer some summaries of the relevant molecular biology. Good moral decisions presuppose a grasp of what is going on, and we all need to learn what is going on and what is proposed in gene therapy and genetic testing, screening, and enhancement. Some polls have found people readily admitting they do not really know much about DNA, genes, genotypes, phenotypes, the genome, germ-line cells, and the issues they generate. But the same people just as readily offer firmly held opinions about genetic testing, screening, engineering, therapy, enhancement, and the like. Opinions based on ignorance are not good. We need to learn something about molecular biology and the ethical, legal, and social implications of genetic information and interventions before we can make morally prudent decisions about how to use the genetic information and how the biotechnology industry should market these discoveries.

SUGGESTED READINGS

The National Information Resource on Ethics and Human Genetics, which is funded by NIH, contains a vast database on ethics and genetics. It is accessible online at bioethics.georgetown.edu/nirehg. See also genome.gov/education and genome.gov/policyethics. Another helpful site with many links is the NIH Bioethics Resources on the Web at bioethics.od.nih.gov. Several classic texts on genetics and bioethics provide good introductions to material in this chapter. See, for example, the 1982 President's Commission Report *Splicing Life* and the 1991 Study Paper of the Law Reform Commission of Canada titled *Human Dignity and Genetic Heritage*. Also helpful are many entries in Thomas Murray and Maxwell Mehlman, eds., 2000, *Encyclopedia of Ethical, Legal, and Policy Issues in Biotechnology*, New York: John Wiley & Sons; Bryan Appleyard, 1998, *Brave New Worlds: Staying Human in the Genetic Future*, New York: Viking Penguin; Mark Rothstein, ed., 1997, *Genetic Secrets: Protecting Privacy and Confidentiality in the Genetic Era*, New Haven: Yale University Press; and Lois Wingerson, 1998, *Unnatural Selection: The Promise and the Power of Human Gene Research*, New York: Bantam Books; Allen Buchanan et al., 2000, *From Chance to Choice: Genetics and Justice*, New York: Cambridge University Press; and John Evans, 2002, *Playing God? Human Genetic Engineering and the Rationalization of Public Bioethical Debate*, Chicago: Chicago University Press.

Clear explanations of molecular biology can be found in G. J. V. Nossal, 1985, *Reshaping Life: Key Issues in Genetic Engineering*, Cambridge, UK: Cambridge University Press, chapters 1–3; and Eve Nichols, 1988, *Human Gene Therapy*, Cambridge, MA: Harvard University Press, chapters 2 and 3. For additional historical background see Daniel Kevles et al., eds., 1992, *The Code of Codes: Scientific and Social Issues in the Human Genome Project*, Cambridge, MA: Harvard University Press, chapters 1–4; Maxim Frank-Kamenetskii, 1997, *Unraveling DNA: The Most important Molecule of Life*, Lev Liapin, trans., Reading: Addison Wesley, chapters 1–7; and Desmond Nicholl, 2008, *An Introduction to Genetic Engineering*, 3rd ed., New York: Cambridge University Press. A simplified overview for those totally unfamiliar with genetics is Tara Robinson, 2005, *Genetics for Dummies*, Hoboken: Wiley, which could be helpful.

For an example of testing embryos for genetic flaws, see Alan Handyside et al., "Birth of a Normal Girl after In Vitro Fertilization and Preimplantation Diagnostic Testing for Cystic Fibrosis," *New England Journal of Medicine* 1992, 327, 905–9. For some ethical background on preimplantation testing see Richard Tasca et al., "The Emerging Technology and Application of Preimplantation Genetic Diagnosis," and Jeffrey Botkin, "Ethical Issues and Practical Problems in Preimplantation Genetic Diagnosis," both in the *Journal of Law, Medicine & Ethics* 1998, 26, 7–16 and 17–28. The possibility of testing children without symptoms for genetic diseases and predispositions for disease has received a great deal of attention. Most professional groups and many authors advocate a cautious approach. See, for example, the position taken by the American Society of Human Genetics and the American College of Medical Genetics in "Points to Consider: Ethical, Legal, and Psychosocial Implications of Genetic Testing in Children and Adolescents," *American Journal of Genetics* 1995, 57, 1233–41; and by the American Medical Association in its *Code of Medical Ethics* 1996–1997, section 2.138. See also Ellen Clayton, "Genetic Testing in Children," *Journal of Medicine and Philosophy* 1997, 22, 233–51; Dena Davis, "Genetic Dilemmas and the Child's Right to an Open Future," *Hastings Center Report* 1997, 27 (March–April), 7–15; Diane Hoffmann and Eric Wulfsberg, "Testing Children for Genetic Predispositions: Is It in Their Best Interest?" *Journal of Law, Medicine & Ethics* 1995, 23, 331–44; and Dorothy Wertz, "Genetic Testing for Children and Adolescents: Who Decides?" *JAMA* 1994, 272, 875–81. For a less cautious approach, see Cynthia Cohen, "Wrestling with the Future: Should We Test Children for Adult-Onset Genetic Conditions?" *Kennedy Institute of Ethics Journal* 1998, *8*, 111–30.

For the medical background of the breast cancer (BRCA) genes see Donna Shattuck-Eidens et al., "BRCA 1 Sequence Analysis in Women at High Risk for Susceptibility Mutations," *JAMA* 1997, *278*, 1242–50. A good analysis of the special considerations for informed consent in genetic testing for mutations can be found in the Consensus Statement of the Cancer Genetics Studies Consortium's Task Force on Informed Consent titled "Genetic Testing for Susceptibility to Adult-Onset Cancer: The Process and Content of Informed Consent," *JAMA* 1997, *277*, 1467–74. The dilemmas generated by the testing are explored in D. Schrag et al., "Decision Analysis—Effects of Prophylactic Mastectomy and Oophorectomy on Life Expectancy among Women with BRCA1 and BRCA2 Mutations," *New England Journal of Medicine* 1997, *336*, 1465–71; and Eric Kodish et al., "Genetic Testing for Cancer Risk: How to Reconcile the Conflict," *JAMA* 1998, *279*, 179–81. For a study on mastectomies in women at high risk of breast cancer and some thoughtful comments, see Lynn Hartmann et al., "Efficacy of Bilateral Prophylactic Mastectomy in Women with a Family History of Breast Cancer"; Andrea Eisen and Barbara Weber, "Prophylactic Mastectomy—The Price of Fear"; and Kelly-Anne Phillips et al., "Putting the Risk of Breast Cancer in Perspective," *New England Journal of Medicine* 1999, *340*, 77–84, 137–38, 141–44.

Many of the risks of genetic testing are outlined in Ruth Hubbard et al., "Pitfalls of Genetic Testing," *New England Journal of Medicine* 1996, *334*, 1192–94. See also the final report of the Task Force on Genetic Testing created jointly by the ELSI group at NIH and the Department of Energy: Neil Holtzman and Michael Watson, 1998, *Promoting Safe and Effective Genetic Testing in the United States*, Baltimore: Johns Hopkins University Press.

For an excellent account of mapping and then identifying the gene for cystic fibrosis, and of the various molecular mutations and clinical manifestations of CF, see Bruce Korf, 1996, *Human Genetics: A Problem-Based Approach*, Cambridge: Blackwell Science, chapter 3. For the study showing that many couples do not think testing for carrier status is a benefit, see Ellen Clayton et al., "Lack of Interest by Nonpregnant Couples in Population-Based Cystic Fibrosis Carrier Screening," *American Journal of Human Genetics* 1996, *58*, 617–27. However, in April 1997 an NIH Consensus Development Conference advocated CF carrier testing for couples planning pregnancy.

For research showing that CF carriers have a genetic predisposition for pancreatitis, see Nicholas Sharer et al., "Mutations of the Cystic Fibrosis Gene in Patients with Chronic Pancreatitis"; Jonathan Cohn et al., "Relation between Mutations of the Cystic Fibrosis Gene and Idiopathic Pancreatitis"; and Peter Durie, "Pancreatitis and Mutations of the Cystic Fibrosis Gene," *New England Journal of Medicine* 1998, *339*, 645–52, 653–58, and 687–89.

The original National Society of Genetic Counselors (NSGC) "Code of Ethics" stressing "nondirectiveness" and the ethics of care for genetic counselors was published in the *Journal of Genetic Counseling* 1992, *1*, 41–43. It is available online at nsgc.org. The latest revision (January 2006) is also available online. It continues to base the counselor-client relationship on "care and respect for the client's autonomy, individuality, welfare, and freedom" and states that the "the primary concern of genetic counselors is the interests of their clients." Virtue ethics would look for an expanded view of the human good that would include the counselor's moral character and societal welfare. The 2007 NSGC Scope of Practice statement does encourage counselors to "recognize and respond to ethical and moral dilemmas arising in practice" but does not elaborate on just how a counselor is to do this. For evidence of the need for new directions in genetic counseling, see Barbara Biesecker, "Future Directions in Genetic Counseling: Practical and Ethical Considerations," *Kennedy Institute of Ethics Journal* 1998, *8*, 145–60; Mary White, "Decision Making through Dialogue: Reconfiguring Autonomy in Genetic Counseling," *Theoretical Medicine and Bioethics* 1998, *19*, 5–19; and Glenn McGee and Monica Arruda, "A Crossroads in Genetic Counseling," *Cambridge Quarterly of Healthcare Ethics* 1998, *7*, 97–100.

For ethical concern about employers or insurers using genetic information in harmful ways, see Karen Rothenberg et al., "Genetic Information and the Workplace: Legislative Approaches and Policy Challenge," *Science*, 1997, *275*, 1755–57; Lawrence Gostin, "Genetic Privacy," *Journal of Law, Medicine & Ethics* 1995, *23*, 320–30; Alan Strudler, "The Social Construction of Genetic Abnormality: Ethical Implications for Managerial Decisions in the Work Place," *Journal of Business Ethics* 1994, *13*, 839–48; Nancy Kass, "Insurance for the Insurers: The Use of Genetic Tests," *Hastings Center Report* 1992, *22* (November–December), 6–11; Larry Gostin, "Genetic Discrimination: The Use of Genetically Based Diagnostic and Prognostic Tests by Employers and Insurers," *American Journal of Law and Medicine*,

1991, *17*, 109–44. See also Deborah Stone, "The Implications of the Human Genome Project for Access to Health Insurance," and Adrienne Asch, "Genetics and Employment: More Disability Discrimination" in Thomas Murray et al., eds., 1996, *The Human Genome Project and the Future of Health Care*, Bloomington: Indiana University Press, 133–57 and 158–72; and Henry Greely, "Health Insurance, Employment Discrimination, and the Genetics Revolution" in Daniel Kevles, *The Code of Codes*, 264–80.

The adult screening programs on Sardinia and Cyprus are described by Antonio Cao, "Molecular Diagnosis and Carrier Screening for Beta-Thalassemia," *JAMA* 1997, *278*, 1273–77. For general background, see the President's Commission Report, 1983, *Screening and Counseling for Genetic Conditions*. See also Amo Motuisky, "Screening for Genetic Diseases," *New England Journal of Medicine* 1997, *336*, 1314–16; and a report of the National Research Council, 1997, *Evaluating Genetic Diversity*, Washington, DC: National Academy Press.

The 1980 letter expressing concern about genetic engineering from the religious organizations can be found in the President's Commission Report *Splicing Life*, Appendix B. The results of the research trial on the two girls with ADA, the first approved testing of genetic therapy in the United States, can be found in R. Michael Blaese et al., "T Lymphocyte-Directed Gene Therapy for ADA-SCID: Initial Trial Results after Four Years," *Science* 1995, *270*, 475–80. Since that time similar research has been conducted on a few more children; some projects failed, but most had varying degrees of success. For the history of RAC (the Recombinant DNA Advisory Committee), see LeRoy Walters et al., 1997, *The Ethics of Human Gene Therapy*, New York: Oxford University Press, chapter 5. Appendix D of Walters' book (pp. 171–85) contains the 1995 "Points to Consider" developed by RAC for researchers seeking support for trials on human subjects. For the need to recognize that only genetic research on human subjects, and not genetic therapy on patients, is now being done, see Larry Churchill et al., "Genetic Research as Therapy: Implications of 'Gene Therapy' for Informed Consent," *Journal of Law, Medicine & Ethics* 1998, *26*, 38–47.

For good summaries of the ethical arguments for and against germ-line therapy, see LeRoy Walters. *The Ethics of Human Gene Therapy*, pp. 76–92; the six articles on human germ-line engineering in Eric Juengst, ed., *Journal of Medicine and Philosophy* 1991, *16*, 587–694; Donald Rubenstein et al., "Germ-Line Therapy to Cure Mitochondrial Disease: Protocol and Ethics of In Vitro Ovum Nuclear Transplantation," *Cambridge Quarterly of Healthcare Ethics* 1995, *4*, 316–39; John Fletcher et al., "Germ-Line Gene Therapy: A New Stage of the Debate," *Law, Medicine & Health Care* 1992, *20*, 26–39; John Robertson, "Oocyte Cytoplasm Transfers and the Ethics of Germ-Line Intervention," *Journal of Law, Medicine & Ethics* 1998, *26*, 211–20; and David Resnick, "Debunking the Slippery Slope Argument against Germ-Line Gene Therapy," *Journal of Medicine and Philosophy* 1994, *19*, 23–40. Most of these authors favor the arguments for germ-line trials; for a more cautious approach, see Erik Parens, "Should We Hold the (Germ) Line?" *Journal of Law, Medicine & Ethics* 1995, *23*, 173–76; and Ruth Hubbard, 1993, *Exploding the Gene Myth*, Boston: Beacon Press, chapter 8. For a survey of the conservative position of European governmental and nongovernmental organizations, see Maurice deWachter, "Aspects of Human Germ-Line Gene Therapy," *Bioethics* 1993, *7*, 166–77. The Council of Europe's statement against germ-line therapy and the complete text of its *Convention on Human Rights and Biomedicine* can be found in the *Kennedy Institute of Ethics Journal* 1997, *7*, 277–90.

The Alliance for Human Research Protection, a nonprofit educational organization, also has a worthwhile anonymous article "Gene Therapy Death Highlights Weaknesses in Patient Safety Net" at ahrp.org and ahrp.blogspot.com. Friedman's article on the Gelsinger tragedy is in *Science* 2000, *287*, 2163–65. He acknowledges that "There is a debate in the medical ethics community whether this distinction to exclude desperately ill newborns was appropriate." For the view that it was not appropriate, see Julian Savulescu, "Harm, Ethics Committees and the Gene Therapy Death," *Journal of Medical Ethics* 2001, *27*, 148–50. Several important documents in the Gelsinger case and other gene transfer litigations can be found under "Bioethics Issues" at the website of the law firm that represented the Gelsinger family (sskrplaw.com). Links to many stories and documents in the Gelsinger case can also be found on the Citizens for Responsible Care and Research (CIRCARE) website (circare.org). See also Paul Gelsinger and Adil Shamoo, "Eight Years after Jesse's Death, Are Human Research Subjects Any Safer?" *Hastings Center Report* 2008, *38* (March–April), 25–27. A series of articles in the *FDA Consumer* magazine, which unfortunately ceased publication in 2007, is available at fda.gov/fdac and has several excellent articles on clinical gene trials. See also information from the FDA's Center for Biologics Evaluation and Research at fda.gov/cber/gene. Dr. James Wilson's 2008 editorial is "Adverse Events in Gene Transfer

Trials and an Agenda for the New Year," *Human Gene Therapy* 2008, *19*, 1–2. See also in the same issue Arthur Caplan, "If It's Broken, Shouldn't It Be Fixed? Informed Consent and Initial Clinical Trials of Gene Therapy," pp. 3–4; and Jeffrey Kahn, "Informed Consent in Human Gene Transfer Trials," pp. 5–6. The emphasis on informed consent in complicated genetic trials is important, but an emphasis on protecting human subjects even if they are informed and willing to give consent is also very much needed.

The proceedings and reports of the RAC (Recombinant DNA Advisory Committee) are now available at nih.gov/oba, and its meetings are available on webcasts. A good source for ongoing clinical trials is clinicaltrials.gov. For an account of Jolee Mohr's death see Christopher H. Evans, Steven C. Ghivizzani, and Paul D. Robbins, 2008, "Arthritis Gene Therapy's First Death," which appeared in *Arthritis Research & Therapy* and is available online at Arthritis-Research.com.

For background on the enhancement debate see Erik Parens, "Taking Behavioral Genetics Seriously," *Hastings Center Report* 1996, *26* (July–August), 13–18, and "Is Better Always Good: The Enhancement Project," *Hastings Center Report* 1998, *28* (January–February), S1–SI7; Eric Parens, ed., 1998, *Enhancing Human Traits: Ethical and Social Implications*, Washington, DC: Georgetown University Press; Manuel Torres, "On the Limits of Enhancement in Human Gene Transfer: Drawing the Line," *Journal of Medicine and Philosophy* 1997, *22*, 43–53; Glenn McGee, 1997, *The Perfect Baby: A Pragmatic Approach to Genetics*, Lanham: Rowman & Littlefield, and "Parenting in an Era of Genetics," *Hastings Center Report* 1997, *27* (March–April), 16–22; and LeRoy Walters, *Ethics of Human Gene Therapy*, chapter 4. One of the researchers who performed the first approved gene therapy trial on the two girls with ADA, W. French Anderson, has taken a strong stand against enhancement. See his classic article "Human Gene Therapy: Why Draw a Line?" *Journal of Medicine and Philosophy* 1989, *14*, 681–93, and "Genetics and Human Malleability," *Hastings Center Report* 1990, 20 (January–February), 21–24, reprinted in Robert Blank and Andrea Bonnicksen, eds., 1992, *Emerging Issues in Biomedical Policy*, New York: Columbia University Press, chapter 13.

For background on the Human Genome Project, see Thomas Murray et al., eds., 1996, *The Human Genome Project and the Future of Health Care*, Bloomington: Indiana University Press; Maxwell J. Mehlman and Jeffrey R. Botkin, 1998, *Access to the Genome: The Challenge to Equality*, Washington, DC: Georgetown University Press; Timothy Murphy et al., 1994, *Justice and the Human Genome Project*, Berkeley: University of California Press; and Daniel Kevles, *The Code of Codes*. Helpful articles include Eric Meslin et al., "The Ethical, Legal, and Social Implications Research Program at the National Human Genome Research Institute," *Kennedy Institute of Ethics Journal* 1997, *7*, 291–98; Thomas Murray, "Genetics and Just Health Care: A Genome Task Force Report," *Kennedy Institute of Ethics Journal* 1993, *3*, 327–31; and Eric Juengst, "The Human Genome Project and Bioethics," *Kennedy Institute of Ethics Journal* 1991, *1*, 71–74.

For some sites on the Internet relevant to genetic research, see the informative CDC site on genetics at cdc.gov/genomics; the NIH has another site on the human genome at genome.gov that has links to the National Human Genome Research Institute (NHGRI) and the Ethical, Legal and Social Implications (ELSI) program. See also Francis Collins et al., "A Vision for the Future of Genomics Research," *Nature* 2003, *422*, 835–47, available online at genome.gov/10001161#overview. For an excellent summary of the 2008 federal law prohibiting genetic discrimination (GINA), see Kathy Hudson et al., "Keeping Pace with the Times—The Genetic Information Nondiscrimination Act of 2008," *New England Journal of Medicine* 2008, *358*, 2661–63. For the impact of genetic nondiscrimination laws in Europe see Ine Van Hoyweghen and Klasien Horstman, "European Practices of Genetic Information and Insurance," *JAMA* 2008, 300, 326–27. Among the worthwhile books on biotechnology is C. Ben Mitchell et al., 2007, *Biotechnology and the Human Good*, Washington, DC: Georgetown University Press, which looks at biotechnology from religious perspectives.

UNESCO's International Bioethics Committee (the IBC) has produced a number of reports relevant to genetic issues, among them, *Genetic Screening and Testing* (1994) and *Pre-Implantation Genetic Diagnosis and Germ-Line Intervention* (2003). UNESCO itself adopted a *Universal Declaration on the Human Genome and Human Rights* in 1997 and the *International Declaration on Human Genetic Data* in 2003. Article 10 of the 1997 Declaration sets respect for (1) human rights, (2) fundamental freedoms, and (3) human dignity above the pursuit of genetic research and its applications. Article 1 of the 2003 Declaration repeats the same values: it states that the aim of the declaration is to "to ensure the respect for human dignity and protection of human rights and fundamental freedoms." The declarations are available at unesco.org/shs/ethics. The World Health Organization (WHO) has also issued a number of documents on genetics. In 2003 it published a draft document titled *Review of Ethical Issues in Medical Genetics* to guide those developing policies and practices in their own nations. In 2005 it published a report on the ethical, legal, social, and health issues raised by patenting of DNA sequences (*Genetics, Genomics, and the Patenting of DNA*), and in 2006 it published *Medical Genetic Services in Developing Countries: The Ethical, Legal and Social Implications of Genetic Testing and Screening*. These documents are available online at who.int/genomics.

SEVENTEEN

Social and Political Issues

PRACTICAL DECISION MAKING in virtue ethics embraces political decisions as well as the personal decisions that we make for ourselves. We are, as Aristotle put it, "social animals," and hence ethical decision making is about what is good for us socially—what some ethicists call the common good and what Aristotle called "politics," as well as about what is good for us individually.

There are many ethical issues embedded in the social and political dimensions of health care in the United States today. In this chapter we consider but four of them: paying for health care, resolving "futility" disputes by legislation, allowing people who are dying to obtain unapproved investigational drugs, and the use of seeding trials and ghostwriters to market new drugs.

PAYING FOR HEALTH CARE

Until the first part of the twentieth century, most Americans paid for health care with their own money. When they were sick, they called a doctor. He charged a fee for his services, and they paid his bill. Often he varied the fee according to the family's ability to pay, sometimes taking care of poor people for little or nothing. If people required hospitalization, the payment system was the same. The hospital billed for its services, and the patient or his family paid it. The general name for this payment system is *fee-for-service* (FFS): the physicians and hospitals set fees for the services they provided and billed the patients.

Health Insurance

This FFS system worked well until the Great Depression of the 1930s left many people unable to pay their medical bills. This economic maelstrom triggered a new development—health insurance. Insurance plans permitted people to pay a small premium at regular intervals for coverage of whatever care they might need from hospitals and doctors. People no longer had to worry about high bills for unexpected problems and expensive treatment. The first major insurance programs were the nonprofit Blue Cross and Blue Shield plans of the 1930s. Blue Cross paid hospital bills, and Blue Shield paid physicians' bills. Soon commercial (for profit) insurance companies entered the heath insurance market.

Insurance plans had one unintended consequence. Once patients began paying insurance premiums instead of their actual medical bills, they no longer focused on how much their medical care cost. Their concern now became the cost of the insurance premiums rather than the cost of services provided by doctors and hospitals.

Before long many people did not even have to worry about the cost of insurance because their employers began paying the premiums. During the early 1940s many large corporations, hampered by wartime controls on wages, tried to attract workers by offering free health insurance as a fringe benefit. When employers began paying for health insurance, working people and their families paid even less attention to the cost of health care. Neither the bills for treatment nor the premiums for insurance were of concern to them.

Some people, of course, were neither working nor were they spouses or children of workers. This meant that no one was paying for their health insurance. Many of these people were elderly, and some were unemployed and impoverished. This left them at risk. Without money or health insurance, they could not afford needed care, which was becoming more and more expensive. By 1960 their needs became obvious, and the government responded.

Medicare and Medicaid

In 1966 two large government programs—Medicare and Medicaid—began covering many people not covered by employer-based health insurance. Medicare is a federal program providing insurance for people over sixty-five and for people any age suffering from disability or end-stage renal disease. Medicare began with two major parts. Part A, financed in large measure by payroll taxes levied on employers as well as employees, helps cover expenses for inpatient hospital and skilled-nursing facility care, whereas Part B, financed largely from general tax revenues as well as from premiums paid by patients, helps cover outpatient hospital care and doctors' services. In January 2006 Part D, which covers some expenses for drugs, was added to Medicare coverage.

Enrollment in Part A is mandatory—employers and employees must contribute to the Trust Fund, and those enrolled are automatically covered for the Part A services. Parts B and D are voluntary, but most eligible people opt to pay monthly premiums and join the programs. In 2007 Medicare Parts A and B covered 44 million people (36.6 million over age sixty-five and 7.3 million disabled).

The second government program is Medicaid, a joint federal-state program providing medical care chiefly for people who are poor. Medicaid covers a broad range of services, notably those provided by hospitals, physicians, nurse practitioners, and nursing homes. It also covers prescription drugs and pays the Medicare premiums and copayments for low-income elderly and disabled people. In 2007 Medicaid covered over 42 million people. The federal government sets guidelines for coverage, but the individual states have wide latitude in determining how low a person's assets and income must be to qualify for assistance. Almost three-quarters of the people covered by Medicaid are adults and children of low income, but they consume little more than one-quarter of its funds. Almost two-thirds of Medicaid expenditures go to elderly, blind, or disabled people.

Thanks to Medicare, Medicaid, and the various other insurance programs, by the last third of the twentieth century most people in the United States were not paying for hospitals and doctors with their own money. They were covered by nonprofit insurance plans such as Blue Cross or Blue Shield, commercial (for profit) insurance plans, or the government plans. All these plans became known as third-party payers. The phrase *third-party payer* means someone other than the patient (first party) or the providers (the second party—doctors, hospitals, pharmacies, etc.) is paying for medical care.

The shift from patient payment to third-party payment did not immediately disturb the basic FFS system. Providers of medical services—hospitals, physicians, pharmacies, and others—continued charging fees for their goods and services. The only major difference was that a party other than the patient or family paid the fees that were billed.

FFS Flaws

Two major structural flaws eventually undermined this combined FFS/third-party payment system. First, the third-party payers had no control over the extent or the cost of the services rendered. Patients decided when to seek treatment, physicians controlled what they would provide and, along with hospitals and pharmacies, what fees they would charge for their services. The third-party payers had no say in the services provided or the fees charged; they simply paid the bills.

The second structural flaw was the incredible built-in incentive for providers to raise their fees rapidly. In the FFS/third-party payer system, the government or the insurance company pays whatever fees are considered customary for the service or medicine. What determines a "customary" fee? Obviously a customary fee is a fee roughly the same as what other physicians, hospitals, and drug companies in the same geographical area are charging. Hence, the faster everyone raises their fees, the faster what is considered "customary" also rises. As long as patients and their families were paying the fees, physicians and hospitals tended to be sensitive to what they charged these people. But when the billing shifted to anonymous government and institutional payers—the third-party payers—it did not take long for everyone reimbursed by these third-party payers to begin to raise their fees rapidly, thereby raising the level of what was considered customary.

Rising Cost Pressures

As if the built-in incentive to raise fees in the FFS system were not enough, other factors conspired to push up health care costs. A peculiar provision of Medicare exerted enormous pressure on cost increases. Medicare not only paid patients' hospital bills but provided money directly to hospitals for the depreciation of their facilities. The more expensive their facilities, the more money the hospitals received for the depreciation. This encouraged hospitals to upgrade and expand their facilities. The more they built state-of-the-art facilities, the more they could receive in depreciation. And the expensive facilities in turn led to more expensive inpatient diagnosis and treatment; there was no incentive to pursue less expensive outpatient diagnosis and treatment.

An additional factor pushing up health care costs was the rising costs of medical education. Medicare, along with Medicaid and the Departments of Defense and Veterans Affairs, underwrites the training of new doctors by paying a share of the faculty and resident salaries and institutional costs. Medicare also allows teaching hospitals to collect higher fees from third-party payers to help cover the added costs of the medical education they provide residents.

Another cost pressure came from the development of new techniques and technologies to cure and control medical problems. The new techniques and technologies push costs up primarily in two ways. First, some new techniques (bypass surgery and organ transplantation, for example) and new technologies (MRIs and PET scans, for example) are expensive.

Second, many new techniques and technologies are not curative but life sustaining. They keep patients alive for months, years, or even decades, often at considerable expense. At one time all people with severe kidney disease soon died; now dialysis keeps many alive in slowly deteriorating health for years. At one time all people with severe lung problems soon died; now ventilators keep many alive for months or years. At one time all people in prolonged comas soon died; now feeding tubes keep some alive for decades in a vegetative state. At one time extremely premature babies or babies failing to thrive soon died; now modern neonatal intensive care units keep some of these infants alive, and they can live for years despite severe damage that requires expensive medical care. Obviously, treatments unable to cure but able to prolong severely damaged lives add a new pressure on the increasing costs of medical care, especially since some of those saved require considerable supportive care.

Another cost pressure came from the development of new and expensive drugs. To stay in business drug companies need to recoup the considerable research and development dollars they put into developing new drugs and getting them approved by the Food and Drug Administration (FDA). They also exist to make money for their stockholders. Their desire to recoup research costs and increase profits is a major reason why some drug prices have become so high.

The net result of the factors making health care more expensive in an era when few incentives existed to hold costs down was, as you would expect, an alarming rise in health care costs. In 1970 the money spent on health care in the United States was 7.6 percent of the gross national product (GNP); by 2008 it was over 16 percent of the GNP, the highest health care/GNP ratio in the world and about double that of other developed countries.

As health care costs rose dramatically in the 1970s, neither patients nor providers (especially hospitals, physicians, and drug companies) were very concerned. After all, most patients were not paying their medical bills, and many were not even paying their insurance premiums. And most providers—the drug companies, hospitals, and doctors—were watching their gross income increase faster than the inflation rates. Not a bad system! Under it, most patients get almost anything they want and pay little or nothing, and most providers see their income increase significantly each year.

Reactions to Rising Costs

Some people, however, were not happy—the people paying the bills. With the rapid escalation in medical costs, the third-party payers were getting hit hard. Legislators became upset as the cost of

Medicare and Medicaid programs consumed more and more tax dollars. Employers providing health insurance for their employees became upset because the insurance companies, both non-profit and commercial, were raising their premiums to cover the skyrocketing costs of treatment. What had begun as a modest fringe benefit during the 1940s was now a significant part of the compensation package they were providing for their employees.

Those looking to control costs realized they had to change the FFS payment system. In the FFS system doctors are paid for treating sickness, and the more they treat, the more they collect in fees. Some suggested an alternative system whereby the payer would cover the cost and also provide the *care*, and thereby have some control over the costs of care. In the alternative system physicians would no longer have a financial incentive to treat, and insurers would have some control over the treatments physicians provided. This alternative system produced what became known as the health maintenance organization, or HMO.

An HMO is an insurance plan, but it works differently from the traditional indemnity insurance plans. Instead of simply paying the fees of doctors, hospitals, and pharmacies after they provide treatment and services, the HMO not only pays for medical care but actually controls how that care is provided. HMOs combine what had been two separate entities under the FFS system into one delivery system—they provide both health insurance and medical treatments. This gives them some control over the delivery and costs of services, something insurers never had under the FFS system. HMOs received a big boost in 1971 when President Nixon and several governors of large states (Governor Reagan of California and Governor Rockefeller of New York) endorsed and encouraged them.

HMOs provide health care in many different ways. Some early HMOs put physicians on salary, set up the medical offices, and provided all the support services including labs, pharmacies, and even hospitals. Today HMOs come in a bewildering array of variations. Some HMOs agree to pay independent physicians a fee instead of a salary to care for their patients. This may sound like the old FFS system, but it is not, because the HMO determines the fee ahead of time by negotiating a reduced fee in return for sending their patients to the physician. Some HMOs hire doctors on salary but only part-time, enabling them to continuing treating patients not enrolled in the HMO. Still others offer groups of doctors a fixed fee that covers all the care for a number of patients in a specified period of time. The latter arrangement is sometimes called *capitation*.

The HMO system also changed the way hospitals were paid. Some HMOs owned their own hospitals. Here the incentive to keep costs down is obvious. Other HMOs used existing hospitals but were able to bargain in advance for lower rates by agreeing to send all or a certain number of their patients to a particular hospital in return for a discount. Many hospitals had to accept the lower rates lest the HMO send their patients elsewhere. They now realized filling their empty beds at a discounted rate was better than nothing.

The ability of HMOs to curb medical costs looked so promising that 1973 federal legislation obliged employers with more than twenty-five people on the payroll to offer an HMO insurance plan along with the traditional FFS insurance plans. Employers who paid their employees' health insurance were happy to do so because the HMO premiums were usually less expensive than those of the traditional FFS indemnity plans. The new HMOs did slow the rising costs, but it was not enough. Medical costs continued to rise much faster than inflation, and the government and employers continued to be concerned.

In 1983 the federal government made another move to cut costs. It introduced a *prospective* payment system for hospital in-patient services covered by Medicare. After more than fifteen years of paying whatever customary fees were billed by hospitals *after* they provided their services, Medicare began telling hospitals what it would pay the hospitals *before* they provide those services. Medicare arranged the services it covered in what it called diagnosis-related groups (DRGs) and began paying a predetermined amount for each service as defined by its DRG designation.

The DRG reimbursement formulas are very complicated and vary geographically, but the general idea of the DRG system is simple. If the hospital can provide care below the predetermined DRG payment rate, it keeps the difference; if the hospital does not complete care at or below the DRG rate, it has to make up the difference itself. Whereas the FFS system encouraged hospitals to keep patients an extra day or so, the DRG system pushes them in the opposite direction—

hospitals improve their income by discharging patients early. The DRG system was so successful that Medicare set up a prospective payment system for physicians' fees in 1992.

The HMOs of the 1970s and the DRGs of the 1980s started the trend whereby third-party payers gained some control over the delivery and the costs of services. In the 1990s they increased this control in a trend known as *managed care*, a complicated phenomenon that tried in many different ways to allow insurance companies to manage care as well as pay for it. The many different managed care plans do this primarily by shifting some of the financial risks of coverage to physicians and hospitals—as treatment costs go up, their income goes down. Today some form of managed care exists in most every insurance system in place in the United States. Allowing third-party payers to manage medical care by deciding what they will pay for has brought both benefits and harms into the insurance system.

Perhaps the greatest social harm in the United States is that more than 45 million people have no health insurance and hence cannot get much in the way of health care. Millions more are underinsured. If employers pay for health insurance, then people who lose their job also soon lose their health insurance. As health insurance costs rise, and they have been rising much more rapidly than the cost of living, more and more companies reduce their costs by not providing health care insurance programs or by providing plans with high copayments.

The moral debate about health care centers on whether or not government should provide a system where everyone has access to basic health care, much as governments now provide access to police protection, fire protection, emergency medical services, and basic education for everyone. All other first-world democracies have some kind of healthcare system covering all their citizens. Although some Americans are covered by government programs such as Medicare, Medicaid, the military health care system, and the Veterans Administration, many Americans still rely on their employers to provide most of their health insurance, and this leaves millions not adequately covered.

What can be done? What politically prudent change would provide good basic health care for all? Given the idiosyncratic way employer-based health insurance developed in the United States; the vested interests that benefit from the current complicated systems and resist radical change; the impact of pharmaceutical companies and their tremendous marketing efforts directed at both consumers and prescribers; and the costs of technologically advanced equipment, new drugs, and expensive new treatments, it is simply not clear what politically feasible modifications of the health care system will better achieve the common human good in the United States. We can do little more here than remind ourselves of the problem and recognize that it is a moral problem because it impacts so significantly on what makes a society good for people.

A hallmark of social morality in virtue ethics is that a country provides for human flourishing by supporting healthy living and taking good care of its sick and dying people. Providing for the basic health of its citizens is no less a good than providing for their basic education. A health insurance system that provides universal coverage is viewed in virtue ethics primarily as a social good, and this social good is not well realized as long as health care is viewed as an economic system of services and goods governed by market forces.

Those promoting continuation of the present fragmented and market-influenced system in the United States need to explain how leaving a large cohort of their fellow citizens without the means to obtain basic health care contributes to the common good of society. The Constitution of the World Health Organization identified the locus of responsibility: "Governments have a responsibility for the health of their peoples which can be fulfilled only by the provision of adequate health and social measures." Government in the United States has done much for public health, but its failure to provide adequate basic health measures for so many of its people is a troublesome social disvalue. The current idiosyncratic health care payment system in the United States is so entrenched that it will require extraordinary political and pragmatic prudence to improve it and make it driven more by concern for the common good than by the forces of the market. The point of this section is to remind us that universal access to basic health care is a moral issue and hence a matter of concern in health care ethics.

LEGISLATION AND THE "FUTILITY" DEBATE

The intractable disagreements that occur when family members demand treatments that hospitals and physicians believe are inappropriate, and perhaps even immoral, have led some to propose a legislative solution: laws that allow hospitals and physicians to withdraw life-sustaining treatments over the objections of family or proxy decision makers without fear of civil or criminal liability.

The ethical questions involved are these: Would such laws be good? Would they create a better society enabling people to flourish as human beings? Certainly they will prevent cases where a family member insists on medically inappropriate life-prolonging treatment for years, cases such as Helga Wanglie, Baby K, and Barbara Howe, for example. Yet there are moral concerns about laws allowing hospitals to withdraw life-sustaining treatments over strong family objections. To see why this is so we will look at two widely publicized cases in Texas, a state that has one of the most controversial "futility" laws in the United States.

Governor George W. Bush signed the Texas Advance Directives Act (ADA) into law in 1999. It was amended in 2003 to cover minors as well as adults. The ADA gives physicians and hospitals the authority to withdraw treatments over the objections of patients or their proxies without fear of criminal or civil liability. The key provisions of the Texas law are as follows:

- The hospital must give the patient or proxy written information about its intent to withdraw treatment and to seek approval for the withdrawal from the hospital ethics committee.
- The hospital must invite the patient or proxy to the ethics committee meeting and give that individual forty-eight hours advance notice of the meeting.
- After the ethics meeting the committee must provide the patient or proxy with a written report detailing its findings, which becomes part of the medical record.
- If the ethics committee meeting fails to resolve the dispute, and if it agrees with the physician that treatment should not be continued, the hospital must notify the patient or proxy that he or she has ten days to find another hospital willing to provide the requested treatments, and the hospital itself must make reasonable efforts to locate such a facility.
- If no alternative provider can be found in ten days after the patient or proxy has received the "ten-day letter" physicians may unilaterally withdraw or withhold the life-support.
- If the patient or proxy requests it, a judge may extend the ten-day time period if there is likelihood of finding a willing provider. However, a judge may not overrule the hospital.
- Hospitals and physicians withdrawing life support in accord with the law have immunity from all civil and criminal liability.

Is the Texas ADA good public policy? Is it a wise law that sets up an environment in the community that fosters human flourishing? In some ways it does, and in some ways it does not. Certainly its main purpose is admirable: it prevents patients or proxies forcing physicians to provide clearly unreasonable life-sustaining treatments, and it protects patients without decision-making capacity from harmful unreasonable treatments demanded by their proxies, usually family members. On the other hand, especially when children are involved, the law raises some serious issues, as the following cases show.

The Case of Sun Hudson

The Story

Sun was born on September 25, 2004, in Houston suffering from a genetic disease known as thanatrophic dysplasia. The disease leaves babies with lungs and a chest so small that they cannot adequately breathe. Afflicted babies seldom live long, although ventilation can temporarily prolong their lives. Sun went into respiratory arrest at birth and physicians, who had no idea what the problem was (his mother had not sought any prenatal care), resuscitated him and started mechanical ventilation.

He was transferred to Texas Children's Hospital, and it soon became obvious that he was slowly suffocating despite the ventilation. Doctors came to believe that the aggressive life-sustaining treatment was inappropriately prolonging a life that could not be saved. They discussed removing the ventilator with Wanda, Sun's mother, but she refused to give consent. Her reasons for refusing were somewhat unusual: She told the physicians that the sun that shines in the sky, not a man, had fathered Sun and that he will live as long as the sun is in the sky. This, and the fact that she had spent several days in a psychiatric facility shortly after Sun's birth, raised some issues about her decision-making capacity. Still, she was Sun's mother and sole spokesperson.

After Wanda refused the physicians' request to withdraw the ventilator, the hospital engaged the dispute resolution process according to the Texas ADA law. The ethics committee approved the withdrawal, and none of the forty hospitals contacted were willing to accept Sun and continue the treatment. Since no hospital would accept Sun as a patient and his mother made no move to ask a judge to extend the ten-day time period, the hospital, after meeting other legal requirements, could withdraw the ventilator without fear of criminal or legal liability. However, aware that withdrawing treatment from a baby whose mother wanted it continued and whose explanations of the pregnancy raised questions about her decision-making capacity, the hospital elected to seek court approval for the ventilator withdrawal, something it did not have to do. The probate judge appointed a guardian for Sun but ruled that the ventilator withdrawal was legal under Texas law. The guardian appealed his ruling to the Texas Court of Appeals in Houston.

Before looking at what happened next, we consider the case from an ethical perspective so we can determine whether the Texas ADA is an example of prudent legislation.

Ethical Analysis

Situational awareness.   We are aware of the following facts in the story of Sun Hudson:

1. Sun suffered from an uncorrectable genetic disorder whereby his body would never develop the capacity to breathe adequately on his own, and he would not live long even with mechanical ventilation. It is not clear whether Sun was conscious. Published reports indicated that the ethics committee was concerned that he was suffering, whereas the hospital said he was not conscious.

2. Sun's mother wanted the ventilation continued but showed some signs that she was not well grounded in reality.

3. Physicians felt that ventilation would be futile and hence the wrong treatment for a baby with this tragic condition.

4. The hospital wanted to withdraw the ventilator and engaged the dispute resolution process in accord with Texas law. Although it was not required to seek court approval for its action, the hospital elected to do so. The hospital argued in court that the ventilation was futile and only prolonged Sun's suffering.

We are also aware of some bad features in the story:

1. Removing the ventilator will play a causal role in Sun's death, and the death of a person is always regrettable.

2. Removing life support from a child against the mother's wishes is a drastic step and will be terribly upsetting for the mother.

3. Continuing ventilation that is causing suffering but doing little more than postponing death for a dying child is not a medically or morally reasonable course unless there are extenuating circumstances.

Prudential Reasoning in the Sun Hudson Story

Proxy's perspective.   Although her reasoning is not well grounded, Sun's mother has taken a position that other mothers might well take. It is not easy for a woman to authorize withdrawal of life support from her infant, and some can never bring themselves to do it no matter how unreasonable the continuation might be. Giving birth and then deciding to stop keeping the child alive goes against the deepest of maternal instincts. It is a horrible predicament for a woman even when she might know intellectually that it is the more reasonable course of action.

Physicians' perspective. If we just focus on the patient, the physicians' perspective is reasonable. At some point it is not reasonable to use advanced life support on babies who are clearly dying, especially if they are suffering. If we focus on the broader picture, however, the physician's perspective is not so obviously reasonable because stopping life-sustaining treatment on a child against the wishes of the mother makes the situation much more complex. In fact some published reports indicate that this was the first time any court approved withdrawal of life support from a child against the parent's wishes

Of course, if the ventilation itself is causing the child significant suffering for no real benefit beyond preventing natural death, then physicians have good reasons for overturning parental wishes. And in this case some did say that Sun was slowly suffocating, not a pleasant experience, and that the ventilation was prolonging Sun's suffering for no good reason. However, this raises an important question: Why was Sun suffering? Physicians have access to sedatives and pain medications to keep patients on ventilators from suffering. Once we recognize that physicians can address Sun's discomfort without withdrawing the ventilator, their decision to remove it against his mother's wishes is no longer so clearly reasonable. At the very least we need to know more before we can conclude that withdrawing the ventilator against the mother's wishes is the better thing to do here.

Judge's perspective. The judge's perspective is rather limited here. Unlike other cases, the Howe case in Massachusetts for example, the judge in Texas, thanks to legislation already in place (the Advance Directives Act), was not being asked to authorize the withdrawal of the ventilator or to remove Sun's mother as the proxy decision maker. His role was simply to rule on whether the ADA applied in this case.

The Decision of the Appeals Court

The Texas Court of Appeals did not address the withdrawal-of-treatment issue because the Texas law clearly allowed it, but it did send the case back to the probate court on a technical issue. The probate court quickly cleared up the technical issue and ruled again that the hospital could withdraw the ventilator under Texas law. This time there was no appeal. On March 15, 2005, the hospital withdrew the ventilator despite Wanda's objections. Sun died almost immediately in his mother's arms.

The Case of Emilio Gonzales

The Story

Twenty-three-year-old Caterina Gonzales gave birth to Emilio on December 3, 2005. According to some reports he was blind and deaf from birth. Physicians soon diagnosed his problem: Leigh disease, a progressive degeneration of the nervous system that, depending on the severity, would cause death within a few years. A year later, on December 28, 2006, Caterina brought Emilio to Brackenridge Children's Hospital of Austin because he was in some distress. Physicians placed him on a ventilator and a feeding tube and explained the poor prognosis to Caterina.

As expected, Emilio got progressively worse. He also experienced discomfort from the necessary thumping on his chest and the suctioning to remove mucus. Physicians believed a tracheotomy was not appropriate, and thus the tube from the ventilator remained through his mouth, an unpleasant experience for anyone. Within a few months, knowing that the life support was simply postponing the inevitable and causing their patient discomfort for so little benefit, physicians talked to Caterina about removing the ventilator.

She adamantly refused to allow ventilator withdrawal, and when it became clear that she was not going to change her mind, the hospital set in motion the procedures of the Texas ADA. On March 12, 2007, Caterina was notified that she had ten days to find another facility that would provide the advanced life support. The hospital also searched for a facility to receive Emilio. Caterina asked the Probate Court to extend the time to find another facility, and it did. Before we look at what happened next, we should consider the ethical reasoning in the case as we consider whether the Texas ADA is an example of prudent legislation.

Ethical Analysis

Situational awareness.   We are aware of the following facts in the story of Emilio Gonzales:

1. Emilio suffered from fatal Leigh disease, was ventilator-dependent for months, and would probably not live long even with mechanical ventilation.

2. Caterina, Emilio's mother, was devoted to his care and wanted the ventilation continued.

3. Physicians felt that continued ventilation would be "futile" and hence would be the wrong treatment for Emilio.

4. The hospital engaged the dispute resolution process in accord with Texas law. The ethics committee approved the withdrawal, and the hospital issued the "ten-day letter" to Caterina explaining that Emilio's ventilator would be withdrawn unless another facility to care for him could be found.

5. Thirty-one facilities had been contacted, but none of them would accept Emilio as a patient. Most of these facilities were at some distance from Austin, which would have caused Caterina, a person of limited means, a severe hardship if he were transferred and she tried to be near her dying son.

We are also aware of some bad features in the story:

1. Removing the ventilator would play a causal role in Emilio's death, and the death of anyone is always something most people consider bad.

2. Removing the ventilator against Caterina's wishes would be a move that would cause a terrible experience for her, a caring mother.

3. Continuing ventilation that providers believed was medically inappropriate and immoral was stressful for the providers.

4. Emilio's discomfort was bad. The ventilation tube ran down his throat, which caused him discomfort as did the procedures to loosen and suction the mucous in his throat. Physicians felt that a tracheotomy was not appropriate in this case.

Prudential Reasoning in the Emilio Gonzales Story

Proxy's perspective.   Caterina's life was difficult. She had given up her job at Wal-Mart to care for her son. She had no health insurance for him; Medicaid was paying for his hospitalization and treatment. Emilio was all she had. She knew he was dying but wanted to provide care for him as long as she could. Removing the treatments that kept him alive went against her deepest feelings.

Physicians' perspective.   In the minds of physicians it makes no sense to sustain with advanced life support the dying life of patients known to be suffering terminal diseases. And in one sense they are right—at some point mechanical ventilation on patients, including infants, who are clearly dying is not a reasonable medical intervention. But sometimes employing an unreasonable medical intervention can be morally reasonable when we consider other values in the wider situation. Once we enlarge the situation and bring Caterina's wishes into consideration, the moral decision making changes. Now it is no longer simply whether it is reasonable to withdraw ventilation from Emilio but whether it is reasonable to withdraw ventilation from Emilio when his mother vigorously opposes the withdrawal.

Once we frame the decision-making scenario in the broader context of family, it is not so easy to conclude that withdrawing the life support from Emilio is the reasonable thing to do. Physicians need to ask other questions before invoking a law that allows them to withdraw life-sustaining treatment from a child against a parent's wishes. Is the parent showing love and concern for her son? Can the hospital provide palliative care so Emilio will not suffer from the interventions that his physicians consider unreasonable or futile? How much longer do they expect Emilio to survive even with life support—is it weeks, months, or many years? Is the expense of providing what we believe is inappropriate medical care causing a major negative impact on the financial resources of our institution and the care we provide for others?

Judge's perspective. As was pointed out in the case of Sun Hudson, there is not much a probate judge can do under the Texas law. He can grant extensions to give people more than ten days to find another facility if he believes it might allow a facility to be located. He can review the process at the hospital to be sure it conforms to the legal requirements. And he can appoint a guardian to represent Emilio and make recommendations. But, as was already mentioned, the law ties his hands: He cannot overrule the hospital if it followed the provisions of the ADA.

The Court Action

Judge Herman extended the March 12, 2007, deadline for finding another facility several times, and he also appointed a guardian *ad litem* to review issues in the case. Finally, he scheduled a hearing for May 8, 2007, to resolve the issue, but as the date approached the hearing was moved back to May 30. Emilio continued to decline, and on Saturday, May 19, 2007, after being kept alive for five months by mechanical ventilation, he died while still on the ventilator. Hence we do not know whether this would have been another example of treatment withdrawal from a child contrary to the mother's wishes. By delaying the legal resolution, the judge rendered the case moot.

Ethical Reflections on the Texas ADA

An important aspect of virtue ethics is the insistence that people live in communities and that their ability to flourish depends greatly on the supportive legislation in those communities. This is why Aristotle insisted that ethics is really a subdivision of politics and that the key virtue of decision making—prudence—is needed by individuals in their personal lives but above all by legislators as they draft laws for the community.

A law such as the Texas ADA provides a process for resolving disputes about care at the end of life when families or patients are demanding what caregivers believe is inappropriate treatment. No caregiver is morally comfortable when inappropriate treatment demanded by families is causing her patient needless suffering. Without something in place like the ADA the dispute over possibly futile care can drag on for years and require the hospital to go to court for authorization to stop unreasonable treatment or to remove the guardian demanding it, something courts are reluctant to do as we saw in the Helga Wanglie, Baby K, and Barbara Howe cases.

A law allowing withdrawal of life support over family objections is a big step, and for it to be morally reasonable one needs cogent reasons. What might they be? One reason would be that the treatment is causing significant suffering for the patient, and it therefore would be morally intolerable for physicians to allow painful treatments to continue when the intervention is doing little more than postponing death. That reason loses force, however, if the suffering can be controlled without resorting to the drastic step of withdrawing life support against family wishes. And normally this can be done for patients on ventilators by the administration of sedatives and analgesics. When parents demand ventilation that is causing discomfort for a dying child, providers can respond by providing whatever palliation is necessary to keep their patient comfortable. The argument that ventilator withdrawal is necessary to relieve suffering loses much of its force once we realize that patients on ventilators can be spared suffering.

A second reason for withdrawing ventilation over family objections is that continuing treatment is so medically inappropriate that it violates the providers' consciences. In other words providers argue that the treatment has become so medically inappropriate it would be immoral for them to continue providing it. If the treatment causes needless suffering, this would be a strong argument, but once the suffering is controlled it is not so much an argument but a difference of opinion. Physicians believe they should stop life-sustaining treatment, but the family believes it should continue. It is often demoralizing for caregivers to care for dying patients on aggressive life support when palliative care is clearly the reasonable goal, but if the patient can be spared suffering and if that is what the patient or family wishes, it is hard to see why they should normally be *morally* uncomfortable with caring for patients in this situation.

A third argument for removing ventilation over family objections is financial. The unreasonable treatment often causes financial losses for the institutions and third-party payers, and this is certainly something to consider, although this reason is often not mentioned lest hospitals and providers be accused of stopping treatment to save money. However, the financial losses are usually an insignificant and rare item in the overall budget of hospitals or insurance plans; hence, the argument is not often convincing. The financial burden to an institution or third-party payer would have to be considerable before it would become a persuasive reason to withdraw life support over family objections.

When families insist on life-sustaining treatments long after these are reasonable, the providers are unfortunately left with an irresolvable predicament: Do we provide unreasonable treatment demanded by the family? In some cases the morally prudent response might be yes provided the patient is not suffering from the unreasonable treatment. Families matter, and their wishes come into play in treatment decisions. The main concern of providers may well be not the withdrawal of unreasonable life-sustaining treatments against family wishes but the prevention of suffering if the family insists on unreasonable life-prolonging treatment.

The cases of Sun and Emilio suggest that a Texas-type legislative solution is not a promising way to foster public trust and shared decision making. It is at least arguable that the law goes too far. The ten-day deadline for transfer unless the patient or proxy can get a judge to extend it, for example, is threatening for people. Moreover, the law gives ultimate power to the hospital ethics committee (and not the courts) without stipulating who should be on such a committee, what constitutes a quorum, how conflicts of interest should be managed, what qualifications the members should have, what constitutes a deciding vote, what constitutes due process in the committee, who may represent the patient or proxy, and so forth. And the Texas ADA does not allow any appeal from the ethics committee decision, not even to the courts. The ability of a person to appeal to the courts if they feel they or their family are not being treated appropriately is an important feature of life in the United States. The Texas legislation rules out seeking judicial relief; it allows the hospital and its ethics committee the final word, not the judicial system. The opportunity to seek relief in court is lost, and this is a major loss despite the reality that the court process is cumbersome and often will not resolve many of these cases.

Perhaps state laws in this area could focus on transferring the patient and, if that is not possible, on preventing the patient from suffering from the inappropriate medical treatments. The law's focus might be better placed on assuring that patients do not suffer as the result of unreasonable family demands rather than on authorizing a procedure whereby treatments can be unilaterally stopped.

EXPERIMENTAL DRUGS FOR DYING PATIENTS

The FDA is responsible for protecting the health of people by assuring that drugs, medical devices, biological products (e.g., blood products, viral vectors in genetic research), and radiation-emitting products (e.g., x-rays, MRIs, CT scans, mammograms) are both safe and efficacious. (The FDA is also responsible for the safety of food, including pet food; veterinary drugs; and cosmetics.)

Normally people can gain access to drugs in two situations: researchers have accepted them as participants in clinical trials, or the FDA has approved the drugs for therapeutic use and their physicians prescribe them. The approval process is rigorous. It usually begins in the laboratories, progresses to animal testing, and culminates finally with clinical research on human beings (often called human subjects or participants) who give voluntary informed consent to become participants in clinical trials that are subject to federal regulations. As we saw in chapter 14, trials enrolling human participants are both approved and monitored by local institutional review boards (IRBs).

Clinical drug trials usually go through three phases. In phase 1 testing researchers give increasingly large doses of the drug to a small number of people (usually fewer than one hundred) to see what dose is safe and what side effects it might cause. Often the people in phase 1 trials do not have the disease in question, although sometimes they do. Researchers frequently perform phase 1 testing with drugs for AIDS and cancer on people with those diseases.

If the drug looks promising after phase 1, researchers move to phase 2 where they enroll more people, all with the disease in question, who receive various doses of the drug. Phase 2 enables the researchers to test more extensively for safety and also provides preliminary data on whether the drug is effective. Often researchers investigate the drug's effectiveness by comparing how well the people receiving it do in comparison with a group not receiving it. Phase 2 trials last typically less than six months and involve a few hundred participants.

If the drug looks promising after phase 2, researchers move to phase 3 where they give many more people, perhaps thousands, even tens of thousands, the drug. In phase 3 the drug under investigation is often compared with approved drugs to see if it is more effective than standard care as well as with a placebo to see how much more effective it is than nothing.

At the end of the trials, which normally take several years, researchers hope to have shown what maximum dosage is both safe and effective for the targeted disease. If they can show this it will enable them to receive FDA approval and begin selling the drug. If the drug is available only by prescription, the FDA approval is only for the targeted disease, although physicians are allowed to prescribe it for other "off label" uses at their discretion. Thus, an oncologist can prescribe "off label" a drug approved for colon cancer to a patient suffering from pancreatic cancer. Of course, the researchers have not tested the drug for pancreatic cancer so there is no scientific evidence that it will work for this cancer, and it will almost certainly cause unwelcome side effects for the patient.

Sometimes researchers conduct studies on humans after the FDA has approved a drug. This is known as phase 4. Pharmaceutical companies sponsor phase 4 studies because they are seeking to expand their sales by having their drug approved for new uses, although sometimes FDA asks for phase 4 studies to gather more data about the already approved drug.

The issue with people trying to obtain unapproved drugs arises because it usually takes several years for new drugs to gain FDA approval, and some terminally ill people cannot wait that long for a drug that might help them. They are willing to try anything that looks promising if standard treatments for their disease are not effective, and they are critical of both the FDA and drug companies for not giving them a chance of extending their lives with the unapproved drugs that have shown some signs of effectiveness in phase 1 or 2 trials.

Actually, the FDA had been informally allowing release of unapproved experimental drugs for groups of patients and, sometimes, even for individual patients who requested them for decades. This informal access had various names, e.g., "compassionate use," "single-patient protocol exception," and "large open protocols."

In 1987 the FDA made access to unapproved drugs more formal by setting forth some clear criteria for the release of unapproved drugs to *groups* of people. For release to *groups* of people these criteria were life-threatening disease, no satisfactory alternative available, and some scientific evidence providing a reasonable basis for believing that the drug might be effective without causing significant risk of illness or injury. The 1987 regulations also allowed unapproved drugs for *individuals* in an emergency situation but did not set forth criteria for this use. This omission became the source of later problems and criticism because, in effect, the FDA was saying it would authorize use of unapproved drugs in individual cases but did not describe the submission requirements and criteria for obtaining them. The result was confusion and a lack of consistency in cases when the FDA responded to requests for unapproved drugs sought for individuals.

In 1997 Congress amended the Food, Drug, and Cosmetic Act to allow physicians to seek better access to unapproved drugs for individual patients in emergency situations by setting forth several criteria for their release. These criteria included the following: there is no satisfactory alternative; the probable risk from the unapproved drug is not greater than the probable risk from the disease; and the use of the unapproved drug will not interfere with the clinical trials the company needs to support its efforts to achieve approval for the drug it hopes to market. The amended Act was trying to balance the need to perform rigorous clinical trials with the requests of terminally ill people who understandably wanted to try an unapproved drug in a desperate attempt to survive a little longer.

In December 2006 the FDA, in response to numerous complaints and mindful of the need to strike a balance between authorizing individual use of unapproved drugs and maintaining the integrity of the drug approval process, proposed additional regulations for various types of access to unapproved drugs. The proposed regulations are detailed and complex, but a helpful addition is that the FDA clarified the criteria for access to unapproved drugs. For both groups and individuals, (1) there must be serious or life-threatening disease and no available satisfactory alternative treatment, (2) the potential benefit justifies risk, and (3) the expanded access will not undermine the clinical trials. In addition for individual requests the FDA set forth two additional criteria: the physician must determine (1) that the risk to the individual is no greater than the risk of disease and (2) that it is not possible for the patient to participate in a clinical trial at this time.

By the beginning of the twenty-first century, then, the FDA was allowing expanded but controlled access to unapproved drugs. Mindful of its mandate to protect people from harm, it usually restricted this access until phase 2 testing was complete or, in case of immediate life-threatening situations, at least under way. The FDA's approach did not satisfy everyone, and a number of highly publicized cases arose where individuals demanded unapproved drugs despite the policies of the FDA.

The controversies raise two very serious and very difficult public policy questions. First, should the FDA, which is charged with protecting public health by assuring as far as possible that drugs are both safe and effective, allow people to use untested drugs that have not been shown to be safe and effective but that might just work? Second, should drug companies, which are legitimately worried about bad publicity if people should be harmed or killed by their untested products, have to provide untested drugs to dying patients who want them?

Perhaps the best way to understand the issues in this difficult debate is to look at a case that received tremendous publicity in recent years: the tragic story of Abigail Burroughs. Then we will try to reflect on the clash of values suggested by these controversies from the perspective of practical political wisdom, i.e., social ethics.

The Case of Abigail Burroughs and the Abigail Alliance

The Story

When Abigail was a 19-year-old college student at the University of Virginia physicians gave her and her parents a devastating diagnosis: life-threatening squamous-cell cancer of the head and neck. After chemotherapy and radiation over the next year had failed to halt the disease, her oncologist at Johns Hopkins thought some new drugs undergoing clinical trials might help her fight her particular type of cancer. One drug was ImClone's Erbitux, which was being tested for colon cancer, and the other was AstraZeneca's Iressa, which was being tested for non-small-cell lung cancer. Abigail did not have these particular cancers, and hence she was not a candidate for trials testing either of these drugs. Nonetheless she and her father asked for the drugs on a "compassionate use" basis.

They were not successful; neither the FDA nor the drug companies thought it wise to give her access to the drugs. The FDA can deny compassionate use (called "treatment use" in 21 CFR 312) if it considers the drug too risky or if it can find no reason to think it will work. At the time there was no evidence that these drugs would work for head and neck cancer, and it was not known if they were safe. Eventually Abigail was accepted in a clinical trial for a third experimental drug called Erlotinib, which was being tested for non-small-cell lung cancer, but she died before enrollment in the trial.

A few months after her death in November 2001, Abigail's father, Frank Burroughs, founded the nonprofit *Abigail Alliance for Better Access to Developmental Drugs*. The Alliance joined forces with the Washington Legal Foundation (WLF), and on June 11, 2003, both groups submitted a joint petition to the FDA asking it to expand the compassionate use of unapproved drugs. At that time the federal regulations allowed compassionate use for serious diseases but only during phase 3 trials or, if the disease was life-threatening, during phase 2 trials. The petition asked the FDA to allow compassionate use for life-threatening diseases earlier—immediately after successful completion of phase 1 trials, that is, before phase 2 trials had even begun provided the patients were not able to enroll in clinical trials.

In July 2003 after not receiving a substantive response to the petition from the FDA, the Abigail Alliance and the WLF sued the FDA and NIH in federal district court alleging that the FDA's restrictive policy on unapproved drugs violated the constitutional privacy and liberty rights of mentally competent terminally ill patients. The lawsuit pointed out that Abigail was not the only dying person left without drugs; it listed several other people who had been denied drugs that might have saved their lives.

The FDA asked the district court to dismiss the law suit, and the judge did so in August 2004. He found no basis for the claim that the Constitution gives terminally ill people a fundamental right to obtain unapproved drugs.

The Abigail Alliance and the WLF appealed this ruling to the federal Circuit Court. In May 2006 much to the surprise of many observers, a three-judge panel of the Circuit Court reversed the lower court ruling in a 2–1 decision. Some of the majority's reasoning seems rather questionable. For example, the majority based one of their arguments on the Supreme Court decision in the Nancy Cruzan case (cf. chapter 9). In *Cruzan* the Supreme Court held that people have a constitutional right to reject life-sustaining treatment. Therefore, the two judges in the majority on the panel argued, "An individual must also be free to decide for herself whether to assume any known or unknown risks of taking a medication that might prolong her life" (*Abigail Alliance for Better Access to Developmental Drugs v. Von Eschenbach*, 445 F3d 470 [DC Circuit 2006], p. 484).

It is difficult to see how one can make a valid legal or moral argument that begins with the premise that people have a right to *reject* life-sustaining treatments and immediately conclude that people therefore have a right to *obtain* risky unapproved drugs that might prolong life. There is no clear logical relation between premise and conclusion, between a right to keep people (doctors) from putting drugs into your body, and a right to force people to give you access to unapproved drugs. The Cruzan case was about *declining* approved life-sustaining treatment; the Abigail Alliance case is about *obtaining* unapproved experimental drugs not known to sustain life.

The FDA appealed the panel's decision to the full Circuit Court. In November 2006 the Circuit Court vacated the panel's decision and reopened the case. Ten months later on August 7, 2007, the Circuit Court issued its decision: There is no constitutional basis for claiming that terminally ill patients have a constitutional right to unapproved drugs. The decision was 8–2; the two dissenters were the two judges who had constituted the majority on the panel. The full court's opinion was written by the judge who had written the dissent on the original panel.

The Abigail Alliance then appealed the Circuit Court's decision to the U.S. Supreme Court. Before looking at what happened next, we consider the case from an ethical point of view.

Ethical Analysis

Situational awareness.   We are aware of the following facts in the Abigail story.

   1. Abigail was a young woman dying from head and neck cancer who had not responded to standard treatments.

2. Her oncologist had reasons for believing that two experimental drugs (Iressa and Erbitux) that were then undergoing clinical trials for other types of cancer might help her. Iressa was undergoing trials for colon cancer, and Erbitux was undergoing trials for non-small-cell lung cancer. The connection with these two drugs and Abigail's head and neck cancer was that these drugs were designed to cripple a natural protein known as EGFR on the surface of cancer cells. This protein causes the cells to grow, and Abigail's head and neck cancer had high numbers of this protein. Hence, her oncologist thought these drugs might work against her cancer.

3. Abigail had tried to enroll in these clinical trials but was rejected.

4. Abigail and her father then tried to obtain Iressa and Erbitux on a "compassionate use" basis. However, in 2001 FDA regulations did not allow "compassionate use" of these drugs at this stage of the clinical trials. Moreover neither ImClone (Erbitux) nor AstraZeneca (Iressa) wanted to release their drugs to people not enrolled in their clinical trials.

We are also aware of the following good and bad features in the case.

1. If Abigail was not able to find a treatment for her advancing cancer she would die. This is obviously a bad outcome, and prolonging her life would be an obvious good.

2. If Abigail were able to take Iressa and Erbitux she would experience deleterious side effects and expose herself to significant risks because the cancer drugs are toxic. However, the chance that Iressa and Erbitux could prolong Abigail's life was very slight.

3. Federal regulations require IRB oversight of human participants in clinical trials, but normally IRB oversight does not extend to people taking drugs on a compassionate use basis. Thus, these people do not have the protection enjoyed by people in clinical trials.

4. If Abigail did not obtain the drugs she and her family understandably would be upset. It is terribly upsetting to be dying, or to see a young member of your family dying, and to know that drug companies are testing drugs that could possibly help but that the policies of the FDA and of the manufacturers do not allow you to get the drug.

5. Many physicians would feel conflicted and upset in cases such as this. Physicians do not want to order unproven interventions that might do nothing more than cause additional suffering for their dying patients. Many physicians will hesitate before giving unproven risky drugs to their patients. Physicians usually are slow to provide interventions that do not meet the standard of care unless their patient is in a clinical trial. Conversely, physicians do want to help their patients live longer despite the risks of treatment if that is what their patients want to do.

6. Releasing unapproved drugs to people not in clinical trials has the potential to undermine clinical trials that are crucial in the development of new drugs. One very possible consequence is that people will opt for the unapproved drug rather then enter a clinical trial where they might receive a placebo rather than the desired drug.

7. If the person taking the unapproved drug suffers a significant setback or dies, the FDA might well suspend or even stop the trials so they can figure out what happened before anyone else is seriously harmed or killed. Any significant adverse events are bad for drug companies and for the advance of scientific research.

Prudential Reasoning in the Abigail Burroughs Case

Patient's perspective. Abigail wanted to try the experimental drugs that her oncologist had brought to her attention. She knew her treatments had failed to halt the disease, and she was willing to try anything that might save her no matter how slim the chance. Her position when looked at from her perspective is not at all irrational. If we face a choice between certain death and an intervention that gives us any chance that we will escape or at least postpone that death, then there is some reason for opting to take that chance if we can tolerate whatever suffering it might cause. After all, it may seem that since we are going to die anyway we have little to lose.

Provider's perspective. Not much is said about Abigail's oncologist in the commentaries on the case except that he apparently advised her about the drugs and helped her seek them. It is difficult to say whether it is morally reasonable for a physician to do this in this type of case. Some would argue that it generates false hopes regarding obtaining the drug or, if it is obtained, that it will result in a benefit that outweighs the burden. The ethical consensus about informed consent, as we saw in chapter 4, is that physicians should communicate treatment options that meet accepted standards of medical care, something that unapproved drugs certainly do not do. Hence, physicians have no responsibility to tell patients about experimental treatments. It is a judgment call whereby the physician has to weigh the good that information about experimental treatments might do against the harms it might cause for the patient and for public health. In any event physicians do face an ethical dilemma when it comes to sharing information about encouraging their patients to consider unapproved drugs or any other interventions that do not meet the current medical standards of care.

Abigail Alliance perspective. The Abigail Alliance alleged in its lawsuit that the FDA restrictions on access to unimproved drugs "amount to a death sentence" (paragraph 14) for patients with life-threatening conditions who have no other treatment options, and thus they violate the Constitution, which prevents the "deprivation of life without due process" (paragraph 32). The Alliance further alleged that the FDA policies interfere with the ability of these "terminally ill patients *to choose the appropriate treatment* for terminal illnesses" (paragraph 30). It is difficult to understand these views. It is a stretch to say restricting access to unapproved and potentially harmful drugs is an action that deprives dying people of life without due process; after all, the unproven drug might actually kill them. It is also a stretch to say that unapproved and potentially harmful drugs are "appropriate treatments." As long as these experimental drugs are in clinical trials they are not treatments but objects of research.

FDA perspective. The FDA's responsibility is to assure that the drugs people ingest are both safe and effective. The FDA has slowly become more open to allowing people access to unapproved drugs outside clinical trials, yet it mounted a vigorous legal battle to prevent a federal court from declaring that terminally ill people have a constitutional right to have access to unapproved drugs in the Abigail Alliance case.

Two things need to be remembered here. First, the primary responsibility of the FDA is public heath and not the health of an individual, and there are good reasons for holding that the FDA better serves public heath by being able to restrict the use of unapproved drugs with unknown risk factors outside of clinical trials. Second, the FDA cannot compel drug companies to give or sell unapproved drugs to people who want them. In fact, the major stumbling block preventing patients from gaining access to unapproved drugs is often not the FDA but the drug companies that want to restrict the use of unproven drugs to clinical trials.

Companies' perspective. In general, pharmaceutical companies are not enthusiastic about releasing experimental drugs for compassionate use. They would rather restrict their unapproved and potentially dangerous drugs to clinical trials with their criteria for eligibility and strict scientific controls. The drug companies have good reasons for their position. First, if they accept people who do not meet the eligibility criteria in their studies, the scientific evidence can be skewed. Second, accepting people not eligible for clinical trials will make it even more difficult to recruit participants for clinical trials because people would rather get the unapproved drug than enroll in a trial and take a chance of being randomized to a placebo arm of the study. Third, if there are adverse events outside a trial, it could generate negative publicity, lawsuits, or investigations that could cause the interruption of clinical trials while the adverse events are investigated to see whether they are related to the drug or some other factor. Hence companies argue, not without reason, that distributing unapproved drugs can actually hurt more people than it helps by delaying the approval of what turns out to be a safe and effective drug.

The Supreme Court action. The focus of the federal court case was on legal issues, most especially in this case a constitutional issue: whether or not terminally ill people have a constitutional right to obtain unapproved drugs. The district court judge did not think the Abigail Alliance had a case, and on appeal the Circuit Court decided 8–2 that the Constitution contained no right to obtain unapproved drugs. In January 2008 the U.S. Supreme Court declined to hear the Abigail Alliance appeal. Thus, it let stand the circuit court decision, namely, that there is no constitutional right giving dying individuals access to drugs not approved by the FDA. The Supreme Court action, however, did not end the efforts of people seeking access to unapproved drugs by passing federal laws authorizing it. Nor does it end the ethical debate about what would be a reasonable public policy.

Subsequent History of Erbitux and Iressa

The history of both Erbitux and Iressa after Abigail died is of some interest. Imclone submitted its first requests for Erbitux phase 3 trials in June 2001, the same month Abigail died, but the FDA could not act on it because important information was missing. The company resubmitted its application to begin phase 3 trials in August 2003. The FDA put the drug on an accelerated program and approved it for colon cancer in February 2004 after reviewing evidence that it shrank tumors and delayed tumor growth (but without evidence that it extended life). Erbitux can cause serious side effects, including difficulty breathing and low blood pressure. More common side effects are a rash, weakness, fever, constipation, and abdominal pain.

AstraZenica had sought fast-track review for Iressa when it began phase 1 clinical trials in 1998, but the FDA had declined approval. Then, in September 2002, more than a year after Abigail died, the FDA did put Iressa on a fast track and approved it for treatment of non-small-cell lung cancer in May 2003. However, in June 2005, after a large study showed Iressa provided no survival benefit, the FDA restricted its use to those patients already taking it whose physicians believed the drug had actually been helping them. Since June 2005, then, doctors can no longer prescribe Iressa for new patients with non-small-cell lung cancer or continue it for patients showing no signs of improvement because it does not extend life and other agents that do extend life are available.

Abigail was accepted in a clinical trial for Erlotinib but died before she could participate. After her death the FDA approved Erlotinib for non-small-cell lung cancer in November 2004 and then for pancreatic cancer in November 2005. As this is being written (2008) there is still no evidence that any of these drugs—Erbitux, Iressa, or Erlotinib—would be effective for head and neck cancer or would have saved or extended Abigail's life, and they certainly would have caused uncomfortable side effects as she died.

Similar Stories

Before sorting out some of the ethical issues involved in reaching a wise position in the matter of regulating unapproved drugs for terminally ill patients, it will be helpful to consider briefly two other well-publicized cases, the stories of Jacob Gunvalson and Penelope London.

Jacob Gunvalson. Sixteen-year-old Jacob was diagnosed with Duchenne muscular dystrophy (DMD), a lethal genetic disease that becomes worse as the child ages, when he was about seven years old. The defective gene causing DMD occurs on the X chromosome; hence, DMD affects mostly boys (about one in five thousand) because males have only one X chromosome. The particular mutation causing Jacob's type of DMD is found in about 15 percent of boys with the disease. DMD causes progressive muscle weakness and bone deformities. Most children with DMD need braces to walk by age ten and eventually are confined to a wheelchair. Cardiomyopathy (enlarged heart) and breathing difficulties, often requiring a respirator, develop in the later years. Most patients die at a young age; it is rare for them to live through their twenties.

In February 2008 a company called PTC Therapeutics began recruiting 165 boys for a late phase 2 clinical trial of its drug then known as PTC124. The primary goal of the trial, as indicated in documents filed with the FDA, was to see whether the drug would improve the distance that boys could walk in a six-minute walk test. To be eligible for the trial the boys had to be able to walk eighty yards unassisted in six minutes. The boys accepted in the study were randomized into three groups: a high-dose group, a low-dose group, and a placebo group. Thus, even if a boy were accepted in the clinical trial, he might not receive the drug or, if he did receive it, he might not receive an adequate dosage. If the trial is successful when it is completed in 2010, the company will make a therapeutic dose of PTC124 drug available to all the participants in the trial. In June 2009 the FDA awarded PTC Therapeutics a $1.6 million grant for the ongoing trial of PTC124, which is now known as Ataluren.

Jacob's mother Cheri had been active for years in support of more research to help children with DMD. She had worked with PTC Therapeutics and knew of its PTC124 clinical trial. Jacob was confined to a wheelchair and hence ineligible for the trial because he could not walk eighty yards, so Cheri asked for the drug on a compassionate use basis. The FDA did not object, but the company refused to release the drug for Jacob. In July 2008 she and her husband John sued PTC Therapeutics in federal court to force the company to provide PTC124 for Jacob. In August 2008 a federal district court judge ruled that PTC should give Jacob the drug, but that ruling was over-turned on appeal in December 2008. The Gunvalsons then dropped the lawsuit in March 2009.

The Gunvalsons were probably aware that PTC124 has shown some promising results in early trials for the type of DMD that afflicts Jacob as well as for another genetic disease, cystic fibrosis. In fact, results were so promising that Genzyme, a major biotechnology company, had agreed to pay PTC Therapeutics $100 million up front to have the right to market PTC124, once it received FDA approval, everywhere in the world except the United States and Canada. More-over, the FDA had agreed to put PTC124 on a fast track to approval.

The case pitting the Gunvalsons against PTC Therapeutics differs from the Abigail Alliance case in several important ways. First, unlike Abigail who was over eighteen, Jacob is a minor, so his parents are the ones who give consent for the unapproved drug. Second, his parents are suing the drug company not the FDA as the Abigail Alliance had done. Third, the patient's mother Cheri has been working with PTC Therapeutics for years and claims that it had promised her son access to the drug. Thus, a key issue in the lawsuit is breach of contract. The company denies it ever agreed to provide the drug for Jacob while phase 2 trials were under way.

Despite these differences, however, the case is typical of this issue. The parents of a minor with a tragic lethal disease want the pharmaceutical company to release an unapproved drug on the "compassionate use" basis for their child before phase 2 trials are completed. Experts are divided in a case such as this. Some would advocate compassionate use in this case, but others would not. Jacob's physician Dr. John Parkin was reported as saying that he would give the drug to Jacob if the company would provide it, but Dr. Richard Finkel, director of the neuromuscular program at Children's Hospital in Philadelphia and the principal investigator in the PTC124 study, was reported as saying that there were not enough safety data at the time to make the compassionate use exception. And PTC officials argued that allowing people to receive the drug before the trials needed for FDA approval had been completed would do great harm because nobody would want to enter the clinical trials and risk being randomized to a control group.

Penelope London. Slightly more than a year before the Gunvalson lawsuit another tragic story had emerged when the *Wall Street Journal* published a story on May 1, 2007, titled "Saying No to Penelope." Penelope had been diagnosed at age sixteen months with neuroblastoma, a rare form of cancer. Chemotherapy, radiation, surgery, and bone marrow transplantation had only slowed the progression of the disease. Her father, John London, a successful Wall Street hedge fund manager, continued to seek treatment after some doctors at the New York University Medical Center advised him and his wife that there was nothing more they could do to combat the disease.

When he heard of a drug being tested by a small company named Neotropix, London sought to obtain it for his daughter. Neotropix refused to release the drug for several reasons. First, the drug had just begun phase 1 testing and at that point had been given to only six participants, all adults. Neotropix estimated that the phase 1 clinical study would not be completed for another year and a half. Second, one of the phase 1 participants had died during the trial, and the FDA then halted the trial for an investigation. Later it allowed the study to go forward after the investigation showed the person had died from cancer, not the drug. Nevertheless, the temporary halt had cost the company money and had delayed the efforts of Neotropix to win FDA approval for the drug. The company did not want any additional complications that might undermine its approval process. Third, the drug involves injecting a virus that invades pigs but is not found in humans, and there are serious safety concerns about injecting a virus not found in humans into humans.

Although Penelope's mother Catherine was willing to focus on palliative care for Penelope, John aggressively pushed Neotropix to release the drug. At one point he convinced House Speaker Nancy Pelosi and Pennsylvania Governor Edward Rendell to lobby the company on his behalf. The executives and the board at Neotropix, as well as a major investor in the firm, steadfastly declined to provide the drug.

After Neotropix refused to release the drug, John found another company, Jennerex, that was also beginning phase 1 trials with a live virus. Jennerex did agree to provide the drug on a compassionate use basis, and Dr. William Carroll, director of pediatric oncology at NYU Medical Center, agreed to provide Penelope with it provided he could get the proper approval from the hospital IRB and also from a biosafety committee because a life virus would be used. Before those committees could consider data that might make a case for saying that the potential benefits outweighed the safety concerns, Penelope died on May 19, 2007.

The ethical concerns in the Penelope story present several unique ethical features. First, morally it is one thing for an adult with decision-making capacity (Abigail) or an older teenager and his parents (Jacob) to choose to assume the risk of taking an unapproved drug, but it is another thing to give experimental drugs to a young child (Penelope) who cannot make the choice or give assent. Second, the intervention of governors and members of Congress in efforts to force companies to release unapproved drugs for individual children raises moral concerns about politicians undermining public policy. This is a move that reminds us of what some people used to do in an effort to obtain organs for their children before a national organ system was put in place. It also reminds us how elected officials tried to force medical treatment on Terri Schiavo against her husband's wishes (and probably against her wishes as well; see chapter 9). Third, unlike the stories of Abigail and Jacob, where the drugs being sought had already received a preliminary safety assessment in completed phase I trials, Penelope's father was seeking a drug that had only just begun its phase I safety studies and had never been given to children.

Ethical Reflections

If we approach these cases from a perspective of virtue ethics, a number of considerations emerge. First, virtue ethics as originally conceived gives high priority to what we call social or political ethics. Aristotle conceived of virtue ethics as a subset of what he called politics—setting up public environments that enable people to flourish and attain happiness. In modern terms, we would say that he made the common good a priority rather than the individual good. In virtue ethics, the question of regulating drugs is seen primarily as a question of the public good, not the good of a particular individual. The key question about the availability of unapproved drugs in virtue ethics will be how the common good is best served, not how people can get what they want. Thus, virtue ethics will ask whether trumping the FDA regulatory framework by granting access to unapproved drugs will contribute to the common good, not whether an individual has a right to demand them without regard to the impact it will have in the community.

Second, in the current debate about access to unapproved drugs the reasoning is often clouded by questionable uses of language, something that needs to be avoided as we saw in chapter 3. For example the American Cancer Society publishes a helpful information sheet online (cancer.org), but it has the misleading title "Compassionate Drug Use." The title obliterates the actual debate; no reasonable person is going to oppose the compassionate use of drugs. A better title· might have been "Compassionate Use of Unapproved Drugs." There are reasonable people opposed to the "compassionate use of unapproved drugs" because safety and efficacy are still unknown, and these drugs can do great harm to dying people. Even the full title of the Abigail Alliance (the Abigail Alliance for Better Access to Developmental Drugs) is misleading. It is premature to call drugs still in clinical trials "developmental" when the great majority of these will never develop into approved treatments. Often the media adds to the linguistic confusion by presenting the stories in terms of the FDA or drug companies denying dying people *treatments* that might save their lives. That sounds cruel, but it is misleading; these drugs are not, and most will never be, approved as treatments. Even the people in clinical trials are not receiving "treatments," although many think they are in what is known as the "therapeutic bias," the assumption by many that whatever pills they receive in clinical trials will likely help them.

Third, the debate about unapproved drugs introduces a host of conflicting issues: private demands versus public health, individual rights versus social good, personal risk taking versus the demands of good science, personal interests versus commercial interests, free markets versus regulations. One needs a rich ethic to move toward a balance that is reasonable. It is not enough to approach the issue with an ethic of individual rights; sensitivity to the common good is an important consideration to achieve balance between compassion for dying people who understandably want to try anything that looks promising and other political and social considerations.

Fourth, we need to keep relevant facts in mind when we try to decide what would be a reasonable policy about unapproved drugs. For example it is a fact that only about 6 percent of cancer drugs that look promising after laboratory and animal testing and then move into phase 1 clinical trials with human participants will ever achieve FDA approval. This means that for every sixteen cancer drugs that begin clinical trials about fifteen will be rejected.

We also need to remember two things that move our thinking about regulating use of unapproved drugs in opposite directions: Some approved drugs are later withdrawn because they are dangerous, and, conversely, some unapproved drugs are safe and could offer significant benefit to people before approval. Two examples illustrate this point: the histories of Vioxx and Gleevec.

Perhaps the most notable recent example of an approved drug being withdrawn was the Vioxx catastrophe. The FDA approved Vioxx in May 1999 for use as an anti-inflammatory pain reliever after a six-month priority review. Studies involving more than five thousand participants indicated it was safe and effective. Two years later in a clinical trial designed to see whether Vioxx prevented recurrence of colon polyps, researchers happened to notice a significantly higher incidence of heart attacks and strokes after participants were on Vioxx for more than eighteen months. The problem was so severe that researchers soon halted that clinical trial, and then, in September 2004, after accumulating more evidence the manufacturer Merck voluntarily withdrew Vioxx from the market. Numerous lawsuits followed, and settlements caused the company huge financial losses.

Vioxx generated about $2.5 billion in annual sales for Merck. During the more than five years it was on the market physicians wrote over ninety million prescriptions for about twenty million Americans, and based on extrapolation of data from studies, the FDA has estimated that Vioxx probably played a role in over 27,000 heart attack deaths. The Vioxx incident shows that even successful phase 3 trials and FDA approval are no guarantee that drugs are ultimately safe for people.

On the other hand a recent notable example of an unapproved drug that could have helped people if it had been made available before FDA approval is Gleevec. The Gleevec story is a kind of poster child for giving people access to unapproved drugs after promising phase 1 trials.

Gleevec targets an abnormal protein that causes chronic myeloid leukemia. In June 1998 researchers began a phase 1 trial, gradually increasing doses in people with leukemia to determine a safe dosage. In December 1999 they reported that a daily dose of at least 300 mg was not only safe with tolerable side effects but had caused blood counts to return to normal in all thirty-one participants in the phase 1 trial. In April 2001 a larger study published in the *New England Journal of Medicine* showed that Gleevec restored normal blood counts in fifty-three of fifty-four people and that fifty-one of these people were doing well after a year. In May 2001 the FDA approved Gleevec for use in leukemia under its accelerated approval program. (Accelerated approval permits doctors to prescribe the drug before phase 3 trials are completed but requires patient follow-up and additional studies to determine whether the drug actually improves survival.) Later the FDA approved Gleevec for other cancers.

Undoubtedly, in hindsight, if some people with leukemia had tried to obtain the unapproved Gleevec in early 2000 and if Novartis, the manufacturer, had given it to them, many would have benefited. Although the Gleevec story is an exception, we need to keep it in mind when we consider whether it is wise to allow greater access to unapproved drugs. Of course, we also need to keep in mind the fact that many drugs that looked so promising after phase 1 trials turned out to be unsafe for people and were never approved.

The Gleevec success points to an important development in phase 1 trials of cancer drugs that is important to note. Typically people think that the main purpose of phase 1 trials is to determine safety. Increasingly, however, researchers in phase 1 cancer trials are also making preliminary determinations about efficacy—whether the drug is showing signs of beneficial impact on the cancer. In fact, a study has shown that most cancer drugs approved in recent years had already shown some clinical benefit in phase 1 trials. How much clinical benefit? In 2005 the *New England Journal of Medicine* published a review of all adult phase 1 cancer trials sponsored by the National Cancer Institute between 1991 and 2002 (460 trials wherein 10,402 participants out of a total of 11,935 were assessed for how the drug impacted their cancer as well as whether the drug was safe) revealed some significant benefit for some participants. Whereas in trials where the experimental drug was tested by itself (20 percent of the phase 1 trials) only 4.4 percent of the people received a clinical response, in trials where the experimental drug was given in combination with at least one approved cancer drug (46 percent of the phase 1 trials) almost 18 percent of the people received a clinical response, and another 34 percent experienced either stable disease or improvement so slight it was considered less-than-partial response.

The authors of the study conclude, "These data suggest that participants may benefit more from current phase 1 oncology trials than previously believed." The authors wisely point out that everyone involved in considering the risks and benefits of phase 1 trials, including ethicists, need to be aware of the complexity and variety of these phase 1 trials and know the specific details about the trial pertinent to their needs. Although the authors focused on persons considering entering phase 1 trials, their data are equally important for people seeking unapproved drugs after phase 1 trials have been completed.

And so access to unapproved drugs remains a thorny ethical issue wherein the understandable desire of some dying patients to try anything to live clashes with the desire of scientists, manufacturers, and the FDA to move forward in a way that helps science advance, protects the company, and contributes to the common good. The recent efforts of the FDA have tried to strike a balance to protect both values. Regulations are needed for the good of society, but they need to be flexible as well.

SEEDING TRIALS AND GHOSTWRITERS

The discovery process in lawsuits involving Vioxx after Merck voluntarily withdrew it from the market in 2004 uncovered a trove of internal documents and company emails that suggest another area where we need to think about ethics and regulations: pharmaceutical marketing that employs seeding trials (clinical trials designed primarily for marketing purposes) and ghostwritten scientific articles in professional journals.

A seeding trial is a clinical trial designed and supervised by the sales and marketing wing of a pharmaceutical company to look like a trial designed to acquire scientific knowledge when in fact its primary purpose is to market the drug. The company does this by recruiting and reimbursing hundreds of primary care physicians as "investigators" in a clinical trial. Companies cannot pay physicians for prescribing their drugs, but they can pay physicians whom they can classify as research investigators.

One sign of a seeding trial is that a large number of doctors are testing the drug, each on a small number of their patients. This is so because the primary purpose of a seeding trial is making many physicians familiar with the drug, not collecting important data about the drug itself. True, if the trial is double-blind, the doctors will not know which patients receive the drug and which receive an alternative drug or a placebo, but they will be aware that half their patients are receiving the company's drug. The clinical trial plants or "seeds" the product in the offices of these doctors. Once the doctors start providing the drug in a trial, marketing studies show that they will likely prescribe it more often than their colleagues after FDA approval.

A ghostwritten scientific article comes to be written in the following manner: A pharmaceutical company designs a clinical trial and then either conducts the research itself or hires a Contract Research Organization called a CRO. After the data are collected and analyzed, the company or the CRO, if the results are favorable, writes up the results in an article for submission to one of the scientific journals. At this point the company or CRO looks for a well-known researcher to review the article in return for reimbursement and being listed as the primary author of the published study.

Listing a "big name" as the primary author of the study, which suggests he or she supervised the research and wrote the article, gives it tremendous credibility in the eyes of physicians seeking to help their patients. In fact, however, the person listed as the lead author was neither the principal investigator nor the author of the article; it was ghostwritten by anonymous writers at the pharmaceutical company or at a CRO under contract to the pharmaceutical company. The role of the lead "author" is usually confined to reading the study and suggesting some editorial changes.

Thanks to documents that surfaced in the discovery process in Vioxx lawsuits, we now have some documentary evidence suggesting that pharmaceutical companies use both seeding trials and ghostwriters to market their products. One example is the clinical trial known as ADVANTAGE (Assessment of Differences between Vioxx And Naproxen To Ascertain Gastrointestinal Tolerability and Effectiveness). It was, according to company emails and records, conceived by the marketing division of the company, and it also involved ghostwritten scientific articles.

The ADVANTAGE Clinical Trial

The Story

Shortly before the FDA approved Vioxx, Merck enrolled about six hundred primary care physicians in the ADVANTAGE trial (earlier trials of Vioxx had enrolled specialists, and now Merck wanted to encourage prescriptions by primary care physicians as soon as the drug was approved). These primary care physicians then recruited about 5,500 patients, which works out to an average of about nine patients for each primary care physician-investigator. The study was blind: About half the patients received Vioxx and the other half received Naproxen. Unlike many clinical trials there was no placebo group; the purpose was not to see how effective Vioxx was but to provide data showing Vioxx was tolerated better than Naproxen, a competing drug made by another company. The three-month trial began at the end of March 1999, two months before the FDA gave the approval that would allow physicians to prescribe Vioxx for their patients.

Ostensibly the company set up the ADVANTAGE trial to see whether Vioxx caused fewer stomach problems than Naproxen, even though an earlier study had already indicated that it did. Yet an internal company document uncovered in preparation for the Vioxx litigation described the real goal of the trial as allowing the physician-investigators to gain "experience with Vioxx prior to and during the critical launch phase." Other internal documents actually identified ADVANTAGE as a seeding trial.

The company withheld the primary purpose of the trial from the physicians, the IRBs, and the participants in the study. Moreover, Merck conducted a study within the study: Without informing the six hundred investigator-physicians, it compared their prescription writing with that of physicians not chosen to participate in the study and gave physicians in the study grades ranging from A+ to D based on their subsequent prescribing history with Vioxx.

The timing was perfect; when the FDA approved Vioxx, the six hundred physicians were already using it in the seeding trial, and many of them would begin prescribing the drug for their patients. A basic ethical concern is apparent here: The trial looked like a scientific trial, but it was not designed to gain knowledge leading to FDA approval; it was designed to get the drug into the hands of hundreds of physicians who would then tend to write more prescriptions for it once it had been approved. It is hard to argue that such behavior is not deceptive.

The seeding trial was not the only ethically questionable issue with the ADVANTAGE trial; it also involved a ghostwritten article. When the results of the seeding trial were published in 2003, this second ethical issue came to light. The ADVANTAGE study published in the *Annals of Internal Medicine* listed Dr. Jeffrey Lisse, a rheumatologist at the University of Arizona, as the lead author. However, Dr. Lisse subsequently denied that he led the study or wrote the paper. He was quoted in the press as saying, "Merck came to me after the study was completed and said 'we want your help to work on the paper.' The initial paper was written at Merck, and then it was sent to me for editing."

Internal company documents in the Vioxx lawsuits show that employees of Merck and of CROs under contract to Merck actually wrote a number of scientific papers and review articles and then recruited academically affiliated researchers who agreed to be listed as major investigators in the scientific papers or as authors of the review articles. Sometimes Merck had completed the clinical trials and analyzed the data before contacting the "guest" authors. Documents showed that Merck contracted with medical publishing companies to ghostwrite review articles and then recruited "authors" that would be listed in the published article.

One e-mail to Merck from a publishing company known as Health Science Communications is a progress report including expected delivery dates on eight papers it was preparing for Merck on Vioxx; it includes the company's recommendations for article titles, for external academic authors who might agree to be listed, and for journals that might accept the articles. One contract example shows that Health Science Communications agreed to provide a twenty-page review article for Merck for $23,841.

Ethical Reflections

Ghostwritten articles in prestigious medical journals have emerged along with seeding trials as a major ethical issue in recent years. Most commentators not connected with pharmaceutical companies believe that the ADVANTAGE study is the tip of the iceberg and that both seeding trials and ghostwritten articles are widespread practices by pharmaceutical companies in the United States. There is concern that such activities undermine both scientific integrity and medical ethics. Seeding trials deceive the physicians, the patients giving informed consent to participate as subjects in trials, and the members of IRBs by disguising the trials as science when the primary intent is really marketing. And the ghostwritten articles deceive people taking care of patients into thinking that the studies have been done and written up by outstanding researchers well known in their fields when in fact companies selling the drugs have managed the studies and written the scientific reports, and the big name authors have entered the picture only after the research is done and the articles are already written.

What to do about these questionable ethical practices? Appealing to the personal moral integrity of the people involved in setting up seeding trials or managing clinical trials culminating in ghostwritten articles is probably not enough to stop the deceptive practices. The practices are deeply embedded in the desire of pharmaceutical companies to make a profit. So deeply embedded are these practices and so powerful the profit motive that the wiser course would be to see the problem as a social and political issue and thus one in need of federal regulation. The federal regulations of the early 1980s that followed the recommendations of the National Commission for the Protection of Human Subjects have unquestionably raised the moral quality of research with human subjects, and this problem with pharmaceutical companies suggests some additional regulations would be in order to curb the deceptions associated with seeding trials and ghostwritten articles.

Suggested Readings

A good overview of the history of health care in the United States can be found in the five chapters of book II in Paul Starr, 1982, *The Social Transformation of American Medicine*, New York: Basic Books.

For a current overview of the health care payment systems, see the series of articles covering Medicare, Medicaid, and employee plans by John Iglehart, "The American Health Care System," *New England Journal of Medicine* 1999, *340*, 70–76, 248–52, 327–332, and 403–8. For an excellent case study showing how decision making in managed care extends beyond the physician-patent (or proxy) relationship to other decision makers, see the Special Supplement "What Could Have Saved John Worthy?" *Hastings Center Report* 1998, *28* (July–August), S1–S17. For a readable account of managed care, see George Anders, 1996, *Health against Wealth: HMOs and the Breakdown of Medical Trust*, Boston: Houghton Mifflin. For a more favorable interpretation of managed care, see Walter Zelman and Robert Berenson, 1998, *The Managed Care Blues and How to Cure Them*, Washington, DC: Georgetown University Press.

One unfortunate consequence of managed care is the breakdown of trust that patients have in their physicians as they worry that doctors will make treatment decisions based on financial incentives rather than on what might help their patients. See Stephen Shortell et al., "Physicians as Double Agents: Maintaining Trust in an Era of Multiple Accountabilities," *JAMA* 1998, *280*, 1102–8; Audiey Kao et al., "The Relationship between Method of Physician Payment and Patient Trust," *JAMA* 1998, *280*, 1708–15; David Mechanic, "Managed Care as a Target of Distrust," *JAMA* 1997, *277*, 1810–11; Edmund Pellegrino, "Managed Care at the Bedside: How Do We Look in the Moral Mirror?" *Kennedy Institute of Ethics Journal* 1997, *7*, 321–30; Edmund Pellegrino, "Interests, Obligations, and Justice: Some Notes toward an Ethic of Managed Care," *Journal of Clinical Ethics* 1995, *6*, 312–17; and Marcia Angell, "The Doctor as Double Agent," *Kennedy Institute of Ethics Journal* 1993, *3*, 279–86. Also compare Marc Rodwin, 1993, *Medicine, Money, & Morals: Physicians' Conflicts of Interest*, New York: Oxford University Press; and Roy Spece, ed., 1996, *Conflicts of Interest in Clinical Practice and Research*, New York: Oxford University Press.

Another unfortunate consequence of managed care is the neglect of pain management. Some MCOs provide little or no place for treating pain that is chronic or resulting from terminal illness. See Diane Hoffmann, "Pain Management and Palliative Care in the Era of Managed Care: Issues for Health Insurers," *Journal of Law, Medicine & Ethics* 1998, *26*, 267–89. Managed care is not upsetting only to patients; physicians are also disturbed and demoralized over some of the more extreme efforts to constrict their medical judgments. See, for example, Kevin Grumbach, "Primary Care Physicians' Experience of Financial Incentives in Managed-Care Systems," *New England Journal of Medicine* 1998, *339*, 1516–21. In 1997 a large group of Massachusetts physicians and nurses issued "A Call to Action" that protested the intrusion of for-profit and market-based mentalities into health care; see "For Our Patients, Not for Profits," *JAMA* 1997, *278*, 1733–38. However, physicians' ethical concerns in managed care differ in important ways from those of ethicists writing about managed care; see Nancy Jecker and Albert Jonsen, "Managed Care: A House of Mirrors," *Journal of Clinical Ethics* 1997, *8*, 230–41.

Managed care issues have moved bioethics from its traditional clinical concern with the rather private clinical encounter between physician and patient or proxy to a more public and organizational ethic. Physicians are seen as caring for populations of patients as well as individuals, and they are embedded in various management arrangements rather than a simple fiduciary encounter. This shift requires new emphases in our ethical thinking; consider M. Hall and R. Berenson, "Ethical Practice in Managed Care: A Dose of 'Realism,'" *Annals of Internal Medicine* 1998, *128*, 395–402; Solomon Benatar, "Just Healthcare beyond Individualism: Challenges for North American Bioethics," *Cambridge Quarterly of Healthcare Ethics* 1997, *6*, 397–415; Ezekiel Emanuel, "Medical Ethics in the Era of Managed Care: The Need for Institutional Structures Instead of Principles for Individual Cases," *Journal of Clinical Ethics* 1995, *6*, 335–38. For some thoughtful cautions about this shift in ethics, see Jerome Kassirer, "Managing Care—Should We Adopt a New Ethic?" *New England Journal of Medicine* 1998, *339*, 397–98.

For background on social justice issues and health care see Rosamond Rhodes et al., eds., *Medicine and Social Justice: Essays on the Distribution of Health Care*, 2002, New York: Oxford University Press; Madison Powers and Ruth Faden, 2006, *Health Care and Philosophy: Adding Justice to the Debate*, New York: Oxford University Press; Gunnar Almgren, 2007, *Health Care Politics, Policy, and Services: A Social Justice Analysis*, New York: Springer Publishing Company; Norman Daniels, 2008, *Just Health: Meeting Health Needs Fairly*, New York: Cambridge University Press; Norman Daniels and James Sabin, 2008, *Setting Limits Fairly: Can We Learn to Share Resources?* 2nd ed., New York: Oxford University Press.

For the Texas Advance Directives Act, see Robert Fine and Thomas Mayo, "Resolution of Futility by Due Process: Early Experience with the Texas Advance Directives Act," *Annals of Internal Medicine* 2003, *138*, 743–46. The article reports cases at Baylor University Medical Center. For a critique of the law generated by the Gonzales case, see Robert Truog, "Tackling Medical Futility in Texas," *New England*

Journal of Medicine 2007, *357*, 1–3. Fine's letter in *New England Journal of Medicine* 2007, *357*, 1558–59 in response to Truog's article defends the law and points out that 93 percent of Texas futility disputes were resolved without the threatening "ten-day letter." Additional support for the law can be found in John Paris et al., "*Howe v. MGH* and *Hudson v. Texas Children's Hospital*: Two Approaches to Resolving Family-Physician Disputes in End-of-Life Care," *Journal of Perinatology* 2006, 26, 726–29. Both the Hudson and Gonzales cases generated a tremendous amount of criticism in the press and on the Internet as the stories unfolded. See also the essay by Geoffrey Miller, "Ten Days in Texas," *Hastings Center Report* 2007, *37* (July–August), back cover. Robert Burt of the Yale Law School argues against the legal system allowing physicians to override treatment demands; he favors negotiation and sees the legal system as ensuring that each side's authority in the situation is recognized. See his "The Medical Futility Debate: Patient Choice, Physician Obligation, and End-of-Life Care," *Journal of Palliative Medicine* 2002, *5*, 249–54.

Important online resources for material on drug approval are provided by the various links at fda.gov. A helpful website is abigail-alliance.org, which contains, among other documents, the text of the ACCESS Act that was introduced in the Senate and House in 2008. See also Benjamin Falit and Cary Gross, "Access to Experimental Drugs for Terminally Ill Patients," *JAMA* 2008, *300*, 2793–95; Susan Okie, "Access before Approval—A Right to Take Experimental Drugs?" *New England Journal of Medicine* 2006, *355*, 437–40; the Society for Clinical Trials Position Paper, *Clinical Trials* 2006, *3*, 154–57; Jerome Yates, "Food and Drug Administration, Partner in Drug Development," *Cancer Journal for Clinicians* 2006, *56*, 321–22; Jerome Groopman, "Should Dying Patients Have Access to Experimental Drugs?" *New Yorker*, Dec.18, 2006, accessed at newyorker.com; John Robertson, "Controversial Medical Treatment and the Right to Health Care," *Hastings Center Report* 2006, *36* (November–December), 15–20; Shira Bender et al., "Access for the Terminally Ill to Experimental Medical Innovations," *American Journal of Bioethics* 2007, *7*, 3–6; Peter Jacobson and Wendy Parmet, "A New Era of Unapproved Drugs," *JAMA* 2007, *297*, 205–8; Razelle Kurzrock and Robert Benjamin, "Risks and Benefits of Phase I Oncology Trials, Revisited," *New England Journal of Medicine* 2005, *352*, 930–32; Geeta Anand, "Saying No to Penelope," *Wall Street Journal*, May 1, 2007; and the case study on Penelope, "All for One, or One for All," *Hastings Center Report* 2007, *37* (July–August), 13–15. For the story of Jacob Gunvalson see Reed Abelson, "Advocating a Treatment, but Denied Access to It," *New York Times*, July 17, 2008. See also "Expanded Access to Investigational Drugs for Treatment Use," *Federal Register* 2006, *71*, 75147–68.

On the Abigail Alliance case see George Annas, "Cancer and the Constitution—Choice at Life's End," *New England Journal of Medicine* 2007, *357*, 408–13; and Abigail Alliance for Better Access to Development Drug v. Eschenbach, 445 F3d 470 (DC Cir. 2006) and No. 04–5350, 2007 WL 2238914 (DC Cir. August 7, 2007).

Evidence that some phase I clinical trials produce information on effectiveness as well as safety can be found in Thomas Roberts et al., "Trends in the Risks and Benefits to Patients with Cancer Participating in Phase I Clinical Trials." *JAMA* 2004, *292*, 2130–40. Steven Joffe and Franklin Miller, "Rethinking Risk-Benefit Assessment for Phase I Cancer Trials," *Journal of Clinical Oncology* 2006, *24*, 2987–90; Elizabeth Horstmann et al., "Risks and Benefits of Phase I Oncology Trials, 1991 through 2002," *New England Journal of Medicine* 2005, *352*, 895–904.

The ADVANTAGE study is described in Jesse Lisse et al., "Gastrointestinal Tolerability and Effectiveness of Rofecoxib Versus Naproxen in the Treatment of Osteoarthritis: A Randomized, Controlled Trial." *Annals of Internal Medicine* 2003, *139*, 539–46 (rofecoxib is the generic name for Vioxx). For commentary on the seeding trials, including the ADVANTAGE trial, see Kevin Hill et al., "The ADVANTAGE Seeding Trial: A Review of Internal Documents," *Annals of Internal Medicine* 2008, *148*, 251–58, and the accompanying editorial on pages 279f by Harold Sox and Drummond Rennie, "Seeding Trials: Just Say 'No.'" Dr. Jeffrey Lisse's statement that Merck listed him as the lead author even though he did not have a role in the data collection or analysis of the ADVANTAGE trial was reported in Alex Berenson, "Evidence in Vioxx Suits Shows Intervention by Merck Official," *New York Times*, April 24, 2005, available online at nytimes.com. It is also cited in Kevin Hill's article. The executive director of the Merck Laboratories Global Center for Scientific Affairs, Jonathan Edelman, posted an online response to Hill's article on the *Annals of Internal Medicine* website (annals.org) on August 21, 2008. He defended the ADVANTAGE study, denying that it was a seeding trial and stating that "the primary intent of the study was to answer scientific questions of importance to primary care physicians." Hill and his co-authors responded to Edelman at annals.org, pointing out that the evidence showing Merck designed

ADVANTAGE as a seeding trial "is clear and is derived from their own internal documents." For a history of seeding trials, see also Bruce Psaty and Drummond Rennie, "Clinical Trial Investigators and Their Prescribing Patterns," *JAMA* 2006, *295*, 2787–90. For evidence that participation in clinical trials shapes physicians' prescribing practices, see Morten Anderson et al., "How Conducting a Clinical Trial Affects Physicians' Guideline Adherence and Drug Preferences," *JAMA* 2006, *295*, 2759–64.

The ghostwritten research articles connected with Vioxx are well described by Joseph Ross et al., "Guest Authorship and Ghostwriting in Publications Related to Rofecoxib: A Case Study of Industry Documents from Rofecoxib Litigation," *JAMA* 2008, *299*, 1800–1912. See also the many letters in response to this article in *JAMA* 2008, *300*, 901–6. See also Catherine DeAngelis and Phil Fontanarosa, "Impugning the Integrity of Medical Science: The Adverse Effects of Industry Influence," *JAMA* 2008, *299*, 1833–35; and Marcia Angell, "Industry-Sponsored Clinical Research: A Broken System," *JAMA* 2008, *300*, 1069–71.

Glossary

Amicus curiae. A Latin phrase meaning "friend of the court." It designates a brief submitted to a court by a party not actually involved in the particular case but interested in the outcome. These briefs give reasons why the court should rule one way or another.

Anovulant. A natural or artificial substance preventing ovulation and thereby preventing pregnancy.

ART. Artificial reproductive technologies, which include the many ways of reproducing human beings.

Autonomy. (1) Self-legislation; people determine their own laws and rules. (2) An action-guiding moral principle proposed by many contemporary ethicists obliging us to respect the particular decisions of adults with decision-making capacity. (3) The right of individuals to make their own decisions and to live their lives as they choose without interference from others. (4) For Kant, autonomy is the universal law of morality, which appears to us as the categorical imperative. Unlike the notions of autonomy in (2) and (3), Kant's notion of autonomy restricts individual choices because only those decisions that can be considered as moral maxims everyone must obey are morally acceptable. Kant considered autonomy objective and universal, not subjective and particular.

Barbiturate. An organic compound providing pain relief and sedation but also affecting respiration, heart rate, blood pressure, and temperature.

Belmont Report. A major report of the National Commission (q.v.) published in 1979. It shaped federal regulations affecting medical research in the United States and promoted the idea that health care ethics is based on action-guiding principles of obligation, specifically the principles of autonomy, beneficence, and justice.

Beneficence. (1) Doing good for others; actions done for the benefit of others. (2) An action-guiding moral principle proposed by many contemporary ethicists, obliging us to help others and to promote their welfare.

Best interests. Whatever promotes the most good for a particular patient without decision-making capacity. When a proxy does not know what the patient without decision-making capacity wants, she must decide about treatment in view of what she thinks is in the overall best interests of the particular patient. This standard is not quite the same as what is sometimes called the "reasonable person standard" because, although it considers what any reasonable person would want, it also considers what is known about how this particular patient lived and thought about life. Best interests is best understood in contrast with substituted judgment (q.v.).

Bible. Literally, the "book." In our culture the word Bible refers to a collection of books written during the millennium before the close of the first century C.E. and accepted as canonical or official by the Jewish or Christian traditions. The early books were written in Hebrew by Hebrews and are called the Hebrew Bible. Later books were written in Greek and include the New Testament. The Bible has made a significant impact on morality in our culture, where it is still widely read and studied. Many of its narratives, commandments, laws, sayings, and parables are ethical in nature.

Brain death. The irreversible cessation of all brain functions, including those of the brain stem. Brain death indicates that the person is dead, even though life-support equipment may be sustaining most biological functions. People in a coma or in a persistent vegetative state are not brain dead.

Capitation. A managed care payment system whereby providers agree in advance to provide care for a number of persons (the "head count") for a specified period regardless of how much care they might have to provide in response to their patients' needs.

Carrier. A person with a genetic mutation that does not affect him but may or will affect his children.

Casuistry. A moral theory making cases rather than principles the guides for behavior. As particular moral questions (the "cases") are resolved, the resolutions gradually fall into typical patterns or categories, which then serve as paradigms for resolving similar cases as they arise. This approach is similar to the appeal to prior cases by lawyers and judges in legal proceedings. Casuistry is more sensitive to circumstances than are moral theories making principles and rules the guides for behavior.

Categorical imperative. The ultimate principle of morality according to Kant. Kant (1724–1804) was influenced by Isaac Newton's seminal *Principia Mathematica* (*Mathematical Principles of Natural Philosophy*, 1687), which not only elaborated the modern laws of physical motion and the universal theory of gravity but formulated rules of reasoning for the scientist as well. Kant, impressed by Newton's work, defined human reason as the faculty of principles, rules, and laws. Unlike the deterministic action-guiding principles of nature discovered by scientific reasoning (every object *must* remain in its state of rest or straight uniform motion unless disturbed), the action-guiding principles and rules of human conduct discovered by practical reason appear to us as imperatives—we *ought* to abide by them, but we can choose to deviate from them. Kant thought that one absolute, incontestable, and universal imperative was the source of all action-guiding moral principles and rules. He called this the categorical imperative and formulated it three ways. The first and best known formulation is: "I ought never to act except in such a way that I can also will that my maxim should become a universal law."

Cloning. When used to produce a new organism it describes a process whereby a somatic cell with its full complement of DNA is put into an ovum whose nuclear DNA has been removed. Almost all the genes of the resulting animal or human would come from the organism contributing the somatic cell, unlike normal reproduction where the spermatozoon and ovum each contribute half the genes.

Coma. An enduring state of total unconsciousness that looks like sleep. Normally one of three outcomes of coma can be expected within months—the patient will die, the patient will recover at least some awareness, or the patient will transition into a persistent vegetative state (q.v.).

Cystic Fibrosis (CF). A genetic disease affecting chiefly the respiratory system and causing chronic difficulties that make it difficult for patients to live beyond their twenties.

Deduction. In moral philosophy, deduction is the reasoning process that applies a general moral principle or rule, or a right considered to be possessed by everyone, to a particular situation in order to determine what ought to be done. It is best understood in contrast with induction (q.v.).

Deontology. Any moral philosophy (*logos*) based on duty (*deon*). Traditional deontological theories are moralities of law (divine law, natural law, or the moral law we give ourselves), but rights-based theories can also be deontological in that one person's natural right creates a duty on the part of others to respect it. Deontological theories usually propose a set of absolute duties or prohibitions; that is, certain actions are always and everywhere immoral regardless of good intentions, extenuating circumstances, or favorable consequences. Deontology is best understood when contrasted with teleology (q.v.)

Diagnosis-related group (DRG). A rigid system based primarily on diagnosis but adjusted for other factors. The DRG code determines what Medicare will pay hospitals for patients it covers.

DNA. Deoxyribonucleic acid, the chemical thread in each cell carrying genetic instructions for that organism.

DNR. Do not resuscitate; a physician's order indicating resuscitation is not to be attempted if the patient suffers cardiopulmonary arrest.

Double effect. A principle developed several centuries ago by moral theologians to justify, under certain conditions, performing actions that have bad as well as good effects. In some cases it produces moral judgments everyone is happy with (for those opposed to all abortion it is used to justify the medically necessary removal of a cancerous uterus despite the loss of an early fetus). In other cases it produces moral judgments practically nobody is happy with (it is used by some theologians to require the medically unnecessary removal of the site of an ectopic pregnancy whenever an ectopic pregnancy is terminated).

ECMO. Extracorporeal membrane oxygenation. A machine that provides oxygen for blood outside the body and then returns the blood to the body.

Electroencephalogram (EEG). A test capable of showing electrical activity in the brain. The absence of electrical activity helps to confirm a clinical diagnosis of brain death.

ELSI. Ethical, Legal, and Social Implications working group sponsored by NIH and DOE (Department of Energy) to consider the impact of the Human Genome Project.

ERISA. The Employee Retirement Income Security Act designed to protect employee benefit funds from burdensome state regulations. Managed care organizations now invoke it to prevent patients from suing them under state law for damages caused by negligence.

Ethics advisory board (EAB). A national ethics committee to review proposals for federally funded research on human subjects. The board ceased to exist when no funding was provided after 1980.

Eudaimonia. A Greek word, literally "good fate." *Eudaimonia* is living a happy and fulfilled life. Eudaimonism is a general term for any ethics whose founding intuition is that ethics is ultimately about the happiness of the moral agent. It stands in contrast to the modern theories whose founding intuition is that ethics is about the obligation and duties of the moral agent. When the word *eudaimonia* is expressed verbally, the accent falls on the second syllable from the end.

Euthanasia. Literally, a good death. The word is now used to describe the intentional killing of a patient by a physician.

FFS. Fee-for-service payment system. Providers provide services and then bill patients or a third-party payer for the services.

Futility. A term not susceptible to a satisfactory definition. In general it means a treatment that will not do any good. Intense debates about whether physicians should provide "futile" treatments demanded by patients or families arose during the 1990s.

Gamete. A sex cell, either a spermatozoon or an ovum.

Genome. All the genes in an organism.

Genotype. The genetic traits of an organism, both dormant and manifest. See phenotype.

GIFT. Gamete intrafallopian transfer. Sperm and ova are retrieved and then placed together in a fallopian tube before fertilization.

G-tube. Gastrostomy tube. A tube surgically inserted into the gastrointestinal system through the abdominal wall.

Guardian *ad litem.* A guardian appointed by a court to represent an incompetent person solely in matters pertaining to the particular case under consideration. The Latin word for a disputed legal process is *lis, litis*; it is the root for the English word litigation. Although almost anyone could be appointed a guardian *ad litem*, judges most often appoint attorneys whom they know. The guardian *ad litem* investigates the case and reports her findings to the judge. In cases involving health care, the guardian *ad litem* usually takes a position for or against the treatment at issue. States without provisions for a guardian *ad litem* have an alternative process whereby someone can speak for the interests of the incompetent person.

HGP. The Human Genome Project, the effort to identify the sequences of all the nucleotides (identified at A, G, C, T) in the DNA of a human cell.

HHS. The Department of Health and Human Services, a successor to HEW, the Department of Health, Education and Welfare. Disbursement of most federal monies for health care (e.g., Medicare and Medicaid) and medical research falls under its oversight.

HMO. Health maintenance organization. An insurance plan that actually delivers, and therefore controls, the health care it provides for its members. HMOs come in many versions and are a type of MCO.

Hospice. An interdisciplinary program of palliative care and supportive services for terminally ill patients and their families. The emphasis is on comforting the dying rather than on using techniques and technologies to extend the patient's life. The care may be provided at home or in a hospice center.

ICSI. Intracytoplasmic sperm injection. An increasingly popular process associated with IVF whereby a spermatozoon is forcibly inserted into an ovum to increase the chances of fertilization. It is not yet known whether forcing the gametes to combine will adversely affect the child.

IEC. Institutional ethics committee. A committee organized in a health care institution to assist providers, patients, and families with ethical issues associated with health care. Often simply called "the ethics committee."

Induction. In moral philosophy, induction is the reasoning process that uses the prevailing particular moral judgments in a society to generate the general principles and rules that serve as obligatory action guides. It is best understood in contrast with deduction (q.v.).

IPA. Independent practice associations. Associations of physicians maintaining their independent practices while contracting with managed care organizations.

IRB. Institutional review board. The federally mandated committee for the protection of human subjects (including fetuses) in medical research; required at all institutions receiving federal funding.

IVF. In vitro fertilization. The fertilization of an ovum in a laboratory. The term is sometimes used in a general way to designate any kind of medically assisted fertilization involving ovum retrieval.

Justice. (1) Fairness; benefits and burdens should be distributed fairly among members of groups, and similar cases should be treated in similar ways. (2) Entitlement; people should receive what is due to them by reason of explicit or implicit agreements. (3) An action-guiding moral principle proposed by many contemporary ethicists, obliging us to behave fairly with others and accord them what is due. (4) A moral virtue; that is, the habit, feeling, and behavior whereby we achieve our happiness by behaving fairly toward others and according them what is due.

Laparoscopy. Abdominal entry and exploration using an optical system inside a tube that can be inserted through a small incision.

Life-sustaining treatment. Treatment directed primarily at preserving life despite the disease rather than at curing the disease. Ventilators, feeding tubes, dialysis, and cardiopulmonary resuscitation are primarily life-sustaining treatments, whereas chemotherapy is a treatment directed primarily at curing disease.

Managed care. The insuring entity not only pays for but controls in various ways some of the health care of the people it covers.

MCO. Managed care organization. An insurance organization that manages in various ways the medical care it underwrites.

Medicaid. A program providing some health care services for people unable to support themselves. It is jointly funded by federal and state monies and administered by the individual states.

Medicare. The federally funded and administered program providing some health care services, chiefly for elderly people, disabled people, and patients with end-stage renal disease.

Minor. In the United States, a child is generally considered a minor until reaching his eighteenth birthday.

NABER. National Advisory Board on Ethics in Reproduction. A privately funded multidisciplinary group concerned with the ethics of reproductive research and practice.

National Bioethics Advisory Commission (NBAC). The commission established by executive order in late 1996 to make recommendations about the ethical issues in genetics and in medical research.

National Commission. The National Commission for the Protection of Human Subjects of Biomedical and Behavioral Research, authorized by Congress and in session from 1974 to 1978. One of its major reports is known as the Belmont Report (q.v.).

Naturalistic decision making. A decision-making tactic that recognizes in a particular situation, thanks to experience, a likely good decision without comparing all alternatives. See rational choice strategy.

Neocortical death. The irreversible cessation of the neocortical functions of the brain. If functions of other parts of the brain or of the brain stem continue, the person is not dead.

NG tube. Nasogastric tube. A tube inserted into the stomach through the nose.

NIH. The National Institutes of Health. The various institutes sponsor most of the government-funded medical research in the United States.

Nonmaleficence. An action-guiding moral principle proposed by some contemporary health care ethicists obliging us not to inflict harm on other people.

Palliative care. Medical and nursing care devoted to comfort rather than to cure or to the prolongation of life.

Partial-birth abortion. A procedure used in some late-term abortions whereby the lower body of a viable or periviable fetus is first pulled out of the uterus, and then its life is intentionally ended.

Patient Self-Determination Act (PSDA). A federal law, effective since 1991, requiring all institutions receiving federal funds to provide written information to patients about their right to make health care decisions.

Persistent vegetative state (PVS). An enduring state of total unconsciousness characterized by phases that alternate between what looks like sleep and what looks like awareness. Most cases of PVS are actually permanent—all consciousness has been irreversibly lost, and only a vegetative body remains. If feeding tubes are used, some vegetative bodies can be kept alive for years, sometimes for decades. Compare PVS with coma (q.v.).

Phenotype. The genetic traits of an organism that actually manifest themselves. Some genetic traits are coded in the DNA but never appear. See genotype.

Phronesis. Aristotle's term for the kind of reasoning suited for moral deliberation. Because there is no real English equivalent, some authors do not translate the word. A close English word is prudence, but it must be used carefully. When the word phronesis is used verbally, the first syllable is the accented syllable.

Physician-assisted suicide. A physician helping a patient to kill him or herself.

PPO. Preferred provider organization. An MCO with a list of preferred providers that allows patients to seek care from providers not on the list if they pay some of the cost.

Premoral evil. The term used by some theologians to designate bad things that are not morally evil. Killing someone is a premoral evil—it destroys human life—but it is not a moral evil unless done intentionally without an adequate reason. Similar terms used by some theologians are ontic evil and nonmoral evil.

President's Commission. The President's Commission for the Study of Ethical Problems in Medicine and Biomedical and Behavioral Research, authorized by Congress in 1978 and in session from 1980 to 1983. The President's Commission produced nine valuable reports, among them *Making Health Care Decisions* (1982) and *Deciding to Forego* [sic] *Life-Sustaining Treatment* (1983).

President's Council on Bioethics (PCB). President Bush established the Council by executive order in 2001, and it is authorized through September 2009. Among its important reports are *The Changing Moral Focus of Newborn Screening* (2008), *Human Dignity and Bioethics* (2008), *Taking Care: Ethical Caregiving in Our Aging Society* (2005), *Reproduction and Responsibility: The Regulation of New Biotechnologies* (2004), *Monitoring Stem Cell Research* (2004), and *Human Cloning and Human Dignity* (2002).

Primitive streak. A dark and thickening band forming on the early embryonic disk about the fifteenth day after fertilization; it marks the future longitudinal axis of the embryo.

Principle. (1) In classical moral philosophies, the very first point of departure for the moral theory; everything else in the theory is derived from the originating principle. Principle in this sense means *beginning* (*principium* in Latin and *arche* in Greek). (2) In most modern moral philosophies, a principle is an action guide derived from a deontological or a utilitarian theory or from experience or from a common morality. Principle taken in this sense means *authority* (in Latin *princeps* means prince or ruler). Moral principles understood as action guides imply moral behavior that is best understood as behavior governed by authoritative principles and rules.

Prostaglandins. Fatty acid derivatives; some cause uterine contractions and are used to cause abortions.

Proxy. (1) The person making a decision on behalf of a person without decision-making capacity. Another term for proxy is surrogate. (2) The document recognized by some states whereby persons can designate a proxy or surrogate to make decisions for them if they ever become incapacitated. Sometimes these documents refer to the proxy or surrogate as the "agent."

Prudence. The intellectual decision-making virtue of practical reasoning managing our natural inclinations so they enhance our life and happiness. Natural inclinations managed well are the moral virtues.

RAC. NIH's Recombinant DNA Advisory Committee that reviews proposals for genetic research on humans.

Rational choice strategy. A decision-making strategy that recommends comparing the benefits and burdens of all options simultaneously or serially before making a choice. See naturalistic decision making.

Rights. (1) Natural or human rights are proposed by many as moral claims enjoyed by all human beings by virtue of being human. Theories of natural rights were first developed as political theories in the seventeenth century by Thomas Hobbes and John Locke. They served as powerful notions supporting the American Revolution in 1776 and the French Revolution in 1789. Three major natural rights are the rights to life, liberty, and property. Advocates of natural or human rights differ on the source of these rights; some say they come from the Creator, others say they simply inhere in human nature. (2) Political, civil, or contractual rights are claims enjoyed by human beings in virtue of their membership in a political or civil society, or in virtue of being parties to a contract. (3) In everyday usage, the word "right" is often used to justify whatever a person wants or needs. Although often abused, the language of rights has been a powerful influence in elevating moral consciousness and securing respect for human beings.

Slippery-slope argument. An argument that claims a proposal is not really morally objectionable in itself but should be rejected nonetheless because it will inevitably, or almost inevitably, lead to morally objectionable actions. The argument is that once you take the first step on a slippery slope, you will not be able to prevent sliding down into a moral abyss. This argument is also known as the wedge argument—once you get the wedge in place, the object can be more easily moved, and as the camel's nose argument—once you let the camel get his nose in the tent, the rest of him will soon follow.

Stoicism. Ancient school of philosophy founded by Zeno in Athens at the end of the fourth century B.C.E. and exerting a major influence on the Greek and Roman worlds until the fourth century C.E. Stoics taught that all nature in the universe is structured and functions in a rational way. Human nature is no exception, and hence our moral task is to live according to nature. Human nature has two components: it is organic (hence, living according to nature means eating, drinking, sex, pleasure, comfort, etc.), and it is rational (hence, living according to nature also means the rational control and transformation of our organic needs and impulses).

Substituted judgment. (1) A proxy knows what the patient without decision-making capacity wants and simply reports this to the physician. Substituted judgment is best understood in contrast with best interests (q.v.). (2) Some courts use substituted judgment in an idiosyncratic way to designate what a judge claims to know never-competent patients—babies, for example—would want if they were competent.

Surrogate. See Proxy.

Teleology. Any moral philosophy (*logos*) based on outcome or end result (*telos*). Traditional teleological theories were eudaimonistic (*eudaimonia*, q.v.) moralities founded on the goal of living a good life—whatever truly constitutes living well for the moral agent is moral. The most popular modern teleological theory, utilitarianism (q.v.), makes the greatest good of the greatest number the desired moral goal—whatever constitutes the greatest social welfare is moral. Teleology stands in contrast to deontology (q.v.).

TPN. Total parenteral nutrition; nutrition meeting all bodily requirements inserted into the venous system rather than the gastrointestinal tract.

Tracheotomy. Also tracheostomy; an incision in the trachea (throat) to open an airway. Many patients on ventilators for an extended period have a tracheotomy to allow insertion of the ventilator tube directly into the throat rather than through the mouth.

Triage. Originally the prioritizing of scarce resources in an emergency by organizing the injured into three groups: those who can do without the resources for now, those who will probably not benefit from the resources, and those who will benefit from the resources and need them to survive. Triage has now come to mean directing patients to appropriate care, i.e., to an emergency room, to an urgent care facility, to a physician's office, etc.

Uniform Determination of Death Act (UDDA). This act serves as a model for accepting two criteria of death—the cardiopulmonary criterion and the brain-death criterion.

Utilitarianism. The moral philosophy based on the greatest good for the greatest number. Whatever actions or, more commonly, whatever principles or rules bring about the greatest good for the greatest number are moral.

Utility. The ultimate moral principle or law proposed by utilitarians as the origin of all morality and as the source of moral obligation. Sometimes it is called the "greatest happiness principle," where happiness is understood as the happiness of everyone. John Stuart Mill formulated it thus: "Utility, or the greatest happiness principle, holds that actions are right in proportion as they tend to promote happiness, wrong as they tend to produce the reverse of happiness." From the principle of utility, most utilitarians derive various moral rules of obligation.

Vasopressor. An agent that stimulates contraction of arteries and veins, thus working to increase blood pressure. The treatments are given to prevent or reverse low blood pressure. For some patients vasopressors are truly life-sustaining treatments because without them they would suffer cardiac arrest.

Viability. The gestational age when a fetus could survive outside the uterus. Once thought to be the beginning of the third trimester (about 26 weeks), viability has now been achieved several weeks earlier in some cases. A viable fetus in the uterus is considered a fetus; a viable fetus expelled or removed is considered a premature baby.

Virtue. Excellence. When a thing or a being functions well, the Greeks called its functioning *excellent* or *virtuous*. When a person manages her natural inclinations well, she is *morally* excellent. Achieving authentic moral excellence requires prudence, the *intellectual* excellence relevant to ethics.

Xenograft. Transplantation of an organ or tissue from one species to another.

ZIFT. Zygote intrafallopian transfer. Placing fertilized ova in fallopian tubes.

Index of Cases

Abigail Alliance v. Von Eschenbach, 495 F3d 695 (2007), cert. denied 128 S. Ct 1069 (2008)
Abigail Alliance for Better Access to Developmental Drugs v. Von Eschenbach, 445 F3d 470 (2007)
Matter of A.C., 573 A.2d 1235 (1990)
City of Akron v. Akron Center for Reproductive Health, 462 U.S. 416 (1983)
Barber v. Superior Court, 147 Cal. App. 3d 1006 (1983)
Bartling v. Superior Court, 163 Cal. App. 3d 186 (1984)
Bellotti v. Baird, 443 U.S. 622 (1979)
Bouvia v. Superior Court (Glenchur), 179 Cal. App. 3d 1127 (1986)
Brophy v. New England Sinai Hospital, 497 N.E.2d 626 (1986)
Buck v. Bell, 274 U.S. 200 (1927)
Canterbury v. Spence, 464 F.2d 772 (1972), cert. denied, 409 U.S. 1064 (1973)
Care and Protection of Beth, 587 N.E.2d 1377 (1992)
Carey v. Population Services International, 431 U.S. 678 (1977)
Matter of Claire Conroy, 486 A.2d 1209 (1985)
Compassion in Dying v. Washington, 79 F.3d 790 (1996)
Cruzan v. Director, Missouri Dept. of Health, 497 U.S. 261 (1990)
Davis v. Davis, 842 S.W.2d 588 (1992)
Matter of Dinnerstein, 380 N.E.2d (1978)
Doe v. Bolton, 410 U.S. 179 (1973)
Doe v. Sullivan, 938 F.2d 1370 (1991)
Matter of Infant Doe, No.GU8204–00 (Cir.Ct., Monroe County, Ind., 1982)
Matter of Jane Doe, 583 N.E.2d. 1263 (1992)
Eisenstadt v. Baird, 405 U.S. 438 (1972)
Gilgunn v. Massachusetts General Hospital, Superior Ct. Suffolk County (verdict) No. 92–4820 (1995)
Gonzales v. Carhart, 550 U.S. 124 (2000)
Gray v. Romero, 697 F. Supp. 580 (1988)
Griswold v. Connecticut, 381 U.S. 479 (1965)
Matter of Howe, No.03 P 1255, 2004 (Mass. Prob.& Fam. Ct. Mar. 22, 2004)
Hudson v. Texas Children's Hospital, No. 01–05–00143-CV (First Court of Appeals, Mar. 1, 2005)
Matter of Jobes, 529 A.2d 434 (1987)
Matter of Baby K, 16 F.3d 590 (1994)
Kass v. Kass, 91 N.Y.2d 554 (1998)
Lane v. Candura, 376 N.E.2d 1232 (1978)
Matter of Baby M, 537 A.2d 1277 (1988)
Maher v. Roe, 432, U.S. 464 (1977)
Matter of Martin, 538 N.W.2d 399 (1995)
Mills v. Rogers, 457 U.S. 291 (1982)
Custody of a Minor, 434 N.E.2d 601 (1982)
Mohr v. Williams, 104 N.W. 12 (1905)
Matter of Mary O'Connor, 531 N.E.2d 207 (1988)
Planned Parenthood v. Danforth, 428 U.S. 52 (1976)
Planned Parenthood Association of Southeastern Pennsylvania v. Casey, 112 S.Ct. 2791 (1992)
Poe v. Ullman, 367 U.S. 498 (1961)
Pratt v. Davis, 79 N.E. 562 (1906)

Prince v. Massachusetts, 321 U.S. 158 (1944)

Quill v. Vacco, 80 F.3d 716 (1996)

Matter of Quinlan, 355 A.2d 647 (1976)

Rennie v. Klein, 720 F.2d 266 (1983)

Rivers v. Katz, 495 N.E.2d 337 (1986)

Roe v. Wade, 410 U.S. 113 (1973)

Guardianship of Roe III, 421 N.E.2d 40 (1981)

Rogers v. Okin, 478 F.Supp. 1342 (1979); 738 F.2d 1 (1984)

Salgo v. Leland Stanford Jr. University Board of Trustees, 317 P.2d 170 (1957)

Satz v. Perlmutter, 362 So.2d 160 (1978), affd., 379 So.2d 359 (1980)

Schindler v. Schiavo, 866 So.2d 136 (2004)

Theresa Schindler Schiavo v. Michael Schiavo, No. 05–11638, U.S. Ct. of Appeals, 11th Circuit, March 30, 2005

Schloendorff v. Society of N.Y. Hospital, 105 N.E. 92 (1914)

Severns v. Wilmington Medical Center, 425 A.2d 1565 (1980)

Skinner v. Oklahoma, 316 U.S. 535 (1942)

Matter of Spring, 405 N.E.2d 115 (1980)

Stenberg v. Carhart, 530 U.S. 914 (2000)

Matter of Storar (Brother Fox), 420 N.F.2d 64 (1981)

Superintendent of Belchertown State School v. Saikewicz, 370 N.E.2d 417 (1977)

Thornburgh v. American College of Obstetricians and Gynecologists, 476 U.S. 747 (1986)

Vacco v. Quill, 117 S.Ct. 2293 (1997)

Matter of Conservatorship of Helga Wanglie, 4th Jud. Dist., PX-91–283 Minnesota, Hennipen County (1991)

Washington v. Glucksberg, 117 S.Ct. 2258 (1997)

Webster v. Reproductive Health Services, 492 U.S. 490 (1989)

Index

Abigail Alliance for Better Access to Developmental Drugs, 471, 473, 477, 482
abortion
AMA on, 266
Aristotle on, 15, 124
Bible on, 125, 265
Catholic Church on, 58, 59, 236, 265–66, 274, 283–84
as contraceptive, 430
in ectopic pregnancies, 59, 274–75, 283–84
and fetal research, 375, 376, 378
and genetic testing, 430
and Hippocratic Oath, 51
historical review, 265–66, 282
Hyde Amendments, 268–69
and informed consent, 79–80, 109, 269–70
late-term, 121–22, 271, 284
medical procedures, 271–72
for minors, 109, 269
and multiple pregnancies, 275, 284
in other countries, 267, 277, 283
and parental consent, 109, 120, 268, 269
partial-birth, 271, 272–73, 488
and premature rupture of membranes, 276
and prenatal life, 64, 121–22, 219, 267
and prenatal testing, 430
and privacy, 109, 332, 333
and public funding, 268–69
rights-based arguments about, 10, 64, 229, 264, 273
and RU-486, 276–78, 284–85
to save woman's life, 122, 265, 266, 272
and seriously defective fetuses, 275–76
as something bad, 273–74
spontaneous, 124, 132, 232, 378
statistics, 264, 266, 282
and stem cell research, 370
Supreme Court decisions on, 109, 155, 239, 266–73, 282–83
trimester framework, 121–22, 269, 270
actions and omissions, 48–49
act-utilitarianism, 382–83
adoption, 243–44, 256

advance directives, 87–91, 92, 95–96, 98
combined, 96
durable power of attorney, 90
Hazel Welch controversy, 93–95
living wills, 88
medical care directives, 88–90
proxy designations, 90–91
PVS patients and, 153, 226, 227, 337
treatment directives, 87–90, 91–92
See also Texas Advance Directives Act (ADA)
ADVANTAGE clinical trial, 479–80, 482–83
Advisory Committee on Human Radiation Experiments, 366–67
African Americans, 359
AIDS/HIV research, 380–86, 392
Alexander, Leo, 390
Alito, Samuel, 272
allele, 421, 431, 432
Alliance for Human Research Protection, 455
altered nuclear transfer (ANT), 371, 372, 391
American Academy of Pediatrics, 120, 282, 296
American Cancer Society, 361, 428, 476
American College of Obstetricians and Gynecologists, 272, 282
American College of Surgeons, 77
American Fertility Society, 248, 260
American Medical Association (AMA)
on abortion, 266
on defining futility, 54, 199
on DNR orders, 187
and genetic research, 434
on interventions by medical students, 83
on organ procurement for transplantation, 416
on physician-assisted suicide, 50, 327
on sedation in end-of-life care, 331
American Neurological Association, 138
American Psychiatric Association, 111
American Society for Reproductive Medicine, 248, 258, 260
amicus curiae briefs, 77, 485
anencephaly, 288–89
and abortion, 275–76

anencephaly (*continued*)
  genetics of, 432
  and infant organ donation, 289, 318, 399–400,
    417
  and ventilator use, 292
  See also Baby K
Angell, Marcia, 383
Angie (Angela Carder) (case), 279–82, 285
Anglican Church, 236
animals
  medical research on, 387–89, 393, 439
  mistreatment of, 14
  and organ transplantation, 409–13
  rights of, 393
anovulants, 108, 236, 240, 485
Antiochus, 9
applied normative ethics, 11, 364–65
Aquinas, Thomas
  and Aristotle, xv, 5, 15, 20, 43, 60
  on direct and indirect behavior, 56, 67
  on ethics of the good, 13, 15, 21, 27
  on fetus and human life, 126, 133
  on immoral actions, 58
  on law, 18
  on life after death, 15, 26
  on love as crowning virtue, 7
  on pride and humility, 30
  on prudence, xiv, xvii, 31, 32, 33, 35–36, 37,
    44–45, 155
  on reason as first principle, 61, 68, 163, 310
  on theoretical and practical intelligence, 31,
    32, 42
Aristippus, 54
Aristotle
  biographical information, xv
  on choosing the "less worse" option, 26–27,
    347
  on happiness and good, 4, 13, 15, 20, 21, 22,
    24, 25, 26, 31, 43–44, 95
  on human body and soul, 123–24, 450
  on importance of religion, 42
  inductive reasoning of, 11
  on infanticide, 60, 287, 322, 352
  on judging immoral actions, xvi, 4, 58, 68
  and naturalistic decision making, 29, 38, 39,
    40
  on need for law, 363
  nonbelief in life after death, 15, 26
  on *phronesis*, 28, 32, 44, 489
  on politics, 14, 23, 458, 467, 476
  on pride, 29–30
  on prudence and prudential reasoning, xiv,
    xv, xvi, xvii, 5, 32, 33, 35, 38, 68, 155
  on reproduction and fetus, 124, 147

  on suicide, 15, 322, 339
  on theoretical and practical intelligence, 31, 32
  on virtue and morality, 7, 20, 26, 29, 30, 31,
    36, 119
ART (artificial reproductive technologies), 258,
    259–60, 485
artificial hearts, 395, 414–16, 418
artificial insemination, 60, 243–44, 430
  Catholic Church opposition to, 59
  and surrogate motherhood, 253, 254
Ashcroft, John, 327
Ashley (case), 312–16, 319–20
Augustine, 57, 388, 450
  on fetus, 125
  on sex and contraception, 234–35, 241
  on suicide, 323
Austria, 401
autonomous moral law, 10
autonomy, principle of, 16–17, 61, 382
  as action-guiding principle, 12, 16–17, 364,
    365, 367, 382, 406, 485
autonomy and self-determination, patient
  defined, 485
  and demands for futile treatment, 54, 170
  and euthanasia, 334, 336–37
  minors and, 109
  nondirective counseling and, 428
  as principle in American bioethics, 12, 27, 97
  vs. medical paternalism, 50–52, 70
  and withdrawal of life-sustaining treatment,
    211
AZT research, 380–82, 392

Baby Doe (case), 298–300, 319
Baby Doe regulations, 293–98, 319
  and "Baby Doe Squads," 294, 295, 300, 303
  enforcement of, 297–98
  ethical issues, 293–94, 300
  history of, 294–95
  reaction to, 296–97
  substance of, 295–96
Baby Fae (case), 410–13, 417–18
Baby Jane Doe (case), 292, 301–4
Baby K (case), 309–12, 319
Babylonians, 4, 8
Baby M (case), 255–56, 260
bad and immoral distinction, 64–65, 68–69
Bailey, Leonard, 410–11, 412, 413
barbiturates, 325, 346–47, 485
Barnard, Christiaan, 394
Bartling, William (case), 158–62, 179
Batshaw, Mark, 437, 438, 443
Bayh-Dole Act of 1980, 440

Beauchamp, Tom
  Principles of Biomedical Ethics, 365
Beecher, Henry, 362–63, 390
  Experimentation in Man, 363
behavior genetics, 449–50
Belgium
  euthanasia in, 325, 339, 354
  organ donation in, 401
Belmont Report
  about, 364, 485
  principle-based approach of, 16, 364, 382
Benedict XVI, Pope, 227
beneficence, 52, 382
  as action-guiding principle, 12, 16–17, 27, 364,
    365, 367, 382, 406, 485
  defined, 485
Bentham, Jeremy
  on animals, 388, 393
  utilitarianism of, 10, 22, 27
best interests standard
  about, 103, 117–18, 485
  limitations of, 118
  in proxy decisions for children, 292–93, 379
  in proxy decisions for mentally ill, 114, 116
  and withdrawing life-sustaining treatment,
    151, 172, 175
beta-thalassemia, 429–31
Beth (case), 102, 119
biases
  in language, 62, 63
  psychological and social, 5, 41, 119
Bible, xvi, 51, 485
  on abortion and fetus, 125, 265
  on animals, 387, 388
  and contraception, 233, 234
  and killing, 58, 322, 339
  miracles in, 55
  on moral living, xviii, 22–23
  on suicide, 322–23
  on surrogate motherhood, 253
  Ten Commandments in, 4, 8, 57, 322, 338
bipolar illness, 112
Borromeo, Charles, 236
Bouvia, Elizabeth (case), 212–15, 230
brain death, 135–44, 147–48, 398–99
  and anencephaly, 289
  in children, 137, 399
  and "conscience clauses," 138
  defined, 136, 485
  determining, 136–38, 397, 398–99
  development of concept, 135–36
  and fetus analogy, 145
  and organ transplantation, 137, 138, 398–99
  problems with determining, 137–39
  See also death

BRCA genes, 425, 454
  testing for, 425–29
breast cancer, 424–29, 432
Breyer, Stephen, 272
Britain, 258, 300, 373
Brophy, Paul, 53
Brother Fox (case), 156–58, 179
Burger, Warren E., 270
Burroughs, Abigail (case), 470–74, 482
Bush, George W., 272, 452, 463
  establishes President's Council, 368, 489
  and Schiavo controversy, 226
  on stem cell research, 370, 372
Bush, Jeb, 225, 226
Buxton, Peter, 358–59

Campbell, A. G. M., 287
Canada, 249, 253
Candura, Rosaria (case), 78–79, 175–78, 180
Canterbury, Jerry (case), 77–78
capital punishment, 15, 323, 324
capitation, 461, 485
Caplan, Arthur, 436, 441, 445
Carder, Angela. *See* Angie
cardiopulmonary criterion of death, 134–35,
    396–97, 417
  problems with, 139–42
Caritas Catholica Vlaanderen, 325
carrier (genetics), 422, 424, 486
  See also genetic testing
Carroll, William, 476
casuistry, 11, 486
categorical imperative, 59, 60–61, 486
Catholic Church
  on abortion, 58, 59, 236, 274, 283–84
  on contraception, 234, 235–38, 259
  on euthanasia, 325
  on in vitro fertilization, 245
  moral theology of, 56, 57–59, 406–7
  on prenatal testing, 431
  on withdrawal of life-sustaining treatment,
    152, 204, 225, 227–28, 231
  See also Christianity
Centers for Disease Control (CDC), 264, 381
  and Tuskegee study, 358–59
chemotherapy
  double effect of, 55
  as restorative treatment, 150, 488
  withdrawing and withholding, 49, 53, 346, 347
child abuse laws, 106, 111, 300
children
  birth defects, 246, 247, 261
  brain death in, 137, 399
  decision making for, 99, 105–11, 119–20

children (*continued*)
  emancipated minors, 108
  genetic research and testing on, 424, 445
  informed consent for, 378–79
  and in vitro fertilization, 258, 261
  legal age for decision making, 106–7, 488
  and medical research, 378–79, 392, 445
  moral development of, 14, 106–7, 119
  and organ transplantation, 104–5, 148–49,
    289, 318, 399–400, 402–6, 410–13
Childress, James
  Principles of Biomedical Ethics, 365
Christianity
  on abortion, 125, 265–66
  on contraception, 233–35
  on divine law, 8
  on euthanasia, 323
  on human soul, 123, 125–26
  on killing, 323–24
  moral theology in, 17, 22–23, 41
  and organ donation, 407
  and pride, 30
  Reformation in, 51
  and Stoicism, 9
  See also Catholic Church
Chrysostom, John, 388
Cicero, 32, 37, 323
  on natural law, 9, 18
"clear and convincing evidence" criterion, 158,
  217, 219
clinical trials, 66, 277, 357, 368, 379–82, 477–78,
  482
Clinton, Bill, 366, 377
  and abortion, 271, 277
  on cloning, 251, 368
cloning
  Catholic Church on, 58, 59
  defined, 249–50, 486
  process, 250–51
  readings, 261–62, 368
  research on, 252–53
  and stem cells, 371–72, 374
Code of Hammurabi, 4
coherentism, 11
coma
  defined, 486
  and PVS, 104, 143, 149
"common morality," xv, 12, 14, 16, 17, 19, 367
compassionate use, 469, 470–71, 472, 473, 475,
  476–77
competence (legal term), 72
Concern for Dying, 88
conflicts of interest
  and experimental procedures, 412

  of IVF clinics, 246
  in physician-assisted suicide, 345–46
  of proxies, 99, 293
  of researchers and drug companies, 435, 440,
    441, 444–45, 447
conjoined twins, 290–91, 318
Conroy, Claire (case), 209–12, 230
contraception
  abortion as, 430
  Bible on, 233, 234
  birth control pill, 236–37
  Catholic Church on, 58, 59, 234, 235–38, 259
  in history, 233–34
  Kant on, 59, 60, 68
  laws against, 233, 238–40, 259
  as medical intervention, 233, 238, 240
  for minors, 108–9, 120, 242
  as moral issue, 232–33, 238, 240–42, 258
  natural family planning method, 236, 241
  readings, 259
Contract Research Organization (CRO), 479
Controlled Substances Act (CSA), 326–27
Convention on Human Rights and Biomedicine, 448
Cooley, Denton, 395, 414
Copernicus, 31
Council for International Organizations of
  Medical Sciences (CIOMS), 383, 385–86
CPR (cardiopulmonary resuscitation)
  defined, 181–82
  distinguishing expected/unexpected arrest,
    189
  on elderly, 183, 189–90
  guidelines for, 184–85
  history of, 182
  learning to withhold, 183–85
  low success rate, 182–83, 200–201
  on newborns, 183, 188, 200
  on organ donors, 139–40, 397–98
  and patient choice, 185
  prudence and, 190
  readings, 200
  during transfers, 188–89
  when inappropriate, 71, 187, 198–99
  See also DNR (do-not-resuscitate order);
    ECMO (extracorporeal membrane
    oxygenation)
CPR controversies
  Catherine Gilgunn, 195–99
  Maria M., 190–93
  Rose Dreyer, 184
  Shirley Dinnerstein, 193–95
C. R. Bard, Inc., 366
Crick, Francis, 420, 451

Cruzan, Nancy (case), 158, 216–20, 230, 471
Cyprus, 431, 455
Cyreanaic school, 43
cystic fibrosis, 422, 429, 435, 451, 454
   defined, 486

Dabis, Mary Sue and Junior (case), 247–48, 261
Danielle (case), 304–9, 319
DCD (donation after circulatory death), 139–42
death
   brain death criterion of, 135–39, 397, 398–99
   cardiopulmonary criterion of, 134–35, 139–42, 396–97, 417
   determination of, 122, 147, 396–97
   intentionally causing/letting die distinction, 49–50, 66–67, 211
   life after, 15, 26
   neocortical, 142–44, 398
   and organ retrieval, 395–99
   "right to die," 10, 16, 229, 324, 334, 341, 349, 352
   when one ceases to be one of us, 13, 134–37, 263
   See also brain death; killing
Death with Dignity Act (DWDA), 326–27, 345, 354, 356
DeBakey, Michael, 414
decision making
   bad, 41
   capacity for, 71, 72–75, 96–97, 99
   clinical/ethical potential conflict in, 72
   by courts, 102, 172, 174, 180, 186, 316
   and expertise, 39
   impairments to, 71, 74, 99
   for mentally ill, 99, 111–17, 120
   naturalistic, 38–39, 45–46, 488
   for older children, 105–11
   paternalistic, 50–52, 70, 74, 78, 95, 116
   for patients of other cultures, 117
   physicians' responsibility in, 70–71, 74, 99
   readings, 45–46
   recognition-primed, 39
   religious faith and, 52, 74
   and younger children, 99, 110–11
   See also proxy decision makers; prudence and prudential reasoning
Declaration of Helsinki, 383–84
deductive reasoning, 17, 31–32, 33, 34, 40, 68
   defined, 486
   in health care ethics, 12
   model of, 10–11
deliberation, 40
deontology, 10, 57, 367, 486
   in health care ethics, 16

Department of Health and Human Services (HHS), 140, 294, 363, 400, 401
   about, 487
depression, 112
Descartes, René, 133
   on animals, 387, 393
   on mind and body, 23, 450
Desert Storm, Operation, 386–87
DeVries, William, 395, 414
diagnosis-related groups (DRGs), 461–62, 486
dialysis, 49, 150, 171
   and Earle Spring controversy, 171–75
   See also life-sustaining treatment
Diane (case), 346–51, 355
diaphragmatic hernias, 291–92
Dickey Amendment, 369, 370
Diekema, Douglas, 313, 314
Dinnerstein, Shirley (case), 193–95, 201
direct and indirect effects, 55–56, 67, 349–50
disabled people
   discrimination against handicapped, 293, 294, 303
   organ transplants to, 419
   vulnerability in medical research, 386
discrimination
   genetic testing and, 423, 450, 452, 454–55, 456
   against handicapped, 293, 294, 303
   against HIV-infected, 385
disseminated intravascular coagulation (DIC), 443
divine law, 6, 8, 18, 41
DNA, 421–22, 434
   defined, 486
   and genetic therapy, 433
   and germ-line genetic research, 447–48
   and Human Genome Project, 451–52
   structure of, 420
DNR (do-not-resuscitate order)
   after discharge, 189
   and anesthesia, 186, 201
   conditions for, 187–88
   court approval for, 102, 186
   decided on by provider, 54, 184
   defined, 182, 486
   ethical elements for, 105–06
   evolution of policy on, 184–85
   overriding of, 189, 200
   by proxy, 187–88, 189, 190, 192–93
   readings, 200–201
   and "slow" and "show" codes, 186, 200
   unreasonable refusal of, 187, 195–99
   See also CPR (cardiopulmonary resuscitation)
Donahue, Phil, 404
donation after cardiac death (DCD), 397, 417

double effect, 55–56, 65, 331–32, 486
Douglas, William A., 238–39
Down syndrome, 22, 290, 299, 300, 432
  See also Baby Doe (case)
Dreyer, Rose (case), 184
Drinker, Philip, 150
drug abuse
  and Controlled Substances Act, 326
  and minors, 105, 108, 109
drug companies
  clinical trials by, 469
  and experimental drugs, 473–74, 475, 476
  and genetic research, 435, 444, 447, 451
  and health care costs, 460, 462
  use of seeding trials and ghostwriters,
    478–80, 482–83
Duchenne muscular dystrophy (DMD), 474
Duff, Raymond, 287
durable power of attorney, 90
Durand, 57–58

ECMO (extracorporeal membrane oxygen-
    ation), 141–42, 188, 201, 291–92, 486
electroencephalogram (EEG), 135, 137, 487
ELSI (Ethical, Legal, and Social Implications),
    452, 456, 487
embryo
  fetus/embryo distinction, 263
  frozen, 247–48, 258
  genetic testing of, 453–54
  as human life, 130, 145, 232, 264
  informed consent for use of, 248, 374–75
  and in vitro fertilization, 247–48
  moral status of, 248–49
  not yet "one of us," 127, 373, 374
  research on, 368–75, 391
  See also fertilization; fetus; stem cell research
emergency medical technicians (EMTs), 84
Emergency Medical Treatment and Active
    Labor Act (EMTALA), 311–12
end-of-life care
  palliative, 331, 356
  physicians and, 92–93
  readings, 98, 180
ends and means, 10, 12, 33
EPEC (Education of Physicians on End-of-life
    Care), 98
Epicurus and Epicureans, 15, 22, 43, 322
Erbitux, 470, 472, 474
ERISA (Employee Retirement Income
    Security Act), 487
Erlotinib, 471, 474
ethics
  changing values, xvii, 4, 60, 338

and choice, 1–2
and clinical decisions, 95
contemporary bioethics, 16–17, 19
and ethical behavior, xvii–xviii
evaluating good and bad in, 2–3, 5
as judgmental, 5–6
as normative, 3–4, 17
as personal, 5–6
principles in, 489
and public policy, 332–33
readings, 17
and reasoning, 4–6
as theoretical, 6
See also principle-based ethics; prudence and
    prudential reasoning; virtue-based ethics
ethics advisory board (EAB), 368–69, 377, 487
ethics of the good. See virtue-based ethics
eudaimonia, xvii, 21, 43, 487
eugenics, 427–28
euthanasia and physician-assisted suicide, 50,
    324–25
  active and passive, 330
  AMA opposition to, 50
  arguments against, 336–46
  arguments for, 334–35
  in Belgium, 325, 339
  case study of Diane, 346–51
  Catholic Church on, 58, 325
  Christian tradition against, 323
  and courts, 327–29, 354–55, 356
  and Death with Dignity Act, 326–27, 345, 354,
    356
  defended as normal medical practice, 335, 338
  defended as relief of suffering, 335, 337–38
  defined, 321, 487, 489
  as divisive for health care providers, 341
  and ethics of the good, 26
  euthanasia/physician-assisted suicide
    distinction, 329–30
  financial incentives for, 345–46, 355
  historical overview, 321–24, 352
  of infants, 60, 287–88, 289, 317, 318, 319, 387
  informed consent to, 337, 355
  intent and causality in, 328–29
  Kevorkian and, 324, 326, 348, 350, 351, 355
  as killing, 332, 333–34, 355
  Nazi Germany and, 229, 343
  in the Netherlands, 317–18, 325, 331, 343–45,
    353
  possibility of mistakes in, 340
  and public policy, 332–33, 340–42
  readings, 352–56
  religious argument against, 338–39
  right-to-life groups and, 92

slippery slope arguments on, 144, 212, 229, 317–18, 329, 342–45, 355
state laws on, 326–27
terminal sedation and, 331–32
voluntary, involuntary, and nonvoluntary, 330–31
Euthanasia Society of America, 88
experimental drugs
clinical trial phase, 469
for dying patients, 66, 445–46, 468–78
politicians and, 476
stories
Abigail Burroughs, 470–74
Jacob Gunvalson, 474–75
Penelope London, 475–76
expertise, definition, 39

fee-for-service (FFS), 458, 487
and rising health care costs, 55, 459–60, 461
feminism, 17
fertilization
and mutations, 432
process, 127, 131–32, 241, 247
and seed theory, 124, 126
See also embryo; fetus; in vitro fertilization (IVF)
fetus
Aristotle on, 124, 147
becoming sentient, 132–33, 145, 263
Bible on, 125
and brain death analogy, 145
early Christianity on, 125–26
embryo/fetus distinction, 263
and fathers' responsibility, 389
fetal-maternal conflicts, 278–82
as human life, 130, 263, 282, 377
research on, 375–77, 391
scientific discoveries about, 127
viability of, 263
when it becomes "one of us," 13, 124, 145, 263
See also abortion; embryo; prenatal care
Feyens, Thomas, 126
Finkel, Richard, 475
Fischer, Alain, 446
Fiske, Jamie (case), 402–3, 417
Food and Drug Administration (FDA)
drug approval by, 468–69, 477–78, 482
and experimental drugs, 469–70, 471, 473, 475
and genetic research, 439, 441–43, 447
and RU-486, 277
and Vioxx, 479–80
Frankena, William, 2–3, 11, 17
Frederick the Great, 324
Freud, Sigmund, 339

Friedman, Theodore, 444
futility
AMA on, 54, 199
definition, 487
difficulties in determining, 53–55, 198, 199
legislation on, 463–68
patient self-determination and, 54, 170
readings, 67
See also Texas Advance Directives Act (ADA)

Gaius, 18
Galen, 147
Galileo, 31, 33, 63, 127
gametes, 59, 249, 258–59, 374
defined, 487
Gelsinger, Jesse (case), 435–46, 455
genes, 420, 423, 449–50
genetic diseases, 422
four classes, 431–33
genetic engineering, 372, 421, 434, 448, 473
genetic enhancement, 449–51, 456
Genetic Information Nondiscrimination Act (GINA), 423, 452, 456
genetic research, 431–49
on children, 445
conflicts of interest in, 440, 441, 444–45, 447
deaths from, 437–38, 446–47
germ-line, 447–49, 455
on human subjects, 434–35
private capital in, 435
public concerns, 433–34
readings, 456
stories
Jesse Gelsinger, 435–46
Jolee Mohr, 446–47, 456
SCID trial in France, 446
genetics
history, 127, 420
human genetic code, 121, 421–22
and Human Genome Project, 451–52, 456
mutations, 422, 425–26, 431–32, 434–35
readings, 453–57
See also cloning
genetic screening, 429–31
genetic testing, 423, 454
for breast cancer, 425–29
of children, 424
and discrimination, 423, 450, 452, 454–55, 456
of embryos, 453–54
for genetic predispositions, 424–25
genetic therapy, 422–23, 431, 433
commercial use, 435
and genetic enhancement, 450
and genetic research, 445, 455

genome, 422, 487
genotype, 422, 424, 433, 451
  defined, 487
Germany, 399, 417
Germany, Nazi
  euthanasia in, 229, 343
  human experimentation in, 359–60, 389–90
ghostwriting, 479, 480, 483
GIFT (gamete intrafallopian transfer), 249–50, 253, 487
Giles, Joan, 360
Gilgunn, Catherine (case), 195–99, 201
Gilligan, Carol, 3
Gleevec, 477–78
Glucksberg, Harold, 327
Goldby, Stephen, 360
Gonzalez, Alberto, 327
Gonzalez, Emilio (case), 465–67, 481–82
goods
  good/bad differentiation, 1–2, 4–5, 33, 65
  noble, 24–25
  potential, 25
  social nature of, 14, 23
  as starting point of ethics, 20–21
  useful, 25
  See also prudence and prudential reasoning; virtue; virtue-based ethics
Gratian, 126
Greer, George, 221–22, 224, 225, 226
Gregory IX, Pope, 126
Groningen Protocol, 317, 318, 320
g-tube (gastrostomy tube), 202–3, 487
guardian, 487
  court appointment of, 101, 111, 152, 162, 167
  responsibilities, 174, 218, 224, 278, 298
Gunther, Daniel, 312–13, 314, 316
Gunvalson, Jacob, 474–75

Hammesfahr, William, 224–25
happiness
  as agent-centered, 22–24
  in ancient Greek philosophy, 4, 20, 21, 22, 24, 25, 26, 31, 42–43, 95
  as collective term, 24–25
  greatest happiness principle, 4, 6, 10, 12, 388, 490
  and moral obligation, 27
  and selfishness, xvi, 22, 23
  and tragedy, 26–27
  and virtue, 25, 27–28
  what it is and isn't, 21–28
  See also goods; virtue; virtue-based ethics
Hardy, James, 410, 411
Harlan, John M., 239

Hatch, Orin, 414
health care
  lack of universal, 345, 462
  in multicultural society, 15
  rising costs, 308, 460–62, 468
  and social justice, 481
health insurance
  ban on discrimination in, 423, 452, 454–55
  history and evolution, 458–59, 480–81
  and life-prolonging treatments, 166, 308
  and managed care, 462
  and medical decision making, 72
  and organ transplants, 402, 411, 412
  rising costs, 308, 461, 462
  uninsured, 55, 340, 411, 462
Hemlock Society, 326
Herbert, Clarence (case), 205–8, 230
"heroic measures," 88
Hippocratic Oath, 265, 321
  and paternalism, 51, 78
HMOs (health maintenance organizations), 72, 166, 487
  development of, 461–62
  See also managed care
Hobbes, Thomas, 9, 22, 228, 489
Homer
  Iliad, 28, 328
homosexuality
  and artificial insemination, 244
  Catholic Church on, 58
  Kant on, 59, 60, 68
  Plato on, 8
hospice, 351–52, 355, 487
hospitals
  Catholic, 228, 325, 339, 354
  interns and residents at, 81–82
  payments to, 55, 461
  refusing to perform abortion and contraceptive procedures, 59, 242
  teaching, 81–83, 95
Howe, Barbara (case), 166–70, 179
Hudson, Sun (case), 463–65, 482
Human Embryo Research Panel, 369, 374
Human Gene Therapy, 443–44
Human Gene Therapy Subcommittee, 434
Human Genome Organization (HUGO), 452
Human Genome Project (HGP), 451–52, 456, 487
human life. *See* death; "one of us"; psychic body concept
Hume, David, 394
Humphrey, Derek
  Final Exit: The Practicalities of Self-Deliverance and Assisted Suicide for the Living, 325

Huntington's disease, 422, 424, 426, 451
Hurlbut, William, 371, 391
Hyde Amendments, 268–69
hypoplastic left-heart syndrome, 404, 413

ICSI (intracytoplasmic sperm injection),
    246–47, 487
    Catholic Church on, 59
inductive reasoning, 11, 17, 31, 487
infanticide. *See* euthanasia and physician-
    assisted suicide
infant mortality, 286–87
informed consent
    and abortion, 79–80, 109, 269–70
    description and origins, 75–76
    documentation of, 81
    in emergencies, 83–85
    ethical significance, 80–81
    exceptions to, 83–87
    and fetal research, 377, 378
    for genetic research, 438, 442, 443, 444
    information needed, 78, 79
    legal history, 76–79, 97
    manipulation to obtain, 80, 116–17
    and medical education, 81–83, 97–98
    in medical research, 374–75, 378–79, 390, 438,
        442, 443, 444
    mentally ill and, 115
    for organ donation and transplants, 395, 398,
        401, 407–8, 415
    and physician-assisted suicide, 337, 355
    and presumed consent, 401, 416
    readings, 96–97
    and refusal of life-sustaining treatment, 217
    and therapeutic privilege, 86–87
    and use of embryos, 248, 374–75
    vs. coerced consent, 79–80
    waivers of, 85–86
informed consent cases
    Candura Decision, 78–79
    Canterbury Decision, 77–78
    Catherine Shine, 84–85
    Salgo Decision, 76–77
    Schloendorff Decision, 76
Innocent III, Pope, 126
Institute of Medicine (IOM), 140–41, 374
institutional review boards (IRB), 378, 379, 447
    defined, 488
    establishment of, 363
    importance of, 316
    purpose, 365
intent and causality, 329
International Bioethics Committee (IBC), 456

intrinsically immoral actions, 57, 67–68
    in Catholic theology, 57–59
    Kant on, 59–61
in vitro fertilization (IVF), 244–49
    cases involving, 247–48
    Catholic Church on, 59, 245
    commercial use of ova, 261, 374
    defined, 488
    ethical considerations on, 232, 248–49, 368
    process, 244–45
Iressa, 470, 472, 474
Islam, 8, 41

Jehovah's Witnesses, 52, 74, 111
Jerome, St., 125, 234
Jewish Chronic Disease Hospital, 361
Jobes, Nancy, 204
John of Naples, 265
John Paul II, Pope, 204, 225, 227, 231
John XXIII, Pope, 237
Jonsen, Albert, 364
Judaism, 8, 41, 137
justice
    as action-guiding principle, 12, 16–17, 364,
        365, 367, 382, 406, 485
    defined, 488
    in virtue-based ethics, 406
    See also principle-based ethics

Kant, Immanuel
    on autonomy, 10, 485
    on categorical imperative, 59, 486
    dualities in, 450
    on homosexuality, 59, 60, 68
    on morality and justice, 4, 7, 10, 16, 18, 27, 34,
        51, 59–61
    on pure reason, 12, 59
    readings, 18, 68
    on sexuality and contraception, 59–60, 68
    on suicide, 59, 60, 68, 324, 339, 352
    on treatment of animals, 388, 393
    underestimation of love, 403
Kantrowitz, Adrian, 394
Kassebaum, Nancy, 295
Katz, Jay, 364
    Experimentation with Human Beings, 363
Kelley, Gerald, 237
Kennedy, Anthony, 273
Kennedy, Edward, 359, 414
Kepler, Johannes, 31
Kevorkian, Jack, 324, 326, 348, 350, 351, 355
Kierkegaard, Soren, 51
killing
    Bible on, 58, 322, 338–39

killing (*continued*)
    capital punishment, 15, 323, 324
    Christian opposition to, 324, 339
    euthanasia as, 332, 333–34, 355
    in self-defense, 49, 56, 57, 323–24, 333
    in war, 49, 323–24, 333
    See also death
Kohlberg, Lawrence, 3, 107
Kolata, Gina, 446
Krugman, Saul, 360

language
    confusion in, 47–48
    descriptive and evaluative, 62–64, 68
    helpful distinctions, 61–66
    misleading distinctions, 48–61
laparoscopy, 244, 249, 250, 488
Leigh disease, 465
L'Enfant, Claude, 414
life-sustaining treatment
    courts and, 102, 172, 174, 180, 193, 194–95,
      211–12
    defined, 488
    ethical reasoning on, 150, 178
    readings, 180
    and reasonable treatment standard, 153, 178,
      310
    right-to-life groups and, 48, 64, 172, 219, 220
    right to refuse, 53, 103, 158, 161, 213, 217, 219
    and rising health care costs, 460
    and substituted judgment standard, 102, 153,
      157, 172, 175
    surgery as, 150, 175–78
    See also dialysis; medical nutrition and
      hydration; ventilators and ventilation
Lisse, Jeffrey, 480
living wills, 88, 160
Locke, John, 128, 450
    on rights, 9, 27, 51, 228, 339, 489
logos, 8, 9, 234, 486, 490
London, Penelope, 475–76
Lorber, John, 287
love
    organ donation as act of, 396, 407
    and sex, 234, 240, 241, 242
    in virtue-based ethics, 7, 29–30, 403, 406, 407
low-birth-weight (LBW) infants, 288

managed care, 462, 481
    defined, 488
    and futility debate, 54
    and pain management, 481
    readings, 481
Maria M. (case), 190–93, 201

marriage, 242
Martin, Michael, 216
mastectomies, 426, 428, 454
masturbation
    and in vitro fertilization, 244, 245
    religious, philosophical condemnations of, 8,
      58, 59, 60, 68, 244
McCormick, Richard, 379
McGee, Tom, 402
Medicaid, 72, 459, 488
    and rising health care costs, 460–61
medical nutrition and hydration, 202, 229–30
    Catholic Church on, 204, 227, 231
    comparisons to abortion, 219
    and ordinary-extraordinary treatment
      distinction, 53
    physicians charged with murder for with-
      drawing, 205, 208
    techniques and technologies for, 202–3
    as treatment or nourishment?, 47, 203–5
medical nutrition and hydration controversies
    Claire Conroy, 209–12
    Clarence Herbert, 205–8
    Elizabeth Bouvia, 212–15
    Mary O'Connor, 215–16
    Michael Martin, 216
    Nancy Cruzan, 216–20, 471
    Nancy Jobes, 204
    Terri Schiavo, 221–26
medical students, 82–83
Medicare, 72, 459, 488
    and rising health care costs, 460–61
Meese, Edwin, 303
Mendel, Gregor, 420, 431
Mengele, Josef, 359–60
mentally ill
    decision-making capacity of, 99, 111–12
    involuntary confinement of, 111, 112–14, 115,
      120
    and medical research, 362, 386
    medical treatment of, 115–17
    proxy decision making for, 99, 111–17, 120
Merleau-Ponty, Maurice, 146
metaphysics, 8, 31
Milgram, Stanley, 361
Mill, John Stuart, 4, 10, 51
miracles, 55
Mohr, Jolee, 446–47, 456
molecular biology, 421–23, 453
Montefiore Medical Center, 365–66
morality. *See* ethics
multiple pregnancies, 245–46
    abortion and, 275, 284

Murray, Joseph, 394
mutations, genetic, 422, 425–26, 431–32, 434–35

NABER (National Advisory Board on Ethics in Reproduction), 261, 488
National Advisory Council for Human Genome Research (NACHGR), 426
National Bioethics Advisory Commission (NBAC), 251–52, 367–68
   about, xiii, 488
   on stem cell research, 373–74
National Breast Cancer Coalition, 426
National Center for Biotechnology Information (NCBI), xiii
National Coalition for Health Professional Education in Genetics, 434
National Commission (National Commission for the Protection of Human Subjects of Biomedical and Behavior Research)
   about, 488
   establishment and role, 364–65
   on ethical principles, 16
   on fetal research, 375–77
National Institute of Neurological Disorders and Stroke (NINDS), 143
National Institutes of Health (NIH), 363, 413, 488
   and genetic research, 439, 441, 451
National Institutes of Health Revitalization Act, 369
National Organ Transplant Act, 400
National Society of Genetic Counselors (NSGC), 454
naturalistic decision making, 38–39, 45–46, 488
natural law
   ethics based on, 8–9, 18
   and opposition to contraception, 235, 237, 259
natural rights, 9–10, 489–90
   See also rights-based theories
neocortical death, 142–44, 398
   and anencephaly, 289
   defined, 488
   See also persistent vegetative state (PVS)
neonatal abnormalities, 288–93
neonatal care
   historical background, 286–88
   readings, 318–19
neonatal care controversies
   Ashley, 312–16
   Baby Doe, 298–300
   Baby Jane Doe, 301–4
   Baby K, 309–12
   Danielle, 304–9

Netherlands
   euthanasia in, 317–18, 320, 325, 331, 332, 343–45, 353
Newton, Isaac, 31, 33, 486
NG tube (nasogastric tube), 202–3, 488
Nietzsche, Friedrich, 51
Nixon, Richard, 461
noncontradiction, principle of, 21
nonmaleficence, 16, 488
Norwood, William, 410
Nuland, Sherwin
   How We Die, 93, 95
Nuremberg Code, 360, 390, 410

O'Connor, Mary, 215–16, 230
O'Connor, Sandra Day, 269
"one of us"
   classical framework for determining, 122–29, 146
   concepts of "self" and "person," 123, 128
   embryos not yet, 127, 373, 374
   establishing criteria for determining, 122, 129–31
   explanation of phrase, 123
   sentience and, 13, 130–31, 132–33, 450
   when something becomes, 13, 121, 124, 132–33, 145, 263
   when something ceases to be, 13, 121, 134–37, 143–44, 220, 263
ordinary and extraordinary treatment, 151, 227
   distinction between, 47, 48, 53, 67, 208
organ donation
   as act of love, 396, 407
   and brain dead individuals, 138, 398–99, 400
   consent for, 104–5, 141, 395, 398, 401, 407–8
   determination of donor's death, 139–41, 396–400
   by infants, 104–5, 148–49, 289, 318, 399–400, 402–6, 410–13
   preservation of organs, 139, 397–98, 400
   readings, 148–49
   sold by living donors, 408–9, 418
   under UAGA, 395–96, 417
   See also transplantation, organ
Organ Procurement and Transplantation Network (OPTN), 400, 408, 416
OTC (ornithine transcarbamylase) deficiency, 435–36
overpopulation, 241
ovum transfer, 250

pacifists, 324
pain management, 352, 355–56, 481
Pakistan, 408, 418

palliative care, 331, 356, 488
Pappworth, M. H.
　Human Guinea Pigs: Experimentation on Man, 363
partial-birth abortion. *See* abortion, partial-birth
paternalism, medical, 70, 74, 95, 116
　in Hippocratic Oath, 51, 78
　vs. autonomy, 50–52, 70
patient-dumping, 311–12
Patient Self-Determination Act (PSDA), 91–92, 98, 488
Paul II, Pope, 58
Paul VI, Pope, 237
Pelosi, Nancy, 476
persistent vegetative state (PVS)
　about, 143, 488–89
　and advance directives, 89
　Catholic Church on nourishing patients with, 204, 225, 227–28, 231
　and current law, 165
　euthanasia and, 325
　and proxy decision making, 104
　readings, 149
persistent vegetative state (PVS) cases
　Clarence Herbert, 205–8
　Helga Wanglie, 162–66
　Karen Quinlan, 152–56
　Nancy Cruzan, 216–20
　Paul Brophy, 306
　Terri Schiavo, 221–26
phenotype, 422, 489
Philippines, 408
Philo, 9, 18
phronesis. *See* prudence and prudential reasoning
physician-assisted suicide. *See* euthanasia and physician-assisted suicide
physician-patient relationship
　disagreements between, 62, 70, 71
　and euthanasia, 341, 348–49
　paternalism and, 51
　and shared decision making, 71
　trust and communication in, 95, 208, 481
Piaget, Jean, 107
Pius XI, Pope, 58, 236
Pius XII, Pope, 152
Plato
　on body and soul, 123, 128, 387, 450
　on infanticide, 287
　on life after death, 15
　on natural law, 8, 18
　on politics and philosophy, 35, 170–71
　on virtue, xvi, 15, 22, 26, 170–71

PPO (preferred provider organization), 489
　See also managed care
pregnancy
　and artificial insemination, 243–50
　ectopic, 274–75
　impact on women's lives, 241–42, 264
　medical supervision of birth, 286
　unmarried women and, 244, 258
　when it begins, 232
　See also abortion; embryo; fertilization; fetus; multiple pregnancies
preimplantation genetic diagnosis (PGD), 371
premoral evil, 64, 489
prenatal care
　case of Angie, 279–82, 285
　historically, 278, 286
　maternal-fetal treatment conflicts in, 278–82
　minors and, 108
　and prenatal testing, 430–31
　See also fetus
President's Commission
　about, xiii, 365–66, 489
　Deciding to Forego Life-Sustaining Treatment, 66–67, 71, 306
　Defining Death, 138, 399
　Making Health Care Decisions, 71
　on patient autonomy and self-determination, 334, 428
　Splicing Life, 434, 448
President's Council on Bioethics (PCB), 252–53, 258, 368
　about, 489
　on stem cell research, 370–72
presumed consent, 401, 416
pride, as virtue, 29–30
primitive streak, 121, 129, 131, 146, 489
principalism, 16, 364–65, 390
principle-based ethics
　action-guiding principles of, 12, 16–17, 364, 365, 367, 382, 406, 485
　and character traits, 2–3
　in contemporary health care, xv, 16–17, 367
　inadequacy of, 46
　moral reasoning in, 10–12
　natural law theories, 8–10
　vs. prudential reasoning, 7–8, 17, 32–33
　See also rights-based theories
prisoners, 386
privacy, right to, 178, 239, 352
profitability
　drug and biotechnology companies and, 435, 440, 444–45, 447, 451
　of fertility treatments, 249
　of organ transplantation, 401

proportionate and disproportionate treatment, 208, 227
prostaglandins, 277, 489
prostitution, 257
proxy decision makers
and "clear and convincing evidence" criterion, 158, 217, 219
conflicts of interest, 99, 293
court-appointed, 101
defined, 489
designation of, 90–91, 99, 100–101, 118–19
and DNR orders, 187–88, 189, 190, 192–93
and futile treatment, 170, 198
importance of designating, 99, 118–19
laws on, 90–91, 166, 168, 169
for mentally ill, 111–16
and older children, 105–11
parental, 105–6, 110, 293, 307–8
for permanently unconscious patients, 104, 153, 155
readings, 119
significant others as, 100–101
standards for, 101–5, 117–18
See also best interests standard; decision making; reasonable treatment standard; substituted judgment standard
prudence and prudential reasoning
Aquinas on, xiv, xvii, 31, 32, 33, 35, 37, 155
Aristotle on, xiv, xv, xvi, xvii, 5, 32, 33, 35, 38, 68, 155
and circumstances, 60, 385
decision making in, 38–40, 41
defined, 489
on ends and means, 33
features of, 35–37
and feelings, 33, 37–38
and formal reasoning, 40–41
and living good life, xvi–xvii, 33, 34–35, 65, 452
and moral judgment, 32–33, 62
origin of word, 32
and principle of double effect, 56
and religion, 41–42
and temperance, 15, 29–30, 34
in virtue-based ethics, xvi, 3, 13, 28
what it is and isn't, 32–35
See also Aquinas, Thomas; Aristotle; virtue-based ethics
psychic body concept, 13, 131, 133–34, 143–44, 146
See also "one of us"
Pythagoreans, 123
on animals, 387
on euthanasia and suicide, 321–22
and Hippocratic Oath, 51, 321

quality of life
as important ethical question, 229
and treatment decisions, 175
undervaluing of, 217, 229
Quill, Timothy, 325, 328, 346–47, 349, 350, 355
Quinlan, Karen (case), 53, 88, 165, 179
case study, 152–56

Ramsey, Paul, 379
Raper, Steven, 436–37, 443
rational choice strategy, 38, 39–40, 45
defined, 489
Rawls, John, 12
Reagan, Ronald, 294, 295, 369, 461
reasonable treatment standard
about, 103–5, 117–18
in deciding on life-sustaining treatment, 153, 178, 310
deciding on research on children, 379
reasonable/unreasonable distinction, 61–62
recognition-primed decision making, 39
recombinant DNA, 421, 433
Recombinant DNA Advisory Committee (RAC), 433, 434, 456, 489
Reemtsma, Keith, 409
Regan, Tom, 393
Rehabilitation Act, 303
religion
belief in miracles in, 55
and ethics, xvii
and healing, 46
and medical treatment, 52, 74, 111, 309, 310
and prudence, 41
See also Catholic Church; Christianity; Islam; Judaism
Rendell, Edward, 476
Reno, Janet, 326
reproduction
fertilization, 127, 131–32, 241, 247
seed theory of, 124, 126
See also artificial insemination; in vitro fertilization; pregnancy
research, medical
on AIDS/HIV, 380–86, 392
on animals, 387–89, 393
on artificial hearts, 414
Beecher's critique, 362–63, 390
on children, 378–79, 392, 412, 413, 445
on cloning, 252–53
conflicts of interest in, 412, 435, 440, 441, 444–45, 447
in developing countries, 379–87, 392–93
on embryos, 58, 368–75, 391

research, medical (*continued*)
  establishing federal guidelines for, 363–64, 390–91
  and "experimentation" term, 357
  on fetuses, 375–77, 391
  genetic, 431–49
  informed consent for, 374–75, 378–79, 390, 438, 442, 443, 444
  participant/subject distinction, 368
  research/treatment distinction, 66, 69, 315–16
  stem cell, 369–73, 391
  therapeutic and nontherapeutic, 357
  on vulnerable population groups, 362, 386–87
research scandals
  C. R. Bard, Inc., 366
  human radiation experiments, 366–67, 391
  Jewish Chronic Disease Hospital, 361
  Montefiore Medical Center, 365–66
  Nazi Germany, 359–60, 389–90
  obedience tests at Yale University, 361–62, 390
  Tuskegee, 358–59, 363, 389
  Willowbrook State School, 360–61, 390
respirators. *See* ventilators and ventilation
right reason. *See* prudence and prudential reasoning
rights-based theories
  and abortion debate, 10, 64, 229, 264, 273
  as dominant in American health care, 16, 252
  and euthanasia and suicide, 229, 324, 334, 352
  inadequacy of, 249, 311
  and organ donation, 401
  philosophical origins, 9–10, 18
  reasoning in, 11, 12, 32–33
  See also natural rights; principle-based ethics
right-to-life groups
  on abortion, 10, 64, 229, 264, 273
  on brain death criterion, 137
  on euthanasia, 92
  on neocortical death criterion, 144
  and quality of life, 229
  on withdrawing life-sustaining treatment, 48, 64, 172, 219, 220
Rios, Mario and Elsa (case), 247
RNA (ribonucleic acid), 421, 433
Roberts, John, 272, 327
Rockefeller, Nelson, 461
Ross, William D., 7, 16–17
RU-486, 276–78, 284–85

Saikewicz, Joseph (case), 53, 175, 193, 194, 195
Salgo, Martin (case), 76–77
Sanchez, Tomas, 265
Sardinia, 429–31, 455

Satcher David, 382
Sauer, Pieter, 317
Scalia, Antonin, 327
Schiavo, Terri (case), 221–26, 231
  political controversy surrounding, 224–26, 476
Schloendorff, Mary (case), 76
SCID (Severe combined immunodeficiency), 446
seeding trials, 478–80, 483
self-determination. *See* autonomy and self-determination, patient
Semb, Bjarne, 414
Seneca, 234
Sepulveda, Jesse (case), 404–6, 417
sexuality
  Christianity on, 58, 234–35, 236
  humanization of, 238
  Kant on, 59–60, 68
  and love, 234, 240, 241, 242
  minors and, 108–9
sexually transmitted diseases
  and HIV transmission, 383–85, 392
  and minors, 108, 109, 110
Shalala, Donna, 400
Sheikh, Abdul, 408
Shine, Catherine (case), 84–85, 97
Silver-Isenstadt, Ari, 82
Sixtus V, Pope, 236, 265
slippery slope arguments
  defined, 490
  and euthanasia, 144, 212, 229, 317–18, 329, 342–45, 355
  and genetic therapy, 448–49
  and treatment of disabilities, 315
Socrates
  on body and soul, 123, 128, 387, 450
  execution of, 15, 328
  on virtue and happiness, xvii, 22, 23, 26
somatic cell nuclear transfer (SCNT), 251–52, 371
Sophists, 338
soul
  Aristotle on, 123–24, 450
  body-soul duality, 146, 450
  Christianity on, 123, 127
  different interpretations of, 122, 129
  and fetus, 125, 126–27
  Socrates and Plato on, 123, 128, 387, 450
Southam, Chester, 361
Spain, 401
Spallanzani, Lazaro, 243
spina bifida, 287, 288, 432
  See also Baby Jane Doe

Spring, Earle (case), 171–75, 179
Starzi, Thomas, 395, 413, 417
static encephalopathy (SE), 312
stem cell research
    and abortion controversy, 370
    clinical trials for, 372–73
    and cloning, 252, 371–72, 374
    destructive, 369–71
    and induced pluripotent stem cells, 372–73, 391
    nondestructive, 371–72
    readings, 391
    See also embryo
sterilization
    Catholic Church on, 58
    as contraception, 109
    forced, 80, 233
Stewart, William, 363
Stoics
    about, 490
    influence on Christianity, 234
    on natural law, 8–9, 18
    on sex and contraception, 234, 235, 238
    on suicide, 322, 339
    on virtue, 15, 26
substituted judgment standard
    about, 101–3, 110, 117–18, 490
    limitations of, 118
    in proxy decisions for mentally ill, 114
    in withdrawing life-sustaining treatment, 102, 153, 157, 172, 175
suicide
    Aquinas on, 15
    Aristotle on, 15, 322, 339
    in Bible, 322–23
    Christianity on, 323
    and human nature, 339
    Kant on, 59, 60, 68, 324, 339, 352
    literary history of, 287, 328
    social arguments against, 339–40
    See also euthanasia and physician-assisted suicide
SUPPORT (Study to Understand Prognosis and Preferences for Outcomes and Risks of Treatment), 92–93, 95, 98
surrogate motherhood, 253–55, 260–61
    Baby M case, 255–56
    ethical problems with, 256–57, 258

Tanenbaum, Melvyn, 302
Task Force on Brain Death in Childhood, 399
Tay-Sachs, 426, 429, 435
teleology, 490
Ten Commandments, 4, 8, 57, 322, 338

Texas Advance Directives Act (ADA), 54, 170, 463, 481–82
    and Emilio Gonzalez case, 465–67
    ethical reflections on, 467–68
    and Sun Hudson case, 463–66
thanatrophic dysplasia, 463
therapeutic misconception, 66, 69
therapeutic privilege, 86–87
Thomas, Clarence, 327
Thomson, James, 369, 372, 391
totality, principle of, 406–7
total parenteral nutrition (TPN), 203
tracheotomy, 150, 490
transplantation, organ
    allocating organs, 400–406, 418–19
    from animals, 409–13
    of artificial hearts, 395, 414–16, 418
    black-market sale of organs, 72, 403, 408
    from cadavers, 395–406
    financial profitability of, 401
    geographical allocation system, 400–401
    history, 135, 394–95
    immune system rejection and, 395
    from living donors, 406–9, 417
    organ shortage, 105, 139, 400, 416
    politics and, 402
    and social justice, 405–6
    waiting list, 400–401, 403, 405–6
    See also organ donation
transplantation controversies
    Baby Fae, 410–13
    Jamie Fiske, 402–3
    Jesse Sepulveda, 404–6
Trapp, Robert, 446–47
triage, 103, 170, 490
Tribe, Laurence, 331
trisomy, 276, 289–90, 432
Tuskegee syphilis study, 358–59, 363, 389

Ubel, Peter, 82
Uganda, 383–85, 392
Uniform Determination of Death Act (UDDA), 136, 141, 142, 395–96
    about, 490
United Network for Organ Sharing (UNOS), 400–401
United States Conference of Catholic Bishops (USCCB), 58
U.S. Public Health Service, 361, 363
    and Tuskegee study, 358–59
utilitarianism, 10, 18, 51, 403
    action-guiding principles in, 367
    defined, 490

utilitarianism (*continued*)
  and ethical treatment of animals, 388
  in health care ethics, 16
utility, definition of, 490

Varmus, Harold, 382
vasopressor, 180, 490
venereal disease. *See* sexually transmitted
  diseases
ventilators and ventilation
  and anencephalic infants, 292, 309–12
  and causing death/letting die distinction, 50,
    151–52
  and life sustaining/prolonging distinction,
    150, 151
  and ordinary/extraordinary treatment
    distinction, 53
  origin of, 150–51
  for PVS patients, 152–56, 162–66
  readings, 179
  and withdrawing/withholding treatment
    distinction, 49, 207
  See also life-sustaining treatment
ventilators and ventilation controversies
  Baby K, 309–12
  Barbara Howe, 166–70
  Brother Fox, 156–58
  Danielle, 304–9
  Emilio Gonzalez, 465–67
  Helga Wanglie, 162–66
  Karen Quinlan, 152–56
  Sun Hudson, 463–65
  William Bartling, 158–62
ventricular assist devices (VADs), 415, 416
Verhagen, Eduard, 317
viability
  defined, 490–91
  of fetus, 263
Vioxx, 477, 479–80
virtue
  and decision making, 3
  defined, 491
  and excellence, 27–28
  and happiness, 25, 27–28
  intellectual, 28, 31–33
  moral, 28–31
  See also goods
virtue-based ethics
  and circumstance, 60, 385
  and good, 3, 7–8, 20–21, 30–31
  and health care ethics, xv, 17
  historical foundations, 13–16

"less worse" choices in, 26–27, 178, 214, 347,
  348, 351, 352, 431
on moral principles and rules, 3, 367, 406
personal responsibility in, 96
prudence as normative in, xv, xvi, 3, 13, 28
readings, 45
vs. principle-based ethics, 7–8, 17, 20–21,
  32–33
See also ethics; prudence and prudential
  reasoning

Wallace, Mike, 161
Wanglie, Helga (case), 162–66, 169, 179
Washburn, Lawrence, 302, 303
Washington Legal Foundation (WLF), 471
Washington Protection and Advocacy System,
  316
Watson, James, 420, 451, 452
Weber, William, 302, 303
Weismann, August Friedrich, 420
Welch, Hazel (case), 93–95, 98
Whitehead, Alfred North, 146
Will, George, 298, 319
Willowbrook State School, 360–61, 390
Wilmut, Ian, 250
Wilson, James, 437, 438, 441, 443
Windom, Robert, 377
withdrawing and withholding treatment
  distinction between, 49, 67, 207–8, 211, 329
Wittgenstein, Ludwig, 47
Wolf-Hirschhorn syndrome, 432
Wolfson, Jay, 225
women
  and control over bodies, 229, 264, 273, 378
  emancipation of, 241–42
  pregnancy's impact on, 241–42, 264
  as subject to exploitation, 254
  unmarried, 234, 244, 245
  See also abortion; prenatal care
World Council of Churches, 236, 238
World Health Organization (WHO)
  on AIDS-HIV research, 381
  on black-market sale of organs, 408
  on genetics, 456–57
  on government responsibility in health care,
    462

xenografts, 410, 413, 491

Yale University obedience tests, 361–62, 390

Zacchias, Paolo, 126–27
Zeno, 8
ZIFT (zygote intrafallopian transfer), 250, 253,
  491